Praise for the I

Using evaluation in today's world is ultimately about humanity's future. The stakes are huge. Evaluation use flows from quality. Quality in today's world requires diversity. Whether evaluation contributes to a more just, equitable, and sustainable world will be determined by how—and how well—evaluators and stakeholders together meet the challenge to respect, promote, and improve quality, diversity, and use. Our collective future rests on those foundational pillars. This book is an outstanding contribution to the evaluation literature.

—Michael Quinn Patton, Utilization-Focused Evaluation

Finally! An evaluation textbook that not only provides information on the mechanics of evaluation practice but also explicitly acknowledges the role of structural racism and its influence on the field of evaluation. This textbook is a timely addition to the evaluation literature, and serves as a meaningful tool to examine and engage the intersections of evaluation, social justice, and privilege.

—Jori N. Hall, University of Georgia

This is the evaluation text I've been waiting for! It weaves together a comprehensive, inclusive history of the evaluation field with issues that face new and experienced practicing evaluators every day. It also brings to the fore topics not covered in other evaluation texts, such as evaluation ethics in practice, the hidden figures and influential women in evaluation, important epistemological shifts in the field, and the intersection of social justice and social programming. This will be a critical resource for all who want to make a difference through high quality evaluation practice.

—Leslie Goodyear, Education Development Center

Very rarely are issues related to race, class, and power discussed so eloquently and effectively within an evaluation text.

—John Ridings, The Institute for Clinical Social Work

Thomas and Campbell have taken topics that are often only alluded to in program evaluation texts and brought them to the forefront, highlighting the importance of understanding the diversity of society when developing effective evaluations.

—Marcus-Antonio Galeste, Arizona State University

This is a much-needed, useful, and relevant text that bridges the evaluation process and methods with our cultural, historical, and political climate. It integrates diverse activities, methods, and applications that will help prepare students to become successful future practitioners and evaluators.

—Karen Tinsley, Guilford College

This text covers the salient features of research and evaluation in clear language and includes the often-overlooked impact of cultural awareness and understanding throughout the research process. In an increasingly multicultural and complex society, the authors have created a resource to help budding researchers evaluate their goals, needs, and biases as they enter this fascinating field.

—Brenda S. Gerhardt, University of Dayton

This is the most comprehensive text on evaluation that I have seen. The section on ethics challenges students to reflect on their own beliefs and values, and how those might cause bias in evaluation.

—Sandra Handwerk, Albany State University

This text provides a strong voice to support the inclusion of social justice issues in evaluation planning, implementation, analysis, and reporting.

—Debra J. Dirksen, Western New Mexico University

Sara Miller McCune founded SAGE Publishing in 1965 to support the dissemination of usable knowledge and educate a global community. SAGE publishes more than 1000 journals and over 800 new books each year, spanning a wide range of subject areas. Our growing selection of library products includes archives, data, case studies and video. SAGE remains majority owned by our founder and after her lifetime will become owned by a charitable trust that secures the company's continued independence.

Los Angeles | London | New Delhi | Singapore | Washington DC | Melbourne

Evaluation in Today's World

In loving memory of my mother (Julia Myers Thomas) and father (Herman Thomas Sr.), who were, in their own quiet and unique ways, my first examples of civil rights warriors and activists for fairness and social justice.

—Veronica G. Thomas

To Jesse J. Campbell-Mortman, who at 10 is a fighter for fairness and justice.

—Patricia B. Campbell

Evaluation in Today's World

Respecting Diversity, Improving Quality, and Promoting Usability

Veronica G. Thomas
Howard University

Patricia B. Campbell
Campbell-Kibler Associates, Inc.

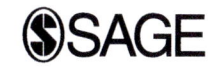

Los Angeles | London | New Delhi
Singapore | Washington DC | Melbourne

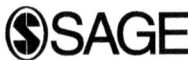

FOR INFORMATION:

SAGE Publications, Inc.
2455 Teller Road
Thousand Oaks, California 91320
E-mail: order@sagepub.com

SAGE Publications Ltd.
1 Oliver's Yard
55 City Road
London, EC1Y 1SP
United Kingdom

SAGE Publications India Pvt. Ltd.
B 1/I 1 Mohan Cooperative Industrial Area
Mathura Road, New Delhi 110 044
India

SAGE Publications Asia-Pacific Pte. Ltd.
18 Cross Street #10-10/11/12
China Square Central
Singapore 048423

Acquisitions Editor: Helen Salmon
Editorial Assistant: Kelsey Barkis
Content Development Editor: Chelsea Neve
Production Editor: Astha Jaiswal
Copy Editor: Melinda Masson
Typesetter: Hurix Digital
Indexer: Integra
Cover Designer: Candice Harman
Marketing Manager: Victoria Velasquez

Copyright © 2021 by SAGE Publications, Inc.

All rights reserved. Except as permitted by U.S. copyright law, no part of this work may be reproduced or distributed in any form or by any means, or stored in a database or retrieval system, without permission in writing from the publisher.

All third-party trademarks referenced or depicted herein are included solely for the purpose of illustration and are the property of their respective owners. Reference to these trademarks in no way indicates any relationship with, or endorsement by, the trademark owner.

Printed in the United States of America

Library of Congress Cataloging-in-Publication Data

Names: Thomas, Veronica G., author. | Campbell, Patricia B., author.

Title: Evaluation in today's world : respecting diversity, improving quality, and promoting usability / Veronica G. Thomas, Howard University, Patricia B. Campbell, Campbell-Kibler Associates, Inc.

Description: Los Angeles : SAGE, [2021] | Includes bibliographical references.

Identifiers: LCCN 2020026040 | ISBN 9781544348162 (paperback) | ISBN 9781544348186 (epub) | ISBN 9781544348193 (epub) | ISBN 9781544348179 (ebook)

Subjects: LCSH: Evaluation research (Social action programs)

Classification: LCC H62 .T4475 2021 | DDC 001.4—dc23

LC record available at https://lccn.loc.gov/2020026040

This book is printed on acid-free paper.

20 21 22 23 24 10 9 8 7 6 5 4 3 2 1

Brief Table of Contents

Preface	xx
About the Authors	xxiv
Acknowledgments	xxv
Chapter 1 Evaluations of Future: Inclusive, Equity-Focused, Useful, and Used	1
Chapter 2 Evaluation Ethics and Quality Standards	27
Chapter 3 Historical Evolution of Program Evaluation Through a Social Justice Lens	65
Chapter 4 Evaluation Paradigms, Theories, and Models	107
Chapter 5 Social Justice and Evaluation: Theories, Challenges, Frameworks, and Paradigms	135
Chapter 6 Evaluation Types With a Cultural and Racial Equity Lens	169
Chapter 7 Social Programming, Social Justice, and Evaluation	205
Chapter 8 Responsive Stakeholder Engagement and Democratization of the Evaluation Process	243
Chapter 9 Planning the Evaluation	273
Chapter 10 Evaluation Questions That Matter	303
Chapter 11 Selecting Appropriate Evaluation Designs	325
Chapter 12 Defining, Collecting, and Managing Data	353
Chapter 13 The Best Analysis for the Data	385
Chapter 14 Reporting, Disseminating, and Utilizing Evaluation Results	415
Chapter 15 Evaluation as a Business	449
Chapter 16 Interconnections and Practical Implications	477

Appendix A	499
Appendix B	502
Glossary	505
References	517
Index	543

Detailed Table of Contents

Preface	xx
About the Authors	xxiv
Acknowledgments	xxv

Chapter 1 Evaluations of Future: Inclusive, Equity-Focused, Useful, and Used — 1

Introduction	1
An Overview of the Book	2
Structure of the Book	2
Chapter Content	2
An Overview of Evaluation	4
Definitions of Evaluation	5
Evaluation Characteristics	6
Evaluative Thinking	7
Race, Racism, Social Justice, and a Racialized Perspective	9
Other Social Justice Issues	10
Objectivity and Bias	13
Objectivity	13
Bias	13
Explicit Bias	*13*
Implicit Bias	*14*
Reducing Bias	16
Culture, Cultural Competence, and Cultural Responsiveness	18
The Impact of Politics	20
The Current Climate	21
Summary	23
Supplemental Resources	23

Chapter 2 Evaluation Ethics and Quality Standards — 27

Introduction	27
A Brief Historical Perspective on Research Ethics	29
The Nuremberg Code of 1947	29
The Tuskegee Syphilis Study of 1932–1972	30
The Radiation Studies of 1940–1960	32
The HeLa Story: 1950s and Beyond	32
Beyond Medical Studies and Physical Harm: The Milgram Study of 1963	32
The National Research Act of 1974	33
The Continuing Importance of Research Ethics	34

Ethics in Evaluation ... 34
    Sources of Ethical Thinking ... 39

Cultural Competence as an Ethical Imperative ... 40
    Ethical Dimension of Racial Bias ... 42

Ethical Sensitivity and Dilemmas ... 44
    Sources of Ethical Dilemmas ... 46
    Handling Ethical Dilemmas ... 47
    Ethics and Conflicts of Interest ... 49

Ethical Challenges and Dilemmas Across the Evaluation Process ... 51

Ethical Principles and Standards for Evaluators and Evaluations ... 52
    The *Evaluators' Ethical Guiding Principles* ... 52
    The *Program Evaluation Standards* ... 56

Evaluation Corruptibility and Fallacies ... 58

Evaluator Role, Power, Politics, and Ethics ... 59

Interplay of Politics and Ethics ... 59

Summary ... 61

Supplemental Resources ... 61

Chapter 3 Historical Evolution of Program Evaluation Through a Social Justice Lens ... 65

Introduction ... 65

History of Evaluation Through a Social Justice Lens ... 66

Evaluation Prior to Modern Times of the 20th Century ... 67
    Intersection Between Education and Evaluation Pre–20th Century ... 68
    Early Social Experiments ... 68

Overview of Evaluation in the 20th Century ... 69
    Evaluation in the First Half of the 20th Century: 1900–1950s ... 71
    Evaluation During the New Deal, Wartime, and Economic Growth: 1930s–1950s ... 72
    The Cambridge-Somerville Youth Program Evaluation ... 73
    Sputnik's Impact on the Growth of Evaluation ... 74
    Prominent Influencers and Users of Evaluation During the 20th-Century Early Years: 1930s–1950s ... 74
        Kurt Lewin ... 74
        Alva and Gunnar Myrdal ... 75
        Ralph W. Tyler ... 75

Hidden Figures and Histories in Early-20th-Century Evaluation ... 76
    Ambrose Caliver ... 78
    Reid E. Jackson ... 79
    Rose Butler Browne ... 79
    Aaron A. Brown ... 80

Leander L. Boykin	81
Journal of Negro Education and Founding Editor Charles H. Thompson	82

Evaluation in 1960–2000 — 84
- Federal Legislation and Great Society Programs — 84
- The Professionalization of the Field — 85
  - *Growth of Evaluation Scholarship* — 85
  - *Establishment of Professional Societies in Evaluation* — 86
  - *Graduate Training and Professional Development in Evaluation* — 86
  - *Establishment of Standards and Codes of Conduct* — 86
- Methodological Approaches and Paradigm Wars — 87
  - *Two Influential Scholars' Contributions to Methodological Approaches of the 1960s–1970s* — 88

Rethinking the Role of Evaluation — 89

Influential Women in Evaluation: 1970s–1990s — 92
- Carol H. Weiss — 92
- Yvonna S. Lincoln — 93
- Eleanor Chelimsky — 94
- Floraline I. Stevens — 95
- Lois-Ellin Datta — 96
- Laura Leviton — 97
- Beatriz Chu Clewell — 98

Influential 20th-Century Evaluator: An Activity — 98

21st-Century Evaluation: Expanding the Focus — 99
- Strengthening Evaluation at the Federal Level — 101
- Shift in the Quantitative–Qualitative Debate — 101
- Increased Emphasis on Social Justice and Diversity — 102
- Support for Capacity Building — 102

Summary — 103

Supplemental Resources — 104

Chapter 4 Evaluation Paradigms, Theories, and Models — 107

Introduction — 107

The Value of Scientific Paradigms and Theories in Evaluation — 108
- The Nature of Scientific Paradigms — 108
- Theories for Guiding and Improving Evaluation Practice — 111

Social Science Paradigms and Theories — 111
- Social Science Paradigms — 111
  - *Application of Social Science Paradigms in Evaluations* — 114
- Social Science Theories — 116

Program Theory of Change — 117
- Evaluating Program Theory — 119

Evaluation Theories, Models, and Approaches — 120
- Why Should We Care About Evaluation Theory? — 121

Distinguishing Evaluation Theories, Models, and Approaches	122
Classifying Evaluation Approaches and Theories	123
Five-Category Classification	123
The Evaluation Tree	125
Mertens and Wilson's Four-Branch Tree of Evaluation Approaches	*126*
Evaluation Theories Within a Cultural Context	129
Evaluation Approaches and Theories: A Summary Description of Selected Examples	130
Summary	132
Supplemental Resources	132

Chapter 5   Social Justice and Evaluation: Theories, Challenges, Frameworks, and Paradigms   135

Introduction	135
Social Justice	135
Definitions of Social Justice	136
Marginalized Groups	137
Impacts of Marginalization	138
Fixing the Group vs. Fixing the System	139
Theories Providing Context for Social Justice Evaluations	141
Critical Race Theory	141
Feminist Research and Theory	142
Queer Theory	144
Disability Theory	145
Race, Racism, and Evaluation	147
Challenges to Social Justice and Evaluation	149
Traditional Definitions of Rigor	149
Deficit Models	149
Cultural Conflict of Interest	150
Efforts to Reduce the Impact of Racism on Evaluation	150
Cultural Competence and Cultural Responsiveness	151
Evaluation Models and Social Justice	153
Social Justice–Oriented Evaluation Frameworks and Paradigms	154
Transformational Evaluation	155
Empowerment Evaluation	157
Feminist Evaluation	158
Participatory Evaluation	159
Deliberative Democratic Evaluation	160
Collaborative Evaluation	162
Equity-Focused Evaluation	163
Summary	165
Supplemental Resources	165

Chapter 6 Evaluation Types With a Cultural and Racial Equity Lens — 169

- Introduction — 169
- Classifying Evaluations — 170
  - An Overview of Formative and Summative Classification — 171
    - *Distinguishing and Coupling Formative and Summative Evaluations* — 174
  - Other Evaluation Classifications — 175
- Different Types of Evaluations — 176
  - Formative and Implementation Evaluations — 179
    - *Needs Assessments* — 179
    - *Evaluability Assessments* — 182
    - *Process Evaluations* — 183
    - *Progress Evaluations* — 185
  - Summative, Outcome, and Impact Evaluation Types — 186
    - *Outcome Evaluations* — 186
    - *Impact Evaluations* — 190
    - *Efficiency Evaluations* — 190
  - Alternative Types of Evaluations — 194
    - *Rapid Evaluations* — 194
    - *Metaevaluations* — 196
- Developmental Evaluations: Another Alternative to Formative–Summative — 198
- Putting It All Together — 201
- Summary — 202
- Supplemental Resources — 202

Chapter 7 Social Programming, Social Justice, and Evaluation — 205

- Introduction — 205
- Understanding Social Problems and Social Programs Through a Social Justice Lens — 206
  - Wicked Problems — 206
  - Social Problems: Definition, Description, and Theoretical Underpinnings — 209
    - *Objective Element of Social Problems* — 209
    - *Subjective Element of Social Problems* — 209
  - Sources of Social Problems — 211
  - Social Problems' Fluid Nature — 212
  - Social Programs Through a Social Justice and Transformative Lens — 213
  - Power, Political, and Economic Nature of Social Problems — 215
  - Equity-Based Social Programming — 217
- Structural Racism, Social Programming, and Evaluation — 217
- Integrating Program Planning and Evaluation Planning — 218
- Social Program Evaluations vs. Social Project Evaluations: Distinctions and Implications — 219

Key Program/Project Components Every Evaluator
Must Understand   219
    Program Mission   220
    Program Goals   221
    Program Objectives   221
    Program Activities   223
    Program Resources   223
    Putting It All Together: Program Mission, Goals, Objectives, Activities,
    and Resources   223

Logic Models: Linking Program Components   225
    Benefits of Logic Models for Program Planning   225
    Limitations of Logic Models   226

Logic Models and Evaluation Planning   227
    Components of Logic Models   227
    Types and Looks of Logic Models   229
        Nested Logic Models   *231*

Beyond Traditional Linear Logic Models   233
    Fuzzy Logic Models   233
    Circular Logic Models   233
    Culturally Relevant Logic Models   233
        Afrocentric-Centered Logic Model Approaches *234*
        Logic Models From an Indigenous Framework   *236*

Summary   240

Supplemental Resources   240

Chapter 8 Responsive Stakeholder Engagement and Democratization of the Evaluation Process   243

Introduction   243

Who Are Stakeholders?   243

Valuing Stakeholders and Diverse Stakeholder Engagement   245

Identifying and Classifying the Right Stakeholders   246
    Stakeholder Classifications   247
    Key and Hidden Stakeholders   249

Democratizing the Evaluation Process With Stakeholders   251

Relationships, Values, and Stakeholder Engagement   254

Responsive Stakeholder Engagement   255
    The Misuse of Responsive Stakeholder Engagement   257

Continuum of Stakeholder Engagement: From
Nonresponsive to Responsive   257

Barriers to Responsive Stakeholder Engagement   259

Benefits of Responsive Stakeholder Engagement   262

Six-Step Process for Responsive Stakeholder Engagement   265

Communicating With Stakeholders ... 268
Summary ... 269
Supplemental Resources ... 270

Chapter 9 Planning the Evaluation ... 273

Introduction ... 273

Dealing With Power Imbalances During Evaluation Planning ... 274

Planning for Culturally Responsive and Social
Justice–Oriented Evaluations ... 277

Evaluation Planning Activities ... 279

Identifying and Involving Stakeholders in Evaluation Planning ... 280
    Identifying Stakeholders and Their Potential Role(s) ... 280
    Involving Stakeholders ... 281

Analysis of the Context ... 282

Identifying and Clarifying Project Goals ... 284

Identifying the Purpose(s) of the Evaluation ... 285
    Varying Stakeholders' Perspectives on Evaluation Goals and Priorities ... 286
        Funder's Priorities ... *286*
        Project Administrators' Priorities ... *287*
        Evaluator's Priorities ... *287*

Defining Success in Evaluation Planning ... 287
    The Problem With "Parity" as Success Definition ... 288
    Beyond Quantitative Definitions of Success ... 288
    Identifying Indicators ... 289
    Understanding Different Types of Indicators ... 290
    Levels of Indicators ... 291

Developing Timelines ... 293

Identifying Resource Needs ... 293

Assembling an Evaluation Team ... 293
    Identifying the Evaluation Team's Roles and Responsibilities ... 294
    Internal vs. External Evaluators ... 294

Evaluation Planning and Management Visualization Tools ... 296
    Gantt Charts ... 296
    Program Evaluation Review Technique (PERT) Charts ... 297
    Time and Task Charts or Data Maps ... 298

Developing a Written Evaluation Plan ... 299

Overcoming Pitfalls in Evaluation Planning ... 300

Summary ... 301

Supplemental Resources ... 301

Chapter 10 Evaluation Questions That Matter — 303

- Introduction — 303
- Why Evaluation Questions That Matter? — 305
  - Questions That Matter Meet Information Needs of Diverse Users — 305
  - Questions That Matter Set the Stage for the Collection of Credible Evidence — 306
- Power and Privilege Issues in Formulating Evaluation Questions — 307
- Characteristics of Good Evaluation Questions: An Overview — 307
  - Good Questions Align With the Funder's Requirements — 308
  - Good Questions Are Useful and Ask About Important Issues — 308
  - Good Questions Are Tailored and Appropriate to Local Needs — 309
  - Good Questions Are Clear, Specific, and Well Defined — 309
  - Good Questions Are Researchable (or Answerable) — 309
  - Good Questions Are Realistic Considering Contexts and Project Realities — 310
  - Good Questions Are Reasonable in Number and Scope — 310
- Sources of Evaluation Questions — 310
- Prioritizing Evaluation Questions for Diverse Audiences — 311
- Inclusion/Exclusion Criteria for Prioritizing Evaluation Questions: Two Approaches — 312
  - U.S. Agency for International Development (USAID) Approach — 312
  - Centers for Disease Control and Prevention (CDC) Approach — 313
- Steps to Identifying, Formulating, and Prioritizing Questions That Matter — 314
- Types of Evaluation Questions — 316
  - Program Theory Questions — 316
  - Context Questions — 317
  - Process Questions — 317
  - Relevance Questions — 318
  - Outcomes Questions — 318
  - Impact Questions — 319
  - Cost-Benefit and Cost-Effectiveness Questions — 320
  - Sustainability Questions — 321
- Summary of Different Types of Evaluation Questions — 322
- Summary — 322
- Supplemental Resources — 323

Chapter 11 Selecting Appropriate Evaluation Designs — 325

- Introduction — 325
- Rigor — 326
  - Bias — 327

Practical Considerations	328
Theoretical and Cultural Considerations	330

Control and Comparison Groups — 333
Ethical Issues — 334
Ethical Use of Control and Comparison Groups — 334

Longitudinal Data — 336

Evaluation Designs — 338
Experimental Designs — 338
Feasibility of Implementation — 340
Quasi-experimental Designs — 341
Feasibility of Implementation — 342
Pretest/Posttest Designs — 343
Feasibility of Implementation — 344
Retrospective Pretest Designs — 344
Feasibility of Implementation — 345
Case Studies/Ethnography — 346
Feasibility of Implementation — 347

Rival Hypotheses and Threats to Validity — 348

The Best Design for the Question — 349

Summary — 351

Supplementary Resources — 351

Chapter 12   Defining, Collecting, and Managing Data — 353

Introduction — 353

Qualitative and Quantitative Data — 353
Sources of Qualitative Data — 354
Interviews — 354
Focus Groups — 355
Observations — 356
Participant-Generated Visual Data — 356
Sources of Quantitative Data — 358
Surveys and Other Structured Questionnaires — 358
Records and Other Archival Data — 359

Strengths and Weaknesses of Qualitative and Quantitative Data — 360

Ensuring Data Quality — 362
Validity — 362
Types of Validity — 363
Reliability — 368
Reliability of Quantitative Data — 368
Reliability of Qualitative Data — 369
Pilot-Testing — 370
Response Rates — 370

Protection of Human Participants	372
Using Existing Measures or Developing New Ones	375
Sources of Measures	375
Assessing Existing Measures	376
Measuring Complex Concepts	376
Modes of Data Collection	377
Data Management	379
Mapping Data Collection to Project Goals and Objectives	379
Timing	380
Electronic Controls and Data Cleaning	381
Privacy	381
Data Management Plans	382
Summary	382
Supplemental Resources	383

Chapter 13 The Best Analysis for the Data   385

Introduction	385
Deductive and Inductive Reasoning	385
An Overview of Deductive and Inductive Reasoning	385
Using Deductive and Inductive Reasoning	387
Quantitative Analysis	388
Levels of Quantitative Data	388
Descriptive Statistics	391
Inferential Statistics and Statistical Significance	392
Parametric and Nonparametric Statistics	*393*
Effect Size	*395*
Decision Error and Statistical Power	*397*
Hypothesis Testing	*398*
Difference-Based and Relationship-Based Analysis	*399*
Disaggregating Data	400
Qualitative Analysis	404
Sources of Qualitative Data	405
Coding and Codebooks	405
Sample Qualitative Analysis Models	409
Summary	412
Supplemental Resources	412

Chapter 14 Reporting, Disseminating, and Utilizing Evaluation Results   415

Introduction	415
Reporting Results	415
The Full Evaluation Report	416
Other Reporting Mechanisms	417

Stand-Alone Summaries	*417*
A One-Page Bullet Point Summary	*417*
A Summary of Conclusions and Recommendations	*418*
Feedback Reports	*419*
Oral Presentations	*420*
Sharing of Raw Data	*421*

Developing High-Quality, Accessible Reports and Presentations — 421
- Readability — 421
- Words Matter — 424
- Images Matter — 426

Visually Representing Data — 427
- Tables — 428
- Figures — 430
- Dashboards — 436

Dissemination — 437
- Why Disseminate — 437
- Dissemination Plans — 437
- Using Websites and Social Media — 439
- Using Mainstream Media — 441
  - Keep It Simple — 441
  - Keep It Interesting — 442
- Creative Dissemination Modes — 442
- Working With Others — 442

Using Evaluation Results — 443

Summary — 446

Supplemental Resources — 446

Chapter 15 Evaluation as a Business — 449

Introduction — 449

Perspectives on Doing Evaluation as a Business — 449

Ethics — 451
- Conflicts of Interest — 451
- Protection of Human Participants — 452
- Nondiscrimination — 453
- Cultural Respect — 454

Business Knowledge and Skills — 455
- Marketing — 455
- Preparing a Proposal — 460
- Making a Budget — 462

Contracts — 466
- Contract Components — 466
- Intellectual Property — 467

Making a Business Financially Viable	468
Selecting a Business Entity	469
Employee	470
Sole Proprietor	470
Partner in a Partnership	471
Limited Liability Company	471
Corporation/S Corporation	471
Nonprofit Organization	471
Bookkeeping and Record Keeping	472
Developing a Business Plan	472
Summary	474
Supplemental Resources	474

Chapter 16 Interconnections and Practical Implications — 477

Introduction	477
Objectivity and Bias	478
Impacts of Bias on Evaluation	478
Acknowledging Subjectivity and Reducing Bias	480
Building Cultural Competence	482
Personalizing a Social Justice Perspective	485
Reflective Practice and Evaluative Thinking	486
Applying to Practice	487
Making Biases Explicit	487
Infusing Cultural Responsiveness in the Involvement/Engagement of Stakeholders and the Development of Evaluation Questions	488
Infusing Cultural Responsiveness in Decisions About Evaluation Designs	489
Infusing Cultural Responsiveness in Decisions About Data Collection and Analysis	490
Data Collection	*490*
Data Analysis	*491*
Infusing Cultural Responsiveness in Decisions About Reports and Presentations	492
Social Justice Evaluation	493
Politics and Evaluation	494
Voices From the Field: Advice for New Evaluators	495
A Final Thought	497
Supplemental Resources	497

Appendix A	499
Appendix B	502
Glossary	505
References	517
Index	543

Preface

Evaluation has never been more important than it is in today's world, and never has evaluation been confronted with so many serious challenges. In addition to having traditional evaluation skills and knowledge, today's evaluators need to understand how to implement high-quality evaluations within different cultural contexts in a world that is increasingly distrustful of science and facts and is being bombarded with deliberate misinformation and "fake news." The goal of our book is to guide students, practitioners, and users of evaluations to understand evaluation purposes, theories, methodologies, assets, and challenges within today's sociocultural and political context. The book, as a whole and in the individual chapters, examines ways power and privilege and social injustices can affect different aspects of evaluation and how an understanding of these issues can help evaluators better design and implement more inclusive and culturally responsive evaluations that will ultimately improve evaluation quality and usefulness.

While designed primarily as a graduate-level textbook, this book also can serve as a reference guide for others and as a tool for professional development and training. Trainers and/or professional developers may want to use the book as a whole or to use individual chapters or groups of chapters. For example, Chapter 2, "Evaluation Ethics and Quality Standards," would be a useful resource for a professional development session as would Chapter 15, "Evaluation as a Business."

As people with different backgrounds and experiences and a common commitment to social justice and a more inclusive evaluation knowledge base than currently exists, we worked together to ensure a balance in coverage of theory, methods, and practice throughout the book to provide readers with the necessary background to understand social programs and the skills needed to successfully plan and engage in inclusive evaluations across diverse settings.

Who We Are

Adding to the uniqueness of the book is who we are. We view ourselves as a "perfect pairing" to bring added value to an evaluation textbook that combines years of academic and real-world experiences. Veronica Thomas (first author) is a professor of human development at Howard University and a part-time practicing evaluator. Patricia (Pat) Campbell (coauthor) is a former associate professor of research, measurement, and statistics at Georgia State University who is president of Campbell-Kibler Associates, Inc., a research and evaluation company, and a full-time practicing evaluator and researcher. There are a variety of reasons we collaborated to write this book. Both of us are longtime workers in pursuit of social justice. As the only African American elementary school student at an all-white elementary school in the South during the civil rights era, Veronica, at a very young age, became keenly attuned to issues of discrimination, marginalization, and social injustice at individual, institutional, and societal levels. Since that time, she has infused social justice agendas in her teaching, research, and service work. The most rewarding work of Veronica's professional career continues to be the training of and collaborations with African American and other students and young professionals of color who are committed to inclusive research and evaluation with (not *on*) marginalized and underserved communities. In the early 1970s, Pat worked with slain civil rights leader Medgar Evers's brother Charles to register African American voters in Mississippi and served as an advisor on his campaign for governor of Mississippi. A decade later, she coauthored the *AERA Guidelines for Eliminating Race and Sex Bias in Educational Research and Evaluation.* Pat's more recent social justice efforts include conducting educational evaluation and research training in South Africa and Uganda and serving as an expert witness in the Citadel sex discrimination case.

We believe that evaluation needs to respond to Melvin Hall's (2018, para. 3) concern "that the training evaluators receive may not provide the skillset necessary to efficaciously handle the thorny issues of race and class when they emerge through an evaluation process." We see not only limitations in addressing issues of race and class but also insufficient guidance for attending to other areas such as disability and gender and sexual orientation. The unwavering commitment that led us to write this book is recognition that training must help evaluators to deal with difficult issues of social injustice, racism, and other "isms" in their reflective practice and to look at the unintended impacts that bias can have on their work and how, as evaluators, they must recognize and make their biases transparent and use that knowledge to improve the work they do.

We finished writing this book in February 2020 and were completing the final edits in April 2020, under self-isolation during the COVID-19 pandemic. By June 2020 with surging protests against racial injustice and police brutality targeting African Americans, we, yet again, are explicitly reminded of this country's sordid past and its continued failure to redress systemic racism and discriminatory laws and practices. During the last few months of editing this book, in many respects, the world has become a very different place. We don't know what the future holds and we remain hopeful for a safe, healthy and equitable society. But we do know there will be an even greater need for evaluation and social justice as the world recovers.

Contents of the Book and Challenging Assumptions

Those using this as a textbook will find much of what they desire and are used to seeing in existing evaluation textbooks, including discussions of evaluation history, frameworks, models, types, planning, and methods. Not only do we cover those areas from a social justice, diversity, and inclusive lens, but we include topics often not covered extensively in evaluation texts, such as

- evaluation ethics and quality with specific focus on ethical sensitivities in settings in diverse cultural contexts;
- social programming, social justice, and evaluation that help readers understand how social problems and social programs get politicized and, sometimes, framed through a racialized lens;
- responsive stakeholder engagement including strategies and benefits of engaging the "right" stakeholders throughout the entire evaluation process;
- reporting, disseminating, and using evaluation results including communicating results in culturally appropriate ways and making evaluation

findings accessible to and usable for a wide variety of stakeholders, including persons with disabilities; and

- conducting evaluation as a business to help readers who wish to do evaluation as a full-time or part-time business be successful.

In this book, we challenge a number of assumptions. Evaluation has traditionally had as its goal to provide objective judgments of the quality and effectiveness of a variety of programs, policies, projects, and interventions. This focus on objectivity has continued, even though for many years researchers and philosophers of science have debunked the illusion of objectivity in science, research, and evaluation. As we rethink the role of objectivity in evaluation, we highlight the roles of subjectivity and bias. To be good evaluators, we have to acknowledge that we all have biases, explore them, examine how they influence us and the work we do, and determine how we can most effectively work with and across our biases. This is not easy to write about or do. We include insights, examples, and lessons learned from our own work and the work of other evaluators wrestling with diversity and social justice issues in evaluation.

Throughout this book, we directly confront issues of power and privilege. The reality is that evaluations are done, generally, at the request of those with power and resources. Government agencies, private foundations, other funders, and program developers are those who either require evaluations or are required to have evaluations done. We are not saying that this is good or bad, but instead, we are acknowledging it as a fact and one that should be taken into consideration when seeking an understanding of the full context of an evaluation.

Those who commission an evaluation influence the evaluation process especially in terms of decisions about the questions that are asked, the variables over which data are collected to determine if a program or project is a "success," and how or even if the results are used. The less powerful, often those whom a program or project is designed to serve, often have little or no voice in shaping the evaluation questions that are asked or how success is defined. This can be a contributing factor as to why so many evaluations are not "on point" or as useful as they could and should be. In the book, readers learn the importance of planning and implementation evaluations that

- engage a broad range of diverse stakeholders;
- identify and minimize ethical issues;
- ask evaluation questions that matter;
- recognize how cultural differences and inequities can impact data and data collection;
- utilize the best design for the questions; and
- employ various modes to communicate evaluation results in culturally responsive ways.

We also foreground "the elephant in the room"—race and racism and how they have impacted evaluation—while also focusing on what evaluators can and should do.

Organization and Pedagogical Features

Each chapter begins with a set of learning objectives or brief statements that describe what readers are expected to know and/or be able to do after reading the chapter and completing the activities. Examples and opportunities for discussion of perceptions and ideas are included throughout the chapters. Important terms are bolded at their first mention in the book and are defined in the glossary as well as in the first chapter in which they are mentioned.

Four features—Reflect and Discuss, Case Study, Activity, and Voices From the Field—build on the book's overarching theme and are designed to pique readers' interest and extend their learning opportunities. Reflect and Discuss features an issue or question that readers critically think about and discuss in small groups. Case Studies present real or hypothetical cases addressing the application of a particular theoretical, methodological, or practice issue in evaluation. Activities ask readers to do something (individually or in small groups, within class or outside class) involving the application of knowledge gained or issues raised in that particular chapter. *Voices* From the Field are commentaries from evaluation scholars, practitioners, and/or users about a particular issue of relevance. Each chapter ends with a brief summary followed by a description of supplemental resources for readers who wish to delve more deeply into the areas covered in the chapter. At the end of the book is a glossary of all bolded terms included throughout the chapters. Additionally, the references cited in the chapters are found following the glossary.

Teaching Resources

This text includes instructor teaching materials designed to save you time and to help you keep students engaged. To access these resources, search for this book on **sagepub.com** or contact your SAGE representative at sagepub.com/findmyrep.

About the Authors

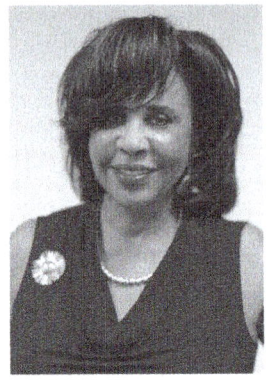

Veronica G. Thomas, PhD, is a Professor in the Department of Human Development and Psychoeducational Studies at Howard University. She also serves as the Evaluation and Continuous Improvement (ECI) Director for the Georgetown-Howard Universities Center for Clinical Translational Sciences (GHUCCTS). Her research interests include culturally responsive evaluation, physical and psychological well-being of Black families, with particular emphasis on women and girls, and the academic and professional development of students of color. Over the years, Dr. Thomas has published work in numerous refereed journals including the *American Journal of Evaluation, New Directions for Evaluation, Journal of Community Genetics, Journal of Black Psychology, International Journal for the Advancement of Counselling* (British spelling), *Family Relations, Adolescence, Educational Leadership, Journal of Adult Development, Review of Research in Education, Journal of Negro Education, Sex Roles, Journal of Social Psychology, Women and Health,* and the *Journal of the National Medical Association*. Her work has been funded by the National Science Foundation, National Institutes of Health, U.S. Department of Education, and the Women's College Coalition. Dr. Thomas major professional associations include the American Evaluation Association (AEA), American Psychological Association (APA), and the American Educational Research Association (AERA). In 2019, she received the AEA Multiethnic Issues in Evaluation Scholarly Leader Award for scholarship that has contributed to social justice-oriented, equity-focused, and/or culturally responsive literature.

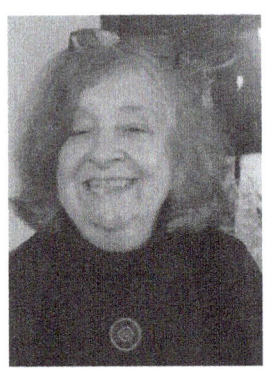

Patricia B. Campbell, PhD, is the president of Campbell-Kibler Associates, Inc. She has been involved in research and evaluation with a focus on issues of race/ethnicity, gender and disability for many years. Formerly an associate professor of research, measurement and statistics at Georgia State University, Dr. Campbell is an Association for Women in Science (AWIS) Fellow and was awarded the Willystine Goodsell Award by the American Educational Research Association (AERA) and the Betty Vetter Award by the Women in Engineering ProActive Network (WEPAN). Dr. Campbell has authored more than 100 publications including coauthoring *Building Evaluation Capacity: Guide I Designing A Cross Project Evaluation and Guide II Collecting and Using Data in Cross-Project Evaluations; A Framework for Evaluating Impacts of Informal Science Education Projects, Good Schools in Poor Neighborhoods: Defying Demographics; Achieving Success"and The AAUW Report: How Schools Shortchange Girls*. Dr. Campbell's websites include www.BeyondRigor.org, which provides easy to use tips to improve the quality of evaluations with diverse populations and www.FairerScience.org which provides researcher and evaluators with tips and tools to more effectively communicate their diversity related research and evaluation findings to the media and the public. In addition Dr. Campbell participates in a variety professional activities include conducting educational evaluation and research training in South Africa and Uganda and serving as an expert witness in the Citadel sex discrimination case.

Acknowledgments

We wish to thank the many individuals who supported the thinking and work behind this book. First, we greatly appreciate the support of our wonderful book editor, Helen Salmon, and the capable SAGE editorial and production staff, especially Chelsea Neve, Megan O'Heffernan, and Kelsey Barkis, for their expert assistance through all phases of the production of this book, and Melinda Masson, for her expert copyediting.

We thank the following reviewers for their critical feedback that certainly helped to expand our thinking and ultimately improved the contents of this book:

Gretchen Arnold, *St. Louis University*

Stephanie Bondi, *University of Nebraska–Lincoln*

Robyn Cooper, *Drake University*

Debra J. Dirksen, *Western New Mexico University*

Marcus-Antonio Galeste, *Arizona State University*

Sebastian Galindo-Gonzalez, *University of Florida*

Brenda Gerhardt, *University of Dayton*

Sandra Handwerk, *Albany State University*

Noriko Ishibashi Martinez, *Loyola University Chicago*

Chad Murphy, *Mississippi University for Women*

Vanaja Nethi, *Nova Southeastern University*

John Ridings, *The Institute for Clinical Social Work*

Marlys Staudt, *University of Tennessee*

John David Tiller, *Tennessee State University*

Karen Tinsley, *Guilford College*

Kasahun Woldemariam, *Spelman College*

Wenfan Yan, *University of Massachusetts Boston*

We both are so very grateful to the many evaluation colleagues, stakeholders, and users, far too numerous to name, who have enriched our thinking and practice, particularly as they relate to cultural competence, social justice, diversity, and inclusion.

I (Veronica) want to thank the (current and former) faculty members, graduate students, and administrators at Howard University who inspired and assisted me in multiple ways, including Peggy C. Carr, Constance Ellison, Lawrence Gary, Brooke McKie, Faun Rockcliffe, Diana Edwards, Kimberly Edelin Freeman, and Dawn Williams. A special thanks to Jennifer C. Greene (University of Illinois at Urbana-Champaign) and Valerie Caracelli (U.S. Government Accountability Office) for their wisdom and for supporting my scholarship and encouraging me to take it to the next level. I thank my family for their support every day, every month of every year. And last, but certainly not least, I wish to extend my heartfelt thanks to Alvin E. Courtney Jr. for his love, motivation, inspiration, and relentless pursuit of excellence.

I (Pat) don't even know where to begin to thank people for their inspiration and support. I am so fearful that I will miss folks. Toni, Eric, Melvin, Lois-ellin, and Lynn and Kathryn, Mort, Pamela, Ann, Seth, Jesse, and—adhering to a tradition started many years ago, in my dissertation—Tonya and Houdini the cats, thank you. And at the beginning and the end, as always, there is Tom. Thank you, my love.

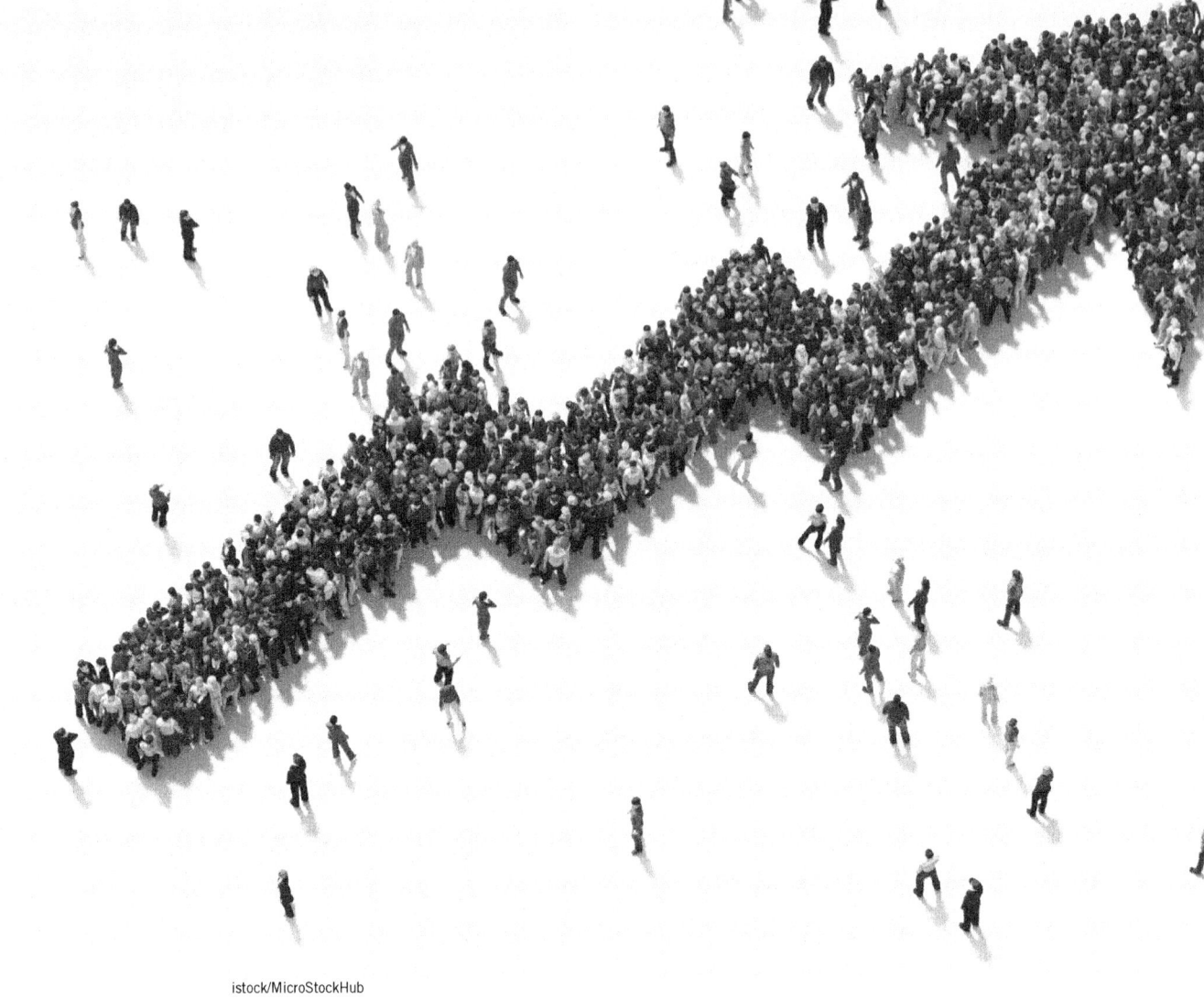
istock/MicroStockHub

Evaluation's ultimate goal is to provide credible evidence that fosters greater understanding and improves decision making, all aimed at improving social conditions and promoting healthy, just, and equitable communities.

CHAPTER 1

Evaluations of Future
Inclusive, Equity-Focused, Useful, and Used

Over the past 20 years, there has been a large increase in the number of evaluations conducted and utilized. During the same time period, there has been an emphasis on the professionalization of evaluation and evaluators and on the skills and knowledge evaluators need to be effective. In today's world, along with having more traditional evaluation skills and knowledge, evaluators need to understand how to implement high-quality evaluations within different cultural contexts in a world that is increasingly distrustful of data and facts. The goal of this book is to provide readers with this knowledge and those skills.

After reading this chapter and participating in the activities, readers will be able to meet the following learning objectives:

- Describe the book's goals and the authors' philosophy underlying the book
- Have a general knowledge of the content to be covered in the book
- Describe what a racialized and social justice perspective is
- Explain the meaning and importance of cultural competence and responsiveness in terms of evaluation
- Explain ways that bias and perceptions of objectivity can skew evaluations
- List some challenges of doing evaluation in today's world

Introduction

This chapter provides an overview of the book, its goals, and its underlying philosophy. It includes an introduction to the content, the major cross-chapter themes, and the framework of the book. In addition, it introduces the concept of **cultural competence**, which is the ability to understand, communicate with, and effectively interact with people across cultures (Make It Our Business, 2017), and **cultural responsiveness**, which is the application of the abilities described in the definition of cultural competence. Along with covering issues of objectivity and bias, the chapter discusses the declining trust in science and data, the rise of fake news and alternative facts, and how this can impact evaluators and evaluation. **Fake news** has been defined as "false new[s] stories, often spread as propaganda on social media. It can also characterize any information that one finds critical about [oneself]" (Dicitionary.com, 2020b, para. 1) while **alternative facts** are the "opposite of reality (which is delusion), or the opposite of truth (which is untruth)" (Dicitionary.com, 2020a, para. 1).

It is expected that after completing this chapter and the activities, the reader will have an overview of the content covered in the book and know its goals and the general themes that cut across chapters, including the influence of a racialized and social justice perspective on the book. Having a **racialized perspective** "means paying attention, even when uncomfortable, to the ways in which race shapes problem definition and solution as well as particular group's access to opportunity" (Thomas, Madison, Rockcliffe, DeLaine, & Lowe, 2018, p. 521).

An Overview of the Book

The focus of this book is to help students and other readers understand both the art and the science of evaluation. It covers theoretical and practical issues related to evaluation of programs, particularly social programs and projects, with an emphasis on viewing evaluation topics through a social justice, diversity, and inclusive perspective. The book provides an approach for evaluators to aim toward being reflective practitioners and culturally competent professionals.

Structure of the Book

Each chapter begins with a series of **learning objectives**, or "brief statements that describe what students will be expected to learn" (Great Schools Partnership, 2014, para. 1 [), and ends with a summary of the chapter. Numerous examples and activities are included for the purpose of illustrating how the information in the book can be applied in actual settings. Within each chapter is commentary from practicing evaluators and evaluation users, called Voices From the Field. Also included is an annotated list of supplemental resources and/or tools for those who would like to delve more deeply into the areas covered. As can be seen in this chapter, evaluation-related terms are bolded the first time they are defined, and at the end of the book is a glossary of the bolded terms. The book as a whole and the individual chapters cover how race and social justice issues affect different aspects of evaluation and how readers can use that knowledge to improve evaluation quality and usefulness.

Chapter Content

The book is composed of 16 chapters. This, the first chapter, provides an overview of the book and its underlying premises. Chapter 2, "Evaluation Ethics and Quality Standards," covers ethical and quality standards for the profession. Building on the American Evaluation Association's (AEA) *Evaluators' Ethical Guiding Principles*, the chapter covers various types of potential ethical dilemmas, including the ethical dimensions of bias. It challenges readers to provide their own solutions to these dilemmas, along with a rationale, and helps readers understand what is and isn't an ethical and quality evaluation, taking into consideration not only culture and context but also the AEA's *Evaluators' Ethical Guiding Principles* and the *Program Evaluation Standards* compiled by the Joint Committee on Standards for Educational Evaluation.

Chapter 3, "Historical Evolution of Program Evaluation Through a Social Justice Lens," covers key events and developments in evaluation practice including the professionalization of evaluation, fundamental and recurring issues in the field, and technological advances. It goes on to discuss emerging trends and key scholars—particularly those little-known or "hidden" figures who contributed to the growth of the field. Chapter 4, "Evaluation Paradigms, Theories, and Models," introduces the reader to the range of evaluation frameworks, models, and theories that make up evaluation while Chapter 5, "Social Justice and Evaluation: Theories, Challenges, Frameworks, and Paradigms," provides an overview of social justice issues and theories. Chapter 5 also builds on the content of Chapter 4 to show how social justice frameworks and paradigms modify and advance more traditional models and theories. Chapter 6, "Evaluation Types With a Cultural and Racial Equity Lens," examines the major categories and types of evaluation, when they typically occur, their purpose or major strengths, and their primary audiences.

Chapter 7, "Social Programming, Social Justice, and Evaluation," moves from the theory, models, and history of evaluation into looking at what will be evaluated. Along with describing social programming and graphically illustrating its components through various types of logic models, the chapter explores the issues, challenges, and complexities of implementing and evaluating social programs in a diverse society.

Chapters 8 through 14 cover the "how to" or practical aspects of doing an evaluation. Chapter 8, "Responsive Stakeholder Engagement and Democratization of the Evaluation Process," discusses the importance of stakeholder engagement and provides a variety of ways to improve the quality and quantity of stakeholder engagement, as well as ways that greater stakeholder engagement can positively influence the evaluation process. Chapter 9, "Planning the Evaluation," and Chapter 10, "Evaluation Questions That Matter," focus on the information that needs to be collected or developed before the evaluation can be designed and implemented. Chapter 9 covers the information and knowledge needed to plan a responsive evaluation and introduces tools that are used in project planning and can be customized for use in evaluation planning. The chapter includes the steps needed to identify project goals and define success including ways of identifying and involving stakeholders. From project goals and definitions of success, the chapter goes on to show readers how to define goals for the evaluation and identify different types of **indicators**, which are "variables that provide evidence that a certain condition exists or certain results have, or have not, been achieved" (Campbell, Thomas, & Stoll, 2009, p. 54). Chapter 10 moves the reader from the goals for an evaluation to the development of the questions the evaluation will answer. Covered in this chapter are ways to develop evaluation questions that matter, including the characteristics and sources of good evaluation questions, and ways of prioritizing those evaluation questions for diverse audiences.

Chapters 11 through 14 target the technical aspects of evaluation including design, data collection, analysis, and reporting. Chapter 11, "Selecting Appropriate Evaluation Designs," describes a variety of experimental, quasi-experimental, and descriptive designs; their strengths and weaknesses; and their appropriateness for different evaluation questions. It also covers issues of rigor, comparison and control groups, and longitudinal data including ethical issues tied to their use with different populations. Chapter 12, "Defining, Collecting, and Managing Data," looks at the strengths and weaknesses of both qualitative and quantitative data, including ways of ensuring data quality including issues of validity and reliability. Also covered are sources of data to be used in evaluations, ways of collecting these data, measures, and ways of managing the data that are collected. Chapter 13, "The Best Analysis for the Data," begins with a discussion of the types of reasoning that underlie analytic decisions and provides an introduction to different types of data analysis. The final chapter in this section, Chapter 14, "Reporting, Disseminating, and Utilizing Evaluation Results," focuses on how to present information visually and textually to different groups in valid and culturally appropriate ways. It also covers different modes for communicating and disseminating results including ways to make evaluation results accessible to people with disabilities as well as ways to make the results more usable.

Chapter 15, "Evaluation as a Business," goes in a very different direction, providing readers who are planning to do evaluations as a consultant or as a part- or full-time business with an overview of the business aspects of evaluation and the knowledge and skills needed to do evaluation as a business. Areas covered in this chapter include evaluation proposal writing, budgeting, interacting with clients, marketing, contracts, and business plans. In the final chapter, Chapter 16, "Interconnections and Practical Implications," we go back to bias and cultural competence and take another look at how bias and a lack of cultural competence can impact evaluation decision making. Also covered are ways that readers can reduce their own biases and increase their cultural competence and how that can lead to evaluators becoming more culturally responsive. Reflecting on what we covered in earlier chapters, we explore some of the impacts of cultural responsiveness on decision making.

An Overview of Evaluation

The Oxford University Press defines evaluation as "the making of a judgment about the amount, number, or value of something" (Lexico.com, 2020, para. 1). As the definition implies, evaluation is an everyday activity. All of us, either consciously or unconsciously, at some point in time consider the value of a thing; take account of the actions we, or others, have taken; and examine the progress (or lack thereof) we have made on the path we are traveling. Individuals evaluate products and prices at a store to determine whether they will buy a product or even continue to patronize that business. People evaluate their relationships, finances, goals, and health to determine where they are and how they can get better in these areas. By engaging in some form of evaluation, individuals try to assess what is good or bad, what option is better or worse, and what conditions are best to nurture and produce the desired outcomes.

Although people make evaluation decisions, this doesn't necessarily make them evaluators. Evaluators are professionals who ask and answer questions regarding projects, policies, and programs through the collection and analysis of data. Evaluators seek to provide information that improves decision making at a variety of levels—funders, policymakers, staff, and actual as well as potential participants. Table 1.1 provides a broad overview of the evaluation process from planning to implementation to reporting and use of results.

Table 1.1 Phases of the Evaluation Process		
Planning→	**Implementation→**	**Reporting/Use of Results**
• Analyze project culture and context • Clarify objectives • Identify questions and indicators • Select measures and an evaluation design • Develop management procedures including a budget	• Conduct pretest or pilot testing as necessary • Gather credible evidence (data collection) • Conduct data analysis, interpretation, and synthesis	• Report findings • Disseminate findings and share lessons learned • Encourage use of results • Determine next steps, if any
↑	↑	↑
Involve and Engage Diverse Stakeholders		

Definitions of Evaluation

While for the general public there is a fairly consistent definition of evaluation, that is not the case for evaluators. As Mark, Greene, and Shaw (2006, p. 6) point out, "If you ask 10 evaluators to define evaluation, you'll probably end up with 23 different definitions. Given that evaluation is diverse, with multiple countenances, it should not be surprising that varying definitions exist."

Definitions of evaluation from leaders in the field, from the 1980s and 1990s, focused on evaluation as a way of determining value. For example, Michael Scriven, in 1991, defined evaluation as "the process of determining the merit, worth, or value of something, or the product of that process" (p. 139). Several years earlier, Yvonna Lincoln and Egon Guba (1985) defined evaluation as "disciplined inquiry" with a goal of determining value for program improvement or refinement. Their definition also made a distinction between formative evaluation (to determine the value of a project, program, or product in order to improve or refine it) and summative evaluation (to determine the worth, value, and/or success of a project, program, or product), both of which are discussed in further detail in Chapter 6. In 1997, Michael Quinn Patton went a step further in his definition, adding that the information collected in evaluation could be used to inform decisions about future programming as well as "to make judgments about the program [and] improve program effectiveness, and/or inform decisions about future programming" (p. 23). Trochim's (1998) definition includes providing evidence in decision making and contexts as well. It also describes those contexts as "inherently political" and as involving "multiple and often conflicting stakeholders, where resources are seldom sufficient and where time pressures are salient" (p. 248).

More recent definitions (e.g., Newcomer, Hatry, & Wholey, 2015; Rossi, Lipsey, & Henry, 2019) refer explicitly to social science methods, with Rossi et al. (2019) including in their definition a reference to context and an explicit goal to "inform social action to improve social conditions" (p. 6). While myriad descriptions of evaluation are found in the literature, consistent across them is the idea that evaluation is a systematic, applied inquiry process for collecting and synthesizing evidence (data) and drawing conclusions about the state of affairs, value, merit, worth, significance, or quality of an entity.

The focus on value is key to understanding what evaluation is. Value is the "feature that distinguishes evaluation from other types of inquiry, such as basic science research, clinical epidemiology, investigative journalism, or public polling" (Fournier, 2005, p. 140). Unlike research, evaluations do not simply report outcomes; they draw conclusions about the value or quality of those outcomes within a particular context and for specific groups. **Program evaluation**, in particular, involves the use of research methods to examine a program's goals, objectives, outcomes, and impact. It can also be used to investigate a program's structure, characteristics, activities, organization, and political and social environment. Evaluation has the potential to enable society to meaningfully learn about its persistent social problems and how to effectively solve them (Cronbach et al., 1980).

Our definition of evaluation encompasses many of the components in the earlier definitions. It includes systematic inquiry, assessing value and awareness of context, and also ethical, quality, justice, and cultural concerns. We define evaluation as a

> disciplined inquiry involving the systematic, contextually responsive, and ethical application of research tools and methods to collect data that assess the effectiveness and operations of programs within the various social, political, and cultural contexts in which they operate. Evaluation's ultimate goal is to provide **credible evidence** that fosters greater understanding and improves decision making, all aimed at improving social conditions and promoting healthy, just, and equitable communities.

Evaluation Characteristics

Evaluation is not simply a scientific endeavor in search of "truth" and "solutions." Evaluation, while complex, is often less concerned with general truths and generalizations because it focuses on specific programs and practices taking place within a specific context. This makes evaluation much more an idiosyncratic activity that must be tailored to the particular circumstances under consideration. "Evaluation is not an examination into the inert, static, and external realities of programs but instead, into the fluid subjective world of people's lives as experienced, interpreted, recalled, and mediated by them and the, oftentimes, racialized contexts of the systems that programs, communities, and individuals are embedded" (Thomas et al., 2018, p. 156). The complexity of social programs makes it critical that anyone who is tasked with evaluating such programs understand the context of the program and the evaluation. Chapter 9 covers this aspect in greater detail.

Evaluation is very much a social enterprise that is best understood by taking into consideration the social, cultural, economic, and political contexts surrounding the program under consideration. Attention to public interest and public good is a critical aspect of the evaluation process. Evaluators cannot ignore the reality that they become a part of the never-ending struggle to make judgment calls about social activities that create the conditions or obstacles for social mobility (Waters, 1998). In 1980, Cronbach et al. pointed out that program evaluation was a process by which society learns about itself. Melvin Hall (2018a) used that point to underscore the need for evaluators to take up more space in the public sphere where institutionalized sources of potential racism and classism should be identified and interrogated. His call was for evaluative thinking, as discussed in the next section, to become more prominent in public debate and policy reviews—an appeal to evaluators to identify and engage the important societal issues embedded in the work we do. Hall's charge is an integral part of the underlying thinking of this book. The social justice focus of this book is not just limited to race and class but includes other social justice issues such as disability, sex or gender, sexual orientation, and socioeconomic status. In the activity that follows, readers begin to develop their own definitions of evaluation.

> ## Activity
> ### Defining Evaluation
>
> In small groups, discuss the characteristics you think should be included in a definition of evaluation.

Evaluative Thinking

The concept of **evaluative thinking** is an increasingly important topic in evaluation and a key component of evaluation capacity and practice (e.g., Baker & Bruner, 2012; Patton, 2008), However as Buckley, Archibald, Hargraves, and Trochim (2015) point out, definitions of evaluative thinking are varied and sometimes ambiguous. They hold that evaluative thinking is, "in essence, critical thinking applied to contexts of evaluation" (p. 376). Other definitions of evaluative thinking describe it as a type of **reflective practice**, which is "a way of studying your own experiences to improve the way you work" (Brightside, 2020, para. 1). Baker and Bruner (2012, p. 1) see evaluative thinking as a reflective practice that "fully integrates systematic questioning, data, and action into an organization's work practices" while Michael Quinn Patton (quoted in Waldick, 2011, para. 13) describes it as "an analytical way of thinking that infuses everything that goes on." After extensive review of the evaluation thinking literature, Buckley et al. (2015, p. 378) proposed the following definition: "Evaluative thinking is critical thinking applied in the context of evaluation, motivated by an attitude of inquisitiveness and a belief in the value of evidence, that involves identifying assumptions, posing thoughtful questions, pursuing deeper understanding through reflection and perspective taking, and informing decisions in preparation for action."

Reflective practice can be an important component of evaluative thinking. Reflection and reflective practice can catalyze evaluators to

- collect information before making up one's mind;
- seek various points of view before coming to a conclusion;
- think extensively about a problem before responding;
- calibrate the degree of strength of one's opinion to the degrees of evidence available;
- think about future consequences before taking action;
- explicitly weigh pluses and minuses of situations before making a decision; [and]
- seek nuance and avoid absolutism. (Stanovich, 2010, p. 36)

Evaluative thinking can start by simply asking some questions and investing in the process of answering them. Sometimes, the reflection and discussion themselves are as important as any answer you might come up with (IllumiLab, 2018a). The following activity provides some questions that readers can ask to help promote reflection and evaluative thinking.

Activity
Applying Evaluative Thinking

Here are three areas and related questions that readers can ask themselves as part of an evaluative thinking process:

Identify and Challenge Assumptions & Assertions

"What are we assuming? Do we actually know that?"

"How do we know that?"

"What makes you say that?"

Seek Out Blind Spots

"What are we missing?"

"Whose perspective isn't represented?"

"What other explanations could there be?"

Capture Musings & Learning Questions

"I wonder if . . ."

"I bet if we . . ."

"If I knew _____, I could _____." (IllumiLab, 2018b, "Asking Questions")

Read the following text about money.

Money can mean so many things to so many people. In evaluation, money can be an outcome, a confounding variable, or even a risk factor. Money is tied to access to resources and power. It is a key component that needs to be considered in evaluations.

Money as defined as annual family income, along with adult educational attainment are the conventional measures of socioeconomic status (SES) or class, although they are not the only ones. Indeed there is no consensus definition of class. . . .

Making assumptions about income based on race, ethnicity or family education is dangerous and should be avoided. While there is a correlation between income and race and ethnicity, as well as between income and educational level in the United States, lower income and higher income families come in all colors and from all educational levels. Race, ethnicity and educational level are not proxy indicators of income or SES and should not be used as such. Indeed, evaluators should consider in their analysis disaggregating by race, ethnicity and educational level to tease out interactions.

Asking about income can be sensitive. Many people don't feel comfortable discussing their income and often students don't know their family income. Many evaluators use ranges the participant can choose such as $0–$25,000 or $25,001–$50,000 rather than asking for exact or even approximate numbers.

When working with lower income participants, particularly if they are in programs that provide them with financial support, evaluators should be sensitive to participant fears that if they don't participate in the evaluation or if they raise concerns, that could impact their continued support from the program. This could impact whether their participation in the evaluation is truly voluntary and if their responses are free from pressure. (Campbell & Jolly, n.d.h, paras. 1–5)

Now, organize in small groups and apply evaluative thinking by asking some of the preceding questions about the text you just read. Discuss your answers with others.

Courtesy of Campbell-Kibler Associates, Inc.

Race, Racism, Social Justice, and a Racialized Perspective

As will be explored more deeply in Chapter 5, race and racism are deeply embedded in the fabric of the United States and have had a complex and destructive influence on the lives of people of color. This influence extends to people's participation in programs and even the very design of the programs being evaluated. It is critical that evaluators work toward unpacking how bias, in general, but racism, in particular, is a complex and destructive force including in evaluations. Thomas et al. (2018) point out that evaluators have both an opportunity and a responsibility to illuminate the potential impact of race and racism on the programs that they evaluate and the environments that they engage. They urge readers "to gain a deeper understanding of racism as a complex interplay of individual attitudes, social values, and institutional policies and practices and to bring these understandings to the work they do" (p. 515).

Race has been defined as "socially constructed differences among people based on characteristics such as accent or manner of speech, name, clothing, diet, beliefs and practices, leisure preferences, places of origin and so forth" (Ontario Human Rights Commission, n.d., para. 3). The process of social construction of race is called racialization: "the process by which societies construct races as real, different and unequal in ways that matter to economic, political and social life" (Ontario Human Rights Commission, n.d., para. 3). There is no fixed definition of racial discrimination. However, it has been described as "any distinction, conduct or action, whether intentional or not, but based on a person's race, which has the effect of imposing burdens on an individual or group, not imposed upon others or which withholds or limits access to benefits available to other members of society" (Ontario Human Rights Commission, n.d., para. 2).

"Racism is a wider phenomenon than racial discrimination. . . . Racism is an ideology that either directly or indirectly asserts that one group is inherently superior to others. It can be openly displayed in racial jokes and slurs or hate crimes but it can be more deeply rooted in attitudes, values and stereotypical beliefs. In some cases, these are unconsciously held and have become deeply embedded in systems and institutions that have evolved over time" (Ontario Human Rights Commission, n.d., paras. 5–6). Racism is pervasive. As entertainer Beyoncé commented, "It's been said that racism is so American, that when we protest racism, some assume we are protesting America" (Nyren, 2017, para. 4).

Racism operates at a number of levels—in particular, individual, systemic, and societal. It is important to note that "stating that racism privileges [W]hites does not mean that individual [W]hite people do not struggle or face barriers. It does mean that [they] do not face the particular barriers of racism" (Akintunde, 1999, p. 24).

A racialized perspective is one that explicitly foregrounds the impacts of society's construction of races in ways that are unequal. This can be a difficult thing to do for members of the **dominant culture**, the group whose members are in the majority or who wield more power than other groups (SparkNotes, 2020). Members of the dominant culture, which in the United States are whites and other people of European origin, can be and often are influenced by the values, or system of thought, in a society that are most standard and widely held at a given time. This is referred to as the **dominant paradigm**. Being a member of the dominant culture with its standard and widely held values can impact one's ability to recognize other, different systems of thought and values (Thomas & Campbell, 2017).

In 2018, Thomas et al. (p. 516) put forth five principled beliefs that explicitly guided their thinking about racism. These principles address concerns about dominant cultures and paradigms and guide the thinking of this text related to social programs, social justice, and evaluation of social programs. The principles are as follows:

1. Race is not a biologically determined reality but instead is a socially constructed phenomenon that continues to differentially shape the allocation of power and distribution of benefits and burden among groups within this country.

2. Racism is real, pervasive, and systematic. Race and racism are timeless, endemic, and permanently entwined within the social fabric of American society (e.g., D. Bell, 1995; Delgado & Stefancic, 2001; Feagin, 2013; C. Lawrence, 1995; Solórzano, 1997). As such, racism is not an aberrant but, instead, the natural order of American life, the usual way business is conducted in this society, and a common everyday experience for most people of color. Short-lived victories for persons of color slide into irrelevance as racial patterns adapt in ways that maintain white dominance (D. Bell, 1992).

3. Individual racists need not exist for institutional racism to persist in the dominant culture (Bonilla-Silva, 2018).

4. Racism is not fluid, meaning that it does not flow back and forth, one day benefiting whites and another day (or even era) benefiting people of color. Instead, the direction of power between whites and people of color is historic, traditional, normalized, and deeply embedded in the fabric of U.S. society (DeAngelo, 2011).

5. Race and racism continue to have tremendous consequences for the work of social and behavioral science researchers, and as such, evaluators are certainly not detached from these socially constructed phenomena.

Other Social Justice Issues

This book has an underlying focus on race and examines evaluation from a racialized perspective, as is covered in detail in Chapter 5. It also focuses on other social justice issues, including those tied to sex and gender where, over time, there has been great change in the ways people are identified and categorized. Traditionally, one identified or was identified as either female or male. When the concept of gender was introduced, it was often used interchangeably with sex, although gender, like race, is a socially constructed phenomenon. It includes how individuals see themselves, how others perceive them and expect them to behave, and the interactions that they have with others (Conger, 2017, para. 21). In terms of both gender and sex, there can be fluidity and change. "Most people—including most transgender people—are either male or female. But some people don't neatly fit into the categories of 'man' or 'woman,' or 'male' or 'female.' For example, some people have a gender that blends elements of being a man or a woman, or a gender that is different than either male or female. Some people don't identify with any gender. Some people's gender changes over time. People whose gender is not male or female use many different terms to describe themselves, with non-binary being one of the most common" (National Center for Transgender Equality, 2018, paras. 1–2).

In the case of race or sex or other areas including disability, sexual orientation, and socioeconomic status, there are those with more or less privilege. Those with less privilege are more apt to be discriminated against. Privilege has been defined as "unearned access to resources (social power) that are only readily available to some people because of their social group membership; an advantage, or immunity granted to or enjoyed by one societal group above and beyond the common advantage of all other groups. Privilege is often invisible to those who have it" (National Conference for Community and Justice, n.d., para. 7). Discrimination can be defined as "the unequal allocation of goods, resources, and services, and the limitation of access to full participation in society based on individual membership in a particular social group; reinforced by law, policy, and cultural norms that allow for differential treatment on the basis of identity" (National Conference for Community and Justice, n.d., para. 4). Table 1.2 defines some common belief systems that negatively affect marginalized groups and lead to privilege for dominant groups.

Table 1.2	Belief Systems Behind Oppression
Ableism	The individual, cultural, and institutional beliefs and discrimination that systematically oppress people who have mental, emotional[,] and physical disabilities.
Ageism	The individual, cultural, and institutional beliefs and discrimination that systematically oppress young and elderly people.
Classism	The institutional, cultural, and individual set of beliefs and discrimination that assigns differential value to people according to their socio-economic class; and an economic system which creates excessive inequality and causes basic human needs to go unmet.
Heterosexism	The belief that heterosexuality is the only normal and acceptable sexual orientation. Now encompasses the individual, cultural, and institutional beliefs and discrimination that systematically oppress lesbian, gay, bisexual, transgender, [and] queer (LGBTQ) people [including] homophobia: An irrational fear of or aversion to homosexuality or LGBTQ people.
Racism	The individual, cultural, and institutional beliefs and discrimination that systematically oppress people of color (Blacks, Latino/as, [Indigenous People], and Asians).
Sexism	The individual, cultural, and institutional beliefs and discrimination that systematically oppress women.

Source: National Conference for Community and Justice, n.d., paras. 12–13, 15–18.

In many of these areas including sex, race/national origin, and sexual orientation there has been **de jura discrimination**—that is, legal discrimination. For example, until the 1967 Supreme Court decision in *Loving v. Virginia*, in some states, Blacks and whites were not allowed to marry (National Constitutional Center, 2019). It wasn't until 2015 and the decision in *Obergefell v. Hodges* that same-sex couples were able to marry anywhere in the United States (Liptak, 2015). Straight women were legally banned from many jobs in the armed services (Pruitt, 2018), and lesbian, gay, bisexual, transgender, and queer (LGBTQ) individuals were not permitted to serve at all (Human Rights Campaign, 2020). In 2019, a ban on transgender individuals serving in the military was enacted (D. Phillips, 2019).

Because of the relentless efforts of many people over time, there have been a number of successful efforts to limit or eliminate de jura discrimination. However, another form of discrimination has been much more difficult to dismantle and is much more apt to impact evaluators and evaluations. That is **de facto discrimination**, or discrimination that is not sanctified by law but happens in fact. For example, racial segregation in schools was allowed by law, but the 1954 Supreme Court decision in *Brown v. Board of Education* determined that segregation in schools was unconstitutional. Today, however, many public schools remain segregated not by law but in fact (Orfield & Frankenberg, 2014). The situation is the same in terms of housing. In 1968, the Fair Housing Act was passed to protect people from discrimination when they are renting or buying a house, but today there is still great segregation in housing (Schuetz, 2017). Discrimination has real consequences for real people in real programs. For example, being in environments that are racially segregated can impact the context in which programs are implemented and the responses of participants to programs. This needs to be a concern to those evaluating programs.

While de jura job segregation by sex no longer exists, de facto segregation does, with men predominating in the more prestigious and more highly paid careers. This has implications for evaluations done in the workplace in terms of the culture and acceptance of women in fields such as engineering and construction where men predominate and in fields like elementary school teaching and nursing where women predominate.

Much of this de facto segregation is based on **stereotypes**, or "preconceived notion[s], especially about a group of people" (Vocabulary.com, n.d., para. 1), and assumptions that people have about others because of their race, sex/gender, disability, and other areas. As will be explained in more detail in Chapter 5, everyone fits into more than one demographic group, some of which are marginalized such as being poor, female, a person of color, and a person with disabilities. Crenshaw (2017, para. 4) calls this **intersectionality**, "a lens through which you can see where power comes and collides, where it interlocks and intersects. It's not simply that there's a race problem here, a gender problem here, and a class or L[GB]TQ problem there. Many times that framework erases what happens to people who are subject to all of these things." Throughout this book are examples of how stereotypes and perceptions about individuals because of their race, sex/gender, disability, and other characteristics can sometimes negatively influence the views of evaluators as well as those of program staff and funders, thus impacting the conceptualization, implementation, and outcomes of evaluations. However, throughout the book we offer some tangible strategies for how this impact can be counteracted.

Objectivity and Bias

Objectivity

For hundreds of years, philosophers of science have commented on the difficulty of attaining scientific objectivity. In 1821, Isaac Watts described the near impossibility of being unbiased: "The eyes of a man in the jaundice make yellow observations on everything; and the soul tinctured with any passion diffuses a false color over the appearance of things" (AZ Quotes, n.d., para. 1). More recently, Nage (1961) wrote about the difficulty of preventing our likes, aversions, hopes, and fears from coloring our conclusions. Looking at the issues of objectivity from a different perspective, Martin, Lee, and Bang (2014, para. 10) suggested that "it is commonly said that scientists should have a professional distance from what they study. But the metaphor of distance is misleading. Science, like a painting, necessarily has a perspective. And that perspective is at least partially shaped by variables such as race, gender and class." When we move past the concept that scientists and evaluators are objective, we are able to look more clearly at biases, including our own.

Bias

Explicit Bias

We all have biases, and we need to pay attention to the biases people have as individuals and as evaluators. Bias has been defined as a particular tendency or inclination, especially one that prevents reasonable, knowledgeable, thoughtful consideration of a question (Harmon, 1973). While bias can be intentional, it often is not. Bias can grow out of one's assumptions—the things one accepts as true without questioning. It can be based on the ways the evaluator thinks things are (or should be). Biases can be explicit—that is, one knows one has a particular bias. For example, we might be biased in favor of people who like Ben & Jerry's ice cream and biased against those who like Häagen-Dazs ice cream. When a bias is explicit, one can accept it or try to counteract it.

Evaluators can, and most often do, have explicit biases. Our biases may be related to methods—for example, being biased against use of online surveys or biased in favor of programs that include a component for participant reflection. Evaluators may also be biased in terms of what they think participants in a program need to be successful. If evaluators have explicit biases that can impact their work, they need to let others know their biases exist and to have others check to see if those biases are impacting the work. It is important for evaluators to remember that, as Hannum (2018, para. 4) points out,

> there is bias and error in all information. Understanding how information can be biased is helpful. Equally helpful is understanding the roots of bias within ourselves. We often think of other people deceiving us, but the best place to begin to whittle away nonsense is within ourselves. The more we know about how to gather, interpret, and use information, the less likely we are to get caught up in assumptions, bias, and outright deception.

The following activity provides an opportunity for readers to reflect on and discuss their own explicit biases.

> ## Reflect and Discuss
> ### My Biases
>
> In small groups, discuss some of the fairly superficial preferences and biases you might have. Then, either speaking in general or personally, discuss preferences that might impact how someone approaches a project.

Implicit Bias

While some biases are explicit, others are implicit. According to the Kirwan Institute at The Ohio State University (Staats, Capatosto, Tenney, & Mamo, 2017, p. 10), **implicit bias** refers to "the attitudes or stereotypes that affect our understanding, actions, and decisions in an unconscious manner." Like explicit biases, they can impact assessments and judgments, both favorably and unfavorably. But unlike explicit biases, implicit biases are "activated involuntarily, without awareness or intentional control" (Staats et al., 2017, p. 10). The following are some key characteristics of implicit biases (Staats et al., 2017).

- Implicit biases are pervasive. Everyone possesses them, even people with avowed commitments to impartiality, such as judges.
- Implicit and explicit biases are related but distinct mental constructs. They are not mutually exclusive and may even reinforce each other.
- The implicit associations we hold do not necessarily align with our declared beliefs or even reflect stances we would explicitly endorse.
- We generally tend to hold implicit biases that favor our own in-group, though research has shown that we can still hold implicit biases against our in-group.
- Implicit biases are malleable. Our brains are incredibly complex, and the implicit associations that we have formed can be gradually unlearned through a variety of de-biasing techniques.

It is difficult to understate the importance of considering the role of implicit bias when analyzing societal inequities. Implicit biases, explicit biases, and structural forces are often mutually reinforcing. Research on implicit bias suggests that many of our decisions regarding racial stereotypes are made at unconscious level (e.g., Greenwald & Banaji, 1995; Staats, 2017). For example, Harvard University's Project Implicit (2011b) has found most Americans have an automatic preference for white people over Black people, and often have automatic preferences for straight people over gay people and for young people over old people. In addition, the Project Implicit researchers have found stronger links between females and family and between males and careers. Similarly, they have found stronger links between females and the liberal arts and between males and science. This does not mean that people are racist or homophobic or believe that a woman's role is in the kitchen, but it does mean that people are influenced, consciously and unconsciously, by the environment around them.

Referring to race, Project Implicit (2011b, para. 17) explains that "implicit preferences for majority groups (e.g., white people) are likely common because of strong negative associations with Black people in American society. There is a long history of racial discrimination in the United States, and Black people are often portrayed negatively in culture and mass media." There are also **implicit stereotypes**, or those that are "relatively inaccessible to conscious awareness and/or control. Even if you say that men and women are equally good at math, it is possible that you associate math more strongly with men without being actively aware of it. In this case we would say that you have an implicit math + men stereotype" (Project Implicit, 2011b, para. 2). One way to explore implicit biases is, as described in the following activity, to take the Implicit Association Test (IAT).

Activity
Take the Implicit Association Test (Optional)

The IAT takes about 10–15 minutes to complete. It measures attitudes and beliefs that people may be unwilling or unable to report and "measures the strength of associations between concepts (e.g., [B]lack people, gay people) and evaluations (e.g., good, bad) or stereotypes (e.g., athletic, clumsy)" (Project Implicit, 2011a, para. 1). The results will be immediately reported to you and will mention possible interpretations that have a basis in research. If you are unprepared to encounter interpretations that you might find objectionable, please do not take the test. You may want to go to https://implicit.harvard.edu/implicit/iatdetails.html for more information about the test.

To take the test, visit https://implicit.harvard.edu/implicit/selectatest.html.

In his 2019 Voices From the Field interview, as follows, Melvin E. Hall discusses objectivity, bias, and why he became an evaluator.

Voices From the Field

Melvin E. Hall: Objectivity, Bias, and Being an Evaluator

I came into evaluation in part because I was aware of the myth of evaluator objectivity. People have built-in biases; we all do. Once you recognize that people have built-in structural biases, you have two choices—you can call them out on their biases, or you can find ways to have those biases balanced with other perspectives. I made the second choice.

The value I bring to evaluation is another worldview, one which will help other people understand their own biases as well as mine. Inherent bias is not only not unavoidable, but you don't even want to try to avoid it—I believe that any knowledge you have biases you. For example, if I know the world is round, it biases me about believing anything contingent to the world being flat. That's a positive bias. I don't see bias as a negative thing. I see it as a necessary thing. The one caveat is not when bias is in the performance of the craft, but when bias is in the assumptions underlying the craft. Bias can be thorny to observe and thorny to deal with when melded into underlying assumptions.

(Continued)

(Continued)

There are little-*b* biases and big-*B* biases. Little-*b* biases impact how you communicate, how you collect data, and how you interpret experiences; it is the little day-to-day stuff. We have to recognize it will be there and be alert to it. I like to think that big-*b* bias is something I will be upfront about and take steps to mitigate. For example, I had a project that I had a positive bias toward. I know I am pro HBCUs [Historically Black Colleges and Universities]. I asked several colleagues to be my sounding board. I would send research briefs to them for their reaction. The process of writing it and thinking about it was one of the best things I could do to be aware of my biases.

Melvin Hall is a Professor of Educational Psychology at Northern Arizona University, Distinguished Scholar in the Marie Fielder Institute of Fielding Graduate University, and AAC&U Senior Scholar, Office of Undergraduate STEM Education, AAC&U He is also a founding affiliate faculty member of the Center for Culturally Responsive Evaluation and Assessment at the University of Illinois, Urbana. He was interviewed by co-author Patricia Campbell, in fall, 2019.

Reducing Bias

There are some ways to reduce explicit bias and to not give implicit bias the chance to operate. One strategy is for evaluators to "blind" themselves from learning a person's gender, race, and other such characteristics when analysis is being done or decisions are being made. It is well known that observers rate the same behaviors differently based on the perceived characteristics of the subjects. For example, observers describe and rate behaviors differently based on a child's race (i.e., Gerwitz & Dodge, 1975; Gilliam, Maupin, Reyes, Accavitt, & Shie, 2016) and on whether they think the child is a girl or a boy. Female musicians are more likely to be hired when a "blind" audition process is used, which means the hiring committee is not aware of the sex of the auditioning musicians. Accents too can make a difference. People view speakers with accents like theirs as more knowledgeable than different-accent speakers, even when the different-accent speaker is actually more knowledgeable. In 1989, Michael J. Zieky concluded that "the potential for bias in the scoring of performance tests is clear. Scorers are human and fallible. Biases both for and against members of certain groups, may be blatant or subtle but they are likely to be present" (quoted in American Association of University Women, 1995, p. 97). His point still holds.

Along with "blind" ratings, which are discussed in detail in Chapter 12, a variety of strategies have been tested to reduce bias. In an analysis of 30 studies of interventions designed to reduce implicit bias, FitzGerald, Martin, Berner, and Hurst (2019) found the most effective categories were intentional strategies to overcome biases, exposure to counter-stereotypical exemplars, identifying the self with the out-group, evaluative conditioning, and inducing emotion. Half of the studies testing appeals to egalitarian values found them to be effective while the other half didn't. The largest number of studies tested an intervention focused on engaging with others' perspectives, but fewer than a third of the studies found it to be an effective intervention. Training may help to reduce bias as well. Morewedge and colleagues (2015) found that research participants exposed to one-shot training interventions, such as educational videos and de-biasing games that taught mitigating strategies, exhibited significant reductions in their biases immediately and up to three months later.

The following are some implicit bias training resources.

The Kirwan Institute has a series of four short, free modules on implicit bias. The modules are Understanding Implicit Bias, Real-World Implications,

Understanding Your Own Biases, and Mitigating Unwanted Biases. See http://kirwaninstitute.osu.edu/special-announcement-implicit-bias-training-available/.

Duke University has an online teachers' workshop on overcoming implicit bias. See https://blogs.tip.duke.edu/teachersworkshop/overcoming-implicit-bias/.

The Institute for Healthcare Improvement also provides information and resources on how to reduce implicit bias in health care. See http://www.ihi.org/communities/blogs/how-to-reduce-implicit-bias.

There are ways to reduce our own biases and those of others, but implementing them can be a challenge. As Tenney (2017, p. 54) explains, "Most white people indicate that they have no racial bias, that they treat everyone equally, that they 'don't see race,' and even that they are better than average at not being racially biased." She asks what it will take for a critical mass of white people to move from being passively not racist to being actively antiracist. In the following activity, readers will hear what three people, two white and one Black, who work to reduce bias and racism say about the challenges tied to working with white people on antiracism, reflect on their response to readings, and if they choose share their responses with others.

Activity
Reflections on Working With White People and Antiracism

Read the following three statements and write a short paragraph about your response to them and any impact they may have on your response to race and racism.

To continue reproducing racial inequality, the system only needs [W]hite people to be really nice and carry on, smile at people of color. Be friendly and go to lunch together on occasion. . . . Niceness will not get racism on the table and will not keep it on the table when everyone wants it off. . . . Where do we go from here? I offer that we must never consider ourselves finished with our learning. Even if challenging all the racism and superiority we have internalized was quick and easy to do, our racism would be reinforced all over again just by virtue of living in the culture. (DiAngelo, 2018, pp. 153–154)

When we shift our focus away from determining whether the intentions of individual white people are "good" or "bad" to instead focusing on the negative effects of white supremacy, we can focus on what matters most in the fight against racism. (Tenney, 2017, p. 55)

Every time I stand in front of an audience to address racial oppression in America, I know that I am facing a lot of [W]hite people who are in the room to feel less bad about racial discrimination and violence in the news, to score points, to let everyone know that they are not like the others, to make [B]lack friends. I know that I am speaking to a lot of [W]hite people who are certain they are not the problem because they are there. Just once I want to speak to a room of [W]hite people who know they are there because they are the problem. Who know they are there to begin the work of seeing where they have been complicit and harmful so that they can start doing better. (Oluo, 2019, para. 16)

If you feel comfortable doing so, share and discuss your responses with others.

Culture, Cultural Competence, and Cultural Responsiveness

Throughout the book, there are many references to culture and the importance of cultural competence.

> While there are almost as many definitions of culture as there are cultures themselves, this definition, from the Center for Advanced Research on Language Acquisition (CARLA) provides a perspective that may be useful to evaluators. They define culture "as the shared patterns of behaviors and interactions, cognitive constructs, and affective understanding that are learned through a process of socialization. These shared patterns identify the members of a culture group while also distinguishing those of another group" [CARLA, 2019, para. 1]. While we often think of culture groups in terms of ethnicity or nationality, they can be any group with shared patterns of behavior and understandings such as evaluators, scientists, or even Boston Red Sox fans (Campbell & Jolly, n.d.d, para. 1).

Culture is a powerful organizing framework that both filters and shapes perceptions, communications, values, and subsequent behaviors. As Table 1.3 shows, response to superficial areas such as what protein to have for dinner can cause strong visceral reactions.

Table 1.3 Cultural Attitudes Toward Proteins to Have for Dinner

Protein	Country	Attitude	Country	Attitude
Cow	United States	Good	India	Bad
Dog	United States	Bad	Korea	Was good but is changing
Bugs	United States	Bad	Thailand	Good
Pork	United States	Good	Saudi Arabia	Bad
Horse	United States	Bad	Poland	Good

Just as many people in the United States, for example, will have a strong visceral reaction to the idea of eating bugs, many people in India will have the same reaction to eating beef. As part of cultural awareness, it is important to learn more about why those in different cultures make the choices they do. As discussed in more detail in Chapter 5, evaluators must have a genuine willingness to learn about the cultures with which they engage within the evaluation context and, as appropriate, a willingness to suspend judgments. They also need to cultivate a belief that cultural diversity is a source of strength and enrichment rather than a deficit or obstacle to overcome (Handford, Van Maele, Matous, & Maemura, 2019). Evaluators need to be aware of the major culture groups that may have relevance for different evaluations. For example, the culture of different institutions of higher education (i.e., Ivy League, large public, historically Black) might be pertinent for an evaluation of a higher education program while the culture of correctional faculty (i.e., maximum, medium, or minimum security) might be pertinent for an evaluation of in-house recidivism programs. Other cultural groups might be important in different evaluations. However, it is important to remember that "accurate predictions of individual behavior based on nationality or other collective-level categories are typically not possible and may even cause offense. We are all members of multiple different groups and these identities become relevant at varying moments of our day" (Handford et al., 2019, p. 45).

As covered further in Chapter 13, how participants in programs and projects being evaluated identify themselves or how they are identified by others is one way to help evaluators understand cultural group memberships that may be salient for the evaluation. Learning about what is currently going on in relevant institutions and the surrounding communities can also help to identify other salient factors. Evaluators need to have ongoing knowledge and understanding of the cultural groups and related factors.

As covered in greater detail in Chapter 5, evaluators need to be culturally competent, and their evaluations need to be culturally responsive. SenGupta, Hopson, and Thompson-Robinson (2004, p. 13) go beyond the relatively simple definition of cultural competence given in the beginning of this chapter to describe cultural competence in evaluation as a "systematic, responsive inquiry that is actively cognizant, understanding, and appreciative of the cultural context in which the evaluation takes place; that frames and articulates the epistemology of the evaluative endeavor; that employs culturally and contextually appropriate methodology; and that uses stakeholder-generated, interpretive means to arrive at the results and further use of the findings." Cultural competence in evaluation takes place through a continuing open-ended series of substantive, ethical, and methodological insertions and adaptations that aligns the inquiry process with the characteristics of the groups/contexts being examined.

It is not enough for evaluators to embrace cultural competence, but as covered in detail in Chapter 5, evaluators must mindfully apply that competence to every aspect of their work from evaluation planning to reporting and use of results. Additionally, cultural competence is important in evaluation scholarship and in evaluation educational and professional development settings.

One of those areas where this was evident for us was in determining the most culturally appropriate terminology to use throughout this book to describe people from different races/ethnicities. There are many different ways to do this, and there is no one right answer. It is particularly difficult because of the practical necessity of using one term to collectively describe diverse subgroups. Our choice has been to acknowledge the complexity and be transparent about the choices we made. Since *Asian American* is the common term for people in the United States of Asian descent, we chose to use that term, knowing that it doesn't acknowledge the great diversity within that group. We were unsure as to whether we should use *American Indian* or *Native American* to collectively identify members of the 562 different tribes in the United States. We asked three people from different tribes who are very active in their tribal communities for advice. While they have used *American Indian* in the past, their preference is for *Indigenous People*, which is the term we are using.

We chose to use the terms *African American* and *Black* fairly interchangeably; however, we tend to use *African American* when we refer to people whose origins are in the African continent but whose history is on the American continent and *Black* when we are speaking more generally. We also chose to use *Hispanic* as a generic collective term because it encompasses people from outside as well as inside Latin America.

The Impact of Politics

In fields like evaluation, where results are used not just for program improvement but for making policy decisions and determining funding, the climate in which the evaluation is done is often challenging and politically driven. In a time when there is increasing distrust of research and evaluation, doing evaluations becomes increasingly difficult. While in recent years the challenges have seemed to be greater, there has always been tension between science, including evaluation, and politics. In 2008, Chelimsky explained that since "our government's need for evaluation arises from its checks and balances structure, evaluations working within that structure must deal not exceptionally, but routinely and regularly, with political infringement on their independence that result directly from that structure" (p. 400). She went on to point out the irony that "what should surprise us would be the absence of pressure on evaluators to make an agency 'look good' or the lack of effort by agency managers to try to manipulate the work of evaluators implementing legislative oversight" (p. 400).

Another way that politics can intertwine with evaluation is the political interest in "quick fixes" and the unwillingness to acknowledge underlying factors. As Thomas et al. (2018, p. 517) point out,

> Evaluators are often asked to assess the effectiveness of social programs that are designed to yield a quick "magic bullet" to fix to problems derived from years of racial oppression. Here, race is and is not the problem inasmuch as racism fuels the disparities we witness. However, this reality is virtually absent in the discourse of numerous commentaries and policy makers who are quick to cite Black failure or pathology without examining the historical root causes. As a result, social programs seek to address outcomes, such as the achievement gap and health disparities, rather than the race-based structural inequalities in the social, economic, and political systems that contribute to these outcomes.

As the following case studies indicate, evaluation results can and at times do lose out to politics.

Case Studies
Evaluation Results vs. Politicians

21st Century Community Learning Centers

An extensive evaluation of the 21st Century Community Learning Centers, a federally funded after-school program, found that the program did not affect student outcomes. Those findings were met with much resistance from those who strongly advocated for the program. For example, then California governor Arnold Schwarzenegger used strong community support and "anecdotal evidence" to justify his support for the program, which continues to exist. Describing the response to the evaluation results, Ron Haskins pointed out "any sentence akin to saying 'Everybody knows this program works' is an enemy of evidence-based policy" (J. White, 2017, p. 11).

> **Project DARE (Drug Abuse Resistance Education)**
>
> Project DARE is one of the most widely used substance abuse prevention programs targeted at school-aged youths. It has been the country's largest single school-based prevention program. Multiple evaluations and meta-analyses have found DARE to be ineffective, yet it continues to be widely used, paid for by federal funds (West & O'Neal, 2004). In 2017, then attorney general Jeff Sessions supported DARE because he "firmly believed" in its effectiveness, regardless of what the data said. Knowing that the program has been found to be ineffective, some school districts continue to use it for a variety of reasons including their belief that no short-term program can change students' drug-taking behavior and that, if it improves student/police relationships, that is enough to keep it going (Ingraham, 2017).

While some of the reasoning behind these examples is political, there can also be what Tom Kibler (personal communication, first quoted in Campbell, Hoey, & Perlman, 2001, p. 34) described as the "pure of heart model" influencing the decisions. The model is based on the premise that "since my heart is pure and my cause is just and I work really hard at it, the change I am seeking will happen." The pure of heart model is often held by caring people who are trying to help others who feel strongly what they are doing is right. If the data don't support that, then the data are wrong. As one program leader explained, "We are doing this on faith and if you don't believe in it, **** you" (Campbell et al., 2001, p. 35).

There can be issues with doing things on faith. Even with the best of intentions, the results of those efforts can be neutral or even negative. For example, one evaluation that I, coauthor Campbell, did found that doing hands-on science activities created by teachers or by after-school leaders caused students to become *more* stereotyped and limited in their opinions of who could do science. A second program to encourage women to continue on in their engineering programs reinforced rather than overcame stereotypes, with some women in the program coming to feel that it existed because women weren't as good as men in engineering. As one participant explained: "[Engineering] theory is easier for boys. That is why they put us together [in the special program]" (Campbell & Hoey, 2000, p. 20). No one wants to hear negative outcomes, but problems can't be fixed unless they are found and acknowledged.

The Current Climate

Of great concern is the onset of a so-called post-truth era, complete with alternative facts, disdain for expertise, and a diminishing reliance on facts and analytic thinking in public life (Hamburg, 2019, p. 563). Evaluators and indeed people in general are living and working in a time where terms like *alternative facts*, *post-facts*, and *post-truth* are used regularly. As indicated earlier in the chapter, traditionally alternative facts have been defined as falsehoods or the "opposite of reality." However, now some are viewing alternative facts as merely a different perspective (Zimmer, 2017). *Post-fact* and *post-truth* both refer to an environment in which objective facts are a thing of the past. In a post-fact society, facts are viewed as irrelevant, and emotional appeals are used to influence public opinion. In 2016, the Oxford University Press named *post-truth* as its word of the year, defining it as "relating to or denoting circumstances in which objective facts are less influential in shaping public opinion than appeals to emotion and personal belief" (para. 2). The idea that "truth no longer mattered. Facts were not just unimportant, but barriers to be smashed through with rhetoric" (Hollo, 2017, para. 3) is increasingly characteristic of today's world. Evaluators need to explore how such constructs impact evaluation work. "Citizens are increasingly asserting their values, hopes and opinions without apparent interest in finding a shared understanding of the actual state of things. Without such a shared understanding, those values and hopes cannot rationally be expressed and realized. Observers speak of 'truth decay,' dismissal of expertise, and neglect of evidence" (Hoit, 2019, p. 433).

The implication of living in a post-truth culture is that science becomes just another perspective with evidence becoming no more valid than personal opinion. This blurring of the distinction between evidence and opinion has a corrosive and delegitimizing effect on evaluation. Evaluation findings become just another kind of opinion (Gauchat, 2012).

There are some strategies and ways to combat this trend. Chapter 14 covers ways that the language and images used can impact readers' or viewers' response to an evaluation and provides strategies to increase the probability that results will be heard. In addition, having everyone, including evaluators, become more critical consumers of information can make a big difference. This can include the application of the aptly named CRAAP Test to help individuals judge the quality and veracity of information. CRAAP stands for

- *currency*—the timeliness of the information, including when it was published and if it requires current information;
- *relevance*—the importance of the information for your needs, including if it answers your question;
- *authority*—the source of the information, including the names and affiliations of authors as well as their qualifications and credentials;
- *accuracy*—the reliability, truthfulness, and correctness of the content, including where it comes from, if it is supported by evidence, and if it has been reviewed or refereed; and
- *purpose*—the reason the information exists, including determining if that purpose is to inform, teach, sell, entertain, or persuade and if there are political, ideological, cultural, religious, institutional, or personal biases (Meriam Library, 2010).

Drawing on the work of Julian Baggini, Eann Patterson (2018b, para. 1) provides some suggestions for ways individuals, can validate "truth":

We need to trust experts because we are unable to verify everything ourselves as life is too short and there are too many things to think about. However, this approach exposes us to the risk of being misled and Julian Baggini has suggested that this risk is increasing with the growth of psychology, which has allowed more people to master methods of manipulating us, that has led to "a kind of arms race of deception in which truth is the main casualty." He suggests that when we are presented with new information then we should perform an epistemic triage by asking:

- Is this a domain in which anyone can speak the truth?
- What kind of expert is a trustworthy source of truth in that domain?
- Is a particular expert to be trusted?

In the following activity, readers apply the CRAAP Test and/or Patterson's three questions to news stories.

Activity
Validating "Truth"

Pick a front-page story on the same topic or a similar one from two different newspapers and apply the CRAAP Test to them and/or ask Patterson's three questions with them in mind. Did doing that change your perceptions of the articles? In small groups, discuss your findings.

SUMMARY

The goal of this chapter was to provide readers with an overview of evaluation, evaluative thinking, and the general themes that underlie the book. These include race, racism, social justice, and a racialized perspective. The chapter also introduced issues tied to objectivity and bias including explicit and implicit bias and ways evaluators can reduce these biases. We also introduced the concepts of culture and cultural competence and the impact of politics and the current political climate on evaluators and evaluation. All of these, and other issues, will be explored, in detail, throughout the remainder of the book.

SUPPLEMENTAL RESOURCES

Bruner Foundation: Effectiveness Initiatives

www.evaluativethinking.org/index.html

This website provides a series of resources on developing and building evaluation capacity as well as on evaluative thinking including a series of four booklets on applying evaluative thinking to data collection.

Equitable Evaluation Initiative

www.equitableeval.org

This website provides principles, frameworks, and resources on equitable evaluation as well as an overview of the equitable evaluation projects in which the organization was involved.

Evaluation Resource Hub: Evaluative Thinking

https://education.nsw.gov.au/teaching-and-learning/professional-learning/evaluation-resource-hub/evaluative-thinking

This website provides a variety of evaluation resources including the mindset, skill set, and values underpinning evaluative thinking.

National Parenting Education Network: Introduction to Evaluation

https://npen.org/resources-for-parenting-educators/evaluating-parent-education-programs/introduction-to-evaluation/

This brief introduction to evaluation includes a definition, standards and guiding principles, logic models, and information about designing an evaluation.

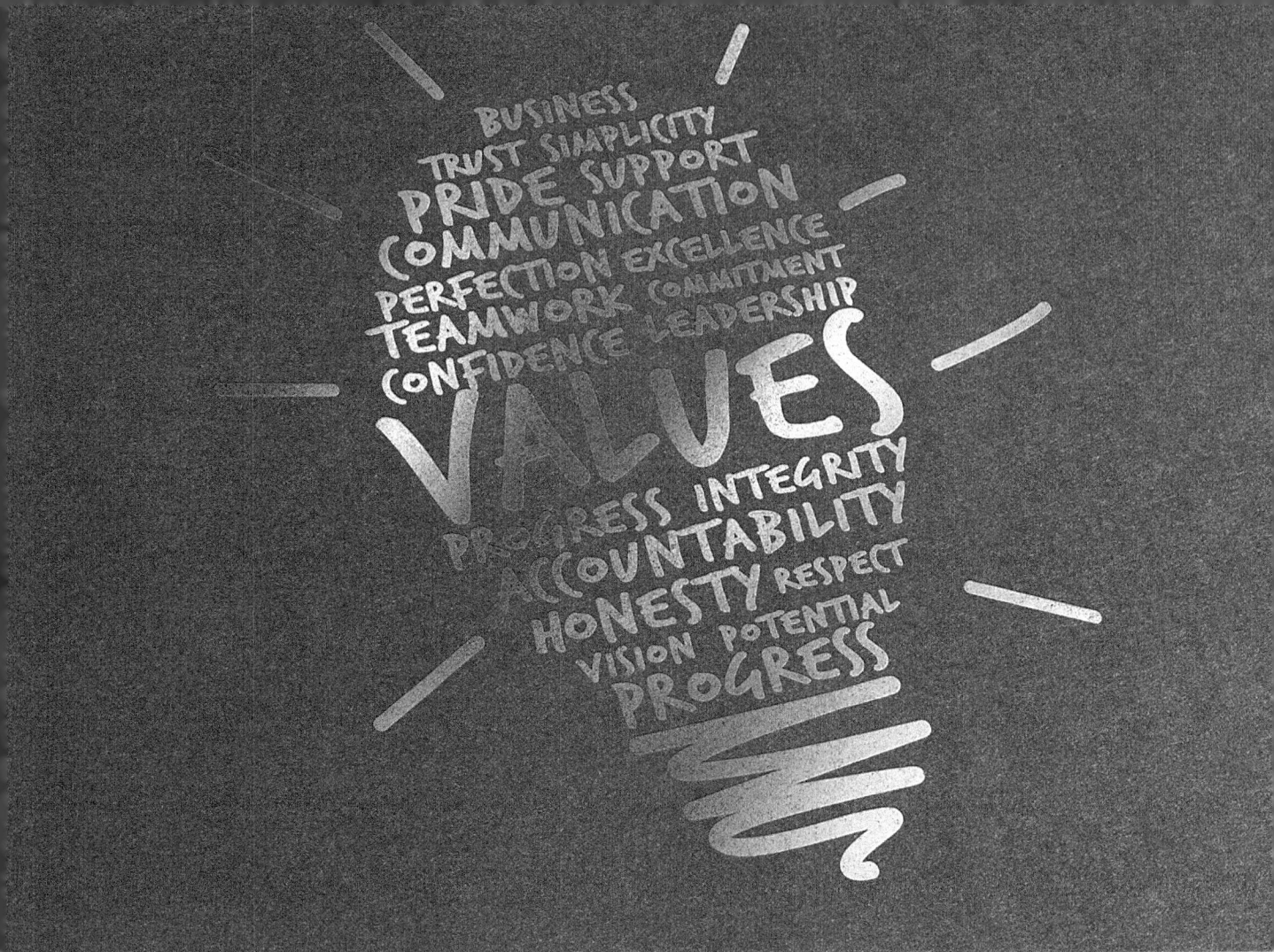

istock/Devrimb

Evaluators must use their own moral compass, in conjunction with the guidance of the profession's principles and standards, to take the most ethical and socially just course of action possible.

CHAPTER 2

Evaluation Ethics and Quality Standards

Making ethical decisions throughout the evaluation process is a relatively easy task when the facts are clear and the choices black-and-white. But it is a totally different story when the evaluation context is clouded by ambiguity, incomplete information, cultural incongruence, biases, multiple points of view and values, conflicting responsibilities, and political pressures. Different stakeholders often prioritize different values and weigh risks and benefits differently. In such situations, which evaluators experience frequently, engaging in ethical behaviors and producing a quality evaluation depends not only on evaluators' methodological skills and experience, but also on their critical insight, integrity, cultural competence, and willingness to take a socially just and defendable course of action in view of the standards and guidelines of the profession and the context in which the evaluation takes place.

After reading this chapter and participating in the activities, readers will be able to meet the following learning objectives:

- Explain the origins of research ethics codes and their relevance to evaluation
- Identify sources of ethical thinking in evaluation
- Demonstrate ethical sensitivities particularly in settings where there might be cultural incongruence and cultural conflicts of interest between the evaluator and the evaluation context
- Discuss and distinguish between the *Evaluators' Ethical Guiding Principles* and the *Program Evaluation Standards*
- Use the *Evaluators' Ethical Guiding Principles* and *Program Evaluation Standards* to support ethical decision making and evaluation quality in diverse contexts

Introduction

It is expected that an evaluator's work results in an evaluation that is ethical, culturally responsive, and high quality. In reality, achieving these important outcomes is more daunting than it appears on the surface. Due to the idiosyncratic, political, and applied nature of social programming, and subsequently the evaluation of those programs, ethical issues can arise that, if not properly handled, will negatively impact the integrity and quality of the evaluation. While the evaluation profession has written, and publically disclosed, ethical principles and quality standards, these represent only a reference point for guiding the attitudes and behaviors of evaluators. Professional evaluators also need to have a keen awareness and deep understanding of contextual factors that may give rise to the complexity and urgency of dealing with ethical concerns in diverse settings.

Ethics is a branch of philosophy focusing on values relating to human conduct with respect to the "rightness" and "wrongness" of actions. It involves standards for responsible conduct prescribed by an external source (e.g., society, businesses, professional organizations) aimed at guiding individual decision making and behaviors. This is in contrast with morals, which stem from within individuals—that is, individuals' own personal boundaries and principles of right and wrong. The following activity provides an opportunity for readers to reflect on and discuss ethics from their own perspective.

> ### Reflect and Discuss
> #### What Ethics Means to You
>
> Most adults have a vision or image in their mind of an ethical business, ethical organization, ethical government, or ethical society. On the individual level, ethics has a specific and oftentimes unique meaning and source. Using the prompts that follow, reflect on and discuss what ethics means to you.
>
> - What does ethics mean to you as a student, parent, spouse/partner, employee, and/or other roles?
> - What is the basis of your own ethical decision making and behaviors?
>
> Questions adapted from Patton, M. (2002). Qualitative research and evaluation methods, (3rd ed.). Thousand Oaks, CA: SAGE

With today's 24/7 cable news cycle, we are frequently bombarded with reports of unethical behaviors engaged in by businesses, politicians, and other professionals. Reported ethical infractions range from cheating (e.g., testing scandals in schools), stealing, and misuse of funds to inappropriate sexual behaviors, abuse of power, misrepresentations, and lying. Reports of these and other unethical behaviors, ultimately, erode confidence and public trust. As social, economic, and political discord manifests in myriad ways throughout the United States, many politicians, educators, activists, practitioners, and researchers, as well as the general public, have become increasingly attuned to the importance of ethics in navigating various aspects of our daily existence.

If evaluations are to be useful to program administrators, staff, participants, sponsors, and the public, the work must be planned, implemented, and disseminated in an honest, objective, and fair manner. In the American Evaluation Association's (AEA, 2018a) *Evaluator Competencies*, the first competency listed under the professional practice domain is

> 1.1 Acts ethically through evaluation practice that demonstrates integrity and respects people from different cultural backgrounds and indigenous groups.

It is essential that evaluators conduct ethically grounded evaluations in the diverse settings in which they work. **Ethically grounded evaluations** are characterized by ongoing critical thinking, reflection, judgment, and decision making. This is squarely aimed at protecting the rights of stakeholders and building daily ethical routines into evaluation planning, implementation, and reporting. There is no separate stage in an evaluation during which ethical issues must be addressed; instead, they arise throughout the entire evaluation process and, thus, must be dealt with continuously. Ethical evaluations require evaluators with more than knowledge of ethics. They also need evaluators with sensitivities, such as the ability to recognize the ethical dimensions of a situation, and a commitment to ongoing ethical self-examination throughout their work. Furthermore, ethical issues in evaluation are not limited to highly egregious acts such as falsification or fabrication of data and violations of confidentiality, but they can also involve seemingly small, everyday decisions and behaviors such as what information or which stakeholders to engage or ignore, what data to collect or dismiss, and how and when to report the evaluative information.

This chapter examines evaluation ethics and quality standards that are expected to govern the behavior of evaluators and the outcomes of an evaluation. While ethical issues in evaluation undoubtedly extend beyond the behavior of the evaluator (to include others such as clients, sponsors, and users), this chapter is primarily concerned with the evaluator's ethics in relation to various stakeholders within the evaluation context. The chapter begins with a brief historical perspective on research ethics, including the origins of our present-day approach to research ethics and ethical principles emerging from the Belmont Report, which serves as the foundation for protection of individuals involved in research and evaluation studies. The importance of ethics in evaluation and the discipline's major professional guidelines and principles are discussed. The chapter's content and activities are designed to help evaluators develop a keen awareness of how ethical issues can manifest themselves across all stages of the evaluation process, particularly in settings where there might be cultural incongruence and a cultural conflict of interest between the evaluator and the evaluation context.

A Brief Historical Perspective on Research Ethics

While research and evaluation serve different purposes, historical knowledge of research ethics can be valuable in helping evaluators understand the state of contemporary evaluation ethics and why ethics remains an important issue. **Research ethics** are core professional behaviors and institutional and federal standards by which every researcher is guided to protect the dignity, rights, and welfare of research participants. However, there have not always been explicit ethical codes and principles to guide the behavior of researchers. In the 1900s, no regulations existed regarding the ethical use of human participants in research. The field of research ethics has largely been built upon disastrous and egregious treatment of research participants, particularly when those individuals were poor or from minority or other vulnerable populations. The sections that follow provide a brief history of research ethics. More detailed historical perspectives can be found elsewhere (e.g., Kitchener & Kitchener, 2009; National Commission for the Protection of Human Subjects of Biomedical and Behavioral Research, 1978).

The Nuremberg Code of 1947

The origins of our present-day approach to research ethics can be traced back to the **Nuremberg Code** established in 1947. This code, including a set of 10 research ethics principles, followed the December 1946 criminal proceedings against 23 leading German physicians and administrators for their willing participation in war crimes and crimes against humanity. Horrifying procedures, such as the breaking and rebreaking of bones to see how many times they could be broken before healing, were conducted for research purposes on thousands of concentration camp prisoners without their informed consent; most of these prisoners either died or were permanently disabled as a result. The first principle of the Nuremberg Code, which was a radical idea at the time, was that voluntary, active consent of the human participant is absolutely essential. Two other principles included the rights of people to withdraw from research and to protect themselves. The Nuremberg Code also included a principle articulating that it is the duty of researchers to act in the best interests of those who take part in research for the good of society.

The Tuskegee Syphilis Study of 1932–1972

Despite the Nuremberg Code being given status of an international code for the ethical conduct of research and its substantial influence on international documents such as the Universal Declaration of Human Rights (adopted by the United Nations General Assembly in 1948), for many years after the introduction of these documents, researchers continued with unethical practices. In the United States, one of the most infamous biomedical research abuse cases, the Tuskegee Syphilis Study, involved experiments, over a 40-year period, on low-income African American males in Tuskegee, Alabama. As part of a research project conducted by the U.S. Public Health Service, 600 low-income (mostly illiterate) African American males were recruited, 399 of whom were infected with syphilis and 201 of whom served as a control group not infected with the disease. The researchers advertised for "colored" participants with the slogan "Last Chance for Special Free Treatment" by the Macon County Health Department and government doctors. Researchers never obtained informed consent from the men and did not inform the men with syphilis that they were not being treated but were simply being monitored and left to suffer with syphilis long after a cure (penicillin) became available in 1947. By the end of the study in 1972, only 74 of the test subjects were still alive. It was not until May 16, 1997, that President Bill Clinton issued a formal apology for the Tuskegee Syphilis Study, denoting that it destroyed the trust many African Americans had for medical institutions. The following activity provides readers with an opportunity to reflect on the lasting impact of the Tuskegee Syphilis Study.

Reflect and Discuss
The Tuskegee Timeline

Review the timeline of the Tuskegee Syphilis Study and then reflect on and discuss the questions that follow.

The Study Begins

In 1932, the Public Health Service, working with the Tuskegee Institute, began a study to record the natural history of syphilis in hopes of justifying treatment programs for [B]lacks. It was called the "Tuskegee Study of Untreated Syphilis in the Negro Male."

The study initially involved 600 Black men—399 with syphilis, 201 who did not have the disease. The study was conducted without the benefit of patients' informed consent. Researchers told the men they were being treated for "bad blood," a local term used to describe several ailments, including syphilis, anemia, and fatigue. In truth, they did not receive the proper treatment needed to cure their illness. In exchange for taking part in the study, the men received free medical exams, free meals, and burial insurance. Although originally projected to last 6 months, the study actually went on for 40 years.

What Went Wrong?

In July 1972, an Associated Press story about the Tuskegee Study caused a public outcry that led the Assistant Secretary for Health and Scientific Affairs to appoint an Ad Hoc Advisory Panel to review the study. The panel had nine members from the fields of medicine, law, religion, labor, education, health administration, and public affairs.

The panel found that the men had agreed freely to be examined and treated. However, there was no evidence that researchers had informed them of the study or its real purpose. In fact, the men had been misled and had not been given all the facts required to provide informed consent.

The men were never given adequate treatment for their disease. Even when penicillin became the drug of choice for syphilis in 1947, researchers did not offer it to the subjects. The advisory panel found nothing to show that subjects were ever given the choice of quitting the study, even when this new, highly effective treatment became widely used.

The Study Ends and Reparation Begins

The advisory panel concluded that the Tuskegee Study was "ethically unjustified"—the knowledge gained was sparse when compared with the risks the study posed for its subjects. In October 1972, the panel advised stopping the study at once. A month later, the Assistant Secretary for Health and Scientific Affairs announced the end of the Tuskegee Study.

In the summer of 1973, a class-action lawsuit was filed on behalf of the study participants and their families. In 1974, a $10 million out-of-court settlement was reached. As part of the settlement, the U.S. government promised to give lifetime medical benefits and burial services to all living participants. The Tuskegee Health Benefit Program (THBP) was established to provide these services. In 1975, wives, widows and offspring were added to the program. In 1995, the program was expanded to include health as well as medical benefits. The Centers for Disease Control and Prevention was given responsibility for the program, where it remains today in the National Center for HIV/AIDS, Viral Hepatitis, STD, and TB Prevention. The last study participant died in January 2004. The last widow receiving THBP benefits died in January 2009. There are 11 offspring currently receiving medical and health benefits.

Source: National Center for HIV/AIDS, Viral Hepatitis, STD, and TB Prevention, Centers for Disease Control and Prevention, U.S. Department of Health and Human Services. (2020, March 20). *U.S. Public Health Service syphilis study at Tuskegee: The Tuskegee timeline.* Retrieved from https://www.cdc.gov/tuskegee/timeline.htm

Now, reflect on and discuss the interplay of ethics and social justice issues raised in the Tuskegee Syphilis Study.

Guiding Questions

- Do you think the Tuskegee Syphilis Study has current and/or lasting societal impact? If so, what?
- Might certain individuals or groups still be suspicious of evaluators and other researchers because of experiments like the Tuskegee Syphilis Study? Elaborate your response.

Courtesy of the Center for Disease Control

The Radiation Studies of 1940–1960

Another example of unethical research practice includes the abuse of human participants during World War II and the early Cold War when U.S. officials studied the effects of radiation through experiments on hospital patients, pregnant women, children with intellectual disabilities, and enlisted military personnel. While officials authorized the wartime experiments to establish health and safety standards for the thousands of workers in atomic bomb plants, few of the participants in the experiments gave informed consent. In fact, most had no knowledge that they were being exposed to radioactive materials. After the war ended, officials justified expanding the study of the effects of radiation on grounds of national security. In the 1990s, following congressional investigations, numerous official reports, scholarly studies, and lawsuits, the government offered apologies and financial compensation to some of the victims of human radiation testing.

The HeLa Story: 1950s and Beyond

Until the *New York Times* best seller *The Immortal Life of Henrietta Lacks* (Skloot, 2010) was published, and subsequently presented as a dramatic television film, Henrietta Lacks was virtually unknown to the general public. At the age of 30, Lacks, a working-class, African American tobacco farmer and mother of five, living near Baltimore, Maryland, was a cancer patient in the "colored ward" of Johns Hopkins Hospital. Lacks died of an unusually aggressive form of cervical cancer in 1951 at 31 years of age. Tissue samples from Lacks were taken during her diagnosis and treatment, and portions were passed along to a researcher without her knowledge or permission, as was common practice at the time (Beskow, 2016). Lacks's cell line, referred to as HeLa (using the first two letters of her first and last names), is the first immortal human cell line in history. HeLa remains viable today and has been used in laboratories around the world for a vast array of biomedical research, contributing to some of the most important medical advances of all time, including the polio vaccine, chemotherapy, cloning, gene mapping, and in vitro fertilization. Further, HeLa cells were the first human biological materials ever bought and sold, which helped launch a multibillion-dollar industry. In 1971, *Obstetrics and Gynecology* (a scientific journal) named Henrietta Lacks as the HeLa source, and this disclosure was subsequently revealed by other scientific publications, including *Nature* and *Science*, as well as the mainstream press. Reportedly, it was not until 1973, two years after Lacks's name was published in a scientific journal as the source of HeLa cells, that her family learned about the HeLa cells. This case, while consent was not required, raises serious ethical concerns about privacy and respect for family members.

Beyond Medical Studies and Physical Harm: The Milgram Study of 1963

Biomedical researchers were not alone in engaging in unethical practices. There, too, are historical examples of horrific ethical violations occurring in social and behavioral science research. Such violations often resulted in psychological or social harm to participants including feelings of shame, embarrassment, loss of self-confidence, and depression. One of the most infamous such studies was conducted in 1961 by Stanley Milgram, a psychologist at Yale University, on the conflict between obedience to authority and personal conscience. Participants were led to believe they were administering real pain through electric shocks to another participant as part of a learning experiment, which was designed to see if ordinary Americans would obey immoral orders as many Germans had done during the Nazi period. Baumrind (1964) noted that participants became distressed and nervous when they thought they were administering severe shocks, but when participants asked for the experiment to be stopped, the researcher in charge insisted that they continue. In the Milgram study, participants sustained no physical harm; however, they suffered shame and embarrassment for having behaved inhumanely toward their fellow human beings. Please reflect upon and discuss the questions presented in the textbox.

> ### Reflect and Discuss
> #### Ethical Considerations and Authority Figures
>
> In contrast to the 1940s and 1950s, in today's society do you think everyday citizens are more aware of ethical behavior related to social and behavioral sciences research—that is, right versus wrong—or do you believe that an authority figure will always be able to sway people's judgment toward unethical behavior? Under what conditions do you believe this is less or more likely to be the case? Provide examples.

The National Research Act of 1974

Due primarily to publicity from the Tuskegee Syphilis Study and after a series of congressional hearings on human subjects research, the National Research Act of 1974 was passed. It authorized federal agencies to develop human research regulations and established the first institutional review boards as a mechanism through which human subjects would be protected. Additionally, the National Research Act created the National Commission for the Protection of Human Subjects of Biomedical and Behavioral Research. Decades after the Nuremberg Code of 1947 and the 1964 Declaration of Helsinki that provided guidance to medical doctors conducting research involving human subjects, the National Commission for the Protection of Human Subjects of Biomedical and Behavioral Research (1978) released the *Belmont Report: Ethical Principles and Guidelines for the Protection of Human Subjects of Research*. This document, known colloquially as the **Belmont Report**, established three basic ethical principles that are the cornerstone for regulations involving human participants:

1. *Respect for persons*, or recognition of the personal dignity and autonomy of individuals, and special protection of those persons with diminished autonomy

2. *Beneficence*, or obligation to protect persons from harm by maximizing anticipated benefits and good outcomes for science, humanity, and the individual and by minimizing or avoiding unnecessary risk, harm, or wrong

3. *Justice*, or ensuring that the benefits and burdens of research are distributed fairly and that research procedures are reasonable, nonexploitative, carefully considered, and fairly administered (pp. 4–6)

The principles identified in the Belmont Report relate both to the participant as an individual and to the participant as a member of social, racial, sexual, or ethnic groups. This means that research participants should not be either favored or disfavored (e.g., more or less likely to be involved in risky research) simply because they are a member of a particular class of people.

The Continuing Importance of Research Ethics

Despite regulations and consciousness-raising regarding ethics in medical, social, and behavioral sciences research, it is an area that still needs attention and monitoring by internal and external bodies. In the article "What Is Ethics in Research and Why Is It Important?" Resnik (2015) cites a number of important reasons for a continued emphasis on ethics in research:

- To promote the goals of research, such as the search for knowledge and truth and the avoidance of error
- To promote essential values for collaborative work, including trust, accountability, mutual respect, and fairness
- To ensure that researchers are held accountable for their actions given policies on conflict of interest, misconduct, and research involving humans or animals
- To build public support for research to the extent that people feel they can trust its quality and integrity
- To support additional important social and moral values, including the principle of doing no harm to others (paras. 7–11)

By introducing evaluators to the history of research ethics and important principles such as "doing no harm," "beneficence," and "respect for persons," they are better positioned to, first, identify potential ethical dilemmas when they emerge and, second, be deliberate about how to address the issue in a manner that is fair and just. Such an understanding can help the evaluator identify **ethical triggers** (Munteanu et al., 2015), or elements that indicate potential challenges during the evaluation, particularly when working with participants who belong to vulnerable or marginalized populations (e.g., persons with disabilities), when dealing with sensitive topics (e.g., abortion services), and when there is the possibility of blurred lines between the evaluator and the end user.

Ethics in Evaluation

Virtually every scientific field or discipline has guidelines that are codified in a set of statements put forth by its relevant professional association. Organizations such as the **American Evaluation Association (AEA)**, National Society of Professional Engineers (NSPE), American Psychological Association (APA), American Sociological Association (ASA), National Association of Social Workers (NASW), and American Nurses Association (ANA) have a publicly disclosed, aspirational set of ethical guidelines for professionals. While the guidelines may differ in content and detail across various organizations, all represent an aspirational set of principles, values, and beliefs that help define the organization and address four overarching issues: (a) *respect others' rights* to act freely and make their own choices while protecting the rights of those who may be unable to fully protect themselves; (b) *do no harm* including both physical injury and psychological harm such as damage to an individual's reputation, self-esteem, or emotional well-being; (c) *act fairly* by treating individuals equitably and without regard to race, gender, socioeconomic status, or other characteristics; and (d) *help or benefit others* through promoting the common good and interests of individuals and society.

In contrast to an organization's code of conduct, which is a directional document focusing on compliance and rules that describe how its members should behave in specific situations (e.g., forbid sexual harassment or racial intimidation), ethical guidelines include broad aspirational values and principles intended to provide an organization's members with a general idea of the types of decisions and behaviors (e.g., treat others with respect) that are acceptable and encouraged by the profession. Individuals must interpret the organization's ethical principles and adapt them in practice. A discipline's ethical statements are used to guide practitioners of that discipline in determining the right course of action in a situation. On the one hand, evaluation shares ethical challenges similar to those of other types of social and behavioral science research. For example, public scrutiny of evaluation, like that occurring in other types of research, has resulted in heightened attention to examining whose views are included or excluded, determining design choices, considering how findings are checked for accuracy, and focusing on how results are reported (Wolf, Turner, & Toms, 2009). On the other hand, evaluation can be challenged by a variety of ethical issues beyond those confronted in other social and behavioral science research. In a presentation on ethical land mines in program evaluation delivered at the 1997 American Educational Research Association (AERA) Annual Meeting in Chicago, Linda Mabry stated that

> evaluation is the most ethically challenging of the approaches to research inquiry because it is the most likely to involve hidden agendas, vendettas, and serious professional and personal consequences to individuals. Because of this feature, evaluators need to exercise extraordinary circumspection before engaging in an evaluation study. (quoted in McDavid, Huse, & Hawthorn, 2013, p. 468)

In 1999, Mabry added that of all the methods of social science inquiry, evaluation occurs in the most intensely political milieu where the heaviest assaults to ethics are threatened. Evaluation, she contended, involves risks that are rare in research such as generating final reports that can lead to expansion of a program or to its reconfiguration, shrinkage, or termination. Furthermore, evaluators are "often flattered, coddled, granted selective access, indoctrinated, misinformed, disregarded, challenged, or discredited according to the interests and opportunities of clients, program personnel, or other stakeholders" (Mabry, 1999, p. 200). Barnett and Camfield (2016) point out that the wholesale adoption of research ethics may not provide the most appropriate solution for evaluation. Instead, they propose a different approach to evaluation ethics that addresses stakeholder relationships, helps rebalance the primary focus on the respondent, and focuses on the duties and responsibilities of evaluation to society more broadly.

Research ethics has a predominant focus on the researcher–research participant relationship. In evaluation, however, other equally important relationships must be considered from an ethical perspective. These include relationships with a host of other stakeholders such as program administrators, service providers, program participants, and community members. Evaluators may experience role conflict with certain stakeholders, such as program staff, funders, or program clients, that raises ethical dilemmas. Happy clients (e.g., program administrators) make for pleasant working conditions for the evaluator, and these stakeholders' favorable comments can generate additional contracts for the evaluator that ultimately enhance both income and professional standing (Mabry, 1999). Thus, client or stakeholder appeasement creates positive bias, which raises not only a validity issue but also an ethics issue. Evaluators who choose to comfort or enrich themselves by providing reports that cheer more than inform may hinder clients' access to the information promised, foreclose on opportunities for program improvement, warp managerial decisions, and yield preventable negative human consequences (Mabry, 1999). The following case study provides an example of a key stakeholder (i.e., the director) attempting to cajole an evaluator in a manner that could present an ethical dilemma depending on the evaluator's action.

Case Study
Identifying Hidden Agendas and Ethical Land Mines

The following description was adapted from one of the Ethical Challenges found in the *American Journal of Evaluation*. Review the case and then respond to the questions at the end of the scenario.

The Case of the Sensitive Survey

The Health Services Center (HSC) at North Central Southeastern State University, a small public institution (popularly known as Where Are U?), has recently engaged you, an external consultant, to conduct an evaluation of its programs and services. Last year, the state legislature mandated that the various administrative units within public colleges and universities be systematically evaluated on a periodic basis, and actually went so far as to allocate funds for this purpose.

The HSC has been included in the "first wave" of offices to be reviewed at Where Are U?, and the HSC director is less than thrilled. He has occupied the director's position for the past 10 years, and he is convinced that (1) several highly placed administrators at the university would like to replace him and (2) these administrators view the evaluation as an opportunity to build a case to support such a move. This afternoon you are meeting with the director to discuss a draft version of a survey that you have prepared, focusing on students' experiences with and opinions of the HSC. One section of the survey contains an extensive list of items that describe both positive and negative encounters that the diverse student body might have had with the HSC, and asks respondents to indicate which ones they have personally experienced.

In previous evaluations, you have found the survey to be an extremely useful, efficient, and comprehensive method for examining stakeholders' perceptions. The survey will also give students an opportunity to rate how important these various issues and experiences are to them in terms of influencing their overall opinion of the HSC.

It is noteworthy to mention that the survey represents just one of the data-gathering strategies that you intend to use in this project. The director is, to put it mildly, unhappy with certain aspects of the survey. He believes that the items focusing on negative experiences will turn the HSC into a "punching bag" (the director's words) for disgruntled students with an "axe to grind," and that it would only be fair to use such a list if comparable ones were employed in the evaluation of other departments on campus. You, of course, are not involved in the evaluation of these other departments.

The director also maintains that many of the negative survey items pertain to matters that are not fully under the control of the HSC (e.g., the hours when certain medical specialists are available at the HSC). As the discussion continues, you become increasingly convinced that the key issue here is not the methodology

> you have proposed for gathering data. Rather, it seems to be the director's intense desire to declare certain domains of the HSC's functioning as "off-limits" in this evaluation. Although you can understand why he might be motivated to take such a position, you also strongly believe that an adequate, professionally respectable evaluation of the HSC cannot omit consideration of the areas that the director wants you to avoid. Interestingly, during the entry/contracting stage of this project, the director had not voiced the "domain concerns" that appear to worry him so greatly now.
>
> Your conversation with the director is cut short when he is called out of the office due to an emergency.
>
> - What do you see as the major ethical issues that the evaluator is facing in this case?
> - What hidden agendas could become ethically problematic for the evaluator?
> - What might be some professional consequences for this evaluator if the ethical issues remain unresolved?
>
> *Source:* American Journal of Evaluation (AJE) Morris, M. (2000). The Case of the Sensitive Survey. American Journal of Evaluation, 21(2), 263 -263. https://doi.org/10.1177/109821400002100216

A number of evaluation-related circumstances could pose ethical dilemmas for the evaluator. Some examples include (a) being contracted to conduct an evaluation on a program not yet ready to be evaluated; (b) being given insufficient time to complete the evaluation, (c) treatment of people associated with the program around issues such as confidentiality, informed consent, and assignment to program groups; and (d) role conflicts facing evaluators (Posavac & Carey, 2016). Ethical issues can also be the result of inappropriate behaviors such as exerting inappropriate influence on program participants, usurping the role of others (e.g., service providers), or having conflicts of interests (e.g., promoting personal interests over those of the client).

Evaluation ethics concerns the responsibility of evaluators to be competent, honest, and respectful to all individuals and groups that are affected by the evaluation. This includes not only evaluators' responsibilities to participants, program staff, and other beneficiaries, whom they must treat with respect, but also their responsibilities to evaluation sponsors to yield a quality and credible evaluation. Because of the different roles (e.g., consultant/administrator, data collector/researcher, reporter, member of profession, or member of society) evaluators fulfill at any given time while in the field, an evaluator may face a variety of circumstances in which ethical dilemmas arise (Newman & Brown, 1996). As a result, evaluators must strike the right balance between what is in the best interest of their client and society (Wolf et al., 2009). Ethics in evaluation does not exist in a vacuum. No set of guidelines or standards can cover every possible situation that evaluators will encounter in the field; thus, evaluators' ethical decision making and behavior must be nuanced to the context with consideration of things such as the values held by the stakeholders, cultural issues, and potential conflicts of interest within the particular setting.

How evaluators make decisions and exercise their ethical and professional judgment in practice will determine the evaluation ethics in context. While professional ethics are designed to protect against the reoccurrence of major atrocities such as the Tuskegee experiments, they also are needed to guard against less obvious, yet still potentially harmful, effects of evaluation when there might be issues such as inaccurate representation of stakeholders' perceptions and viewpoints, invasion of privacy, deception, and insensitivity to those being studied, especially when they represent minority and other vulnerable populations. Evaluators, like other individuals, are likely to overestimate how ethical they are, which, in turn, can be a barrier against behaving ethically, especially in ambiguous situations. Ethical behavior is not just making the easy ethical choices between right and wrong, but also working through the more complex decisions that involve hierarchies of values, prioritized according to circumstances, and deciding what is, and is not, valid and credible information (Mabry, 2004).

Ethics in evaluation can be considered at both the individual and professional levels—both affecting evaluation quality. At the individual level, ethics is concerned with the behavior of an individual evaluator. The evaluator is expected to act with integrity throughout the entire evaluation process from conceptualization and design through dissemination and use of findings. Ethical issues can exist in the way the evaluator presents (or misrepresents) him- or herself during planning and recruitment, data collection, and dissemination activities; ethical issues can arise due to how an individual evaluator interacts and shares responsibility with stakeholders.

Evaluators are presented with an array of messy, complicated issues in the field requiring them to think quickly and ethically in a given situation. They may face what Guillemin and Gillam (2004) refer to as a number of "ethically important moments." These are the difficult, often subtle, and usually unpredictable situations that arise in the practice of doing all kinds of research, including evaluations. During the course of the evaluation, important moments arise without warning, and the evaluator must be prepared to respond in an ethically defensible manner at the time the situation occurs. Sometimes, ethically important moments arise and must be addressed immediately. In such cases, the evaluator must decide what action to take in real time. For example, in a situation where a project administrator offers a new evaluator a gift, the evaluator has to make an immediate decision whether to accept or refuse the gift. On one hand, and in some cultures, a gift conveys a great deal of respect and is a sign that the relationship is valued by the giver. If there is a problem, it may rest with the evaluator who may not trust the program director's motives. On the other hand, when gift giving is intended to favorably influence the evaluator's judgment, acceptance of the gift is ethically problematic. In this case, the evaluator must immediately decide, in real time, his or her course of action—accept or decline the project director's gift.

Ethics in evaluation at the individual level is not only restricted to the behavior of the evaluator. It is also related to the rights, responsibilities, and behaviors of various evaluation stakeholders. For example, program staff, clients, sponsors, and other relevant stakeholders (e.g., users, community members) have an ethical responsibility for acknowledging unique entry and access issues, as well as particular community habits, customs, and values that determine suitable conduct in the evaluation process (Yarbrough, Shulha, Hopson, & Caruthers, 2011).

Over the past three decades, the evaluation profession has undergone major developments that have served to highlight the importance of ethics in the discipline. Probably most notable among these include the development and multiple subsequent revisions of both the AEA's *Evaluators' Ethical Guiding Principles* and the Joint Committee on Standards for Educational Evaluation's *Program Evaluation Standards* (discussed in the next section). Additionally, there have been published books on program evaluation ethics (e.g., Morris, 2008; Newman & Brown, 1996), research on evaluation ethics, and numerous journal articles and book chapters on the topic. Through publication of the Ethical Challenges section of the *American Journal of Evaluation*, the AEA has sought to promote evaluators' understanding of ethical challenges, enhance evaluators' sensitivity to the ethical dimensions of their work, and translate the *Evaluators' Ethical Guiding Principles* and the *Program Evaluation Standards* into everyday practice.

Sources of Ethical Thinking

Most individuals have a set of fundamental beliefs or principles that guide their ethical behavior. However, people differ on the sources they draw upon for ethical decision making. Newman and Brown (1996) point to several sources as guidelines for evaluators' ethical thinking. As outlined in the following activity, these include evaluator intuition, past experience, observations of behavior among colleagues, personal values and beliefs, and ethical rules as presented in ethical codes.

> ### Reflect and Discuss
> #### Evaluator Sources for Ethical Thinking
>
> Consider the five sources of ethical thinking described as follows and the examples provided. Now, provide additional examples of instances when an evaluator should avoid or rely on one or more of these sources while working in the field. Reflect on and discuss your responses with others.
>
> - *Intuition:* An evaluator may have an intuitive feeling that something is wrong when a program director demands a summary of an interview with a particular staff member.
>
> - *Past experience:* Because of a previous bad experience, the evaluator makes sure that the evaluation contract explicitly states the purpose and scope of the evaluation, who has input into the evaluation planning, expected deliverables, and how the results will be used.
>
> - *Observations of or consultation with colleagues:* An evaluator may observe a colleague's use of a particular methodology when conducting focus groups with Indigenous populations that would be most responsive to use in another evaluation. In yet another instance, an evaluator might consult with trusted colleagues about an ethical dilemma in order to get the perspective of other evaluators before taking action.
>
> - *Personal values and beliefs:* Evaluators use their personal values, visions, and beliefs to make a decision about the right course of action to take when mistreatment of clients was observed while visiting the program site for the purpose of meeting with the program staff.
>
> - *Rules and codes:* Evaluators refer stakeholders to guidelines and standards provided by the AEA's *Evaluators' Ethical Guiding Principles* and the Joint Committee on Standards for Educational Evaluation's *Program Evaluation Standards* to justify their behavior.
>
> Source: Adapted and updated from Newman and Brown (1996).

Any one, or a combination, of these sources can be appropriate (or inappropriate) under certain circumstances. For example, evaluators can have "educated intuition," making them more sensitive and alert to the nuances of potential ethical conflicts if they have thought through conflicts before either in simulations or in real life (Newman & Brown, 1996). However, overreliance on one particular source can become problematic. Evaluators who, for instance, primarily rely on intuition or past experience to guide their ethical thinking might inappropriately generalize what was seemingly ethical behavior in a previous setting to a different context that might render that behavior problematic. Evaluators who exclusively use their own personal values and beliefs to make ethical decisions may be on ethically shaky grounds, particularly when they are from the dominant group and working in a setting that primarily serves persons of color and other marginalized groups such as people with disabilities and the elderly. For example, sometimes the values, beliefs, and experiences of the dominant group are used as the yardstick, point of reference, norm, or standard by which persons from the dominant group judge the values, beliefs, and behaviors of marginalized groups. Since values and beliefs are influenced by individuals' cultural background, the use of a dominant standard by the evaluator can be inappropriate and lead to faulty conclusions. For example, as shown in the following case study, the fact that an instrument has demonstrated validity in a dominant setting does not automatically make it ethical to use that same instrument in another setting.

Case Study
Moving Beyond Past Experience

In the Centers for Disease Control and Prevention's (CDC, 2014, p. 16) *Practical Strategies for Culturally Competent Evaluation*, the following scenario is presented:

> An existing validated instrument was piloted as part of an evaluation that assessed risk factors related to heart disease and stroke. Some of the items in the instrument dealt with sensitive issues (e.g., cultural eating practices, cultural perceptions of attractive body images, cultural views on prescribed medications). Respondents were offended by some of the items, which they viewed as racial stereotypes. The inappropriate items led evaluators to conclude that participants would be reluctant or refuse to complete the evaluation protocol. Consequently, the evaluation team members discussed these issues, which resulted in a revised protocol for culturally appropriate communication and the subsequent revision of the data collection instrument.

Cultural Competence as an Ethical Imperative

Evaluators oftentimes work in settings that represent a very different cultural context than their own. The updated AEA (2018b) *Evaluators' Ethical Guiding Principles* highlight the need to mindfully and proactively attend to diversity, equity issues, and common good as prerequisites for ethical practice. Evaluators have an ethical obligation to be culturally competent and to create an inclusive climate in which everyone invested has an opportunity to fully participate in the evaluation process. In the updated preface to the *Evaluators' Ethical Guiding Principles*, a culturally competent evaluator is described as one who

> draws upon a wide range of evaluation theories and methods to design and carry out an evaluation that is optimally matched to the context; the evaluator reflects the diverse values and perspectives of key stakeholder groups. (AEA, 2018b, p. 1)

The AEA (2011) has also issued a *Public Statement on Cultural Competence in Evaluation*. This statement challenges evaluators to deepen their self-awareness and sensitivity in terms of their own cultures and those of others and to acquire the necessary skills to bridge the cultural gaps between themselves and those in the evaluation context.

Cultural competence in evaluation is a reflective activity requiring evaluators to achieve and maintain a high degree of self-awareness and self-examination to better understand how their own cultural backgrounds and life experiences can serve as either assets or limitations in the conduct of an evaluation. Specific examples of ethical practice related to cultural competence offered by the AEA in its *Public Statement on Cultural Competence* include the following:

- Use approaches that are appropriate to the context; for example, verbal consent can be used in communities with oral traditions, high levels of concern about privacy, or low levels of literacy.

- Engage issues of culture directly, respectfully, and fairly when collecting data, making interpretations, and forming value judgments.

- Incorporate ways to make findings accessible to all stakeholders, including forms of communication beyond written texts and the use of languages other than English.

- Consider unintended consequences when reporting findings; for example, in some cultural contexts, participants in evaluations who are proud of their accomplishments may want to forgo anonymity and have their names attached to their stories. While this may be appropriate in some instances, in other situations the identification of participants may infringe on the rights of people who have not given informed consent.

Reflect and Discuss
Self-Exploration

- Consider diverse cultural experiences that have led you to further "self" exploration. What did you learn about yourself that you were not consciously aware of prior to this self-exploration?

- After reviewing the AEA's (2011) *Public Statement on Cultural Competence* (available at www.eval.org/ccstatement) in full, discuss how exploring the "self" can improve one's work as an evaluator.

In **culturally incongruent** settings, ethical issues can arise relative to the evaluator's respect (or lack thereof) for local customs, values, and belief systems. Three types of ethics are particularly relevant in the evaluation of programs serving nonmajority and culturally diverse populations. These include procedural ethics, situational ethics, and relational ethics (Ellis, 2007; Guillemin & Gillam, 2004). **Procedural ethics** involve those mandated usually by institutional review boards to ensure that the study's procedures adequately address the ethical concerns of informed consent, confidentiality, right to privacy, freedom from deception, and protection of participants from harm.

While institutional review boards certainly have tremendous value and are entrusted with ensuring the ethical conduct of research, scholars vigorously pushing for use of antiracist methodologies often cite problems with traditional institutional review boards' ethics review procedures based in positivism, which separates thought from action and subject from object and assumes that research can and should be value free (Chavez, Duran, Baker, Avila, & Wallerstein, 2003). Further, it has been argued that institutional review boards generally give emphasis to assessing risks to individuals without paying attention to risk to communities (Minkler, 2004), a condition that has ethical implications for evaluations focusing on marginalized communities. Institutional review boards and the protection of human participants are covered in more detail in Chapter 12.

Situational ethics, or ethics in practice as it is sometimes referred to, include concerns involving the day-to-day unpredictable, often subtle, yet ethically important periods that arise while conducting research and evaluations. Situational ethics often reveal vulnerability, and the evaluator must decide what to do and how far to probe the situation at hand. Relational ethics, another type of ethics relevant to the evaluator, situates ethical action explicitly in relationships recognizing and valuing mutual respect, dignity, and the connectedness between the researcher and the researched and between researchers and the communities in which they live and work (Ellis, 2007).

Ethical Dimension of Racial Bias

Race is only one of many cultural constructs. However, it is a powerful one in American society and one that deserves special attention. Race, as a socially constructed phenomenon, continues to differentially shape the allocation of power and distribution of benefits and burdens among groups within the United States. When considering the prominent ills (e.g., poverty, crime, education gaps, health disparities) of the country, race is always a factor in the equation. Over two decades ago, Patton (1999) questioned how the lens of race shapes and affects evaluators' understanding and actions. This question still has relevance today.

Racism can be a complex and destructive force in the evaluation context. Evaluators have an ethical obligation to eliminate, or at least mitigate, racial (and other) biases in their work. In 2018, Thomas, Madison, Rockcliffe, DeLaine, and Lowe called for evaluators to use their power and privilege to advance a more equitable society by "calling out" racial biases, policies, and practices and unmasking power inequities and outcomes of people in programs within the context of their racialized environments. Racial bias, particularly as it relates to African Americans, is due in large part to their unique historical position in the United States, and it can be present in both evaluators and evaluation stakeholders such as funders, policymakers, program staff, and others.

Biased conceptions of race can hinder an evaluator's ability to evaluate culturally and socially different worlds and realities. This, in turn, can prevent an evaluator from rendering ethical, honest, and fair evaluations. As discussed in Chapter 1, implicit bias, or unconscious attitudes and stereotypes, can affect evaluators' understanding, decisions, and actions in a manner that lends itself to questionable ethical conduct. Such biases are activated involuntarily and without an individual's awareness or intentional control. Many people do not deliberately discriminate against others, but when they offer preferential treatment to those who are like them, whom they know, and/or whom they like or feel most comfortable with, the resulting outcome can be unconscious bias and discrimination against those who are different. Individuals typically fail to recognize the harm that implicit favoritism of in-group members causes to members of the social out-groups (Sezer, Gino, & Bazerman, 2015). Evaluators, like other professionals and laypersons, are not immune to implicit biases. In the article "Evaluation and the Framing of Race," House (2017, p. 188) pointed out that

> a common error of evaluations is that the conclusions of the study don't fit the data on which they're based. This is more likely when the evaluations involve minorities. We need to weigh the empirical evidence carefully against the conclusions.

Inferences from data to conclusions are particularly susceptible to bias because they're based on more background knowledge than just the study.

Evaluators should be prepared for racial biases (House, 2017). As House and others point out, majority evaluators are often poorly informed and even misinformed about minorities and thus ill equipped to evaluate projects serving communities of color. As a result, various scholars have called for use of evaluation approaches, such as those that are culturally responsive, contextually responsive, culturally competent, and transformative and that emphasize inclusiveness, pluralism, and better understanding of minority cultures on the part of majority evaluators (e.g., Frierson, Hood, Hughes, & Thomas, 2010; Hood, Hopson, & Frierson, 2005, 2015; Hopson, 2009; Mertens, 2009; Samuels & Ryan, 2011; Thomas & Stevens, 2004; Thompson-Robinson, Hopson, & SenGupta, 2004). House (2017) calls for (majority) evaluators to check their own predispositions, arguing that no white person growing up in this country can be entirely free of racial framing. He also stresses that evaluators should check the work of their colleagues for such dispositions. Evaluators can be "critical friends" and look for biases that evaluators might harbor in their beliefs, dispositions, and behavior given that such biases can significantly affect evaluation findings (House, 2017, p. 187). This is indeed an ethical responsibility for evaluators.

The following case study describes an example of how evaluators noticed and highlighted racism inherent in a particular project. Even though Mathison (1999) admits that racism likely did not diminish as a consequence of the evaluation, she contends that at least the evaluation resulted in a range of stakeholders discussing the issue.

Case Study
Raising the Issue of Racism in Evaluation of a Program

Mathison (1999) describes how external evaluators working with a group of doctoral students to evaluate an after-school program for inner-city teens was able to raise the issue of racism. She contends that it was much easier for the external evaluator, in contrast to an internal evaluator, to raise issues of racism that were subtle and insidious within the program.

Mathison's Description of the Case

> The program focused on a transition-to-work program and, as such the [inner-city African American] teens were responsible for finding their own internships within the organizations, in this case a museum. This organization provided a vast array of potentially valuable experiences for them [the teens], but for the most part they either floundered about looking for work or worked in menial jobs, such as cleaning the cafeteria. Underlying the program's inability to provide positive, meaningful work experiences for these teens was a deficit model of inner-city, African American teens—one that presumed they weren't very able, by definition had psychological problems, and couldn't really be counted on in things that mattered. The program itself was ethically flawed. As external evaluators we could much more easily raise these issues of racism than could an internal evaluator. We were not seen as having a vested interest (although the staff did feel betrayed by us for raising these issues, and the teens were grateful for being given an opportunity to reveal their perceptions) and were presumed by our expertise to be doing a fair job.

Source: Mathison (1999, p. 33).

Ethical Sensitivity and Dilemmas

Ethics in evaluation is not simply related to doing the right thing or wrong thing, but is also related to ethical sensitivity. One of the early decisions that an evaluator may be confronted with is when a particular configuration of conditions, circumstances, and available choices should be framed and addressed as an ethical problem (Duggan & Bush, 2014). **Ethical sensitivity** includes an evaluator's ability to recognize and respond to the ethical dimensions of diverse evaluation contexts. Evaluators with ethical sensitivity continuously anticipate and seek to address ethical dimensions in their work rather than be surprised by them or simply ignore them.

In practice, ethical sensitivity in evaluation involves three aspects: the evaluator's awareness of or ability to determine whether a situation related to the evaluation or the *evaluand* involves an ethical issue, the evaluator's ability to identify the particular ethical value(s) underlying the issue under consideration, and the evaluator's awareness of the intensity of the issue.

First, the evaluator must be able to determine whether a situation related to the evaluation or the evaluand involves an ethical issue (i.e., awareness). This is a critical skill since oftentimes ethical issues go unnoticed because of their complexity or because of a particular cultural lens or unconscious bias on the evaluator's part. There is a large body of research arguing that unethical behavior often stems from actions that individuals do not even recognize as unethical (Banaji, Bazerman, & Chugh, 2003; Chugh, Bazerman, & Banaji, 2005; Sezer et al., 2015; Tenbrunsel & Messick, 2004). Individuals have an "illusion of objectivity" by acting against their ethical values without conscious awareness of such behaviors (Bazerman & Tenbrunsel, 2011; Epley, Caruso, & Bazerman, 2006). For example, an evaluator may fail to realize that the perspectives of the most vulnerable program participants are being ignored by the funder or project director. Here, ethical insensitivity may occur due to the evaluator's prejudices and biases toward the relatively powerless stakeholder group and favoritism toward the more powerful stakeholders. Evaluators can maintain what Bazerman and Tenbrunsel (2011) refer to as "ethical blind spots" as a result of seeing the world in a way that obscures one to the fact that a wrong or an unethical action (e.g., ignoring the perspective of the powerless) is occurring. In such instances, evaluators fail to see their own biases and subsequently fail to detect ethical dimensions in certain situations as a result. The activity that follows summarizes three sources of ethical blind spots evaluators might face: implicit bias, temporal distance, and failure to notice others' unethical behavior.

Activity
Ethical "Blind Spots" in Evaluation

Sezer and colleagues (2015) delineated various sources of ethical blind spots. After a review of these sources of ethical blind spots, summarized as follows, organize into small groups. Then discuss them as sources of evaluator blind spots. Give specific examples of how these sources might affect evaluators' sensitivities and course of action in practice.

- *Implicit biases:* These include attitudes or stereotypes that affect individuals' understanding, actions, and decisions in an unconscious manner and can lead those individuals to act against their ethical values.

- *Temporal distance:* Individuals overestimate the extent to which they will behave ethically in the future; therefore, temporal distance from decisions with ethical dimensions can be a source of unintentional ethical behavior.

- *Failure to notice others' unethical behavior:* Certain factors lead people to ignore the unethical behaviors of others including self-serving biases (e.g., if unethical behavior benefits them), outcome bias, the presence of intermediaries, and gradual erosion of ethical behavior; actions that produce negative outcomes are perceived as more unethical than similar actions that produce positive outcomes.

Another aspect that Sezer et al. (2015) discussed was the *slippery slope effect* or the gradual deterioration of ethical behavior. Here, individuals are more likely to justify small ethical indiscretions than major ones; however, over time, as they justify more and more, they can be led to justify even big indiscretions. When faced with abrupt and large dilemmas (rather than those that gradually increase), individuals are less likely to be unethical.

There are strategies that an evaluator can use to overcome ethical blind spots and be able to better identify ethical issues in real time. Among these are **active listening** (i.e., hearing a speaker and avoiding premature judgment, asking questions, reflecting understanding, clarifying information by restating a paraphrased version of the speaker's message, and summarizing the conversation), imagining the perspectives of others, and practicing **cultural humility** and openness to others' points of view.

A second aspect affecting evaluators' ethical sensitivity is their ability to identify the particular ethical value(s) underlying the issue under consideration. After gaining awareness of a potential ethical issue, evaluators need to reflect by asking themselves what ethical values are being compromised. In other words, an evaluator must first recognize there is an event to react to and then define an event as having an ethical dimension. Identify any ethical issues that might be facing the evaluator in the case study that follows.

Case Study
The Compromised Evaluator?

In an effort to become the long-term evaluator of a five-year project, an evaluator presents the project in a *slightly more* favorable light in the Year I Annual Report than in her original draft report submitted to the project administrator.

What ethical violations are present in this case, and how might such violations actually hurt (not help) the project being evaluated?

The third aspect affecting evaluators' ethical sensitivity is their awareness of the intensity of the issue. Evaluators do not treat all ethical issues the same. A decision must be made whether the ethical dimension is significant or important enough for the evaluator to do something about it. Ethical intensity often plays a role in how an evaluator will act. Intensity pertains not only to the awareness of an ethical issue but also to how important such issues are to various stakeholders. Thomas M. Jones (1991) argues that ethical decision making in organizations is generally a function of six factors, each of which we view as relevant to program evaluation:

- *Magnitude of consequences:* the total harm or benefit that participants or the evaluator can derive from an ethical action
- *Social consensus:* agreement among evaluators or the evaluator, client, and other stakeholders whether a behavior is "good" or "bad"
- *Probability of effect:* the chances that something will happen and result in harm to others
- *Temporal immediacy:* the time between the act and the consequences the act produces
- *Proximity of effect:* the social, psychological, cultural, or physical distance of the decision maker (e.g., evaluator) from the beneficiary or victim (e.g., program stakeholders) of the course of action
- *Concentration of effects:* the number of people affected or how much an action affects the average person (pp. 374–378)

All six factors represent characteristics of the ethical issue itself and are expected to have interactive effects. Jones (1991) theorizes that if any factor increases, it is generally expected that the overall level of intensity will also increase, and vice versa, assuming all remaining components are constant. For example, depending on the extent to which evaluators believe that their unethical behavior will result in an immediate impact (i.e., temporal immediacy), they are more or less likely to engage in such behavior.

Sources of Ethical Dilemmas

There are multiple sources of ethical dilemmas for the evaluator. Mathison (2007) identified three sources of ethical dilemmas in evaluation that are not mutually exclusive. One source includes *ethical issues that arise from doing the evaluation*. These, she argues, are manifested in various ways such as delivering evaluation findings or reports that (a) are laundered to omit negative findings, (b) exaggerate successes and positive findings, (c) are suppressed altogether, (d) are released belatedly so they are no longer relevant, and (e) are prematurely released or leaked to the public. Reducing complex evaluation findings into sound bites can become an ethical issue when they are misleading. For example, based on some positive findings from the evaluation, a program administrator can post flyers or hold press conferences claiming "our treatment works." This fails to communicate the complexity of the findings that "treatment worked" only for certain groups of participants and not others.

A second source of evaluation dilemmas identified by Mathison (2007) includes *ethical issues that are created by the evaluator*. Relevant examples include the evaluator's (a) personal or financial interest in the evaluand (i.e., conflicts of interest), (b) lack of knowledge or skill in the evaluation technique or method being used, (c) lack of cultural competence and sensitivity (such as lack of knowledge and respect for local culture and values), (d) ideological positions or values that can bias the evaluation outcome, and/or (e) propensity to deliver positive evaluations to increase job security. When evaluators make promises that they cannot deliver such as agreeing to totally unrealistic timelines just to secure a contract, another ethical dilemma arises as a result of their behavior. Ultimately, ethical evaluators have a responsibility to be honest, independent, impartial, credible, and accountable for their work and to the public. They also have the ethical responsibility to respect the rights, dignity, and diversity of participants; to do them no harm; and to maintain their dignity and confidentiality.

The third source of ethical dilemmas identified by Mathison (2007) includes *ethical issues that do not arise from the conduct of the evaluator or from doing the evaluation, but instead exist within the context of the evaluand and are discovered when planning or conducting the evaluation.* When such an issue is uncovered by the evaluator, it unexpectedly places the evaluator in an ethical dilemma. Examples include uncovering (prior to any data collection activity) that program administrators are engaging in illegal activities (e.g., theft) and malfeasance (e.g., misappropriation of program funds). Uncovering program activities that are knowingly harmful to clients or to public health or safety (e.g., poor food-handling practices) can also pose an ethical dilemma for the evaluator. Here, evaluators must determine whether there is an ethical imperative to "blow the whistle" on the activity in order to protect the public (Mathison, 2007).

It is noteworthy to mention that evaluators do not always agree whether a particular situation represents an ethical dilemma. Many times, the lines between ethical and unethical ways of responding can be blurred or ambiguous. In such situations, the evaluator must make a judgment call, which, of course, is done through his or her own cultural lens. In ambiguous situations, the course of action taken will be a function of how the evaluator interprets the situation. Morris and Jacobs (2000) had a national sample of evaluators respond to a case vignette in which the evaluator assembles a widely representative advisory group for a project but does not actively involve group members in the evaluation process. Their findings indicate that 39 percent of the sample regarded the evaluator's failure to involve stakeholders actively in the advisory group as "definitely" or "probably" ethically problematic; 49 percent of the sample believed that the evaluator's behavior was "definitely not" or "probably not" ethically problematic; and 12 percent were "unsure." Thus, one evaluator's ethical dilemma may be viewed by another evaluator as a political problem, a philosophical disagreement, or a methodological concern (Morris, 2008).

Handling Ethical Dilemmas

Evaluators are frequently faced with ethical dilemmas at some or all parts of the evaluation process. An **ethical dilemma** occurs when the evaluators have uncertainty about the proper or right thing to do because there is conflict between two or more valid and morally acceptable options such that making one choice prevents selection of the other. The complexity of an ethical dilemma arises out of a situational conflict or paradox between two possible ethical imperatives, in which obeying one would result in transgressing another. For example, focusing on the common good might result in failing to reveal malfeasance that could result in the elimination of a program and job loss for community-based staff who were not at fault. Here, there is not a definitive, clear correct response—as may become evident to readers after reviewing the dilemma in the following case study.

Case Study
Revising the Evaluation Report

This case was taken from work reported by Morris and Jacobs (2000). It involves a request for an evaluator to tone down the negatives of a report in order to make the program appear more flattering. The evaluation's sponsor and primary client is a philanthropic foundation that is the major source of funding for the program. Review the scenario and answer the five questions posed at the end of the case.

Scenario

An evaluator has recently shared the draft of a final report with the director of the program being evaluated. After reviewing the draft, the program director asks the evaluator to tone down one section of the report that describes some operational problems within the program. The director believes that the findings in this section, although accurate, are presented in a way that could cause readers to overlook the overall success of the program's implementation.

The evaluator reexamines the draft and concludes that the findings on operational problems have been reported in a fair and balanced fashion. Nevertheless, the evaluator wishes to be responsive to the director's concerns. The evaluator revises the section in question, mainly by deleting a number of harshly worded quotes concerning operational difficulties that were voiced by interview and survey respondents.

What is the ethical course of action?

Imagine that you are the evaluator referred to in this case. First, identify why this situation poses an ethical dilemma for the evaluator.

Answer the following questions, adapted from Newman and Brown (1996, p. 52), that will assist you (as the evaluator) in deciding how to respond to the potential ethical dilemma being posed in the case:

1. What are the consequences of the evaluator's choice? What would happen, for example, if every evaluator made the same decision?
2. What duties and obligations do evaluators have to themselves, the funder, project stakeholders, and society at large?
3. What would be just or fair in this situation?
4. What would be the caring response or course of action? Is that the ethical response? Justify your position.

There is no perfect solution when faced with ethical dilemmas since these situations require the evaluator to make a decision that requires placing certain ethical values over others. In theory, acting in an ethical manner may seem quite simple—that is, just do the right thing! But, in practice, identifying an issue, making decisions, and acting in ethical ways is not so straightforward for evaluators. In the following activity, readers are provided an opportunity to identify potential ethical issues for an evaluator working in the field.

> ## Reflect and Discuss
> ### You Didn't Hear It From Me!
>
> Identify the potential ethical issues the evaluator faces in the activity that follows.
>
> ### The Situations
>
> During a confidential interview with a disgruntled (white) female staff member, an evaluator was told of an (alleged) incident of inappropriate sexual behavior by a program administrator (middle-aged white male) toward program clients (mostly poor women of color). The disgruntled staff member, while clearly wanting the conversation to remain confidential, stated to the evaluator, "I'm just saying; but you didn't hear it from me."
>
> In another situation, during several confidential interviews, an evaluator learned that program administrators may have falsified the program's accountability reports. However, no one who made these allegations wanted to go on record.
>
> ### Questions for Discussion
>
> - Which potential ethical dilemmas exist for the evaluator in the two situations described?
> - Should the evaluator do anything? If so, what, and why?

Both of these scenarios require the evaluator to weigh the principles of the common good against promises of confidentiality made to the interviewees. Given the possible hidden agendas and complexities embedded in these cases, the evaluator should examine the situations from multiple perspectives, reflecting on whether the situations represent an ethical, legal, or professional problem or a combination of the three. Unless evaluators are forced to take an immediate course of action, they should pause to seek out different points of view and review and troubleshoot options with a more experienced, knowledgeable, and culturally competent colleague for this particular setting while remaining open-minded and reflective. Evaluators who are not culturally competent and who do not know and respect the unique cultural values operating in the evaluation context might inadvertently use culturally insensitive and incongruent methods that damage, instead of support, the community under study. This raises ethical issues related to the value of doing no harm.

Reviewing case studies, such as those found in *Evaluation Ethics for Best Practice: Cases and Commentaries* (Morris, 2008), is a useful way to help evaluators think about, analyze, and organize their thinking about real-life ethical dilemmas that they may face when conducting evaluations. Reflecting on evaluation cases, and discussing them with others, can better prepare evaluators for effective evaluation practice by developing the understanding, skills, and confidence necessary to confront ethical dilemmas in a thoughtful and coherent manner.

Ethics and Conflicts of Interest

A major concern that has serious ethical ramifications is conflict of interest. A **conflict of interest** refers to a set of conditions in which professional judgment concerning the primary interest (i.e., the evaluation) might be influenced by a secondary competing interest such as financial gain (Tobin, 2003). Evaluators must always be concerned with actual and potential conflicts of interest and must deal with them openly and honestly so that they do not compromise the evaluation process and results. Conflicts of interest in evaluation are inevitable, and they emerge in and affect all groups of stakeholders, including evaluators (Yarbrough et al., 2011).

A conflict of interest, in particular, occurs when two or more competing or contradictory interests relate to an activity by an individual or an institution. In evaluations, conflicts of interest include situations in which financial or other personal considerations may compromise, or have the appearance of compromising, an evaluator's judgment in conducting the evaluation and/or reporting the findings. When evaluators are caught in conflicts of interest, biases often distort findings (House, 2016). Conflicts of interest are distinct from bias, inasmuch as conflicts of interest occur when evaluators' judgment concerning their primary interest (i.e., the production of valid and useful evaluations) is clearly influenced by some secondary and competing interest. Here, conflicts of interest exist regardless of whether the evaluator's judgment and behavior can be demonstrated to have adversely influenced the evaluation. Instead, the conflict exists simply as a condition of the evaluator having competing interests (Tobin, 2003).

Currently, there are two major conflict of interest areas generally considered in the evaluation field that can negatively impact the ethical integrity of the evaluator and the resulting evaluation. These include financial conflicts of interest (e.g., monetary arrangements with sponsors) and professional conflicts of interest (e.g., personal friendships, professional relationships). In evaluation, conflicts of interest extend beyond simple personal or financial interest; they can also occur when different individuals or groups try to influence when evaluations are commissioned, which purposes and questions are addressed, who can serve as evaluators or evaluation staff, when data are collected, which methods are used, who can provide or later access information, who has primary access to findings, and how findings are interpreted (Yarbrough et al., 2011). Examples of conflicts of interest in evaluation include

- any personal benefit the evaluator (or the evaluator's spouse, child, etc.) might gain in a direct or predictable way from the developments of the program or projects the evaluator is reviewing or asked to review in the future;
- any previous involvement the evaluator has had with the program or projects he or she has been asked to review, such as serving on the advisory board or having an undisclosed relationship with the program administrators or staff; and
- financial interest held by the evaluator (or the evaluator's spouse, child, etc.) that could be affected by his or her evaluation.

In addition to financial and professional conflicts of interest, we propose a third conflict of interest area; that is, **cultural conflict of interest** is about evaluator power, status, knowledge of, and identification with the goals and values of the dominant culture and how these factors become a secondary yet competing interest, with the primary interest of the individuals and communities under consideration. This secondary interest might impact the evaluator's questions, methods, measures, definitions of success, and interpretations. Evaluators, particularly those from the dominant culture, are at risk of experiencing a cultural conflict of interest because they think the world is the way they see it or, if not, it ought to be that way. The evaluators may be well intentioned but still demonstrate cultural arrogance or lack of respect. Here, they need to work to educate themselves about relevant cultures in the evaluation context.

A cultural conflict of interest may be unconscious and thus not recognized as a conflict by the evaluator. Such unrecognized conflicts can result in ignoring important perspectives and rendering some important (yet marginalized) stakeholders and communities as relatively invisible.

Ethical Challenges and Dilemmas Across the Evaluation Process

Scholars have researched and written extensively on ethics and evaluation (e.g., Barnett & Camfield, 2016; House, 2011; Mathison, 1999, 2007; Morris, 2008, 2015; Newman & Brown, 1996). Morris and colleagues (Morris, 2015; Morris & Cohen, 1993) identify common ethical challenges evaluators face at various stages of the evaluation. The following case study provides a list of commonly reported ethical challenges faced by evaluators across various phases of the evaluation process.

Case Study
Ethical Challenges Commonly Reported by Evaluators

Entry/Contracting Phase

- A stakeholder has already concluded what the findings "should be" or plans to use the findings in an ethically questionable fashion (e.g., to support a decision previously made).
- A conflict of interest exists.
- The type of evaluation to be conducted is not adequately specified or justified.
- A stakeholder declares certain research questions "off limits" in the evaluation despite their substantive relevance.
- Legitimate stakeholders are omitted from the planning process.
- Various stakeholders have conflicting expectations, purposes, or desires for the evaluation.
- The evaluator has difficulty identifying key stakeholders.

Designing the Evaluation Phase

- The evaluator fails to gain acceptance of the overall design from all relevant stakeholders.
- The evaluator believes evaluation design is fundamentally flawed.
- Insufficient time and resources are available to conduct a credible evaluation.

Data Collection Phase

- The rights or dignity of those providing data are compromised in some fashion (e.g., violations of confidentiality, anonymity, informed consent).
- The evaluator discovers behavior that is illegal, unethical, or dangerous while conducting the evaluation.
- The evaluator discovers staff incompetence.

Data Analysis and Interpretation Phase

- The evaluator fails to distinguish between findings and his or her opinions in data analysis.
- Methodological choices highlight some findings while downplaying others of equal or greater importance.

(*Continued*)

(Continued)

Communication of Results Phase

- The evaluator is pressured by a stakeholder to misrepresent findings.
- The evaluator is pressured by a stakeholder to violate confidentiality.
- Although not pressured to violate confidentiality, the evaluator is concerned that reporting certain findings could represent such a violation.

Utilization of Results Phase

- Findings are suppressed or ignored by the stakeholder.
- Disputes or uncertainties develop concerning ownership/distribution of the final report, raw data, and so on.
- Findings are used to punish the evaluator or someone else.
- Findings are deliberately modified by a stakeholder prior to release.
- Findings are misinterpreted by a stakeholder.
- Plagiarism/misrepresentation of authorship occurs.
- Information gathered for one purpose is used for another.

Source: Morris, M. (2015). Research on evaluation ethics: reflections and an agenda. In Paul R. Brandon (Ed.), Research on evaluation. New Directions for Evaluation, 148, 31–42.

Ethical Principles and Standards for Evaluators and Evaluations

One of the best ways evaluators can avoid and resolve ethical dilemmas is to know both what their ethical obligations are and what resources are available to them. In the evaluation field, there are explicit principles and standards for guiding the ethical behavior of evaluators and achieving quality evaluations. This section summarizes and discusses two major sources of guidance for evaluators: the AEA's (2018b) *Evaluators' Ethical Guiding Principles* and the *Program Evaluation Standards* developed by the Joint Committee on Standards for Educational Evaluation (Yarbrough et al., 2011). Both of these sources were developed in the United States and represent the longest-standing professional principles and standards in the evaluation profession. Many other regions of the world have also developed their own statements of standards. Notable examples include the Canadian Evaluation Society's *Guidelines for Ethical Conduct*, the African Evaluation Association's *African Evaluation Guidelines*, and the Australasian Evaluation Society's *Code of Ethics* (links to these guidelines are provided in the additional resources section at the end of the chapter). It is imperative that evaluators become intimately familiar with the *Evaluators' Ethical Guiding Principles* and the *Program Evaluation Standards* to be better positioned to understand how they should respond in the evaluation context in order to produce the most ethical and highest-quality evaluations possible.

The *Evaluators' Ethical Guiding Principles*

The AEA's *Evaluators' Ethical Guiding Principles* (referred to as the *Guiding Principles for Evaluators* until 2018) were first adopted in 1994 and have subsequently undergone multiple revisions. They are intended to proactively guide and inspire the ethical conduct of evaluators at all stages of the evaluation process. These guidelines build, implicitly and explicitly, upon the three principles (respect for people, beneficence, and justice) in the *Belmont Report*. The *Evaluators' Ethical Guiding Principles* stress that it is the primary responsibility of the evaluator to initiate discussion and clarification of ethical matters with relevant parties to the evaluation. (See Appendix A for a full presentation of the *Evaluators' Ethical Guiding Principles*.)

There are five major *Evaluators' Ethical Guiding Principles*. Each of these ethical principles is accompanied by several directives or subprinciples to amplify the meaning of the overarching five principles and to provide guidance for their application. The five guiding principles, briefly described as follows, do not imply priority among them, but instead, priority will vary by situation and evaluator role.

- *Systematic inquiry:* Evaluators conduct data-based inquires that are thorough, methodical, and contextually relevant. This principle focuses most directly on methodological decisions made during the evaluation, although it renders no judgments favoring some methodologies over others. There are six subprinciples under systematic inquiry.

- *Competence:* Evaluators provide skilled professional services to stakeholders. The principle of competence focuses on issues of the evaluator's education, experience, relevant expertise, cultural competence, and professional development. This guiding principle includes four subprinciples.

- *Integrity:* Evaluators behave with honesty and transparency in order to ensure the integrity of the evaluation. Here, evaluators must cultivate openness and full disclosure with stakeholders throughout the entire evaluation process. There are seven subprinciples under integrity.

- *Respect for people:* Evaluators honor the dignity, well-being, and self-worth of individuals and acknowledge the influence of culture within and across groups. At all times, evaluators must demonstrate respect in terms of their interactions with stakeholders (regarding ethnicity, class, gender, orientation, etc.), including not judging them; not discrediting them; ensuring that their views are faithfully recorded, as appropriate; and giving them due consideration in the evaluation process. This guiding principle includes four subprinciples related to the overarching respect for people principle.

- *Common good and equity:* Evaluators strive to contribute to the common good and advancement of an equitable and just society. Prior to the August 2018 *Evaluators' Ethical Guiding Principles* revision, this principle was labeled "responsibilities for general and public welfare." Because the revised principle places more explicit focus on common good and equity, it was renamed as such. There are five subprinciples under common good and equity.

The five *Evaluators' Ethical Guiding Principles* are not independent, but instead, they overlap in many ways. For example, being honest and transparent (*integrity principle*) overlaps with honoring the dignity, well-being, and worth of individuals (*respect for people principle*). Conversely, sometimes these principles will conflict, and so evaluators will have to choose among them. When this occurs, evaluators must use their own values and knowledge of the evaluation context to determine the appropriate course of action. The following case study involves the external evaluation of a health program and was developed in 2006–2007 by the AEA Ethics Committee Professional Development Task Force. The first author, Veronica Thomas, was a member of that task force, and this case has been used as part of a training package on the *Evaluators' Ethical Guiding Principles*.

Case Study
Application of the *Evaluators' Ethical Guiding Principles*

Read the following case example, keeping in mind the AEA's (2018b) *Evaluators' Ethical Guiding Principles*. Then, organize into small groups and discuss the case. Complete the worksheet and question at the end of the case.

Evaluation Context. The Health Care Collaborative program grew out of a multiyear effort funded in many sites by a national foundation. That initiative promoted local collaboration among health care providers and residents in poorly served or underserved neighborhoods. The Health Care Collaborative office uses trained residents as outreach health workers to raise health-issues awareness among residents and to give them options for accessing health care. Health care providers who are collaboration partners deliver a range of services to neighborhood residents. A local funding source supports the Health Care Collaborative, which has a program director, administrative staff, and a small network of outreach workers. The Health Care Collaborative Board of Directors consists of a small group of health care providers.

The Health Care Collaborative serves an economically challenged neighborhood in a small metropolitan area: Average income is one-third to one-half of its metro and national counterparts. The neighborhood is quite diverse along many dimensions, including age, household composition, sexual identity, education, religious preference, race, and ethnicity. The neighborhood has a large African American population, an increasing population of refugees from African and Eastern European nations during the past 20 years, and a rapidly growing Hispanic population in recent years.

Entry, Contracting, and Design. The Health Care Collaborative Board and local funders found that they needed more information than the program's reporting system alone could provide about how program participants viewed the Health Care Collaborative, how the staff viewed the program and the neighborhood, and how the program met or did not meet identified service needs. The funder provided $20,000 for this purpose, and the Board established a one-year schedule for completing an evaluation. The funder and the program director approached a local faculty member, an evaluator who also teaches evaluation, to ask for a proposal. The faculty member has previously served on the Health Care Collaborative Board. Discussions with the funder, the program director, and some members of the Board identified key expectations and constraints.

The faculty evaluator proposed a multimethod approach for a formative evaluation. The design included surveys of participants (brief), program staff, and other health care provider partners. The surveys would include questions about racial and ethnic identity. Selected program participants would be asked to keep journals and to participate either in a focus group or in an observed service delivery for a small group. Three focus groups were proposed: one for senior citizens; another for adult, nonsenior males; and a third for adult, nonsenior females. The Health Care Collaborative focus group participants would be offered a $25 gift card for their time. The institutional review board's approvals would be obtained for informed consent to voluntarily participate in the evaluation.

A graduate student would do most of the data collection, under the evaluator's supervision. The student was fluent in Spanish and English, and this project would be the subject of the student's master's thesis. The evaluation's final product would be a presentation of results, in PowerPoint format, with the slides and notes delivered to the program director and funder.

Data Collection. The student administered the staff surveys in person. These surveys asked for how long the staff members worked with the Health Care Collaborative, what they did in the program, how they viewed the participants, and what difference the program made in the neighborhood. Surveys of other providers involved with the Health Care Collaborative were web-based. The questions concerned what kinds of interaction the providers had at the Health Care Collaborative, with whom, and how often; how that relationship affected both organizations; and what services the responder brought to resident-participants in the Health Care Collaborative.

The Health Care Collaborative staff administered surveys to program participants during ongoing program contact. The student also conducted a small number of interviews of people identified for their longevity in working with this particular neighborhood, and added open-ended historical questions.

The student observed both staff and participants in health care awareness sessions for small groups to better enrich the evaluator's and student's understanding of the program, its staff, and the participants. Participants' journals provided inspirational stories of their experiences in navigating the health care maze.

Data Analysis and Interpretation. From the surveys, some data were aggregated and reported descriptively (e.g., comparisons of the racial and ethnic composition of the Health Care Collaborative participants for the neighborhood). Scaling and cluster analyses were used to structure and analyze the results of the focus groups, and some journal entries and responses to open-ended questions from interviews also were analyzed.

All in all, the program served a disproportionate number of Hispanic adults (compared to the neighborhood's composition) and disproportionate numbers of people without health insurance and without other known ways to access health care. Participants and staff were very positive about the program and its value in their neighborhood and lives. The Health Care Collaborative program participants overwhelmingly credited the use of racially and ethnically diverse staff, from the neighborhood itself, as the main reason for the Health Care Collaborative's success.

Younger adults placed more concern on financial issues related to health care, compared with older adults. Hispanic participants in focus groups were all female, and most were unemployed. From all three focus groups, whether participants were treated fairly and had access to insurance and to health care was more important than waiting times or actually getting to appointments.

When the evaluator and student felt comfortable with their work, they shared draft findings informally with the program director, funder, and Board members—through in-person as well as telephone conversations and through email. Some feedback was given and considered in reviewing those findings and in developing the final product.

Dissemination and Utilization of Results. The final evaluation briefing was delivered at a meeting of the Health Care Collaborative Board, to which the funder and some residents were invited. The funder could not make this meeting, accepted the electronic PowerPoint file, and asked no further questions. Only one resident—a regular attendee of Board meetings—was present for the briefing. Two or three questions were asked, more of apparent curiosity than any other cause or purpose. No future plans for the findings were discussed at this meeting.

The student completed the thesis based on this project, and it was very well received by the faculty committee. The evaluator adapted the evaluation for use in an advanced evaluation course for graduate students.

The student and evaluator also proposed a poster session focusing on the evaluation findings to an annual, national professional conference in their discipline. The proposal was accepted and a large poster developed, which covered the basics of the evaluation. Those who stopped to read and talk about the evaluation expressed admiration for its scope and methods.

As the evaluator, what are some things that you would do differently to better ensure that your actions are ethically defensible?

Case Study Worksheet to Be Completed

Guiding Principle	Issues or Questions Raised Related to the Principle
Systematic Inquiry	
Competence	
Integrity	
Respect for People	
Common Good	

Source: This case is republished with permission of the American Evaluation Association (with minor edits).

The *Program Evaluation Standards*

In addition to the *Evaluators' Ethical Guiding Principles*, the ***Program Evaluation Standards*** is another document that provides guidance and direction for those in the evaluation field. It includes much more specificity regarding what to do and not do in program evaluation than the *Evaluators' Ethical Guiding Principles*. Whereas the *Evaluators' Ethical Guiding Principles* are concerned specifically with the ethical conduct of the evaluator, the *Program Evaluation Standards* pertain to the quality of the evaluation. Initially established in 1981 by the Joint Committee on Standards for Educational Evaluation[1] with multiple editions since then, the *Program Evaluation Standards* provide guidance for improving evaluation quality and accountability. The *Program Evaluation Standards* contain 30 standards organized around five central attributes of evaluation quality. These quality attributes include (a) utility ($N = 8$ standards), (b) feasibility ($N = 4$ standards), (c) propriety ($N = 7$ standards), (d) accuracy ($N = 8$ standards), and (e) evaluation accountability ($N = 3$ standards). A full description of the 30 *Program Evaluation Standards* is provided in Appendix B. An overview of the five central attributes discussed in the *Program Evaluation Standards*, as adapted from Yarbrough et al. (2011), include the following:

- **Utility** standards are concerned with evaluation use, usefulness, influence, and misuse. Utility is supported by standards that provide guidance to increase the likelihood that the evaluation will have positive consequences and substantial influences such as contributing to stakeholders' learning, informing decisions, leading to improvements, or providing information for accountability judgments.

- **Feasibility** standards are intended to increase evaluation effectiveness and efficiency by ensuring that an evaluation is practical, efficient, and contextually viable. These standards highlight the logistical and administrative requirements of evaluations that must be managed, bring the world of possible evaluation procedures into the world of practical procedures for a specific evaluation, and serve as a precondition for other attributes of quality.

- **Propriety** standards support what is proper, fair, legal, right, and just in evaluations. These standards cover three overlapping domains: (a) the evaluators' and participants' ethical rights, responsibilities, and duties; (b) systems of laws, regulations, and rules that regulate the conduct of people and organizations, such as federal, state, local, and tribal regulations and requirements, institutional review boards, and local/tribal constituencies that authorize consent to work in and with respective communities; and (c) the roles and duties inherent in evaluation professional practice.

---

[1] The Joint Committee on Standards for Educational Evaluation (JCSEE) is supported by 17 sponsoring organizations and has been a member of the American National Standards Institute (ANSI) since 1989. During its history, the mission of the JCSEE has remained to develop and implement inclusive processes producing widely used evaluation standards that serve educational and social improvement. To learn more about the history and organizational support of the JCSEE, visit www.jcsee.org.

- **Accuracy** standards seek to increase quality in data collection and analyses and to increase the truthfulness and dependability of evaluation representations, propositions, and findings by urging that evaluations strive for as much accuracy (i.e., validity, reliability, reduction in error and bias) as is feasible, proper, and useful to support sound conclusions and decisions in specific situations. Ignoring nondominant cultural perspectives and assuming that certain methodologies (e.g., experimental designs) are the only factor necessary for justified conclusions and decisions is a barrier to adherence to the accuracy standards.

- Evaluation **accountability** standards encourage adequate documentation of evaluations and a **metaevaluation** (evaluation of the evaluation) focuses on improvement and accountability for evaluation processes and products. Attention to accountability guides improvement during all phases of the evaluation, and it encourages reflection and a metaevaluative perspective in evaluators and evaluation users.

In his Voices From the Field interview, Michael Morris stresses that evaluators must uphold the *Evaluators' Ethical Guiding Principles* and the *Program Evaluation Standards* and resist pressure to act unethically. This sometimes takes, as he points out, consideration of potential ethical challenges during evaluation planning, moral courage, and just the willingness to do the right thing.

Voices From the Field

Michael Morris: Ethical Considerations in Evaluation

Evaluators must act with integrity and see themselves as more than just methodological technicians as they uphold the *Evaluators' Ethical Guiding Principles* and the *Program Evaluation Standards*. They should strive to understand the organizational and other cultures in which a project is embedded, because they cannot do justice to the evaluation without such an appreciation. Before the evaluation is designed and implemented, evaluators should consider the ethical challenges that might arise and find a way to introduce these topics into discussions with stakeholders during the contracting and negotiation phase, in addition to soliciting the stakeholders' concerns. Having mildly uncomfortable conversations with stakeholders early on can reduce the likelihood of having to engage in much more difficult interactions later in the project. Doing this will also enable the evaluator, at a later point, to bring stakeholders' attention back to those initial discussions, increasing the chances that the latter will act in accordance with whatever guidelines had been agreed upon. For example, pressure to misrepresent or ignore (unflattering) findings is frequently encountered by evaluators. Early discussion of how to deal with potentially unwelcome results in the evaluation report is a worthy investment of everyone's time. Ultimately, moral courage is key for evaluators, particularly internal ones. Doing the right thing can put an evaluator at risk. Sometimes, however, the only reason for doing the right thing is that it is the right thing to do.

Michael Morris is emeritus professor of psychology at the University of New Haven and a former chair of the AEA Ethics Committee. He is the author of Evaluation Ethics for Best Practice: Cases and Commentaries *(Guilford Press, 2008). Veronica Thomas interviewed Dr. Morris in the fall of 2019.*

Evaluation Corruptibility and Fallacies

It is often said by numerous scholars and practitioners in the evaluation community that "evaluators must be able to speak truth to power." Evaluation corruptibility and evaluation fallacies are two factors that can put an evaluator at risk of unethical decision making, jeopardizing evaluation quality, and, thus, an inability to "speak truth to power." Fitzpatrick, Sanders, and Worthen (2004) use the term *evaluation corruptibility* to describe ways that evaluators may be convinced to go against ethical standards, thus engaging in ethical compromises or distortions. They point to five specific areas of evaluation corruptibility (Fitzpatrick et al., 2004, pp. 423–424):

- *Conflict of interest:* a willingness to twist the truth and produce positive findings due to conflict of interest or other perceived payoffs or penalties (such willingness may be conscious or unconscious)
- *Unsubstantiated opinions:* an intrusion of unsubstantiated opinions because of sloppy, capricious, and unprofessional evaluation practices
- *Prejudices and biases:* "shaded" evaluation "findings" as a result of intrusion of the evaluator's personal prejudices or preconceived notions
- *Inducements:* obtaining the cooperation of clients or participants by making promises that cannot be kept
- *Not honoring commitments:* failing to honor commitments that could have been honored

To avoid corruptibility, evaluators must be transparent and disclose any relationships (e.g., previous organizational ties or ties with program staff) that might predispose them to bias or give the appearance of bias. Further, they should in no way profit from the outcome of an evaluation. Familiarity with and adoption of the *Evaluators' Ethical Guiding Principles* and the *Program Evaluation Standards* can provide much-needed guidance for dealing openly with situations that can impact ethical decision making and quality evaluations.

House (1995) considered the issue of evaluator corruptibility from a different perspective than Fitzpatrick et al. (2004). He suggested that evaluators can have the best intentions and may not be corrupt, per se, but, at times, may have a misunderstanding about their responsibilities. House referred to these misunderstandings as *evaluation fallacies*. A fallacy is a mistaken belief based on unsound argument deriving from reasoning that is logically inaccurate. House (1995, pp. 29–30) identified five evaluation fallacies that can have negative ethical consequences:

- *Clientism:* the fallacy that doing whatever the client requests or whatever will benefit the client is ethically correct
- *Contractualism:* the fallacy that the evaluator must follow the written contract without question, even if doing so is detrimental to the public good
- *Methodologicalism:* the belief that following acceptable inquiry methods ensures that the behavior of the evaluator will be ethical, even when some methodologies may actually compound the evaluator's ethical dilemmas

- *Relativism:* the fallacy that opinion data the evaluator collects from various participants must be given equal weight, as if there is no basis of appropriately giving less priority to the opinions of peripheral groups than to those of more pivotal groups
- *Pluralism/elitism:* the fallacy of allowing powerful voices to be given higher priority because the evaluator feels they hold more prestige and potency than the powerless or voiceless

Evaluator Role, Power, Politics, and Ethics

Ethical issues can arise centering on the evaluator roles, power imbalances between the evaluator and key stakeholders, and evaluator privilege. Politics can also have ethical dimensions that impact an evaluator's work. As discussed throughout this book, power and privilege are concepts that extend far beyond an individual evaluator or a particular evaluation. Frequently, relationships between the evaluator and stakeholders and between/among stakeholders are enthralled in power imbalances and hierarchical struggles. Hierarchical arrangements and power imbalances in the evaluation context exist long before the evaluator is on the scene since oppressive systems often shape the conception, design, and implementation of the program that the evaluator is tasked with studying. Evaluators are often asked to assess the effectiveness of social programs that are designed to yield a quick "magic bullet" fix to problems (e.g., racial achievement gaps, poverty) derived from years of racial and other oppressions (Thomas et al., 2018). In order to accomplish this, evaluators must develop a critical consciousness of how institutional, historical, and systemic forces limit and promote the life opportunities for particular groups. Instead of, for example, identifying delinquency, substance abuse, and violence as problems, evaluators should emphasize the root causes by examining the larger political, economic, and social forces that create persistent poverty, thus jeopardizing healthy development (Thomas et al., 2018).

In any given evaluation, the evaluator occupies multiple roles, including those of expert, knower, judge, and educator. For example, an evaluator can be an expert or program facilitator during the program implementation, a researcher when collecting and analyzing evaluation data, a judge during the reporting phase when making an assessment of program merit and worth, and an educator or advisor throughout the entire evaluation process. The roles that evaluators assume are generally all positions of tremendous power with opportunities to exercise that power in either ethically "just" or "oppressive" ways. Power in evaluation is more distributed toward the evaluator since it is, in fact, the evaluator who is studying others and generating knowledge (and not vice versa). While evaluators do not generally own the knowledge generated from their evaluations, it is still the case that their perspectives and interpretations are often privileged over those being studied in the evaluation context.

Interplay of Politics and Ethics

It is also worth distinguishing ethical considerations from political issues, although they are oftentimes closely intertwined. Ethical considerations relate to issues of right and wrong, good and bad, whereas the central focus of political issues relates to power and control. Political issues can undermine the integrity of an evaluation and certainly have ethical ramifications by silencing voices and perspectives of the less powerful and rendering these individuals invisible. For example, politics is likely operating when an evaluator is only allowed to evaluate what project administrators or funders believe to be model or successful sites while more troublesome sites are hidden or excluded from consideration. This is a power play that has definite ethical implications related to excluding certain perspectives from consideration.

Power plays, or attempts to gain an advantage by using certain tactics to magnify one's influence or power, can be exhibited by the evaluator, as well as by various stakeholders. For example, power plays by those being evaluated (e.g., program staff) include denying the need for an evaluation, claiming the evaluation will take too much time away from their normal workload, and/or intentionally providing the evaluator with huge amounts of information so it is difficult to sort out what is relevant and what is not (International Program for Development Evaluation Training [IPDET], 2009). Power plays by the evaluator might include using the "experts know best" line, applying unstated criteria to decision making, and/or applying unstated values and ideological filters to the data interpretation (IPDET, 2009). Other stakeholders, such as community members, can also engage in power plays with ethical ramifications (see the following case studies for additional examples).

Case Studies of
Political Power Plays in Evaluation With Ethical Ramifications

Political Power Plays Engaged in by Evaluatees

- Denying the need for the evaluation
- Claiming the evaluation will take too much time away from their normal workload
- Claiming the evaluation is a good thing, but introducing delaying tactics
- Providing the evaluator with huge amounts of information so it is difficult to sort out what is relevant and what is not
- Omitting or distorting information they are asked to provide so they do not look bad
- Coming up with new data at the end
- Arguing that the evaluation findings are irrelevant because things have changed

Political Power Plays Engaged in by Evaluators

- Using the "experts know best" line to exclude the perspectives of others
- Insisting evaluations should only be quantitative in nature since statistics do not lie
- Not stating or shifting the measurement standards
- Applying unstated criteria to decision making
- Applying unstated values and ideological filters to the data interpretation
- Ignoring certain evaluation findings

Political Power Plays Engaged in by Other Stakeholders

- Giving their own conclusions to meet their own agenda
- Trying to get the media (or powerful others) to criticize (or praise) the organization being evaluated in order to sway opinion

Source: Adapted from International Program Development Evaluation Training (2009).

SUMMARY

A critical task for evaluators in any evaluation is to identify issues, including those of an ethical nature, that might hamper the conduct of a fair, honest, and accurate evaluation. This chapter examined evaluation ethics and the quality standards that are expected to govern the behavior of evaluators and the outcomes of an evaluation. Evaluators must take necessary steps to equip themselves with the knowledge, skills, and dispositions to accomplish this goal. This means having the sensitivity to identify and deal with the ethical challenges in the evaluation context. This chapter highlighted some common ethical challenges and offered possible solutions. Special consideration was given to how conflicts of interest, cultural issues, racial bias, and political issues impact evaluation ethics. The origin of research ethics, why they are important, and the three ethical principles from the Belmont Report were discussed to provide readers with a foundation for better understanding current evaluation ethics. The AEA's *Evaluators' Ethical Guiding Principles* and the Joint Committee on Standards for Educational Evaluation's *Program Evaluation Standards*, although unable to cover every possible scenario that an evaluator might face, were discussed to provide a framework that gives guidance to evaluators.

In conclusion, the following is a set of reflective questions, adapted from Patton (2003, pp. 408–409), that evaluators can ask themselves to help them think through some ethical issues that might arise during their work.

- How will the evaluation contribute to society, the community, and/or the world?

- Why should individuals participate in your project? What are the benefits to them?

- How will you explain the purpose of the inquiry and methods to be used in ways that are accurate and understandable to those you are researching?

- In what ways, if any, will conducting this research or program evaluation put people at risk? (Consider psychological, legal, and political issues and the possibility of people becoming ostracized by others.)

- If you uncover controversial information, how should it be shared?

- What are reasonable promises of confidentiality that can be fully honored?

- What information can you *not* promise to keep confidential?

- What kind of informed consent, if any, is necessary for mutual protection?

- Who will have access to the data, and why?

- How will you and your respondent(s) likely be affected by conducting this research or program evaluation?

- Who will be the researcher or evaluator's go-to person(s) during the study regarding ethical issues that might arise?

- How hard will you press participants for data? Where will you draw the line?

- What ethical framework and philosophy informs your work and ensures respect and sensitivity for those you study, beyond whatever may be required by law?

In the final analysis, evaluators must use their own moral compass, in conjunction with the guidance of the profession's principles and standards, to take the most ethical and socially just course of action possible.

SUPPLEMENTAL RESOURCES

Practical Strategies for Culturally Competent Evaluation

www.cdc.gov/dhdsp/docs/cultural_competence_guide.pdf

Provided on the website of the Centers for Disease Control and Prevention (CDC), this document includes a crosswalk table in Appendix A, listing each of the *Program Evaluation Standards* in column 1 with suggested strategies an evaluator can engage in to increase cultural competence relative to that standard in column 2. It also includes other appendices of resources and tools and tips for integrating cultural competence into evaluation.

The *Belmont Report*

www.hhs.gov/ohrp/humansubjects/guidance/belmont.htm

Part of the U.S. Department of Health and Human Services Office for Human Research Protections, this website provides a link to the full *Belmont Report: Ethical Principles and Guidelines for the Protection of Human Subjects of Research*.

"Human Subjects"

www.nsf.gov/bfa/dias/policy/human.jsp

This website of the National Science Foundation (NSF) has information concerning the basic principles of protection of human subjects as well as information about institutional review boards.

Protection of Human Subjects in Research

www.ed.gov/about/offices/list/ocfo/humansub.html

This U.S. Department of Education web page includes links to general information concerning human subjects in research and the regulations/legalities surrounding using human subjects in research.

Human Subjects Research (HSR)—CITI Program

https://about.citiprogram.org/en/series/human-subjects-research-hsr/

Human Subjects Research (HSR) basic content is organized into two courses: Biomedical (Biomed) and Social-Behavioral-Educational (SBE). They are intended for anyone involved in research studies with human participants, or who have responsibilities for setting policies and procedures with respect to such research, including institutional review boards (IRBs). Additional modules of interest within HSR allow for exploration of several important topics and may be selected to meet organizational needs. HSR includes additional stand-alone courses for institutional/signatory officials, IRB chairs, and public health researchers, as well as a revised Common Rule course that covers the regulatory updates to the Common Rule. These courses were written and peer-reviewed by experts.

Web Links to Ethical Principles and Quality Standards

AEA's *Evaluators' Ethical Guiding Principles*

www.eval.org

Joint Committee on Standards for Educational Evaluation's *Program Evaluation Standards*

https://jcsee.org/program/

Canadian Evaluation Society's *Guidelines for Ethical Conduct*

www.evaluationontario.ca/membership/standards-guidelines/

African Evaluation Association's *African Evaluation Guidelines*

https://afrea.org/the-african-evaluation-guidelines/

Australasian Evaluation Society's *Code of Ethics*

www.aes.asn.au/images/stories/files/membership/AES_Code_of_Ethics_web.pdf

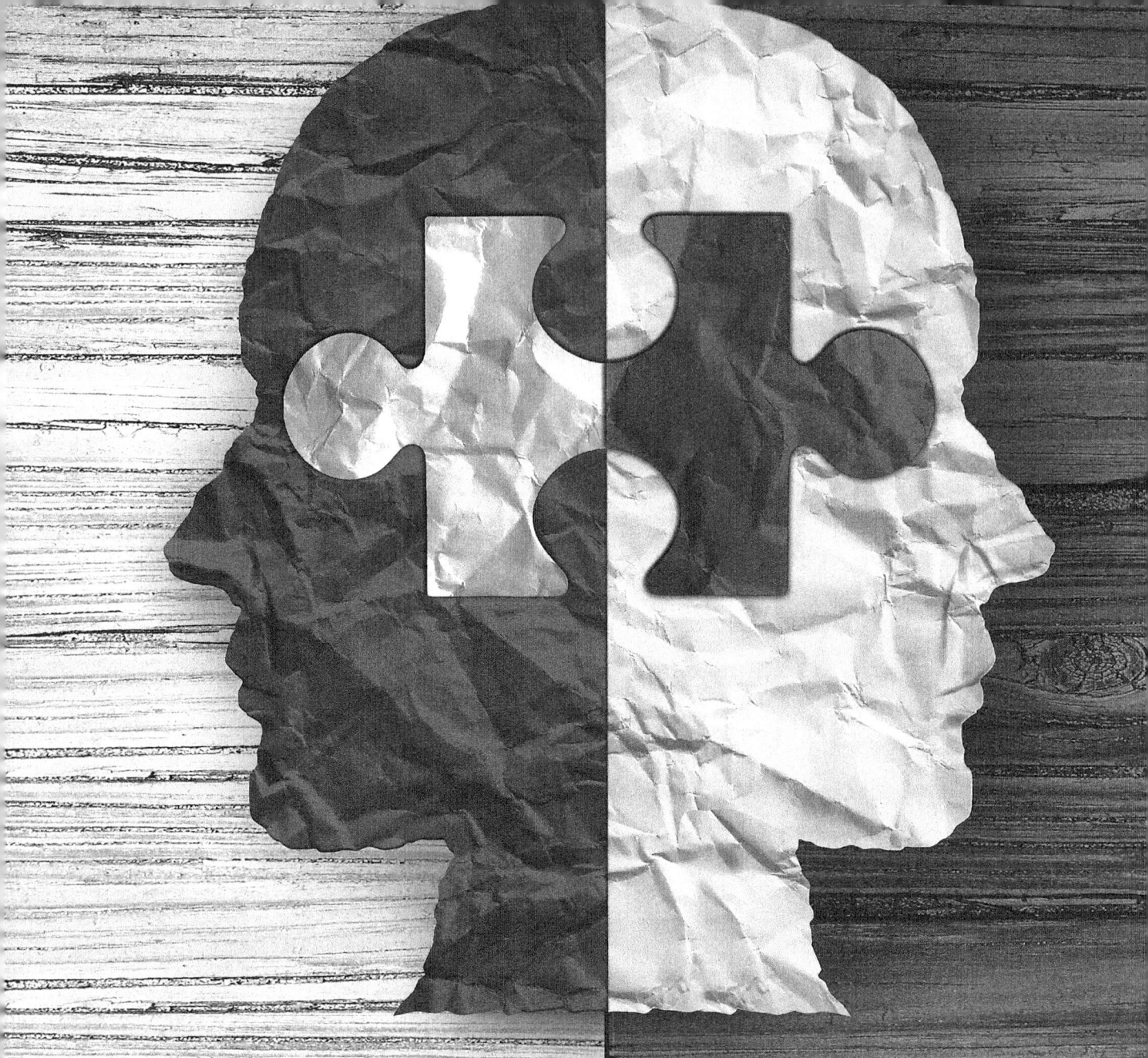
Shutterstock/Lightspring

Tracing evaluation's history must be more inclusive than it has been in the past, uncovering and acknowledging a broad range of events, influential figures, and "multiple truths" that left an indelible footprint on the field, especially aspects that moved us closer toward a more equitable society.

CHAPTER 3

Historical Evolution of Program Evaluation Through a Social Justice Lens

The history of evaluation matters but only when it is an inclusive history of evaluation that is both critical and contextual and not just a celebratory and ceremonial account of ideas, methodological perspectives, and dominant figures of the past. A history of evaluation that matters includes letting readers know that evaluation, in some form, has been around since antiquity; that evaluation in the modern times has been powerfully influenced by the social, economic, political, and racialized climate of the day; and that there are "hidden histories" and prominent evaluators of color who made substantial, but often unrecognized, contributions in the field toward social justice aims as early as the 1940s and 1950s.

After reading this chapter and participating in the activities, readers will be able to meet the following learning objectives:

- Describe evaluation activities taking place prior to the 20th century
- Connect political, economic, and other societal conditions to the growth, and sometimes decline, of evaluation in the 20th century
- Identify "hidden histories," "hidden figures" of color, and influential women who contributed to evaluation's theoretical, methodological, and equity agendas
- Explain 21st-century trends in the evaluation profession

Introduction

To date, there have only been modest efforts to comprehensively chronicle the historical evolution of evaluation. Historical knowledge of evaluation provides greater clarity on how and why the field has evolved as it has today. Additionally, historical knowledge enables one to discern the conditions, at particular points in time, in which evaluation flourished or stagnated and, ultimately, may stimulate thinking that shapes the progression of theoretical perspectives and practices, especially related toward working more effectively in diverse and vulnerable communities.

Over 40 years ago, Glass and Ellett (1980, p. 211) stated that "evaluation, more than any science, is what people say it is; and people currently are saying it is many different things." Even today, we contend that if you ask a sociologist what program evaluation is, you will likely get a very different answer, focusing on different things, than if you ask an economist; and their answers both likely differ from how an epidemiologist, educator, or psychologist defines program evaluation. Our definition of evaluation has elements of many of the various definitions of evaluation provided in Chapter 1 but also includes distinctive features:

> Evaluation is a disciplined inquiry involving the systematic, contextually responsive, and ethical application of research tools and methods to collect data that assess the effectiveness and operations of programs within the various

social, political, and cultural contexts in which they operate. Evaluation's ultimate goal is to provide credible evidence that fosters greater understanding and improves decision making, all aimed at improving social conditions and promoting healthy, just, and equitable communities.

Because multiple disciplines contributed to evaluation as currently understood and practiced, unifying its historical roots is not an easy task. The history of evaluation, like histories of many topics, differs depending on who is telling the story and the disciplinary background of the writers (Mertens & Wilson, 2019). A common misconception in writing a history chapter is that it simply involves finding out what happened and then documenting those events in chronological order. Undoubtedly, documenting notable evaluation-related events in temporal sequence can be useful because knowing the order in which events occur can help us understand potential causes (or influences) and effects of those events. This, in turn, allows us to step back and view the "big picture" of evaluation history. In this chapter, we seek to present a more inclusive history of evaluation than is generally presented in other evaluation books and to weave together a story of consequential events in the growth of evaluation.

History of Evaluation Through a Social Justice Lens

Published accounts of evaluation's historical roots and evolution are relatively scant. The few existing histories were written in the 1990s or early 2000s, and they often covered narrow aspects of evaluation's evolution such as theories or 20th-century developments. Shadish and Luellen (2005) wrote a brief history of evaluation in the *Encyclopedia of Evaluation*. Probably the most comprehensive and frequently cited historical overview is Madaus and Stufflebeam's (2000) chapter characterizing evaluation over seven periods from 1792 to 2001. Stufflebeam and Coryn (2014) extended this historical overview to also include accounts of events from 2005 to 2014. Accounts of how evaluation has continued to evolve during the 21st century are still quite limited.

Since evaluations, in some form, have taken place over the many centuries in various arenas, chronicling the full history of evaluation in a single chapter is virtually impossible. There exist far too many events, theoretical and methodological perspectives, influential figures, and evolving trends to cover. In this chapter, we seek to provide a historical account of evaluation that infuses a social justice lens within our synthesis by situating evaluation within the political, sociocultural, and racialized contexts of the times. Existing published historical accounts virtually ignore the early contributions of persons who were engaged in evaluative efforts to advance social justice agendas. Hopson and Hood (2005, p. 88) argue that "the rich intellectual history of the evaluation profession may be improvised as a result of an overemphasis by those who some have anointed as 'fathers' (or 'mothers', in recent history) of the field." We seek to redress this by providing a historical account that is more inclusive of important, but often ignored, events and people who utilized evaluation as a tool to ameliorate prominent social inequities of the time.

Evaluation Prior to Modern Times of the 20th Century

If one thinks of evaluation simply in terms of assessing the value of something, then there is clearly no single moment in time that we can pinpoint when individuals began to use evaluative judgments to draw conclusions. During ancient times, individuals were faced with making determinations (i.e., evaluations) about the best course of action for securing the essentials of life (i.e., food, clean water) and avoiding and treating diseases. In this sense, as Scriven (1996, p. 395) stated, "evaluation is a very old practice yet a very young discipline."

Evaluations of people, programs, and events have a long history that has been loosely documented. While certainly not exhaustive, Table 3.1 highlights notable evaluation activities taking place in various settings and across different fields prior to the modern times of the 20th century. Some of these events are elaborated in more detail in the text that follows.

Table 3.1 A Brief History of Evaluation Activities Prior to the 20th Century: Selected Listings

Time Period	Significant Evaluation-Related Events
5000 BCE	Ancient Egyptians conducted regular tracking of the government's outputs in grain and livestock production.
2200 BCE	Performance evaluations were used in China by officials when conducting civil service examinations to select the most talented government employees; the examinations, built on a rigid essay format, tested the applicants' rote-learned knowledge of Confucian philosophy.
500 BCE	The Socratic method of asking questions to teach and evaluate students' performance was first used.
1601 CE	Concerned about scurvy among his crew, British captain admiral James Lancaster conducted an experiment by serving daily dosages of lemon juice to men on one of four vessels sailing from England to India while the men on the other vessels did not receive this treatment.
1747 CE	Concerned about scurvy among his crew, Scottish doctor James Lind purportedly conducted a controlled experiment on the *Salisbury* by dividing the men on his ship, half of whom consumed citrus fruit in addition to their regular diet while the other half continued with their regular diet only.
1800s CE	The first request was made by the U.S. government for external inspectors to evaluate public facilities such as prisons, schools, hospitals, and orphanages.
1800s CE	Initial focus was placed on accreditation in U.S. schools and colleges; the first regional accrediting agencies were formed with particular focus on educational standards and admissions procedures.
1815 CE	The U.S. military sought to evaluate arms supplies; the Ordnance Department devised a system of regulations for the uniformity of manufacture of all arms ordnance.
1845 CE	In Boston, Massachusetts, Horace Mann led the first documented use of student test scores to evaluate the instructional quality of school effectiveness.
1897 CE	One of the first implemented educational evaluations in the United States occurred when progressive education advocate Joseph Mayer Rice conducted a 16-month experimental comparative study of spelling performance of nearly 33,000 students in grades 4–8.

Mosteller (1981) argues that the earliest known evaluation is described in the Old Testament book of Daniel. It spoke of what can be essentially viewed as a nutrition evaluation study based on what Daniel (Belteshazzar), Hananiah (Shadrach), Mishael (Meshach), and Azariah (Abednego) ate, in comparison to the diet of other males, during their time in Babylon as captives. According to the Old Testament, Daniel said to the guard over him and others: "Please test your servants for ten days: Give us nothing but vegetables to eat and water to drink. Then compare our appearance with that of the young men who eat the royal food, and treat your servants in accordance with what you see." The guard agreed, and at the end of this trial period, Daniel and his mates looked healthier and better nourished than any of the young men who ate the royal food. While clearly not meeting scientific standards, this is still loosely an example of an evaluation study during ancient times.

Intersection Between Education and Evaluation Pre–20th Century

Evaluation, in large part, as practiced today evolved from pre-20th-century work in two areas of education: student assessment and measurement and the accreditation of schools and colleges. Many contemporary evaluation methods and procedures, such as the use of comparison groups, standardized testing, and surveys, are built on systematic strategies and techniques that were applied in the 1600s in the field of education.

The first evidence of formal educational program evaluation recognized in the United States took place between 1897 and 1898 when Joseph Mayer Rice evaluated the spelling performance of 33,000 students in relation to their spelling instruction (Madaus & Stufflebeam, 2000). Because of this groundbreaking work, Rice is recognized as a pioneer of educational research and the originator of comparative methodology in the field. Further, Rice's work remains critical in the history of evaluation because it began a long tradition of using achievement test scores, or standardized testing, as a key indicator for judging the effectiveness of a school or instructional program (Madaus & Stufflebeam, 2000; Morra-Imas & Rist, 2009).

Educational accreditation in this country represents another major and long-standing influencer on educational evaluations (Kellaghan, Stufflebeam, & Wingate, 2003). The first regional accrediting agencies formed in the 1880s with particular focus on educational standards and admissions procedures. Accreditation of educational institutions was conceived of as a quality assurance process whereby educational institutions, programs, services, and operations are evaluated and verified by an external body to determine if recognized standards are met. It became (and continues to be) a means of conducting nongovernmental peer evaluations of educational institutions and programs.

Early Social Experiments

As Rossi, Lipsey, and Freeman (2004, p. 2) pointed out, one of the technically challenging forms of contemporary evaluation research, "social experiments," is not hardly a recent invention. Probably one of the most-cited areas of evaluation taking place in the 1600s includes the experiments with scurvy (a disease resulting from lack of vitamin C) (Mosteller, 1981; Rossi et al., 2004). In the early 1600s, British captain admiral James Lancaster, in an effort to address the incidence of scurvy among crews on ships, ran an evaluation experiment by serving daily dosages of lemon juice to men on one of four vessels sailing from England to India while the men on the other vessels did not receive this treatment. During the 1700s, even more systematic controlled evaluations were carried out to determine the impact of citrus intake on the prevention of scurvy.

In the United States, with the wartime activities of the 1800s, it may not be surprising to note that perhaps the earliest formal evaluation occurred in 1815 when the military sought to evaluate arms supplies (Madaus & Stufflebeam, 2000). Additionally, during the 1800s, U.S. cities faced substantial problems related to poor sanitation and the lack of piped water. This meant that incidences of disease such as cholera were high among the population in cities. It was during this time when the U.S. government first asked for external inspectors to evaluate public facilities such as prisons, schools, hospitals, and orphanages (cited in Mertens & Wilson, 2019).

Overview of Evaluation in the 20th Century

Widespread implementation of evaluation, with its extensive use of social science methods, is a relatively modern 20th-century phenomenon. Many events and influential leaders through their scholarship and/or practice throughout the 20th century impacted the evaluation field and/or utilized evaluation to spotlight and redress social injustices. While not exhaustive, Table 3.2 highlights key individuals, agencies/organizations, studies, federal policies, and programs that stimulated the growth and use of evaluation during the 20th century. It should be noted that Table 3.2 is not limited to specific evaluation studies or evaluators, per se, but also highlights specific incidents (e.g., launch of Sputnik) that contributed to the implementation of new programs

Table 3.2 Key Events in the Evolution of Program Evaluation During the 20th Century

Time Period	Significant Evaluation-Related Events
1921	Two U.S. government agencies were established, taking the lead in evaluations at the federal government level: the General Accounting Office (GAO) and the Bureau of the Budget (BOB).
1930–1945	Ralph Tyler conducted his Eight-Year Study (1932–1940), a groundbreaking study in evaluation and education; prominent African American scholars conducted important surveys and evaluation studies to illuminate inequalities in African American educational resources and outcomes.
1932	The *Journal of Negro Education* was launched, including publication of important (some large-scale) evaluation studies conducted by African American scholars that remained largely unread by the white scholarly community during that time.
1933	President Franklin D. Roosevelt launched the New Deal, including a series of programs, public work projects, financial reforms, and regulations; application of social science research grew rapidly after the launch with an increasing demand for evaluating program effectiveness.
1935	The Cambridge-Somerville Youth Study, one of the earliest attempts at building evaluation into a community-based treatment program to prevent juvenile delinquency, was launched.
1939	African American scholar Rose Butler Browne became the first African American woman to earn a doctorate in education from Harvard University; she is acknowledged as the first African American woman who had the word *evaluation* in her dissertation, *A Critical Evaluation of Experimental Studies in Remedial Reading*.

(Continued)

Table 3.2 (Continued)

1944	As the third African American to receive a PhD from the University of Chicago, Aaron Brown completed a dissertation (under the general supervision of Ralph Tyler) that consisted of a historic evaluation of the 93 accredited secondary schools for African Americans in the South.
1946–1957	The Educational Testing Service (ETS) was established in 1947, prompting considerable development in the technical aspects of evaluation, particularly in relation to the growth in standardized testing.
1950s	Program evaluations rooted in the social sciences were expanded, including studies in areas such as education, public health, employment, delinquency prevention, public housing, and international initiatives.
1950	As the first African American to receive a PhD from Stanford, Leander L. Boykin completed evaluation research that was the first comprehensive examination of differentials in African American education stemming from inequalities in the resources available for and the effort put forth to support education for African Americans.
1957–1958	After Russia launched Sputnik in 1957, the U.S. government subsequently approved $1 billion to enact the National Defense Education Act of 1958, funding curriculum development; new educational programs in mathematics, science, and foreign language; and large-scale evaluations.
1960s	Implementation of War on Poverty and Great Society included numerous social programs aimed at providing for the well-being of the nation's citizens, more equitably serving persons of color and those with disabilities, and protecting national prosperity. There was an increase in evaluations as the federal government called for a systematic approach to evaluating these social programs.
1960s	The federal government pushed for new achievement tests to evaluate instructional methods and schools.
1965	The Elementary and Secondary Education Act was passed, designed to improve educational equity for students from lower-income families along with required evaluation of program results.
1969	The first successful conduct of the National Assessment of Educational Progress (NAEP) began under the leadership of Ralph Tyler; NAEP remains the only assessment that measures what U.S. students know and can do in various subjects across the nation, in individual states, and in some urban districts.
1970–1979	Evaluation began to crystallize and be recognized as a legitimate professional field.
1975	The two-volume *Handbook of Evaluation Research* (edited by Marcia Guttentag and Elmer Struening) was published, and is thought to have helped establish evaluation as a distinct field of applied social science scholarship and practice.
1976	Two U.S.-based professional societies were formed to foster evaluation as a profession and a science: the Evaluation Research Society and the Evaluation Network.
1978	Initial publication of *Utilization-Focused Evaluation* (Michael Patton) focused attention on the importance of intended users and uses of evaluation information.
1980–1990s	Many federal programs were reduced or eliminated during the Reagan administration in the 1980s; a rethinking of both the role and methods of evaluation occurred.
1981	Standards for educational evaluation were first presented by the Joint Committee on Standards for Educational Evaluation.
1986	The Evaluation Research Society and the Evaluation Network merged to form the American Evaluation Association (AEA).

1988–1989	Noted educational psychologist Asa Hilliard became one of the first African Americans to provide a keynote at the AEA conference (in 1988); his presentation, which focused on structural racism in evaluation, was later published in *Evaluation Practice*.
1990	Yvonna S. Lincoln became the first woman president of the AEA.
1993	The Government Performance and Results Act was originally passed into law with intent to provide a framework for government to plan, implement, and evaluate.
1993	The *User-Friendly Handbook for Project Evaluation*, a National Science Foundation (NSF) document, was published and has since been updated over the years and is still in use in professional development and training activities.
1994	AEA president Karen Kirkhart selected "Evaluation and Social Justice" as the conference theme.
1994	Initial approval was granted to the AEA's *Guiding Principles for Evaluators*.
1995	The first joint International Evaluation Conference was held in Vancouver, Canada, and included the coming together of five evaluation associations and evaluators from 66 countries and five continents.
1999	African American scholar John Stanfield delivered a plenary address (subsequently published in the *American Journal of Evaluation*) at the annual meeting of the AEA, calling on the field to acknowledge the role that white supremacy plays in evaluation and fundamental problems with researchers who do not understand or value the context or life experiences of people of color.
1999	The Centers for Disease Control and Prevention (CDC) developed and published its *Framework for Program Evaluation in Public Health*, which was designed to be a practical tool, comprising steps in program evaluation and standards for effective program evaluation; this framework is extensively used across various areas of evaluation beyond public health fields.
1999	The Federal Evaluators Network, an informal association of evaluation officials in the legislative and executive branches of the U.S. government, was organized to share information and concerns about evaluation methodology, policy, and practice at the federal level.

and evaluations of those programs, as well as people who promoted or engaged in evaluation research to advance social justice agendas. The sections following the table elaborate on some of these individuals and factors, placing them into the sociopolitical and cultural context of the time.

Evaluation in the First Half of the 20th Century: 1900–1950s

Evaluation in the modern times of the 20th century was influenced tremendously by the social, economic, and political climate of the day. Conditions such as social inequities, escalating poverty rates, unprecedented growth and recession, political perspectives toward deficit reduction and balanced budgets, and funding for social programs all impacted interest in and the demand for program evaluation. During the early part of the 20th century, evaluation and measurement studies were occurring in various areas such as public health, mortality and morbidity from infectious diseases, housing, worker productivity and occupational training programs, and standardized educational testing (Morra-Imas & Rist, 2009; Rossi et al., 2004). Many of these studies were small-scale efforts conducted by government agencies and social services.

In 1921, two U.S. government agencies, the General Accounting Office (GAO), renamed the Government Accountability Office in 2004, and the Bureau of the Budget

(BOB), which in 1970 became the Office of Management and Budget (OMB), were established, and they took the lead in conducting evaluations at the federal government level. Most of the GAO's work involves auditing, program evaluations, policy analysis, and legal opinions and decisions on a broad range of government programs and activities both at home and abroad. While the OMB's most prominent function is to prepare the president's budget, it also evaluates the effectiveness of agency programs, policies, and procedures; assesses competing funding demands among agencies; and sets funding priorities.

Evaluation During the New Deal, Wartime, and Economic Growth: 1930s–1950s

Franklin D. Roosevelt, elected U.S. president in 1933 during the midst of despair and impoverishment of the Great Depression, enacted the New Deal. This included a series of social programs, public work projects, financial reforms, and regulations focusing on providing relief for the unemployed and poor, recovery of the economy back to normal levels, and reform of the financial system to prevent a repeat depression (Berkin et al., 2011). With the New Deal, there was rapid growth of the federal government, and new agencies were created to manage and implement these new large-scale programs. At this time, there was also great demand for evaluating these programs' effectiveness in stimulating the economy, creating jobs, and instituting social safety nets (Morra-Imas & Rist, 2009). By the 1930s, social scientists were routinely engaged in evaluations of social programs using social science methods.

The first half of the 20th century, in particular, was characterized by extreme and explicit racial prejudice and legal discrimination in the United States. African Americans continued to be marginalized through enforced segregated and diminished access to facilities, housing, education, and opportunities. **Jim Crow laws**, a set of repressive regulations and customs affecting virtually every section of daily life, made it legal for legislators to racially segregate everything including schools, public parks, swimming pools, theaters, residential areas, jails, asylums, phone booths, residential homes for the elderly and persons with disabilities, and even cemeteries. Further, some states required the use of separate textbooks for African American and white students; some courts even provided African Americans and whites separate Bibles for their swearing in.

The New Deal, although far from ideal, featured some of the most antiracist policies in U.S. history up to that time. Prior to 1933, assistance to African Americans, particularly in the South, was virtually nonexistent. However, the New Deal did bring some federal assistance. For example, New Deal work-relief programs were open to unemployed people of all races, although whites got the better jobs and higher wages. While African Americans received fewer benefits than their white counterparts, on average, from many New Deal programs, they did receive some benefits. Although African Americans (and white women) experienced some limited advancement during this time, many New Deal programs were still able to discriminate against African Americans since many of these federal programs were administered through local authorities or community leaders whose racial biases influenced their program administration. In public assistance programs, for example, African Americans generally received substantially less assistance than their white counterparts, and some charitable organizations even excluded African Americans from their soup kitchens. In another example, the Agricultural Adjustment Administration offered white landowners cash for leaving their fields fallow, which they happily accepted; they, however, did not pass on their government checks to the Black sharecroppers and tenant farmers who actually worked the land (Leuchtenburg, n.d.). Virtually no attention was paid to evaluating programs, through a social justice lens, to document the (known) harsh realities faced by persons of color in accessing and benefiting from existing social programs of the time.

The Cambridge-Somerville Youth Program Evaluation

As more large-scale programs were being implemented in various areas, such as for the military, urban housing, jobs, juvenile delinquency, occupational training, and health, there was increasing interest in evaluation to assess the success, or lack thereof, of these programs. The Cambridge-Somerville Youth Study is a notable example of a social program, and its accompanying evaluation, that was initiated in the 1930s. It is one of the earliest experiments of a social program (Forsetlund, Chalmers, & & Bjørndal, 2007). This experimental evaluation was deemed to be a comprehensive attempt to determine if helpful interventions would deter delinquency and produce other important changes in the behavior and personalities of a cohort of boys, many of whom seemed headed for difficulty (Geis & Dodge, 2003).

The following case study provides an opportunity for readers to briefly review and reflect on the Cambridge-Somerville Youth Study.

Case Study
Example of Experimental Evaluation in the 1930s: The Cambridge-Somerville Youth Study

The Cambridge-Somerville Youth Study, which began in 1935, is one of the earliest attempts at building evaluation into a community-based treatment program to prevent juvenile delinquency. One contribution of this study to evaluation's history was its early success in combining large-scale social program evaluation with longitudinal design. It also highlighted some potential hazards in executing and drawing evaluative conclusions built on longitudinal designs. Several follow-up evaluations have been conducted over the past 70 years to assess the impact of the program.

Program Description

The Cambridge-Somerville Youth Study involved mentoring boys placed at risk, ages 5–13 from low-income backgrounds, who lived in facilities in eastern Massachusetts in an effort to prevent or lower rates of juvenile delinquency (Cabot, 1940; Powers, 1951).

Method and Procedures

A randomized, experimental trial of the program was conducted in 1939 and lasted for 5 years on average. Six hundred and fifty boys (later reduced to 506) of average and difficult temperament between the ages of 5 and 13 years (median = 10.5 years) from Cambridge and Somerville, Massachusetts, who were considered at risk were placed in matched pairs, and one member of each pair was randomly assigned to the treatment group. Referred to as directed friendship, the preventive intervention involved individual counseling through a range of activities and home visits with the families. Counselors talked to the boys, took them on trips and to recreational facilities, tutored them in reading and arithmetic,

(Continued)

(Continued)

encouraged them to participate in the YMCA and in summer camps, played games with them at the project's center, and encouraged them to attend church. Boys in the control condition received no special services.

Selected Results

In the initial and 10-year follow up, there was either no difference or a higher rate of negative results as reported by the authors (Cabot, 1940; McCord, 1978). A 30-year follow-up evaluation found that the program had no impact on the delinquency of juveniles or when children in the program aged into adulthood (McCord, 1978). Likewise, the program had no positive effects on health of either juveniles or, later, adults. In fact, those in the program were more likely to be rearrested for crimes as youth and adults. Some negative impacts on physical and psychological health were found.

Reflect and Discuss

1. What do you see as important contributions of the Cambridge-Somerville Youth Study to the field of evaluation?

2. What are some issues raised by this study, particularly in relation to its longitudinal experimental approach? (Longitudinal studies will be covered in more detail in Chapter 11.)

Sputnik's Impact on the Growth of Evaluation

Russia's launch of Sputnik, the first artificial satellite to reach space and orbit the Earth, in 1957 was a major coup for the Soviet Union. It resulted in many U.S. policymakers feeling that the country was falling dangerously behind its Cold War rival in science and technology. The launch of Sputnik was so serious that then president Dwight D. Eisenhower appeared on national television to apologize to the country for its failure, and he promised a boost to U.S. science efforts. As a result, there was sizable investment in educational reform (especially science and technology), and the federal government approved $1 billion to enact the National Defense Education Act of 1958. This act funded curriculum development and new educational programs in mathematics, science, and foreign language. Additionally, funds were provided to evaluate these new initiatives.

Prominent Influencers and Users of Evaluation During the 20th-Century Early Years: 1930s–1950s

In the first half of the 20th century, there were a number of individuals whose philosophy, values, and research work helped to shape how evaluation evolved during that time and in subsequent years. There were also individuals whose evaluation work may not have impacted the evolution of evaluation theory and practice, per se, but who instead used evaluation as a tool to expose major social injustices of the time. Some of these influential scholars were not identified as evaluators during their time, yet their work made contributions to evaluation as theorized and practiced today. While they are too numerous for our coverage to be exhaustive, we highlight a few well-known, and a few lesser-known, early contributors to the evaluation field.

Kurt Lewin

In their book *Social Psychology and Evaluation*, editors Melvin M. Mark, Stewart I. Donaldson, and Bernadette Campbell (2011) explored the relationship between social psychology and the evaluation of programs, policies, and practices. They stress that Kurt Lewin, one of the most prominent social psychologists of the early 20th century, made important historical contributions—more than are often recognized—to evaluation. Considered the father of social psychology, Lewin contributed to evaluation most notably through his **action research** movement (Mark et al., 2011). He described action research as comparative research on the conditions and effects of various forms of social action, and research leading to social action, that uses a spiral of steps, each of which is composed of a "circle of planning, action and fact-finding about the result of the action" (Lewin, 1946, p. 38). This movement, taking place during the 1940s, led to the application of social psychology to social problem solving coupled with the need to evaluate those efforts in field settings. Another important area of Lewin's work that was groundbreaking during his time (and became an important focus in contemporary evaluation approaches) is his focus on context. His field theory approach focused on studying behavior but without separating it from its natural context.

Mark et al. (2011) cited a number of contemporary approaches that were influenced by Lewin's action research perspective. These include, for example, Fetterman's (1998) empowerment evaluation, Rothman's (1997) action evaluation research, Cousins and Whitmore's (1998) practical participatory evaluation, and Patton's (2008) developmental evaluation.

Alva and Gunnar Myrdal

The 1930s and 1940s work of Swedish scholars Alva and Gunnar Myrdal had an enormous influence on social science research, policy, and social justice perspectives in evaluation. Alva Myrdal was one of the most influential social reformers of the 20th century, seeking to end inequalities among all peoples. Gunnar Myrdal, an economist and sociologist, made an international reputation with his study and 1944 book, *An American Dilemma*, which provided deep insight into the contradictions of American democracy and its treatment of African Americans. It is worth noting that Ralph Bunche, the first African American to win the Nobel Peace Prize and a longtime distinguished member of the United Nations diplomatic corps, collaborated with Myrdal between 1938 and 1940 in the monumental study of U.S. race relations. The American Evaluation Association (AEA) bestows an annual award named in honor of Alva and Gunnar Myrdal. The Alva and Gunnar Myrdal Evaluation Practice Award is presented to an evaluator who exemplifies outstanding evaluation practice and who has made substantial cumulative contributions to the field of evaluation through the practice of evaluation and whose work is consistent with the association's *Evaluators' Ethical Guiding Principles*.

Ralph W. Tyler

For more than 60 years in the early part of the 20th century, Ralph Tyler was undoubtedly one of the most influential figures, both nationally and internationally, in education and evaluation. Tyler is credited with coining the term *educational evaluation* (Stufflebeam & Shinkfield, 2007), and his contributions to education, in general, and to testing and evaluation, in particular, have been extensively documented (e.g., Bloom, 1986; Madaus, 2004; Madaus & Stufflebeam, 1989). One of Tyler's most notable achievements is his role as head of evaluation in the monumental Eight-Year Study of 1932–1940. This research is considered the second major landmark in educational evaluation (after Rice's spelling performance evaluation in the 1800s), and it introduced educators throughout the United States to a new and broader view of educational evaluation than that which had been prevalent at that time (Madaus & Stufflebeam, 2000). Tyler viewed this comprehensive study as having multiple evaluation-related purposes including grading, grouping, and guiding students; reporting to parents on their children's attainment; reinforcing teachers; reporting to school boards on the attainment of students, schools, and classrooms; validating the assumptions under which the institution operates; and providing feedback for public relations (Madaus & Stufflebeam, 1989).

In comparison to the work of others of his time, Tyler's work offered a greater variety in evaluation procedures including the use of examinations, questionnaires, interviews, observational evidence, checklists, rating scales, anecdotal records, pre- and posttests, and various other types of evidence and records (Bloom, 1986). The National Assessment of Educational Progress (NAEP)—still the only assessment that measures what U.S. students know and can do in various subjects across the nation, in the states, and in some urban districts—was first successfully conducted in 1969 under Tyler's leadership.

Hidden Figures and Histories in Early-20th-Century Evaluation

Across many fields, too often, the historical contributions of persons of color are dimmed in the limelight of white males, at best, or totally omitted, at worst, from accounts of significant events in this country. Increasingly, there are efforts to tell the untold accounts and hidden stories across various fields. For example, the nonfiction book *Hidden Figures: The American Dream and the Untold Story of the Black Women Who Helped Win the Space Race* (Shetterley, 2016) tells the incredible untold story of four brilliant African American female mathematicians, Dorothy Vaughan, Mary Jackson, Katherine Johnson, and Christine Darden, who worked at the National Aeronautics and Space Administration's (NASA) Langley Research Center as "human computers" in the 1940s, 1950s, and beyond. In some respects, accounts of the historical evolution of evaluation, too, share the problem of ignoring the early contributions of persons of color and omitting critical evaluation studies that examined issues aimed toward ameliorating discrimination and social injustice. For example, between 1935 and 1951, 25 African Americans received their doctorates in education and conducted evaluations for their dissertations, but their work was, for the most part, unrecognized in its social and educational significance for African Americans (Hood, 2001; Hopson & Hood, 2005).

In critiquing Marvin Alkin's (2004) historical assessment of evaluation theory and practice published in his *Evaluation Roots* volumes and depicted as an evaluation tree with three limbs (discussed in more detail in Chapter 4), Hood (2017) states that

> Alkin's historical contribution to evaluation theory and practice has consistently been discussed in my evaluation courses over the years. However, as I looked at the illustration of Alkin and Christie's (2004) "evaluation tree," I found no disagreement with roots. . . . Yet, what stood out to me was that Chen [Asian] was the only evaluator of color to be identified on this evaluation tree. As I looked at this evaluation tree and its branches, I could not help but

think that there were other mighty trees in this evaluation forest which were either hidden from view or simply outside the view of this illustrator. (p. 265)

As Stafford Hood states in his Voices From the Field interview, it is important that evaluation history is told in a manner that is more diverse and inclusive than it has been in the past.

Voices From the Field

Stafford Hood: Toward a More Inclusive History of Evaluation

If we are going to tell the history of evaluation, then we must tell the whole story. A more inclusive evaluation history is critically important because it lets evaluators, particularly young evaluators of color, know that the field has a rich history and that their work stands on the shoulders of lots of other folks. I started by looking from the vantage point of my own heritage and roots as an African American and saw that we were truly part of the story of evaluation history, and that story needed to be told. In doing this work, what I found was fascinating inasmuch as during the early years of the 1930s and 1940s, African Americans were conducting evaluations using sophisticated methods such mixed methods, although they didn't name it as such. There were African American scholars, such as Leander L. Boykin, Reid E. Jackson, Aaron Brown, and others, navigating the community, having a cultural reference, and providing examples of how to conduct large-scale evaluation studies. The work of early African American pioneers in evaluation illuminated stories of social injustice during that particular time through their evaluation work especially related to segregated schools. They were committed to doing work that was for "the cause" and work that was culturally responsive and socially responsible. Such evaluations provide examples of the struggles faced by African Americans to get this work done and the impact of that work. However, uncovering untold stories of evaluation's early history does not stop here. We must continue uncovering the footprint of African Americans and other people of color in the history of evaluation.

Stafford Hood is the Sheila M. Miller Professor of Curriculum and Instruction and a professor of educational psychology at the University of Illinois at Urbana-Champaign, and founding director of the Center for Culturally Responsive Evaluation and Assessment (CREA). Veronica Thomas conducted the interview in the fall of 2019.

Hood and colleagues, in the evolving *Nobody Knows My Name* project, continue to research the historical contributions of African Americans who engaged in evaluation in the early years (prior to the 1954 *Brown v. Board of Education* Supreme Court decision). The title of his project was borrowed from Baldwin's (1961) collection of essays under the title, *Nobody Knows My Name: More Notes of a Native Son*, because, as Hood (2017) points out, "it spoke more directly to what I felt after being told there were no early African American evaluators or simply that no one knew of any" (p. 263). The Nobody Knows My Name project was conducted to "retrieve, from near obscurity, the work of early contributors and pioneering African American scholars who have been excluded from what is taught as the history of educational evaluation research in the United States" (Hood, 2017, p. 263). In the sections that follow, we discuss some of the scholars that Hood and colleagues refer to in the *Nobody Knows My Name* project. Borrowing from the title of Shetterly's (2016) book, we refer to these individuals as "hidden figures" in the field.

During the 1930s–1950s, African American scholars used their platform as a vehicle to carry their message of social inequalities and social responsibility to the research and evaluation community, in particular, and society, more generally. While the work of such scholars may not have had an impact on the evaluation theory and practice of their time, their work did "respond to a social agenda that addressed the intentional disentranchement and undereducation of African Americans during the period between *Plessy v. Ferguson*, where the Supreme Court declared the concept of separate but equal legal, and *Brown v. Board of Education*" (Hopson & Hood, 2005, p. 89). Work by these scholars also paved the way for the development, recognition, and use of more culturally responsive approaches to evaluation. Some of these scholars, such as Charles H. Thompson and Reid E. Jackson (both highlighted in this section), received doctoral degrees from elite centers for training in educational research and evaluation such as the University of Chicago and Ohio State. One common thread among such scholars is that they conducted and disseminated research and evaluation studies that offered evidence for the negative impact of racism, inequities, and legal sanctioning of segregation on the life outcomes of African Americans.

As part of our effort to highlight the identified "hidden figures" in this chapter, we included a photo for each.

Ambrose Caliver

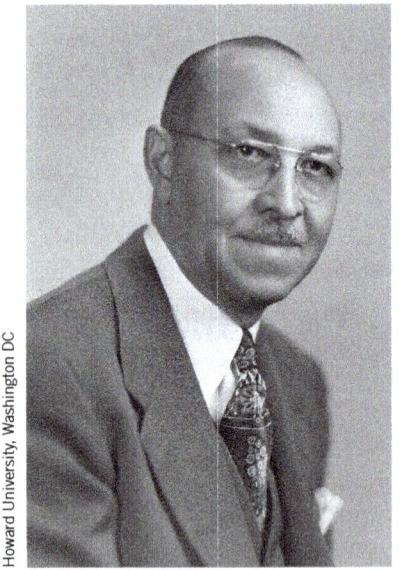

Courtesy of the Moorland-Spingarn Research Center, Howard University Archives, Howard University, Washington DC

Ambrose Caliver was the first African American to earn a PhD (in 1930) in education from Columbia University. He taught at Fisk University, where he also became the university's first African American dean in 1927. In 1930, Caliver was appointed to the new position of Senior Specialist in the Education of Negroes in the U.S. Office of Education by President Herbert Hoover. In 1932, when Franklin D. Roosevelt was elected president, Caliver remained in his post and became a member of Roosevelt's "Black Cabinet," being the first African American to receive a permanent appointment to the federal service on a professional level. Subsequently, Caliver advanced to other positions within the U.S. Office of Education including (a) a 1946 promotion to specialist of Negro higher education, (b) a 1950 promotion to assistant to the commissioner in the Office of Education, and (c) a 1955 promotion to chief of the adult education section. Because this was the first time African Americans had been employed in the Office of Education, Caliver and his staff were objects of curiosity. They were sometimes tolerated, ignored, and rarely accepted (Wilkens, 1962).

Despite systemic racism, during his 32-year tenure in the U.S. Office of Education (1930–1962), Caliver made significant contributions to federal evaluative inquiry of African American education during the pre-*Brown* era. He worked tirelessly to raise national awareness about the inequities and disparities in education between Blacks and whites, especially in the rural South, by traveling extensively throughout the country surveying and documenting the funding failures of public schools.

Perhaps Caliver's most influential works were the national studies that he headed in the 1930s that provided data that illuminated educational inequalities in 20th-century U.S. education. These include the (a) National Survey of Teacher Education, (b) National Survey of Secondary Education, (c) National Survey of the Vocational and

Educational Guidance of Negroes, and (d) National Survey of the Higher Education of Negroes. Further, Caliver compiled the national *Statistics of the Education of Negroes* from 1933 to 1934 and again from 1935 to 1936. Caliver's work is credited with opening the door to systematic inquiry by African American researchers and evaluators (Hopson & Hood, 2005).

Reid E. Jackson

Reid E. Jackson has been identified as "the first bright light of the African American evaluation community" (Hopson & Hood, 2005, p. 90). In 1938, Jackson received his PhD in education from The Ohio State University, being the fourth African American to achieve this status. He held various positions over his career including, for example, secretary of the Southern Negro Conference for Equalization of Educational Opportunities (1944–1946), administrative dean at Wilberforce University (1949), and professor at several Historically Black Colleges and Universities (HBCUs) including Talladega, Alabama State, West Virginia State, Central State, and Morgan State. Hood (2001) identified Jackson as one of the earlier pioneers in educational evaluation, and later, Hopson and Hood (2005) described the significance of Jackson's work as providing "one of the earliest glimpses of culturally responsive evaluative judgments" (p. 96).

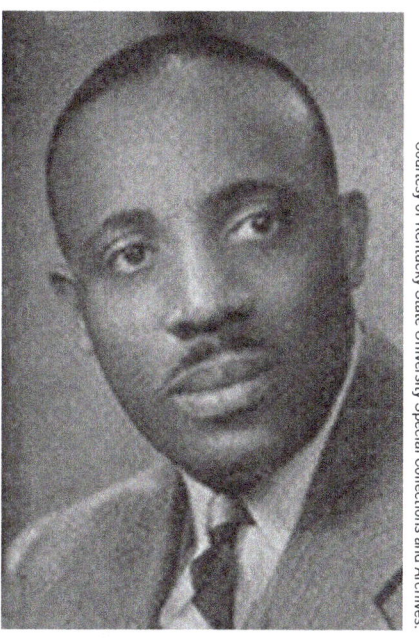

Jackson's evaluations of segregated schooling for African Americans in Kentucky (R. Jackson, 1935), Florida (R. Jackson, 1936), and particularly Alabama (R. Jackson, 1938, 1940a, 1940b) provide concrete examples of an evaluator designing and implementing evaluations where race and culture are central considerations. Between 1935 and 1940, he published 14 scholarly articles focusing on evaluation of secondary schools for African Americans and teacher training programs, both of which he argued should serve as vehicles to further democracy. One of Jackson's conclusions from the evaluation of segregated schooling for African Americans in Kentucky was that the "curricula of the public high school do not adequately meet the demands for a proper vocational preparation of the student" (R. Jackson, 1935, p. 191). Similarly, Jackson (1940b, p. 207) concluded from his evaluation of Alabama segregated schools that "the challenge to secondary education for the Negro in Alabama includes not only preparation for existing vocations but also the development for latent possibilities of the Negro as a contributing factor in a democratic society." From these selected examples, it is clear that Jackson's work provided significant insights to educational evaluations aimed toward social justice ends.

Rose Butler Browne

Rose Butler Browne was the first African American woman to graduate (in 1921) from Rhode Island College (now the University of Rhode Island) and the first African American woman to receive a doctorate in education (in 1939) from Harvard University. She is the first known African American woman to have had an evaluation project as the focus of her dissertation (Hood, 2001) and, as a result, is acknowledged as an early African American female pioneer in evaluation (Frazier-Anderson & Bertrand Jones, 2015). Browne was deeply concerned about African American children's failure

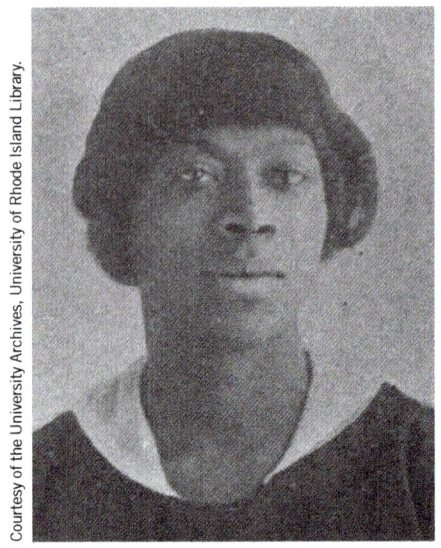

to reach their age norms in reading proficiency. Because of this concern, she evaluated the effectiveness of the Craig Method, which adapted many of the teaching strategies of the Montessori program to the specific needs of children in American culture. Browne believed that the Montessori tools would introduce children living in poverty to materials that supported their development and encouraged their curiosity.

During her career, Browne was on the faculty at various colleges including Virginia State College (Richmond), West Virginia State College (Institute), and Bluefield State College in (Bluefield) West Virginia. As a pioneer for social justice, Browne obtained national publicity when she refused to send students for teaching in West Virginia because the state's board of education was paying African American teachers less than white teachers. The publicity and subsequent shortage of teachers led to a change in the policy. In 1969, Browne coauthored (with James W. English) her autobiography, *Love My Children: The Education of a Teacher*.

Aaron A. Brown

As the third African American to receive a PhD in education from the University of Chicago, Aaron A. Brown, and his work toward social justice ends, places him among the African American scholars who contributed to the educational evaluation literature during the 1940–1960 Tyler years (Hood, 2001). Later in his career, Brown served as president of Albany State College (1943–1954), one of three HBCUs in the university system of Georgia. Eleven years after his presidential installment, Reid was fired by the Board of Regents of the university system because of his involvement in the voter registration drives for Albany's African American citizens. Brown's dissertation (in 1944), "An Evaluation of the Accredited Secondary Schools for Negros in the South," included

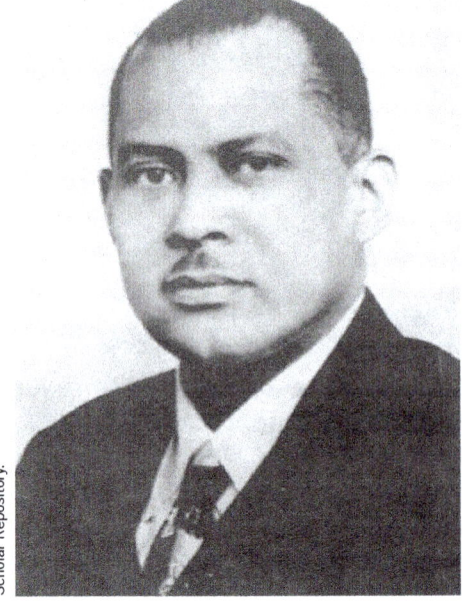

an evaluation of the 93 accredited secondary schools for African Americans living in the South. He sought to find out how well the schools were performing when measured by the best objective criteria available during that time by comparing data on the accredited secondary schools for "Negroes" with normative data on other types of secondary schools.

That in 1931 the Southern Association of Colleges and Schools agreed to accept the responsibility for the accreditation of colleges and secondary schools for African Americans and subsequently supported an evaluation of the school's status was historic. Brown's (1944a; 1944b) dissertation was carried out under the general supervision of Ralph Tyler and others, and it was considered an outstanding contribution that was subsequently published into a book (Brown, 1944c) by the University of Chicago Press. Wright (1945) pointed to an important evaluative question of the time that Brown sought to answer: What is the quality of work being done by these schools, which represent the best among such institutions for Negroes in the Southern region? Brown conducted analysis of his evaluative findings against the backdrop of the socioeconomic setting of schools for African Americans. His evaluation has been hailed as a needed contribution to the literature concerned with providing optimal educational advantages for the African Americans in the country, the majority of whom were living in the South (Wright, 1945). Hood (2005) stressed that, more than 60 years ago,

> Aaron Brown called for cultural responsiveness in educational evaluation but his plea was unheeded. Brown persuasively argued that African Americans had special and critical needs due to their unique experiences in American society. He appropriately raised the question in the 1940s of whether there should be special consideration given when evaluating schools for African Americans. (p. 96)

Leander L. Boykin

Earning a PhD from Stanford University in 1948, Leander L. Boykin became the first African American to achieve this distinction. After postdoctoral work at Harvard University in 1957 and 1958, Boykin served in various positions including, among others, professor of education at Southern University in Baton Rouge, Louisiana, and dean and researcher at Florida A&M University in Tallahassee. Boykin's dissertation and subsequent publication, "Negro Differentials in Education" (1950), was probably one of the most notable and comprehensive evaluative contributions of an African American researcher in the pre-*Brown* era. In this evaluation study, Boykin examined the 17 Southern states, which required completed separation of schools for Black and white populations.[1]

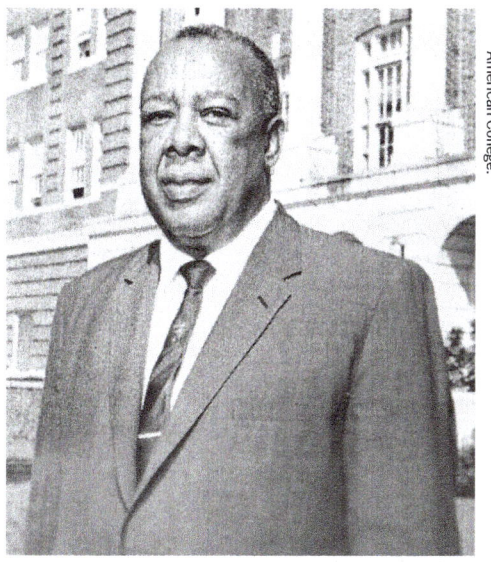

Across his various studies, Boykin (1949, 1950, 1954) evaluated differentials in financial resources, teacher salaries, and interpretation of quantitative data for segregated schools. Interestingly enough, Boykin (1950) indicated that

> in sharp contrast to the usual procedure of evaluating one's findings in terms of practical implications, or attempting to establish a general set of principles, the data and not the findings on differentials in Negro education are evaluated and interpreted. The purpose of evaluating the data rather than the findings is to determine the adequacy of Negro education. By educational adequacy is meant (1) what the state is doing, what activities it is engaging in to provide education for the average child in that state; (2) the educational benefits that the average child of the nation receives as a result of educational activities of the nation; [and] (3) the extent to which Negro education is supported and maintained in terms of ability. (p. 536)

After the *Brown v. Board of Education* decision of 1954, Boykin continued his work. In his 1957 article, "Let's Eliminate the Confusion: What Is Evaluation?," he argued that the ultimate purpose of evaluation is to improve an educational program and offered a set of

---

[1] These 17 states included Alabama, Arkansas, Delaware, Florida, Georgia, Kentucky, Louisiana, Maryland, Mississippi, Missouri, North Carolina, Oklahoma, South Carolina, Tennessee, Texas, Virginia, and West Virginia.

guiding principles, characteristics, and functions of effective evaluation. Boykin (1958) also viewed evaluation as a "group endeavor" or cooperative process involving multiple stakeholders and an endeavor that "strengthens democracy because it is dependent upon the use of democratic procedures for its successful fulfillment" (p. 532).

Furthermore, being somewhat ahead of his time in this respect, Boykin (1958) stressed that a sound program of evaluation requires the use of both quantitative and qualitative data. He used evaluation and evaluative data as a vehicle to argue for equity and social justice during a time in this country when overt racism and legal discrimination were acceptable. Through his work, he concluded that in the future the problem of "Negro" education would be viewed no longer as a race problem or a Southern problem, but as a problem of American democracy in which Negroes are regarded as citizens along with all other Americans (Boykin, 1950, p. 540).

Journal of Negro Education and Founding Editor Charles H. Thompson

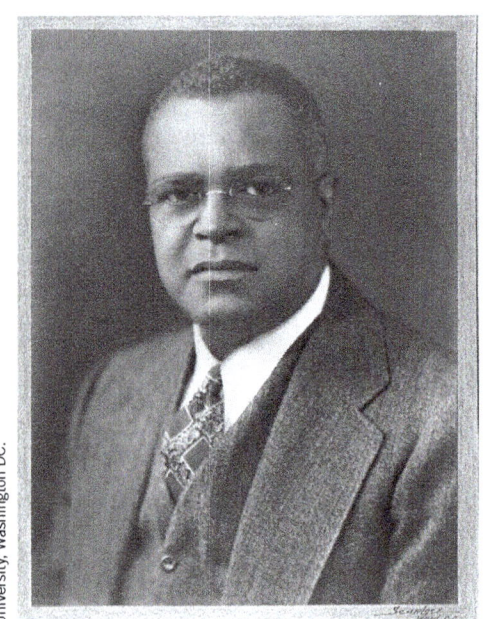

Courtesy of the Moorland-Spingarn Research Center, Howard University Archives Howard University, Washington DC.

The launching of the *Journal of Negro Education* in 1932 was quite significant, and it included important scholarship that was influential and social justice oriented but essentially ignored in the documented evaluation work of the early 20th century. Charles H. Thompson founded the *Journal of Negro Education* as a vehicle for documenting the persistent and substantial problems facing African Americans in this country.

Thompson was the first African American to receive a PhD in educational psychology (in 1925) from the University of Chicago. He joined the faculty at Howard University in 1926 and remained there for the next 40 years in continuous service to the university until his retirement in 1966.

After founding the *Journal of Negro Education* in 1932, Thompson served as its editor-in-chief for 30 years. His passion for policy research and his recognition of its significance in opposing segregation undoubtedly fueled his desire to launch the journal as a means of fully documenting the conditions of "Negro" schools and exploring the implications of segregation. Thompson authored well over 100 scholarly publications and editorials. He served as an expert educational witness in many of the major desegregation cases in the field of higher education argued before the U.S. Supreme Court including the 1950 *Sweatt* case in Texas and the 1948 *Sipuel* case and 1950 *McLaurin* case in Oklahoma. Further, Thompson was a consultant in developing the legal strategies that led to the 1954 *Brown v. Board of Education* decision.

At the time of the *Journal of Negro Education*'s inception, there was no publication that systematically or comprehensively addressed the enormous problems that characterized the education of Blacks in the United States and elsewhere. Mainstream educational journals (e.g., the *Journal of Educational Research*) rarely published articles during the 1930s by African American scholars or studies pertaining to Black education. So, the *Journal of Negro Education* was a response to the urgent and critical need for a scholarly journal that would identify and define the problems, provide a forum for analysis and solutions, and serve as a vehicle for sharing statistics and research on a national basis.

During the 1930s and several decades thereafter, the *Journal of Negro Education* was a primary vehicle for scholars and legal advocates to voice their opposition to segregation and oppression. These included, for example, writings of W. E. B. Du Bois (sociologist, historian, civil rights activist); E. Franklin Frazier (sociologist, author); James Weldon Johnson (poet, novelist, civil rights leader); Alain Locke (philosopher, writer, first African American Rhodes Scholar); Ralph Bunche (scientist, academic); Mamie and Kenneth Clark (psychologists, researchers); and Kelly Miller (mathematician, sociologist, newspaper columnist).

Important research and evaluation work by African American scholars and legal advocates and/or about African Americans that remains largely unread by the white scholarly community found an outlet in the *Journal of Negro Education*. In its very first issue, an evaluation study was published by Mary Crowley (1932), "Cincinnati's Experiment in Negro Education: A Comparative Study of the Segregated and Mixed School." This early study, conducted in 1929–1930, included a methodology using four mixed schools and two segregated schools with groups equated by grade, age, mental age, and intelligence quotient obtained in Binet intelligence tests. At the end of the article, the author poses interesting contextual questions for further consideration including, for example, (a) What are the differences between the curricula and extracurricular activities of "Negro" pupils in segregated and mixed schools? (b) What are the differences between the two types of schools with respect to their interest in community affairs, their cooperation with community leaders, and their influence on the social, moral, and political life of their communities? and (c) What are the cultural influences of the two types of schools (i.e., their influence on the art and the refinement of living)?

See the following feature for examples of evaluation-related publications in the *Journal of Negro Education* prior to the 1954 *Brown v. Board of Education* decision. Readers are encouraged to reflect on and discuss the activity at the end of the listing.

Reflect and Discuss
Pre–*Brown v. Board of Education* (1954) Evaluation Publications in the *Journal of Negro Education*

The following table is a listing of evaluation studies published in the *Journal of Negro Education* between its founding year, 1932, and 1950.

Article Title	Author(s)	Publication Information
Cincinnati's Experiment in Negro Education: A Comparative Study of the Segregated and Mixed School	Mary Crowley	1932, *1*(1), 25–33
Evaluation of Business Curricula in Negro Colleges	V. V. Oak	1938, *7*(1), 19–31
An Evaluation of Educational Opportunities for the Negro Adolescent in Alabama, I	Reid Jackson	1940, *9*(1), 59–72

(Continued)

(Continued)

Article Title	Author(s)	Publication Information
An Evaluation of Educational Opportunities for the Negro Adolescent in Alabama, II	Reid Jackson	1940, *9*(2), 200–207
A Negro College Examines Its Curricula by Measuring Improvement in Reading	Roy R. Davenport	1941, *10*(2), 178–184
An Evaluation of the Accredited Secondary Schools for Negroes in the South	Aaron Brown	1944, *13*(4), 488–498
An Experimental Study of Workshop-Type Professional Education for Negro Teachers	William H. Brown	1945, *14*(1), 48–58
An Evaluation of Industrial Education Programs in Secondary Schools for Negroes in Louisiana	E. C. Harrison	1950, *19*(1), 38–46

Reflect on the works of African American evaluators of color during the pre-*Brown* era and the founding of the *Journal of Negro Education* discussed in the preceding sections. Now, organize into pairs and discuss the potential impact of the omission of such early works on our historical understanding of evaluation and evaluators' role during the early part of the 20th century.

Evaluation in 1960–2000

The 1960s and early 1970s represent the "Golden Age" of evaluation (Rossi & Wright, 1984) with a vision of the federal government being a major patron of large-scale social experimentation. The government passed legislation that required recipients of federal funds to set aside monies for evaluation of program results. In 1978, the federal government passed an act requiring all federal cabinet departments to establish high-level evaluation units, known as Offices of Inspector General, and many agencies had created internal evaluation offices and units (Datta, 2003). During the 1980s, however, there were major reductions in evaluations, especially at the federal level, under the Ronald Reagan administration with budget cutbacks in human services and entitlement programs. By 2000, there was a renewed interest in program evaluation, particularly at the federal level. The sections that follow highlight some of the major legislations, events, and people influencing the evaluation field between 1960 and 2000.

Federal Legislation and Great Society Programs

During the 1960s, under Presidents John F. Kennedy and Lyndon B. Johnson, numerous social programs were initiated aimed at providing for the well-being of the nation's citizens and protecting national prosperity. In response to a (then) national poverty rate of 19%, during his January 1964 State of the Union address, President Johnson announced the War on Poverty/Great Society programs, which included legislation that provided billions of dollars for reforms aimed at eliminating poverty and racial injustice via reducing unemployment, crime, urban deterioration, and inadequate access to medical care and mental health treatment. Systematic evaluation was mandated in several of the most important pieces of Great Society legislation. The Elementary and Secondary Education Act (ESEA) of 1965, for example, was passed as part of the Johnson administration's War on Poverty, and it was designed to improve educational equity for students from lower-income families. This provided, for the first time, federal funds to school districts serving poor students. This legislation mandated that the government evaluate standards for student performance and teacher quality with resources set aside to undertake these activities. Legislative authorization also required evaluation of both the housing allowance program in the U.S. Department of Housing and Urban Development and the U.S. Department of Labor's Comprehensive Employment and Training Act programs (Rossi & Wright, 1984).

Within five years, Johnson's vision included the enactment of nearly 200 pieces of legislation and an unprecedented bold set of programs aimed at improving Americans' everyday lives. Concomitant with the increase in social programs during the 1960s, there was also a rise in the demand to impose accountability requirements in order to determine how the funds were being used and the effects of these programs. As a result of the proliferation of these programs, by the end of the 1960s, evaluation research had become a growth industry (Rossi et al., 2004), and its applications grew substantially beyond government-financed programs and educational settings to other areas such as corporations, faith-based organizations, and foundations.

The Professionalization of the Field

The 1970s, in particular, were an important time in the evolution of evaluation research as an independent branch of study. With this growing independence, evaluation was emerging as an independent profession related to, but quite distinct from, its forebears of research and testing (Madaus & Stufflebeam, 2000). Various activities were taking place in the 1970s and 1980s that characterized evaluation's independence as a profession. These included a growth in evaluation scholarship, the establishment of professional societies in evaluation, development of evaluation standards and codes of conduct, and an increase in graduate training and professional development.

Growth of Evaluation Scholarship

In 1967, the first full-scale description of the application of research methods to evaluation was published in a text, *Evaluative Research: Principles and Practices in Public Service and Social Action Programs*, by Edward Suchman. In the introductory chapter of his book, Suchman says that

> the growing demand for evaluation constitutes the rationale for this report [book]. Unfortunately, the theory and method of evaluative research have lagged far behind the development of the scientific method. . . . Today, as modern man [sic] turns more and more to basic research for his answers to practical problems, a great need exists for the methodological development of evaluative research as a reliable and valid means of testing the degree to which scientific knowledge is being successful put to practical use. (p. 6)

Other notable texts published in the 1970s include Carol H. Weiss's *Evaluation Research: Methods for Assessing Program Effectiveness* (initially published in

1972); Elmer L. Struening and Marcia Guttentag's *Handbook of Evaluation Research* (initially published in 1975); Peter H. Rossi and Howard E. Freeman's *Evaluation: A Systematic Approach* (initially published in 1979); and Michael Q. Patton's *Utilization-Focused Evaluation* (initially published in 1978). These texts are currently still in use, and some have been revised numerous times such as *Evaluation: A Systematic Approach*, now in its eighth edition (Rossi, Lipsey, & Henry, 2019). Additionally, during the 1970s–1980s, various journals dedicated to program evaluation were launched. *Evaluation Review*, published in 1977 by SAGE, became the first journal designed to advance the practice of evaluation and to publish the results of high-quality evaluations. By the end of the 1990s, there were numerous journals dedicated to scholarship-related evaluation theory, methods, practice, and research (see supplemental resources at the end of the chapter).

Establishment of Professional Societies in Evaluation

Two U.S.-based professional societies were formed to foster evaluation as a profession and a science. The Evaluation Research Society was established in 1976 to serve the professional needs of the growing number of people engaged in program evaluation and was composed primarily of academic and quantitative researchers. The Evaluation Network, also founded in 1976, consisted mostly of practitioners (e.g., school-based evaluators) who were more interested in conducting evaluations than concerned about theory and methods issues. As indicated in Table 3.2, in 1986, the Evaluation Research Society and Evaluation Network merged to form the AEA. The association currently has over 7,000 members representing all 50 states in the United States as well as over 80 foreign countries (www.eval.org).

Graduate Training and Professional Development in Evaluation

In the 1960s, there was only a paucity of well-trained evaluation specialists with broad training or experience. With the increasing demands for accountability and documentation of the effectiveness of government-financed programs, there was a need for more skilled evaluators to complete this work. By the mid-1970s, evaluation was recognized as a legitimate professional field that possessed its own core of knowledge, specialized concepts, methods of inquiry, and particular strategies that could be taught in graduate-level courses. To address the void in evaluation training, in the 1980s, graduate-level evaluation specializations and/or courses were flourishing and being taught in many university departments such as education, psychology, public policy, sociology, and health administration. In addition to graduate courses in evaluation, there were increased opportunities for professional development to enhance practicing evaluators' knowledge and skills.

Establishment of Standards and Codes of Conduct

Another indicator of the growth and professionalization of a field is the development of standards, guiding principles, and codes of conduct for individuals engaged in the profession. By the end of the 1960s, program developers, sponsors, and evaluators recognized the need for rigorous standards to guide program evaluation. In 1974, representatives from three national professional associations joined together to form the Joint Committee on Standards for Educational Evaluation. The committee developed and disseminated three sets of standards including the *Program Evaluation*

Standards, the *Personnel Evaluation Standards*, and the *Student Evaluation Standards*. In 1994, the membership of the AEA Board approved the *Guiding Principles for Evaluators* intended to be a guide to the professional ethical conduct of evaluators. (The *Program Evaluation Standards* and the *Evaluators' Ethical Guiding Principles*, a later version of the *Guiding Principles for Evaluators*, were discussed in greater detail in Chapter 2.)

Methodological Approaches and Paradigm Wars

Evaluation in the 1960s and 1970s was undoubtedly a quantitative enterprise. During the 1960s and 1970s, new developments in techniques and methodologies appeared that promised to raise the overall quality of evaluations. Perhaps the most impressive and substantial achievements during this time were those of large-scale field experiments. Each of the country's major federal departments that operated social programs had at least one large-scale field experiment taking place during the 1970s, including, for example, (a) housing allowance experiments (U.S. Department of Housing and Urban Development); (b) experiments on transitional aid to release prisoners and on supported work (U.S. Department of Labor); and (c) enhanced police patrolling (U.S. Department of Justice) (cited in Rossi & Wright, 1984).

Leaders in the field at that time, such as Donald T. Campbell, Peter H. Rossi, and Carol H. Weiss, generally argued for evaluation to take advantage of the methods of research and analysis being utilized in the most prestigious domains (mostly **quantitative methods**) of social science such as psychology and sociology. As stated earlier in this chapter, Suchman (1967) published one of the earliest textbooks in evaluation, *Evaluative Research: Principles and Practices in Public Service and Social Action Programs*, which also placed emphasis on use of the experimental design (discussed in greater detail in Chapter 11).

In evaluation, like other social and behavioral science fields, during the 1970s and 1980s the dominant use of quantitative methods came under attack as part of the **paradigm wars**. There was increasing recognition that while experimental design may work in small-scale evaluation studies, it is more "difficult" or "unworkable" in the context of large-scale social and educational programs, resulting, in part, in findings showing program failure (Brandon & Sam, 2014). The 1978 meeting of the Evaluation Research Society devoted substantial program time to consideration of **qualitative methods** (Patton, 1980). With the initial publication of *Qualitative Evaluation Methods,* Michael Quinn Patton (1980) provided evaluators with a reference for expanding their methodological approaches to include qualitative methods. In his book, Patton argues that

> the issue of selecting methods is no longer one of the dominant paradigm versus the alternative paradigm of experimental designs with quantitative measurement versus holistic-inductive design based on qualitative measurement. The debate and competition between paradigms [are] being replaced by a new paradigm—*a paradigm of choices*. The paradigm of choices recognizes that different methods are appropriate for different situations. (p. 20)

By the mid-1980s, the evaluation literature was beginning to reflect the potential value of integrating quantitative and qualitative methods for the purposes of both **triangulation** (L. Smith & Kliene, 1986) and enhancing the rigor and credibility of evaluations (Silverman, Ricci, & Gunter, 1990).

Two Influential Scholars' Contributions to Methodological Approaches of the 1960s–1970s

Many scholars contributed to discourse on evaluation methodologies in the 1960s and 1970s. In the sections that follow, we focus on probably the two most prominent individuals of the time: Donald T. Campbell and Lee J. Cronbach. They are among the most influential figures who first advocated different methodological views of evaluation methods in their writings.

Donald T. Campbell. Shadish and Luellen (2004) refer to Donald T. Campbell as the "accidental evaluator" given his central importance in the field of evaluation. While Campbell did not start out intending to be an evaluator, his dedication to understanding causality behavior and how to solve social questions led him to this field. The evaluation field came to embrace Campbell's works, including "Reforms as Experiments" (1969) and *Experimental and Quasi-Experimental Designs for Research* (D. Campbell & Stanley, 1963), which were probably his most influential writings on evaluation methods (Rossi et al., 2004; Shadish & Epstein, 1987). According to Campbell (1994), "Reforms as Experiments" was his first publication targeting a program evaluation agenda. Campbell and Stanley's (1963) work on research designs created an entirely new vocabulary for the taxonomy of research designs and illuminating validity issues (Rossi & Wright, 1984). Campbell introduced issues that made their way into thinking about evaluation findings. As is covered in detail in Chapter 11, these include concepts such as internal validity, external validity, and threats to validity. Campbell's work was instrumental in making the randomized controlled trials (or designs), with their emphasis on **net effects**, the design of choice in program evaluations throughout the 1970s and 1980s. It is worth noting that Campbell and Stanley did put forth the quasi-experimental design option when that was all the situation allowed, thus allowing evaluators and other researchers to test hypotheses in less-than-ideal field settings.

Numerous scholars and practitioners have challenged Campbell's "experimenting society" approach that called for use of experimental methods in evaluation. The major points of contention and conclusions, as summarized by Shadish and Luellen (2004), are that

> experimental methods were insufficient to address social problems in a world where policy practice is entangled with politics, economy, and social pressures; questioned the importance of noncausal questions and nonexperimental methods; complained that experimentally based knowledge was not fully implemented in solving social problems; and pointed out limitations of experimental methods. Eventually, the field of evaluation rejected Campbell's Experimenting Society as too narrow and Utopian, preferring a broader vision of the role of evaluation. Even so, because bias remains a central problem for evaluation, the solutions Campbell offered will be his greatest legacy. (pp. 82–83)

Lee J. Cronbach The work of Lee J. Cronbach also was influential in evaluation and a contrast to the approach of Donald T. Campbell. As early as 1963, Cronbach challenged the evaluation community and pointed out that the current level of evaluation practice was wholly inadequate to meet the needs of the newly developed, federally sponsored curriculum reforms (O'Sullivan, 2004). He was skeptical of the view of evaluation as sterile, detached, objective scientific activities.

Cronbach did not champion a particular methodology for evaluation, and he valued methodological pluralism in evaluation centered on "better understanding society's enduring social problems and the ways in which the specific policy and program being evaluated are meaningfully addressing one such problem" (Greene, 2004, p. 172). Cronbach's work emphasized the limitations of randomized field trials, the importance of local contexts on performance, and the social and political aspects of program evaluation. As such, he focused not on the technical aspect of measurement in evaluation, but on the policy-oriented nature of evaluation. Cronbach's evaluation research influenced program evaluations across various fields such as health and criminal justice reform, from health programs to juvenile delinquency programs. Cronbach coauthored two influential books in the evaluation field: *Toward Reform of Program Evaluation* (1980), which was written by a team of consortium faculty led by Cronbach, and a parallel volume, *Designing Evaluations of Educational and Social Programs* (1982).

Rethinking the Role of Evaluation

The proliferation of ambitious new social programs beginning with the Great Society initiative in the 1960s begged the important questions "Does this program work?" and "Does this program work better than something or nothing?" Many believed that requiring evaluation of initiatives would help build a body of knowledge regarding which policy ideas and programs are effective. The Perry Preschool Project, a high-quality preschool program for African American children from disadvantaged backgrounds carried out from 1962 to 1967, has been characterized as a social program that worked based on evidence from experimental evaluation design. The following activity invites students to reflect on and discuss an evaluation of the Perry Preschool Project.

Reflect and Discuss
The Perry Preschool Project

Read the following description of an evaluation of the Perry Preschool Project. Then answer the questions that follow.

Program Description: A high-quality preschool program for children from disadvantaged backgrounds, the Perry Preschool Project was conducted from 1962 to 1967 but led to a longitudinal study.

Evaluation Purpose: The Perry Preschool Project evaluation sought to determine whether access to high-quality education could have a positive impact on preschool children and the communities where they live.

Methodology: The Perry Preschool Project was a small, but well-conducted, randomized controlled trial with a sample of 128 three- and four-year-old African American children living in poverty and assessed to be at high risk of school failure.

(Continued)

(Continued)

The preschool children were randomly divided into two groups: One group entered a high-quality preschool program, and a comparison group received no preschool education. Investigators continued to follow the Perry Preschool Project participants throughout their lives in this landmark study.

Selected Key Findings: Evaluation results yielded large effects on educational attainment, income, criminal activity, and other important life outcomes, sustained well into adulthood.

At age 27, the participants who experienced the preschool program

- completed an average of almost 1 full year more of schooling (11.9 years vs. 11 years);
- spent an average of 1.3 fewer years in special education services—for example, for mental, emotional, speech, or learning impairment (3.9 years vs. 5.2 years); and
- had a 44% higher high school graduation rate (65% vs. 45%).

At age 40, the participants who experienced the preschool program

- had fewer teenage pregnancies;
- were more likely to have graduated from high school;
- were more likely to hold a job and have higher earnings;
- had committed fewer crimes; and
- were more likely to own their own home and car.

Source: Adapted from https://highscope.org/perry-preschool-project/

Brainstorming Questions

1. What social, political, economic, and racial issues were happening in the country that might have influenced the conceptualization, design, and outcome of the evaluation?
2. If you were the evaluator of this project in 1969, what would be the top two historical factors that you would consider during your work? Why?

Unfortunately, evaluation findings from many other high-profile social programs yielded dismal measurable results. This resulted in some rethinking of evaluation and its purpose, methodologies, and problems. Edwards, Guttentag, and Snapper (1975) offer what they refer to as five complaints about folkways of evaluation research that were the prevailing sentiment of the time and resulted in more rethinking of evaluation's purpose and methodology. These include reification of programs; insistence on causal inference; conducting pseudo-experiments; planning the formative, then summative, evaluation in a stage-by-stage sequence; and a baseball statistical approach to handling lots of data. Table 3.3 elaborates on their complaints.

Despite some successes, one of the most important lessons to be learned from all the evaluations initiated during the 1960s and 1970s was the difficulty in carrying out randomized controlled experimental designs in field settings. Due, in large part, to the dismal findings from large-scale randomized controlled trial evaluation studies

Table 3.3 Five Complaints About Evaluation Research in the 1970s

Complaints	Description
Reification of programs	Programs are thought to be fixed and unchanging objects, which can be observed in various times and places
Insistence on causal inference	Evaluations that insist that if "why" (e.g., why are some people prone to criminal acts?) cannot be answered, then "what" (e.g., what would reduce criminal acts of certain people?) should not be asked
Pseudo-experiments	Researchers attempt to use control groups that are not comparable, or insist that the program studied remain invariant while data about it are being collected
Planning vs. formative vs. summative evaluation	The assumption that programs develop in a stage-by-stage sequence and should be evaluated accordingly. Thus, one evaluates the planning stage, evaluates the monitoring apparatus, and then does a final evaluation of whether stated goals or objectives have been reached
Baseball statistician's approach	Researchers engage in the gathering and reporting of voluminous amounts of data that describe the program's operation in a manner analogous to the box scores of baseball games

Source: Edwards, Guttentag, & Snapper (1975).

of the late 1960s through the end of the 1970s, many evaluators became disheartened with the traditional approaches to evaluation. In fact, a reasonable summary of the large-scale field experimental evaluation findings of the 1960s and 1970s is that the expected value of the effect of any program hovered around zero (Rossi & Wright, 1984). Of course, such a conclusion was quite disheartening to the social reformers who had hoped that the Great Society programs would result in significant improvements in the lives of poor people and marginalized communities. Given this reality, evaluators had to contend with two possibilities: (a) that the implementation of social programs of the day truly had little to no impact on the intended outcomes for their participants, or (b) that the existing evaluation models and methods being used were inadequate to capture the outcomes of interest.

With the evaluation challenges of the 1970s and 1980s, there were increasing concerns among evaluators, particularly around how evaluation was viewed and its methodology. L. Ross and Cronbach (1976), for example, emphasized moving away from the mainstream view of evaluation that characterizes evaluation as an event that begins, runs alongside a program for a time as the evaluator makes observations and collects data, and ends rather abruptly with a report to an all-powerful decision maker (usually someone outside the program under consideration). In this mainstream view, the evaluator, essentially, enters the picture only after the initial events in the life of the program have begun. Instead, they argued for a better approach to evaluation, whereby evaluation becomes a component of the evolving program itself rather than simply providing "disinterested monitoring undertaken to provide ammunition to the warring factions in a political struggle" (L. Ross & Cronbach, 1976, pp. 18–19).

Influential Women in Evaluation: 1970s–1990s

Since the 1970s, numerous (mostly white) women have contributed to evaluation scholarship and practice. Based on our review of the AEA's listing of past presidents, from its founding in 1986 through 2020, the association, unlike many other professional organizations in this country, had about equal proportion of men and women presidents (i.e., 17 female presidents and 18 male presidents). So, women certainly have been represented in the leadership of the discipline's major professional association.

In the section that follows, we focus on some of the women that made significant contributions in evaluation between the 1970s and the early 1990s. In particular, we highlight the contributions of seven women who contributed directly to evaluation theory, method, policy, and/or practice through their work in academia, government, and evaluation practice communities. We highlight Carol H. Weiss, Yvonna S. Lincoln, Eleanor Chelimsky, Lois-Ellin Datta, Floraline I. Stevens, Laura Leviton, and Beatriz Chu Clewell. Similar to the earlier section on "hidden figures," we also included a photo of each woman featured in this section.

Carol H. Weiss

Carol H. Weiss was probably the most prominent female evaluation theorist and practitioner of her time. In the mid-1960s, Weiss evaluated a Harlem-based training project as part of President Johnson's War on Poverty. This yielded invaluable lessons that Weiss later disseminated through her scholarship. Her 1972 book, *Evaluation Research: Methods for Assessing Program Effectiveness*, provided an in-depth analysis of many of the crucial and complex issues that plague evaluators and public managers. While many of the criticisms of the time focused on methodological inadequacies, Weiss (1986) also pointed to issues related to the lack of fit between evaluation and the sociopolitical context of the program world. She noted that

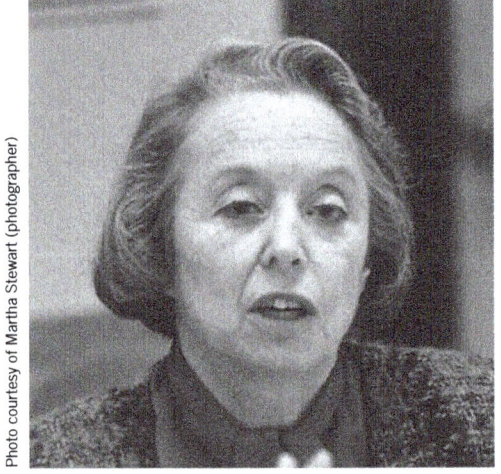

Photo courtesy of Martha Stewart (photographer)

> evaluation is narrow because it focuses on only a small set of questions of importance to program people; unrealistic because it measures the success of programs against unreasonably high standards; irrelevant because it provides answers to questions that no one really cares about; unfair because it is responsive to the concerns of influential people, such as bureaucratic sponsors, but blind to the wants of others lower in the hierarchy, such as front-line staff and clients; and unused in councils of action where discussions are made. (p. 149)

Weiss (1993) called for a reconceptualization of the purpose of evaluation from simply judging program merit and worth, to also generating reliable knowledge that could guide improvement. She also stressed the need for evaluators to gain a better understanding of the political context and its influence on their work:

> Now I have more understanding how difficult it is to bring about improvement in long-standing stubborn problems, like poverty and violence. The experience of the 1960s and 1970s showed us that even under relatively favorable

conditions, progress was slow and uneven. To change social conditions in the swift, massive fashion that we yearned for was much harder than we expected. I have come to have more respect for the incremental changes that evaluation helps to bring about. If evaluation contributes to making small continuing improvements in current policy, as I think it does, this is no small beans. It is well worth our time and effort. (Weiss, 1993, p. 109)

Probably Weiss's major contribution to the historical evolution of evaluation is her sustained effort to push the field toward better recognition of programs as not neutral, antiseptic, laboratory-type entities but instead as entities that emerge from the "rough and tumble" of political support, opposition, and bargaining—attached to which are the reputations of legislative persons, the careers of administrators, the jobs of program staff, and the expectations of clients. Even rigorously documented evidence of outcomes, Weiss (1993) adds, may not outweigh all other interests and concerns, and only with sensitivity to the politics of evaluation research can evaluators be as creative and strategic as they can be. Insights from Weiss's 11 published books and more than 100 articles continue to shape how evaluators think about theory and practice evaluation.

Yvonna S. Lincoln

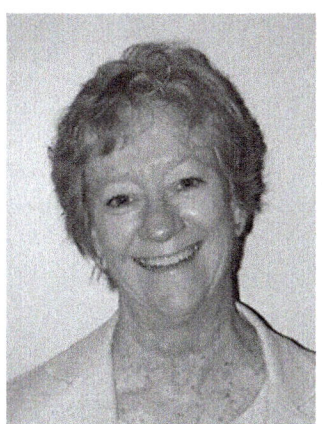

Yvonna S. Lincoln, the first female president of the AEA, is probably best known in social science research, more generally, and evaluation, in particular, for her contribution to qualitative methodology. Lincoln, often in collaboration with her husband, Egon Guba, championed a constructivist, qualitative approach to understanding human phenomena. Their publications, *Naturalistic Inquiry* (Guba & Lincoln, 1985) and *Fourth Generation Evaluation* (Guba & Lincoln, 1989), especially the latter book, were written, in part, to address what they believe to be the inadequacies of previous evaluation methodologies. In *Fourth Generation Evaluation*, the authors point out that it was their intention to define an emergent, but mature, approach to evaluation that goes beyond mere science, or just getting the facts, to include the myriad human, political, social, cultural, and contextual elements involved (Guba & Lincoln, 1989, p. 8).

A major contribution that Lincoln made to the evaluation field during the 1980s and 1990s was to highlight the limitation of the field in its focus primarily on methods (i.e., how we come to know something) and rigor (i.e., how much trust we have in what we know). In her 1990 AEA presidential address, Lincoln (1991) focused on aspects of science that the profession had failed to notice, including the science of locating interested stakeholders; the science of getting information—good, usable information—to those same stakeholders; the science of teaching various stakeholder groups how to use information to empower themselves so they can participate more fully in democratic life and in decision making; and the science of communicating results. She moved the field beyond thinking only of the "sciences of evaluation" (i.e., methods and rigor) to also thinking more seriously about the "arts of evaluation" (summarized in Lincoln, 1991, pp. 4–6). Aspects of the arts of evaluation that Lincoln focused on in much of her work, and something she urged the evaluation community to consider, include

- *judgment*—for evaluators to be able not only to render their own judgments in such a way that they can back them up, but also to elicit the judgments of stakeholders such that both evaluators and stakeholders are clear about the values, belief systems, and community mores undergirding those judgments;

- *appreciation*—cultivating the art of appreciating in both evaluators and stakeholders and comprehending meaning within context, understanding the social and cultural milieu from which a program draws its particular expression, and seeing something fully and in its wholeness;
- *cultural analysis*—paying attention to rituals, symbols, and meanings that coalesce when groups of people are engaged in a common pursuit;
- *"hearing secret harmonies"*—or learning to listen for the meanings and not just searching for the one-to-one correspondence between objectives and their achievement; and
- *dealing with people very different from ourselves*—for evaluators to get out on the front lines more, to rely on stakeholders who want to speak for themselves, to give voice to those who cannot be heard, and to see those who have been invisible.

Lincoln is the author or coauthor of more than 100 chapters and journal articles on aspects of higher education or qualitative research methods and methodologies. Her contributions to the field of evaluation continue and have provided insight for some more contemporary approaches such as transformative evaluation (see Chapter 5) and culturally responsive evaluation.

Eleanor Chelimsky

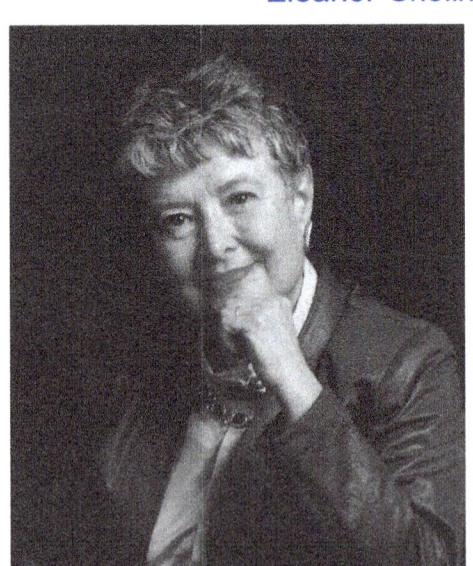

Eleanor Chelimsky has been described as a guiding light in the field of evaluation since its inception as a profession, with several decades of experience conducting evaluations of government policies and programs, developing methodologies to respond to complex questions meaningfully, and transferring her knowledge to the evaluation community at large both domestically and internationally (Oral History Project Team, 2009). From 1966 to 1970, she was an economic analyst for the U.S. Mission to NATO, charged with statistical, demographic, and cost-benefit studies. Subsequently, from 1970 to 1980, she worked at MITRE Corporation, where she directed work in evaluation planning and policy analysis, criminal justice, and research management. Between 1980 and 1994, Chelimsky directed the Program Evaluation and Methodology Division of the U.S. GAO whose mission was to serve Congress through evaluations of government policies and programs and through the development and demonstration of methods for evaluating those policies. Chelimsky's influence on evaluation, particularly at the federal level, has been enormous. In her position at the GAO, she pioneered the use of meta-analysis as a tool for providing program evaluation and other legislatively significant advice to Congress (Chelimsky, 1994). Chelimsky received many awards for her work, including the GAO's top honor, "the Comptroller General's Award," for contributions in developing innovative approaches to evaluate the effects of government programs and fostering their use by the GAO and other decision makers in the United States and abroad.

Chelimsky has been a leader in the evaluation profession serving as president of the Evaluation Research Society in 1980 and of the AEA in 1995. She has been credited with producing nearly 300 evaluations of government policies and programs for Congress, as well as developing and demonstrating new methods for evaluation. In response to a question about evaluation's future, Chelimsky responded that she would stress two things:

> We [first] should not be producing so many "johnny-one-notes," . . . evaluators who show up for work knowing only one methodology (usually survey research or the randomized field experiment). . . . [E]valuators need to know how economists, engineers, and political scientists . . . deal with evaluation questions in their different disciplines. . . .
>
> [Second] I would stress the study of context. . . . [S]o long as we try to force-fit evaluative ideas into political or social milieux without understanding those milieux we'll never get them in. . . . [W]e need to understand bureaucracy if we want government to listen to us, we need to understand other evaluative professions both to borrow their methods and let them borrow ours. . . . Evaluation really has to fit in . . . and we must find partners, even though speaking truth to power is not calculated to bring us advocates. Perhaps the best way to do this is by avoiding zealotry, whether about methods or anything else. . . . If we can remember that there is no such thing as perfection, I think we'll survive, find allies, flourish, and do an amazing job in helping to make government more transparent, more effective, and more publicly accountable. (Oral History Project Team, 2009, p. 244)

Floraline I. Stevens

Floraline I. Stevens served as the director of the Research and Evaluation branch of the Los Angeles Unified School District (LAUSD) from 1979 to 1994. She was also a senior research fellow for the National Center for Education Statistics (NCES) in Washington, DC (1991–1992), and a program director for the National Science Foundation (NSF) in the Education and Human Resources Directorate (1992–1994). While at NSF on an interagency personnel assignment from the LAUSD, Stevens conceived the idea for the NSF's seminal publication, *User-Friendly Handbook for Project Evaluation: Science, Mathematics, Engineering, and Technology Education*. This handbook was developed to provide principal investigators and project evaluators with a basic understanding of selected approaches to evaluation. Further, the handbook 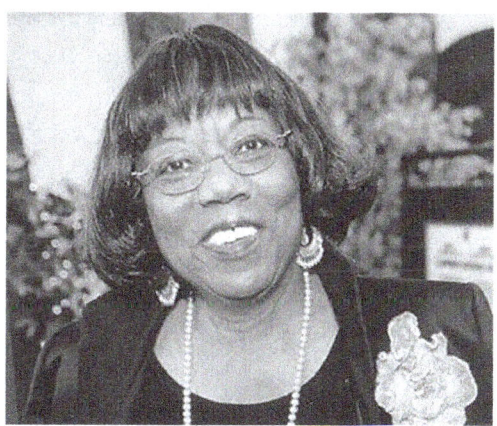 builds on firmly established principles, blending technical knowledge and common sense to meet the special needs of NSF programs and projects. This handbook has been updated several times and is still currently in use.

Stevens (2000) indicated that she became an evaluator in 1965 when the Elementary and Secondary Education Act (ESEA, now referred to as the Every Student Succeeds Act, or ESSA) Title I legislation was enacted and federally funded education programs were being implemented in the LAUSD:

[T]here were no evaluation types in the school district. However, in response to the federal guidelines, the school district recruited a cadre of persons who had training in counseling because of their coursework in test and measurement, statistics, and research design. . . . We knew nothing about evaluation theories and evaluation procedures. (p. 42).

Stevens described how she and her colleagues overcame difficulties attendant to being responsive to culture during an evaluation project in this large, diverse metropolitan school district, noting that their extensive knowledge of the culture in the classroom and cultural background of the students helped them overcome difficulties in collecting accurate data in the schools where the ESEA Title I programs were operating. She said she (and her colleagues of color) knew how to gain access to people and information in schools, a critical element in evaluation. But equally important, Stevens indicated that she knew when the information provided did not make sense.

It was from those early experiences that Stevens later became an evaluator of her first science education project, an ESEA Title III, K–12 ecology- and biology-focused project. Subsequently, she evaluated many K–12 science education and science-focused programs. As the director of the Research and Evaluation branch of the LAUSD, Stevens developed ongoing programs of professional development to assist the evaluation staff to become better qualified. She played a significant role in focusing attention to issues of race, culture, and context in program evaluation. In situations where programs involved ethnically diverse participants and stakeholders, Stevens (2000) called for the creation of multiethnic evaluation teams to increase the chances of really hearing the voices of underrepresented students. Stevens was also a major champion of evaluation capacity building, especially in relation to increasing the number of minorities in the evaluation field. In the 1990s, she argued that the NSF should step forward to train minority evaluators of science and technology projects.

When Stevens retired from the LAUSD in 1994, she formed Stevens and Associates, an independent evaluation and research consulting firm. Her early work and involvement with various NSF minority capacity-building efforts had a visible impact on the developing scholarship related to culturally responsive evaluation.

Lois-Ellin Datta

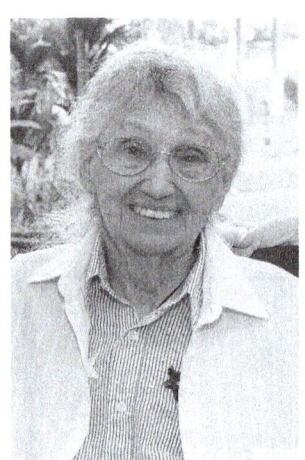

For decades, Lois-Ellin Datta has been a leading evaluation researcher and international consultant. Datta also served in many other roles during the course of her distinguished career in government, working 30 years in Washington, DC. For example, she was director of program evaluation in the human services area at the U.S. GAO's Program Evaluation and Methodology Division and director for teaching, learning, and assessment at the U.S. Department of Education's National Institute of Education. Over the years, Datta has also done work with the Maori in New Zealand and with Native Hawaiians.

In the 1960s, Datta served as the national director of evaluation for Project Head Start and the U.S. Children's Bureau. Some years later while reflecting on that time, Datta (2018a) noted that Head Start's immediate popularity was overwhelming and that increased the stakes for evaluation, while also pointing to the program's obvious face validity and demand validity. For her, a major takeaway from those pioneering evaluation days was the importance of mixed methods, multiple approaches, and diverse designs and analyses to address the complexities and multiple dimensions of a major program like Head Start. This is a position that she has urged for the field. Datta (2018b) has stated that

> In the years and evaluations that followed [after Head Start] every study was a new opportunity to think through what approaches seemed good fits with the contexts, complexities, evaluation questions, stakeholders, demining, costs, and, yes, new ideas to try out. (p. 20)

Datta's numerous contributions to the field of evaluation include serving as editor-in-chief of *New Directions for Evaluation* and serving on the editorial boards of the *American Journal of Evaluation*, the *Encyclopedia of Evaluation*, and the *International Handbook of Educational Evaluation*, among others, and her publications have significantly advanced thinking and practice in evaluation particularly in the areas of case study methodology, evaluations in nontraditional settings, and mixed-methods evaluation approaches (Oral History Project Team, 2004). The author of numerous books and over 100 articles about evaluation, she has always been keenly focused on achieving social justice and mindful of the importance of policy.

Laura Leviton

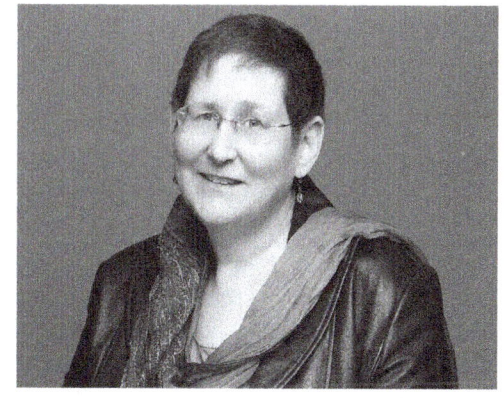

Laura Leviton is the coauthor of *Foundations of Program Evaluation* (Shadish, Cook, & Leviton, 1991). This was one of the first comprehensive assessments of evaluation theories providing both insightful analysis of the current state of evaluation theory and suggestions for improving evaluation practice. From 1999 to 2017, Leviton served as special advisor for evaluation at the Robert Wood Johnson Foundation, an organization that seeks to improve the health and health care of all Americans. This position was created for Leviton at the foundation to advise and consult on evaluations across its many initiatives and national programs. In this position, Leviton describes her role as striving to represent the quality and consistency of the foundation's research and evaluation and its impact on health and health care nationwide. During her time at the foundation, since 1999, Leviton has overseen more than 80 national and local evaluations. She is interested in all aspects of evaluation methodology and practice. Leviton has been recognized as a leader in the field of evaluating community health promotions (Francisco, Butterfoss, & Capwell, 2001). She collaborated on the first randomized experiment on HIV prevention, and later on two large place-based randomized controlled experiments on improving medical practices.

In an interview conducted by Francisco et al. (2001), Leviton provided an interesting (and still timely) insight that about evaluation:

> Regarding evaluation, I learned how incredibly important it is to take culture into account. When I was in Pennsylvania, we had a project in the central mountain region of the state, and we all thought we understood their Appalachian culture. We found out quickly that we were quite wrong. One should never assume that one knows enough about this. Go into the situation with an open mind and learn what you can from the community. Secondly, I also

learned how important it is to remain flexible about evaluation methods. We really need to have the questions drive the methods we use, and not vice versa. (p. 204)

Leviton was president of the AEA in the year 2000. She has been a scholar on evaluation methods and practice, particularly in the area of disease prevention, publishing over 100 articles and books and providing oversight on more than 100 evaluations.

Beatriz Chu Clewell

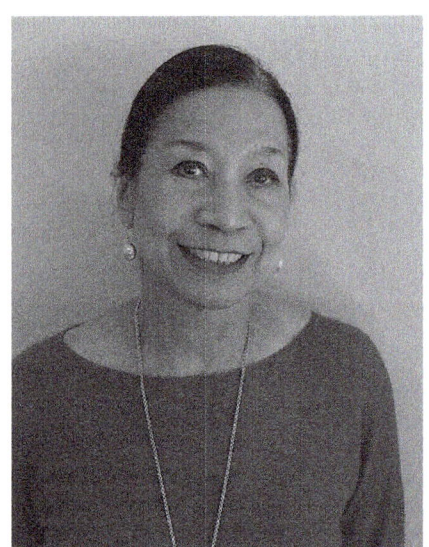

Beatriz Chu Clewell has been involved in evaluation practice over several decades. Much of her work has focused on breaking barriers and moving more women and underrepresented minorities into the technology and science workforce. While Clewell may not be well known in the academic evaluation community, she is very well known in the NSF, STEM (science, technology, engineering, and mathematics), and evaluation practice communities. Clewell spent over 20 years conducting research on the access of underrepresented groups—specifically, racial/ethnic minorities and women—to science, mathematics, and engineering fields. She was a principal research associate at the Urban Institute, from 1994 to 2008, where she directed the Evaluation Studies and Equity Research Program in the Education Policy Center and led several large-scale research projects and program evaluations.

Clewell has conducted a number of evaluations of teacher recruitment programs, including the Pathways to Teaching Careers Program, for which data on 42 programs and close to 3,000 participants over a six-year period were collected. The aim of many of these evaluations was to identify the policies and practices that characterize schools where all students achieve. She has also conducted multiple evaluations of national programs to increase the participation of women and underrepresented minorities in STEM.

Further, Clewell led an analysis of data to determine the effect of teacher race/ethnicity on student achievement in mathematics and reading, an evaluation of the NSF's Louis Stokes Alliances for Minority Participation (LSAMP) program involving 27 alliances of approximately 200 institutions nationwide. The aim of many of Clewell's evaluations was to identify policies and practices that inhibited or encouraged access of women and minorities to fields where they were underrepresented. Her impact on the STEM evaluation community is immense.

Influential 20th-Century Evaluator: An Activity

The previous sections highlighted a few of the prominent evaluators of the 20th century, particularly those doing important work from the 1940s to the late 1990s. The following activity gives readers an opportunity to research an influential 20th-century evaluator and learn more about his or her life, professional experiences, and contributions to the field.

Activity
Research an Influential Person or Event

Organize into groups of two or three and work toward giving a 10- to 15-minute presentation on a historical event or influential figure in evaluation during the 20th century. First, identify an influential person or event relevant to the evolution of program evaluation. Provide a biographical sketch of the person or an overview of the event, identifying key contributions that were added to the evaluation field. Among the contributions discussed, which does your group feel are the most significant, and why?

Discuss what you learned during your inquiry. Why was this person or event important to evaluation practice, scholarship, and/or society? Finally, consider the implications of these contributions in today's context.

21st-Century Evaluation: Expanding the Focus

At the start of the 21st century, evaluation was in a boom period with increasing diversity in theoretical and methodological options available to evaluators. Stufflebeam and Coryn (2014, p. 39) referred to the period of 2005–2014 as the "age of global and multidisciplinary expansion" with several characteristics: (a) over 50 professional evaluation societies throughout the world, (b) a growing evaluation profession encompassing a wide range of disciplines and evaluators from various disciplinary perspectives and backgrounds who are increasingly exchanging information, (c) studying in interdisciplinary degree programs, (c) more collaboration on evaluation projects and publications, and (d) meeting together in broadly focused evaluation conventions and meetings. With Congress under increased pressure to balance the federal budget, new calls for accountability resulted in an escalating demand on social programs to demonstrate their worth. Evaluation in the 21st century can be described, in part, as a profession and practice influenced by the strengthened legislation for evaluation at the federal level; expansion of evaluation approaches, paradigms, and methodologies; and increased emphasis on social justice and diversity.

The new millennium began with a vision of (large- and small-scale) evaluations taking place in a wide range of settings with more diverse evaluators (or evaluation teams) than in earlier decades. There was greater buy-in across various audiences of the value of evaluation, in part, due to the increasing demand of funders for evidence of program process and outcomes. There were also calls for evaluation to more accurately represent the voices of the less powerful and marginalized in an increasingly diverse society and a changing political and policy context. There was an expansion of capacity-building efforts, particularly in relation to increasing the pipeline for more ethnically diverse evaluators. The 21st century also began with greater respect for methodological diversity—that is, being more inclusive in the types of methods and approaches needed to establish rigor and credibility. There was increased focus on expanding evaluation use and limiting misuse. These, and other issues, are discussed in the following sections.

Table 3.4 highlights some key evaluation-related events and people of the 21st century. Similar to Table 3.2 reflecting significant issues in the 20th century, Table 3.4 also includes events and people not limited to specific evaluation studies or evaluators, per se, but highlights specific individuals and activities that contribute to the current thinking in evaluation scholarship, methodology, and practice.

Table 3.4 Key Events in the Evolution of Program Evaluation During the 21st Century

Time Period	Significant Evaluation-Related Events
2000s	Debates in the field intensified regarding using randomized controlled trials in evaluations, particularly their limitations in including the complexity of program participants' experiences and issues related to gender, race, class, and other cultural and contextual factors.
	There was recognition and considerable growth of culturally responsive evaluation and, to a lesser degree, culturally responsive indigenous evaluation as holistic approaches for centering evaluation within culture.
	Substantial efforts were made to diversify the pipeline and talent pool of competencies (e.g., the AEA's Building Diversity Initiative and Graduate Education Diversity Internship and Robert Wood Johnson Foundation's Evaluation Fellowship Program from 2008 to 2013).
	There was an increased emphasis on evaluation use, data visualization, and use of mixed methods in evaluation.
2001	Daniel Stufflebeam published, in *New Directions for Evaluation*, a descriptive and evaluative review of 22 different evaluation approaches that had been used over the past 40 years.
2002	The No Child Left Behind Act (NCLB) was passed and signed into law mandating annual student (grades 3–8) testing in reading and mathematics (and later science).
2002	The Diversity Committee of AEA's Board of Directors engaged in a "cultural reading" of the second edition of the *Program Evaluation Standards* with respect to coverage of cultural diversity, treatment of cultural concerns, and attention to cultural competence.
2003	The U.S. Department of Education issued a notice of proposed priority for scientifically based evaluation methods; in response, the AEA, along with other professional association such as the American Educational Research Association (AERA) and the National Education Association (NEA), issued a response with criticism and suggestions for revising the proposed priorities.
2010	The Centers for Disease Control and Prevention (CDC) created the first evaluation officer position.
2011	The AEA released a *Public Statement on Cultural Competence in Evaluation*.
2012	Rodney Hopson became the first African American elected president of the AEA.
2016	The AEA published *An Evaluation Roadmap for a More Effective Government*, which provides a vision for the role of evaluation within the federal government and a road map for improving government through evaluation.
2017	The AEA hosted a series of national dialogues on race and class, bringing together evaluators, policy analysts, and applied researchers.
2018	The AEA released the *Evaluator Competencies* that provide a set of expected competencies in the two domains of professional practice and methodology.
2018	Revision of the *Guiding Principles for Evaluators*, now referred to as the *Evaluators' Ethical Guiding Principles*, was conducted to include more explicit attention to culture, cultural competence, social justice and common good.
2019	The Foundations for Evidence-Based Policymaking Act (PL 115–435) was signed into law mandating that federal agencies expand their capacity for engaging in program evaluation, including designating evaluation officers, developing learning agendas, producing annual evaluation plans, and enabling a workforce to conduct evaluations.

Strengthening Evaluation at the Federal Level

The Government Performance and Results Act (GPRA), originally passed in 1993 (PL 103–62) and signed into law by President Bill Clinton, was strengthened by the GPRA Modernization Act of 2010, signed into law by President Barack Obama. The law's intent was to provide a framework within which that government plans, implements, and evaluates its programs. In January 2019, the Foundations for Evidence-Based Policymaking Act (PL 115–435) was signed into law. Under this law, federal agencies are expected to expand their capacity for engaging in evaluation, including designating evaluation officers, developing learning agendas, producing annual evaluation plans, and enabling a workforce to conduct evaluations. As the following case study illustrates, there has also been a strengthening of program evaluation at the level of particular various federal agencies.

Case Study
Evaluation Activities of the Centers for Disease Control and Prevention

The Centers for Disease Control and Prevention (CDC) incorporated evaluation into its programs earlier than many other federal agencies. Some notable activities that moved evaluation forward at the CDC, as well as expanded to the field, include

- publication of the widely used *Framework for Program Evaluation in Public Health* (1999), which was designed to be a practical step-by-step tool for conducting effective program evaluation;
- creation of the first chief evaluation officer position in 2010;
- development of the Program Performance and Evaluation Office, which consolidated program evaluation, performance measurement, and planning, previously dispersed across the CDC, under a single high-level office;
- creation of the CDC Evaluation Fellowship Program (under auspices of the Program Performance and Evaluation Office); and
- implementation of an annual CDC Evaluation Day (under auspices of the Program Performance and Evaluation Office).

Source: www.cdc.gov/eval/

Shift in the Quantitative–Qualitative Debate

In the spring of 2002 *Evaluation Exchange*, Coffman summarized a conversation that she had with Michael Quinn Patton where he stated that one major recent breakthrough in evaluation over the past 15–20 years was the end to the qualitative–quantitative debate. Since 2000, there has been considerably more emphasis on the use of **mixed methods** or integrating qualitative and quantitative approaches in a single evaluation study or series of studies to understand an evaluation problem. While qualitative and quantitative approaches, in isolation, each have strengths and weaknesses, evaluators have argued that a stronger, more comprehensive account of what is happening within a program can be ascertained when combining the methods in comparison to the conventional evaluation approach of relying only on one method (e.g., Greene, Benjamin, & Goodyear, 2001; Mertens & Hesse-Biber, 2013). Chapter 11 covers mixed methods in detail.

Increased Emphasis on Social Justice and Diversity

Probably one of the most notable shifts in the evaluation field that gained increased prominence in the 21st century is more attention to issues of culture, social justice, and, to a lesser degree, race/racism in both evaluation theory and practice (e.g., Hood, Hopson, & Frierson, 2015; Kirkhart, 2005; Samuels & Ryan, 2011; Thomas, 2011; Thomas & Stevens, 2004; Thompson-Robinson, Hopson, & SenGupta, 2004). Even beginning in the late 1990s on into the 2000s, the AEA put forth a number of initiatives to expand attention to issues of culture, social justice, and, to a lesser degree, race/racism that will undoubtedly have a historical impact on the future of evaluation. Many of these initiatives are summarized in Table 3.4 or are discussed throughout this book and, therefore, are not presented again in this section.

An important milestone in relation to culturally responsive evaluation was the creation of the Center for Culturally Responsive Evaluation and Assessment (CREA), founded in 2013 by Stafford Hood and located in the College of Education at the University of Illinois at Urbana-Champaign. This includes an international community of scholars/practitioners who promote a culturally responsive stance in all forms of systematic inquiry including evaluation, assessment, policy analysis, applied research, and action research. The CREA hosts an annual international conference, as it seeks to produce a body of informed practitioners, published scholarship, professional development opportunities, technical assistance resources, and advocacy advancing cultural responsiveness across inquiry platforms and settings. See https://crea.education.illinois.edu/# for more information.

Culturally responsive Indigenous evaluation is another area that gained momentum in the 21st century. The culturally responsive Indigenous evaluation contribution to the field is that it provides theoretical, methodological, and practical evaluation designs and strategies for carrying out a culturally responsive evaluation of services and programs provided for and/or designed by Indigenous peoples. It began as a practical method and strategy used to include culture, language, community context, and sovereign tribal governance when conducting research, policy, and evaluation studies and emerged as a paradigm that is situated within and a partner to culturally responsive evaluations (Bowman, 2006). Culturally responsive Indigenous evaluation is intended to be a transformative evaluation model that provides flexibility to be implemented in diverse Indigenous contexts. Over the last decade, culturally responsive indigenous evaluation resources have become more readily available to academia and evaluation practitioners within the mainstream literature (Waapalaneexkweew [Bowman] & Dodge-Francis, 2018).

Support for Capacity Building

There are too numerous examples of federal and foundation support for evaluation capacity building to discuss in this chapter. The NSF is one federal agency that has substantially contributed to the evolving status of the evaluation field, having funded evaluator training centers, institutes, and programs in STEM areas to address the shortage of evaluators. These included collaborations and/or support for university degree programs and short-term professional programs for faculty and advanced graduate students. Some centers that received substantial federal funding and devoted part of their efforts to evaluation include facilities at Northwestern University, the Evaluation Center at Western Michigan University, and the Center for Instructional Research and Curriculum Evaluation at the University of Illinois. In early 2000s, the NSF funded an

Evaluation Training Institute at Howard University for midlevel evaluators designed to broaden their knowledge of evaluation models, methods, standards, and guiding principles, as well as raise their awareness and understanding of the influence of culture and context. The Centers for Disease Control and Prevention (CDC), W. K. Kellogg Foundation, Robert Wood Johnson Foundation, Colorado Trust, and Annie E. Casey Foundation have also played a major role in efforts to diversify both the talent pool of evaluators and the theories and methods utilized by evaluators through either its funding to professional associations or its own initiatives.

SUMMARY

Clearly, evaluation in some form has evolved over the entire history of people's existence, although systematic program evaluation began to come into its own in the early to mid-20th century. Program evaluation is very much rooted in the sociopolitical and legislative climate of its time. Although there were many explicit racialized experiences (e.g., racism, Jim Crow laws) for persons of color, particularly African Americans, during evaluation's early history, such events were not adequately reflected in the social programming or evaluations of that time. Further, there has been little discussion of the evolution of evaluation through a social justice lens when recounting its history.

Over the years, the federal government has played an enormous role in the historical evolution of evaluation. Datta (2003) identifies eight influences of the government on the evaluation profession and of evaluation on the government, including increasing the

- demand for internal evaluation within the federal government;
- demand for internal evaluation among the recipients of federal support;
- demand for external evaluation among the recipients of federal support;
- specification of methods, designs, and measures to be used;
- support for the development of evaluation as a profession;
- creation of opportunities for employment of evaluators;

- leadership for evaluation emulated by nongovernmental entities such as private foundations; and
- support of evaluation capacity such as evaluation training, development of standards and definition of evaluation, and a professional infrastructure.

Foundations have also made substantial contributions to evaluation over the years through funding demonstration projects and evaluation efforts.

There is much to trace in the evolution of evaluation, and it is impossible to neatly fit it into a single chapter. Our attempt was to trace the historical evolution of evaluation to the present time through a more inclusive and social justice lens. We covered notable, and sometimes ignored, events and people contributing to this evolution. Other noteworthy events and influencers not mentioned in this chapter are found elsewhere throughout this text. Currently, there are numerous professional evaluators, with diverse perspectives, around the world conducting evaluations in a variety of areas such as health, education, and criminal justice. These evaluators are employed in a myriad of settings including universities, research institutes, government agencies, K–12 school districts, and private industry. Knowledge of the evolution of program evaluation, its various traditions, and key figures/events within a sociocultural context can better help these and aspiring evaluators appreciate current evaluation perspectives, recurring issues, and persistent gaps.

The evaluation of programs designed to ameliorate social problems is not going away. And, undoubtedly, program evaluation will continue to evolve in a changing and increasingly diverse society. The challenge to the profession as it evolves into the future is to continue its push to make evaluations more socially just, inclusive, methodologically sound, and useful to intended users.

SUPPLEMENTAL RESOURCES

Major Evaluation Journals

American Journal of Evaluation, launched in 1981, publishes original, peer-reviewed, often highly cited articles that explore the decisions and challenges related to conceptualizing, designing, and conducting evaluations including issues ranging from choosing program theories to implementing an evaluation to presenting the final report to managing an evaluation's consequences. https://journals.sagepub.com/home/aje

Canadian Journal of Program Evaluation, first published in 1985, publishes full-length articles (in both French and English) on all aspects of the theory and practice of evaluation, real-life cases written by evaluation practitioners, and practice notes that share practical knowledge, experiences and lessons learned. https://journalhosting.ucalgary.ca/index.php/cjpe/index

Educational Evaluation and Policy Analysis, established in 1979, publishes rigorous, policy-relevant original research of interest to those engaged in educational policy analysis, evaluation, and decision making from multiple disciplines, theoretical orientations, and methodologies. https://journals.sagepub.com/home/epa

Evaluation: The International Journal of Theory, Research and Practice is an interdisciplinary, international peer-reviewed journal launched in 1995, whose purpose is to promote dialogue internationally and to build bridges within the expanding field of evaluation. www.tavinstitute.org/what-we-offer/journals/evaluation-the-international-journal-of-theory-research-and-practice/

Evaluation and the Health Professions, established in 1978, is a peer-reviewed, quarterly journal that provides health-related professionals with state-of-the-art methodological, measurement, and statistical tools for conceptualizing the etiology of health promotion and problems and developing, implementing, and evaluating health programs, teaching and training services, and products that pertain to a myriad of health dimensions. https://journals.sagepub.com/home/ehp

Evaluation and Program Planning, initially published in 1978, has as its primary goals to publish articles that assist evaluators and planners to improve the practice of their professions, develop their skills, and improve their knowledge base. www.journals.elsevier.com/evaluation-and-program-planning/

Evaluation Review: A Journal of Applied Social Research, published since 1977, seeks to bring together the latest applied evaluation methods used in a wide range of disciplines. https://journals.sagepub.com/home/erx

Journal of MultiDisciplinary Evaluation, initially published in 2004, is a free, online journal published by the Evaluation Center at Western Michigan University focusing on the profession and discipline of evaluation. http://journals.sfu.ca/jmde/index.php/jmde_1

New Directions for Evaluation, a quarterly thematic journal first published in 1978 by the AEA, publishes empirical, methodological, and theoretical works on all aspects of evaluation. https://onlinelibrary.wiley.com/journal/1534875x#pane-01cbe741-499a-4611-874e-1061f1f4679e01

Practical Assessment, Research, and Evaluation is a peer-reviewed online journal, first published in 1999, whose purpose is to provide free access to articles that can have a positive impact on assessment, research, evaluation, and teaching practice. https://scholarworks.umass.edu/pare/

The Evaluation Exchange, the Harvard Family Research Project's evaluation periodical, launched in 1995, publishes brief articles addressing current issues facing program evaluators and highlights innovative methods and approaches to evaluation. https://philanthropynewsdigest.org/connections/harvard-family-research-project-the-evaluation-exchange

CDC Evaluation Resources

www.cdc.gov/eval/resources/index.htm

www.cdc.gov/eval/tools/index.htm

These links include a variety of evaluation manuals, tools, self-study guides, and other evaluation-related resources.

University Programs in Evaluation

www.eval.org/p/cm/ld/fid=43

This AEA website provides a listing and description of university graduate programs or certificate programs either directly in evaluation or with available concentrations in evaluation. To be listed, a program must include a sequence of at least three courses focusing directly on evaluation supported by other coursework in appropriate methodologies.

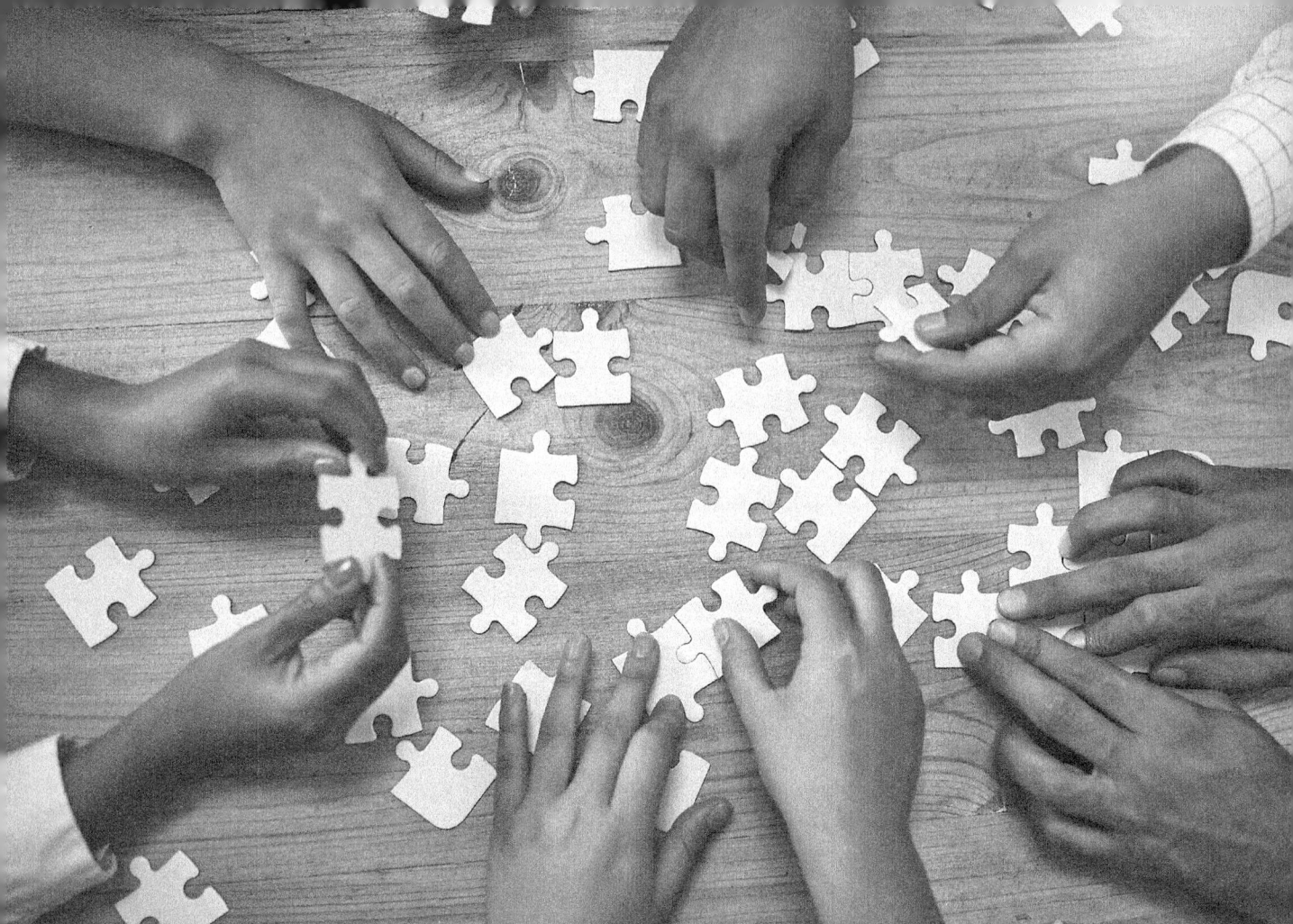
istock/ PeopleImages

Evaluators must not accept a paradigm, theory or model simply because it has been extensively used. Instead, they should interrogate values and assumptions espoused and the extent to which they include or exclude perspectives from nondominant communities.

CHAPTER 4

Evaluation Paradigms, Theories, and Models

There are many researchers who conduct evaluations with little to no knowledge of evaluation theory and think that's absolutely fine because of their methodological prowess. However, evaluation is more than a methodological enterprise. Over the past 25 years, there has been increasing interest in creating, promoting, and using theories and models in evaluation. Proponents argue that social science and program theories, more generally, and evaluation theories and models, in particular, can play a major role in enhancing our understanding of how programs work and how to engage in effective evaluation practice. Evaluations grounded in coherent theories are more explicitly driven by intentionality, purpose, and values rather than simply by methods and methodological tools.

After reading this chapter and participating in the activities, readers will be able to meet the following learning objectives:

- Describe the major paradigms that inform research and evaluation

- Identify the three most popular types of theories (social science theory, program theory of change, evaluation theory) used to guide and improve evaluation practice

- Explain the differences between social science theory and evaluation theory along with recognizing the relationship between them

- Discuss evaluation theories available for evaluating programs and projects

- Reflect on the fit, or lack thereof, between selected evaluation theories, models, and approaches and their attention to issues of equity and social justice

Introduction

This chapter examines some of the major paradigms, theories, and models that inform the evaluation field. Attention will be given to the extent to which the paradigms, theories, and models discussed reflect the dominant paradigm that is limited in its applicability or appropriateness to members of society who are not part of the dominant culture. Readers are encouraged to interrogate each of the approaches presented in this chapter with an eye toward asking themselves about the values and assumptions espoused as well as what questions about reality, knowledge, and power are reflected in the perspective.

Paradigms are grounded in big assumptions about the world, essentially seeking to discern what is real and how we create knowledge, while theories, on the other hand, describe more specific phenomena often grounded within a larger paradigm. The latter assist us in organizing different observable events, making sense of these events, asserting predictions about these events, and coherently connecting them to some comprehensive principles. "There is nothing so practical as a good theory" is a frequently cited quote and one originally stated by German American social psychologist Kurt Lewin, who was making the argument that psychology was thin on good theories but benefited substantially when they existed. Evaluation scholar and practitioner Carol H. Weiss (1995) extended Lewin's thinking to the field of evaluation, arguing that evaluation should surface theories and lay them out in as fine a detail as possible, identifying all the assumptions and sub-assumptions built into the program.

As we discussed in Chapter 1, evaluation is a disciplined inquiry involving the systematic, contextually responsive, and ethical application of research tools and methods to collect data that assess the effectiveness and operations of programs within the various social, political, and cultural contexts in which they operate. Its goal is to provide credible evidence that fosters greater understanding and enhances decision making aimed at improving social conditions and promoting healthy, just, and equitable communities. This is done, in part, through evaluation's focus on assessing the (intended and unintended) consequences of deliberate social actions (e.g., programs and policies) put in place to eliminate or reduce a variety of social problems such as homelessness, the racial achievement gap, substance abuse, and unemployment. To achieve this goal, evaluation relies on paradigms, theories, and models to assist in the process of understanding programs, planning evaluations, implementing evaluative studies, and disseminating results. Paradigms, theories, and models all play an important role in shaping what evaluators think about and study, how they ask about it, and, in some cases, even what they are likely to find. After reading this chapter, readers will have a better understanding and appreciation for the major paradigms, theories, and models that have influenced evaluation practice over the years.

The Value of Scientific Paradigms and Theories in Evaluation

Paradigms exist in virtually every area of human life. For example, most individuals have a paradigm, or personal frame of reference, related to political, cultural, and religious affairs. Similarly, every evaluation, either explicitly or implicitly, is guided by a set of values, beliefs, and assumptions that may also be underpinned by theory. These values, beliefs, and assumptions, along with methodology, reflect a particular paradigm. Evaluators have a plurality of paradigms, theories, and models to select from when approaching an evaluation.

The Nature of Scientific Paradigms

Often taken for granted, paradigms are assumptions and expectations about how the world works and/or what we value. American physicist and philosopher of science Thomas Kuhn (1962) was the first individual to use the word *paradigm* in his very influential book, *The Structure of Scientific Revolutions*. He used it to mean a conceptual worldview or philosophical way of thinking. Kuhn argues that when we look at scientists who are working under the same paradigm, we can find common methods, common standards, common aims, and fundamental agreement about the nature of the world and the nature of the processes in it. In a similar definition, Filstead (1979) defined a paradigm as a "set of interrelated assumptions about the social world which provides a philosophical and conceptual framework for the organized study of the world" (p. 34). A paradigm is essentially the analytic lens through which researchers view things, including their worldviews about reality, knowledge, and methods.

The following activity provides an example of how paradigms shape individuals' everyday view of the world, including how they both perceive and interpret things. It also gives readers an opportunity to reflect on and discuss their own paradigm(s) in specific areas.

Reflect and Discuss
Paradigms Shaping Your Everyday Worldview

Paradigms are our lens or a way of framing what we know, what we can know, and how we can know it. Individuals operate under a set of assumptions about the way the world does, or at least should, work. For some individuals, their assumptions or paradigms are rooted in their religious, political, or cultural perspectives, which, in turn, shape their views on the issue at hand. For example, individuals have different paradigms regarding how they think about capital punishment (i.e., the death penalty). For some, the death penalty is a violation of human rights, regardless of whether or not the person has been found guilty of a crime. Many of these individuals who oppose the death penalty believe, first and foremost, that any person, including the government, has no right to take a life for any reason. Further, they often believe that living with one's crimes is a worse punishment than dying for them. Also, opponents maintain that the historical application of capital punishment demonstrates that attempts to single out certain kinds of crime (and certain criminals) as deserving death will continue to be arbitrary and discriminatory, thus precluding the possibility that capital punishment will be fairly applied. They note in particular that the poor and ethnic and religious minorities often do not have access to good legal assistance and, thus, are more likely to receive death sentences. For those who favor capital punishment, they argue that it has a uniquely potent deterrent effect on potentially violent offenders for whom the threat of imprisonment is not a sufficient restraint. They also say that capital punishment is just retribution for victims and families, bringing them closure. Another common argument for the death penalty is that death is cheaper than feeding a murderer for life. As evident, people can have very different paradigms about certain issues yet be equally confident in the "truth" of their perspective.

Now, reflect on your own personal paradigm in relation to one of the following broad areas:

- Health and wellness
- Child-rearing
- Gender and gender roles

Organize into small groups and discuss your paradigm in terms of your views and assumptions about the topic and how you arrived at those views.

As was covered in Chapter 3, during the 1980s, the social sciences focused on paradigms fairly narrowly and mostly in terms of method (i.e., the quantitative vs. qualitative debate). Quantitative research was the generally accepted research paradigm until the early 1980s when the "paradigm wars" between advocates of quantitative and qualitative research reached a new peak. During the 1980s, however, many quantitative and qualitative researchers argued that their approach was superior. The selection of a particular method, quantitative or qualitative, was not simply methodology but was also equated with a particular philosophical stance (Guba & Lincoln, 1994). The paradigm wars, as related to methodology, were a major catalyst in the development of mixed methods as a distinct third methodological movement (Teddlie & Tashakkori, 2003).

Paradigms frame what we know, what we can know, and how we can know it. There are several dimensions and belief systems through which they are differentiated from each other. Scholars primarily discuss four dimensions—**axiology**, **ontology**, **epistemology**, and **methodology** (e.g., Guba & Lincoln, 2005; Mertens & Wilson, 2019). Ponterotto (2005) included **rhetorical structure** as another paradigm dimension. These dimensions of paradigms are described in Table 4.1 in terms of their meaning and the types of questions relevant to each dimension.

Keeping these dimensions in mind, an evaluator's paradigm will, in large part, dictate (a) the phenomena observed (and ignored), (b) the questions asked (and not asked) about those observations, (c) how the questions are formulated, (d) what is measured (or not measured) and how it is measured, (e) the procedures of the research, and (f) how the results are interpreted.

Table 4.1 Dimensions of Various Paradigms

Dimensions	Meaning	Examples of Relevant Questions
Axiology	Role and place of values in the research process	• What does the evaluator value? • What does the evaluator feel is ethical?
Ontology	Belief about the nature of reality, being, or existence	• What exists? • What do we view as the nature of truth and reality? • What can be known about that reality?
Epistemology	Study of knowledge (how we come to know what we know) and the acquisition of knowledge (theory of knowledge)	• How do we come to know what we know? • What is the relationship between the knower (evaluation participant) and the would-be knower (evaluator)?
Methodology	Processes, procedures, and strategies of research (theory of method)	• What methods or systematic approaches (e.g., surveys, interviews) do we use to gather information about something to be known?
Rhetorical structure	Language and presentation of research	• How do we present the procedures and results of our evaluation to the intended audiences (e.g., is rhetoric presented as "precise," "scientific," and "objective" or first person, often personalized, and detailing comprehensively the evaluator's own experiences, expectations, biases, and values)?

Sources: Descriptions adapted from Guba & Lincoln, 2005; Mertens & Wilson, 2019; Ponterotto, 2005.

The historical exclusion and marginalization of nondominant communities in knowledge production activities has a long history. Stanfield (1999) pointed out the racialized conventional wisdoms and academic traditions that impede the ability of social scientists to adequately explain and evaluate the colorization of the lifeworlds around them, particularly in terms of explanations involving power, privilege, and empowerment. Trainor and Bal (2014) argued that researchers contribute to the reproduction and obfuscation of structural inequalities when they rely on certain paradigms and methodological tools that are promoted as the most effective way to answer all research questions or when the quality indicators of any given methodology fail to acknowledge research as a "situated practice." Later, Bal and Trainor (2016) stressed that

> universalist, culture-free perspectives that do not critically consider disabled, racialized, gendered, or classed experiences and enduring structural inequalities are products of culture and history through local performances of researchers, participants, and consumers of research. The significance and implications of research results can be fully understood if and when the specific contexts of the researchers, the participants, and scientific fields frame the work. (p. 327)

Over the past several decades, we have certainly witnessed an increase in the number of scholars interrogating many long-standing scientific paradigms in terms of the treatment of marginalized groups and the extent to which they, intentionally or unintentionally, contribute to the status quo that perpetuates disparities and inequalities.

Theories for Guiding and Improving Evaluation Practice

A paradigm acts as a frame of reference for a theory. There can be a number of theories within the framework of a particular paradigm. Theories, important in virtually every discipline, include an interrelated set of concepts, definitions, and propositions. Theories help one better understand events, behaviors, or situations and provide a framework for thinking about those things. In this chapter, we discuss three popular types of theories used to guide and improve evaluation: (a) social science theory, (b) program theory of change, and (c) evaluation theory. These theories inform thinking about social processes, social problem solving, program development, and subsequently the development of evaluation models and approaches. They all can play an invaluable role in informing the practice of evaluation and can enhance evaluators' planning as they discern in which paradigm they will work and which evaluation model or approach they will utilize in their practice. Evaluation practice grounded in coherent theories ensures that evaluations are more explicitly driven by intentionality, purpose, and values rather than simply by methods and methodological tools.

Social Science Paradigms and Theories

Social Science Paradigms

Program evaluation and social science are intimately intertwined. They select from the same repertoire of methodological techniques, they operate in the same milieu, and they are indeed often conducted by the same people (A. Ryan, 1988). Several social science paradigms—each with its own unique axiology (what is valued), ontology (nature of reality), epistemology (study of knowledge and how to achieve it), and methodological perspective—have been used to guide the thinking of evaluation and evaluators. These different paradigms begin with different philosophical assumptions and lead to different methodological assumptions and methods choices (Guba & Lincoln, 2005). How one evaluates a project will vary depending on the social science paradigm or lens used to frame the evaluation.

Evaluators' worldview about the nature of knowledge informs their basic beliefs about who informs (or should inform) the evaluation process, who are (or should be) the primary beneficiaries of inquiry, questions asked, and favored research traditions and strategies (e.g., ways in which questions are formulated and how data are collected, analyzed, and disseminated). The major social science paradigms that have influenced evaluation include positivism/postpositivism, interpretivism/social constructivism, pragmatism, and critical theory (Creswell, 2014; Guba & Lincoln, 2005; Mertens, 2020; Mertens & Wilson, 2019).

Positivism dominated much of the early social science research. This is based on the rationalist, empiricist philosophy that originated with Aristotle, Francis Bacon, John Locke, Auguste Comte, and Immanuel Kant (cited in Mertens, 2020, p. 11). Positivism purports that the world is external and objective, that it exists externally to ourselves, and that we can discover the singular truth about it. It is rooted in the belief that one can investigate the social world in the same way as the natural world with a method of studying the social world that is "value-free." Positivists assert the existence of an objective reality, or truth, out there waiting to be discovered and that the use of particular methods will accurately illuminate that objective reality (Guba & Lincoln, 1994).

Around the middle of the 20th century, there was a shift in thinking from positivism to postpositivism. Postpositivism argues that external reality is something that we can understand and capture using the right tools, but we can never achieve perfect knowledge of that reality because of the researcher's human limitations. Postpositivism revises earlier assertions that reality exists independent of the observer and can be apprehended accurately by objective processes (Guba & Lincoln, 1994). While positivists believe that the researcher and the researched person are independent of each other, postpositivists accept that theories, background, knowledge, and values of the researcher can influence what is observed (Reichardt & Rallis, 1994).

Postpositivism considers context as an important—and, in some cases, necessary—component to social science research. This paradigm has emphasis on causal explanation with the recognition that "social causality is inherently complex" (Greene & McClintock, 1991, p. 14). Postpositivism favors the use of quantitative methods; thus, postpositivist evaluations are expected to have an experimental, quantitative core buttressed by critique from varied analyses, theoretical perspectives, and values frameworks (Greene & McClintock, 1991).

Interpretivism, rooted in philosophies such as hermeneutics and phenomenology, postulates that reality is constantly renegotiated, debated, and interpreted. From this perspective, the world exists according to how it is experienced, interpreted, and perceived by individuals. Interpretivists believe that reality is multiple and relative (Hudson & Ozanne, 1988), and these multiple realities depend on other systems for meanings (Lincoln & Guba, 1985), which, in turn, makes it even more difficult to interpret in terms of fixed realities (Neuman, 2000). Interpretivists view knowledge as based on understanding and interpretation of individuals' experience (not universal laws), and, as such, knowledge is highly context specific and inherently time and place bound (Greene & McClintock, 1991).

Interpretivism favors the use of qualitative methods (especially interviews and observations), which places the researcher in direct interaction with the phenomena being studied (Guba & Lincoln, 1981) and allows for close interactions between the researcher and research participants. An evaluation embedded in the interpretivist paradigm is likely to involve (a) a case study of a single program at a single site, with the evaluator developing detailed descriptions of key features of that context; (b) an emergent understanding of how different participants viewed their experience, what it meant to them, and why; and ultimately (c) an integrated portrayal of these diverse experiences, meanings, and values and their connections to a specific context (Greene & McClintock, 1991).

Social constructivism is an interpretive framework whereby individuals seek to understand their world and develop their own particular meanings that correspond to their experience (Creswell, 2013). The paradigm, originating in sociology, argues that reality is socially constructed based on individuals' knowledge that is influenced by values, interactions, experiences, and context. An evaluation from a social constructivist paradigm might ask program participants open-ended questions that allow them to fully and freely describe their own experiences. Hence, the evaluator's role is to listen carefully to the participants' views and interpret the findings based on their background and experiences (Creswell, 2013).

Pragmatism, as a social science paradigm, emphasizes the practical uses and effects of any conception of knowledge, ideas, beliefs, and values rather than just focusing on how this conception increases our understanding of reality and truth. The utility of knowledge, and not knowledge per se, is emphasized. Pragmatism is a diverse philosophical tradition, with contributions from classical pragmatists (e.g., William James, Charles Peirce) and neo-pragmatists (i.e., Richard Rorty, Cornel West) (J. Hall, 2013).

Pragmatists believe that reality is not static but is grounded in the environment that changes and can only be encountered through human experience. Pragmatist philosophy sees inquiry as a natural part of life aimed at improving our condition by adaptation and accommodations in the social world in which we live (Cronen, 2001). As a social science research paradigm, this approach emerged as a method of inquiry for more practical-minded researchers who orient themselves toward solving practical problems in the real world. As a research paradigm, pragmatism is based on the proposition that researchers should use the philosophical and/or methodological approach that works best for the particular research problem being investigated (Tashakkori & Teddlie, 1998).

An evaluation conducted from a pragmatic paradigm would likely focus on data that are found to be useful for stakeholders, and it would lean toward the use of mixed methods as the most appropriate way to address the evaluation questions (Mertens & Wilson, 2019). From this paradigm, the value of the evaluation is primarily determined through how it is used to solve problems or guide decision making toward such ends.

The critical theory paradigm assumes multiple realities that are produced through historically based social and political processes (Guba & Lincoln, 1988) and the values associated with them. The historical roots of critical theory are grounded in the Western European Marxist tradition. As this paradigm evolved in the United States, it was not tied to a particular disciplinary field but, instead, drew ideas from various academic disciplines. Critical theory is aimed at challenging and destabilizing established knowledge with the goal of raising consciousness of social conditions and promoting emancipatory values such as equity, social welfare, justice, and political liberty (Hammersley, 2005). The critical paradigm focuses on issues of power, inequality, and social change, and it seeks to illuminate the historical, structural, and value bases of social phenomena and, in doing so, to catalyze political and social change (Greene & McClintock, 1991).

An underlying assumption of the critical paradigm is that social science can never be truly value-free and should be conducted with the express goal of stimulating social change. Critical researchers consider the moral and ethical issues within the context of their work through an examination of the historical problems of domination, alienation, social struggles, and how social inequities arising from racism and other forms of oppression continue to privilege certain groups and disadvantage others (Thomas, 2009). Newer forms of critical theory have emerged related to racism (critical race theory), sexism (critical feminist theory), and the intersection of racism and sexism (critical race feminism). The transformative paradigm is embedded in the critical paradigm "focusing on viewpoints of marginalized groups and interrogating systemic power structures through mixed methods to further social justice and human rights" (Mertens & Wilson, 2019, p. 42). Evaluation following a critical paradigm amplifies respect for cultural diversity, human rights, and social justice. This paradigm argues that knowledge is of no value unless it empowers and transforms people, particularly the marginalized, during its construction. (Chapter 5 discusses the transformative social justice paradigms in greater detail.)

Application of Social Science Paradigms in Evaluations

The following case study illustrates what an evaluation focusing on the same topic might look like under each paradigm.

Case Study
Evaluating the Same Project Using Different Social Science Paradigms

Project Description

This project focuses on eliminating and/or reducing illicit drug use among unemployed or underemployed urban men of color.

Positivism/Postpositivism

An evaluation conceptualized from a positivist/postpositivist paradigm will focus on "objective," observable, and measurable aspects (or predetermined variables) of the project, requiring the gathering of predominantly quantitative evidence. For example, the evaluation might attempt to precisely measure illicit drug use and abuse (e.g., quantity of use, frequency of use, number of using days per hundred days, duration of periods of total abstinence, and periods of low-volume use or low-problem use) and look to determine the key causes of illicit drug use among the unemployed and underemployed urban men of color. Factors of interest are converted into quantitative variables that can be ascertained and subjected to statistical analysis.

Interpretivism/Social Constructivism

An evaluation conceptualized from an interpretivist or constructivist paradigm would not be so focused on the notion of objectivity (as would the positivist/postpositivist evaluation), but instead might focus on the subjective truth of each participant in the evaluation. Here, the focus would be on generating knowledge about how urban men of color who use illicit drugs understand their lives, their social context, and their relationships with their illicit drug(s) of choice. The emphasis is on the use of qualitative methods given the need to construct meaning in context and the evaluator's role in seeking the subjective truth of each participant in the evaluation. Here, more personal, interactive modes of data collection (e.g., interviews, observations) will be favored.

Pragmatism

An evaluation based in the pragmatism paradigm would focus primarily on data that are found to be useful by stakeholders. For example, the evaluation might be aimed at collecting data that inform planning decisions needed for substantial revision to the existing substance abuse project or for planning new projects. Yet, on the other hand, an evaluation from a pragmatist paradigm might look at the men's outcomes for the purposes of program funders and administrators. Such an evaluation is judged by the extent to which it achieves it purpose. Both qualitative and quantitative data collection techniques are used.

Critical Theory

An evaluation based in a critical theory paradigm would examine how the urban men of color who have illicit drug use problems are part of an oppressed group in society and would seek to liberate them from external sources of oppression, such as punitive drug and sentencing laws, racism, and internal sources of oppression (e.g., internalized fear and shame). The value of this evaluation would be determined primarily by the extent to which it reciprocates power with marginalized drug-abusing men of color and improves the conditions for flourishing within such groups. A variety of methodological approaches are used, combining qualitative and quantitative techniques.

The following activity can help readers enhance their understanding of the various social science paradigms, their characteristics, and the extent to which they would favor or disfavor a particular paradigm.

Activity
Applying Paradigms to Evaluation Study

Review the following rationale and overview of a gender equity intervention in science, technology, engineering, and mathematics (STEM). Then select two paradigms from among the ones discussed (i.e., positivist/postpositivist, interpretivist/social constructivist, pragmatist, critical) that might be applied in framing the evaluation of the intervention described. Write a short description of the two paradigms you chose, including why you selected them to help frame the evaluation and what you hope to learn by using these particular paradigms.

Project Rationale and Overview

Results of both correlational and experimental research suggest that gender bias remains problematic within STEM fields. These biases have persisted over time, with more recent work indicating that elite male faculty in the biological sciences are less likely to hire female postdoctoral researchers and graduate students in their laboratories (Sheltzer & Smith, 2014). Additionally, researchers have found that journal articles with female first authors are less likely to be cited than those with male first authors (Lariviere, Ni, Gingras, Cronin, & Sugimoto, 2013). Thus, given this and other evidence, an intervention is developed that seeks to reduce gender bias in STEM.

Social Science Theories

Social science theories seek to understand how social processes work and under what conditions they change or remain stable. As such, social science theories have an important role in informing decisions about programs and evaluation practice. Social science theories provide a framework for thinking about the interrelationships of constructs important in theory-based program development and evaluation studies. These theories, as Leeuw and Donaldson (2015) point out, are capable of contextualizing and explaining the consequences of policies, programs, and evaluators' actions, including their impact on society and behavior and the role of social and institutional domains in evaluations.

Social science theory enables program planners and evaluators to identify the relevant disciplinary theory in the context of the intervention being planned and/or evaluated. Social learning theories (Bandura, 1977) and social-cognitive theories (Bandura, 1986) are two social science theories that have been used considerably in risk prevention and health programs. For example, in health promotion programs, the underlying theoretical assumption, based in social learning theory, is that the program provides knowledge (e.g., about methods to break a smoking habit), which leads to modification in individual motivation and intentions to change (e.g., willingness to try to reduce smoking), which leads to change in behavior or the desired outcome (e.g., cessation of smoking) (Weiss, 1997). Evaluations then follow the anticipated sequence of change (Weiss, 1997). The health belief model (Rosenstock, 1974), which derives from psychological and behavioral theory, is another popular approach used in health intervention social programming. It is based on the premise that people's willingness to change their health behaviors is primarily due to several factors: perceived susceptibility (individuals will not change their health behaviors unless they believe that they are at risk), perceived severity (the probability that individuals will change their health behaviors to avoid a consequence depends on how serious they consider the consequence to be), perceived benefits (individuals do not want to give up something they enjoy if they don't also get something in return), and perceived barriers (individuals do not want to change their health behaviors if they think that doing so is going to be hard). Working with tested and robust explanatory theories from the social sciences can add crucial insights about mechanisms and contexts underlying programs and policies, including evaluation interventions (Leeuw & Donaldson, 2015). Here, mechanisms refer to the things that intervene between the delivery of services and the outcomes achieved. Mechanisms of change are not a program activity but a response to a program activity (Weiss, 1997).

Donaldson and Lipsey (2006) point out that social science theory can also be useful to evaluators in multiple ways. These include (a) helping evaluators assess the likelihood that programs will be able to accomplish certain objectives, (b) guiding evaluation measurement and design decisions, and (c) providing a context for interpreting evaluation findings. From the social science literature, evaluators may be able to identify relevant and valid measures of constructs of interest or feasible designs that can be applied in their work. Social programs are generally conceptualized and implemented around a theory, explicit or implicit, about how the change will or should occur. In the activity that follows, readers are provided an opportunity to identify the social science theory that underlies a particular social program.

> ## Activity
> ### Interface Among Social Science Theory, Social Programming, and Evaluation
>
> Find a report or journal publication of a social intervention that has been evaluated. A few examples include the following:
>
> Dierendonck, D., Dirk, W. B., Schaufeli, W. B., & Buunk, B. P. (1998). The evaluation of an individual burnout intervention program: The role of inequity and social support. *Journal of Applied Psychology, 83*(3), 392–407.
>
> Phillips, G., Lindeman, P., Adames, C. N., Bettin, E., Bayston, C., Stonehouse, P., . . . Greene, G. J. (2019). Empowerment evaluation: A case study of citywide implementation within an HIV prevention context. *American Journal of Evaluation, 40*(3), 318–334.
>
> Thomas, V. G., Gaston, M. H., Porter, G. K., & Anderson, A. (2016). Prime Time Sister Circles II: Evaluating a culturally relevant intervention to decrease psychological and physical risk factors for chronic disease in mid-life African American women. *Journal of the National Medical Association, 108*(1), 6–18.
>
> Identify the social science theory that helped frame the conceptualization of the intervention identified in the publication. Give specific examples of how the particular social science theory and its accompanying research informed the intervention described.
>
> Describe how the evaluator utilized this particular social science theory to design the evaluation?

Program Theory of Change

While social science paradigms and theories can be useful in providing broad guidance in various areas, they do not reflect the specific contextual and cultural conditions of stakeholders. A **theory of change** describes the processes of change by outlining causal linkages in an initiative and its shorter-term, intermediate, and longer-term outcomes (Leeuw & Donaldson, 2015). The theory of change gives the big picture, including issues related to the environment or context that are not under the control of the creator of the theory of change, and shows all the different pathways that might lead to change. To develop a theory of change, a fundamental theoretical and practical understanding of the social problem to be addressed is needed. Theories of change should be grounded in, or at least be informed by, relevant social science theory, empirical research, previous evaluations, good practice, and the perspectives of those with lived experience of the program or the situation it is intended to address. Doing this will better ensure that the program is built on a solid knowledge base of what is perceived to be working in both theory and practice.

Program theory (sometimes used interchangeably with theory of change) is a theory of change applied to a specific program. It is the thinking behind how a particular program or intervention will bring about results. Program theory (not to be confused with social science theory) has been described as the process through which program components are presumed to affect outcomes and the conditions under which these processes are believed to operate (Donaldson, 2001, 2003, 2007). Whether expressed in detail as an **articulated program theory** (one that is explicitly stated) or as an **implicit program theory** (one that is not explicitly stated but is presumed to work in a certain way) (Weiss, 1997), the program theory explains why the program does what it does and provides the rationale for expecting that doing so will achieve the desired results. It generally includes a sequence of sets or logical chain of if–then relationships that link investments to activities to results.

Program theory can be developed at any time during the program's life cycle. However, it is generally developed during the planning stage of a new intervention. Program theory can assist an evaluator in a variety of ways including in managing and engaging stakeholders, monitoring and evaluation, and generating evidence-based practice by documenting innovative practices and supporting adaptation of program elements (Funnell & Rogers, 2011). When an evaluation is being planned, it can be quite useful to review the program theory to get an understanding of how the intervention is understood to contribute to a chain of results that is to produce the intended or actual impacts. It can play an important role in helping evaluators understand the evaluand and subsequently determine which evaluation approaches and methods are most appropriate for evaluating the project under consideration.

The program theory also should identify assumptions underlying the model. Assumptions are preconditions or resources that are most critical for successful implementation of the program and needed for achieving desired outcomes. Assumptions are often unvoiced. Transparency around assumptions, however, makes explicit the beliefs that underlie chosen actions. Two examples of assumptions that underlie a theory of change for a hypothetical employment program designed to increase low-income women's entry into nontraditional blue-collar jobs (e.g., electrician, welder, carpenter, plumber, mechanic) include (a) If women have the requisite knowledge and skills, they will be hired in nontraditional blue-collar jobs, and (b) Employment in these nontraditional areas of work for women is more likely to pay livable wages, more likely to be unionized, and more likely to provide job security.

An evaluator may be contracted to assist with the development of the program theory as well as evaluating the appropriateness of the existing program theory. This latter generally entails determining how well the program theory is conceptualized and the extent to which it presents a feasible and plausible plan for achieving the intended outcomes.

The following activity provides an example of a program theory of change for an after-school violence prevention program. Readers have the opportunity to reflect on and discuss questions posed at the end of the case.

Activity
School Violence Reduction Program Theory of Change

Review the following components of a generic program theory (left column) and an example of a school violence intervention program theory (right column). Then, reflect on and discuss the issues posed after the table.

Components of Generic Program Theory	Sample Program Theory
• *If* a certain set of resources (such as staff, equipment, and materials) is available, *then* the program can provide a certain set of activities or services to participants. • *If* participants receive these services, *then* they experience specific changes in their knowledge, attitudes, or skills. • *If* individuals change their knowledge, attitudes, or skills, *then* they will change their behavior and usual practice. • *If* enough participants change their behavior and practice, *then* the program may have a broader impact on the families or friends of participants or on the community as a whole.	An after-school violence prevention program could have the following theory: Qualified counselors provide violence prevention training to children. Children gain knowledge of nonviolent conflict resolution and coping strategies. Children practice nonviolent conflict resolution and coping strategies. Children reduce their violent behavior and demonstrate improved social skills. As a result of the reduced violent behavior of individual children, violent behaviors in schools will decline.

Source: Holsey, C. (2005, October). What's your theory? Tips for conducting program evaluations. Tips for conducting program evaluation. (Issue 4 Newsletter) Wilder Research: Minnesota Office of Justice Programs.

Identify two assumptions you believe underlie the causal links in this program theory.

What do you think are the most important assumptions for successful implementation and outcomes inherent in this sample program theory?

Identify three risks that threaten the accuracy of the theory of change. These can include things (e.g., cultural, political, economic) beyond the organization's control that can derail program outputs and outcomes.

Program theories that focus solely on the assumptions and goals of policymakers are oftentimes conceptualized from the dominant paradigm. In such cases, the theories may fail to attend to issues of equity and social justice. There is a need for theories and programs that accommodate the perspectives of different stakeholders (Leeuw & Donaldson, 2015). In **culturally responsive evaluations**, evaluators go beyond simply attending to the funder's agenda in evaluation to also hearing and infusing the perspectives of the target community in determining the evaluation's purpose.

Evaluating Program Theory

Program implementation involves putting the program into effect using real people and diverse stakeholders in a specific sociocultural context where real-world issues can creep in to facilitate or impede successful implementation. When a program fails to achieve its intended results, it is usually due to one of two failures: program theory failure or implementation failure. Evaluating program theory can help distinguish between the two, but such an evaluation can only be done *after* the program theory is complete and clearly expressed enough to be reasonably reviewed.

Program theory failure results when the program is implemented in the intended manner, but the program theory was inadequate or incorrect, and therefore the program failed to achieve its intended outcomes. **Implementation failure** occurs when the implementation of the program is not carried out properly within that context. This can occur when real-world issues creep in and unanticipated problems can occur that prevent fidelity in program implementation.

Evaluation Theories, Models, and Approaches

While building their **explanatory framework**, in large part, from social science theories, evaluation theories are distinctly different from social science theories. Unlike theories of science, which provide empirically testable hypotheses, evaluation theories are conceptual positions or arguments posing a resolution to some fundamental question about evaluation practice (N. Smith, 2010). They can provide guidance in determining the purpose for evaluation and define what is acceptable evidence for decision making.

Evaluation theories reflect thinking about why we engage in evaluation—that is, whether evaluation is done for purposes of validation, accountability, monitoring, or improvement and development, and whether evaluation is a form of knowledge production, client service, social reform, or political control (N. Smith & Brandon, 2008). In contrast, a social science theory attempts to provide generalizable and verifiable knowledge about the principles that shape social behavior (such as social-cognitive theories, as described earlier). Using a military metaphor, Shadish, Cook, and Leviton (1991) characterized evaluation theories as follows:

> Evaluation theories are like military strategies and tactics; evaluation methods are like military weapons and logistics. The good commander needs to know strategy and tactics to deploy weapons properly or to organize logistics in different situations. The good evaluator needs theories for the same reasons in choosing and employing methods. (p. 34)

H. T. Chen (1990) emphasized the importance of distinguishing between descriptive and prescriptive theories. Simply put, **descriptive theories** characterize what is, while **prescriptive theories** describe what should be. Evaluation theories are primarily prescriptive in nature, offering a "set of rules, prescriptions, prohibitions, and guiding frameworks that specify what a good or proper evaluation is and how evaluation should be done" (Alkin, 2004b, p. 5). Evaluation theories are not predictive, nor do they offer an empirical theory or offer testing.

As the field began to judge the merits of evaluation theory, quality characteristics emerged for assessing evaluation theory. Shadish and colleagues (1991, p. 32) identified five general criteria for judging evaluation theory, asserting that a comprehensive evaluation theory should include a description of all these elements:

> *Criterion 1: Social programming*—the nature of social programs, their role in social problem solving, and the ways social programs and policies develop, improve, and change
>
> *Criterion 2: Knowledge construction*—ways researchers learn about social action

Criterion 3: Valuing—ways values can be attached to program descriptions

Criterion 4: Knowledge use—ways social science information is used to modify programs and policies

Criterion 5: Evaluation practice—things that evaluators do or should do (tactics and strategies) in conducting evaluation

The discipline's professional standards also represent a way to judge evaluation theory. Evaluation theories, like evaluations, can be judged according to the five attributes in which the 30 *Program Evaluation Standards* (Yarbrough, Shulha, Hopson, & Caruthers, 2011) are organized: utility, feasibility, propriety, accuracy, and accountability. The *Program Evaluation Standards* are discussed in greater detail in Chapter 2.

Why Should We Care About Evaluation Theory?

Many eminent scholars agree that **evaluation theory** is essential and should play a crucial role in guiding evaluation practice (e.g., Alkin, 2004b; H. Chen, 1990; Christie & Alkin, 2013; Donaldson, 2003; Mark, 2003; Shadish, 1998; Weiss, 2004a, 2004b). In his presidential address at the American Evaluation Association (AEA), William Shadish (1998) urged that

> all evaluators should know evaluation theory because it is central to our professional identity; it is what we talk about more than anything else, it seems to give rise to our most trenchant debates, it gives us the language we use for talking to ourselves and others, and perhaps most important, it is what makes us different from other professions. Especially in the latter regards, it is in our own self-interest to be explicit about this message, and to make evaluation theory the very core of our identity. Every profession needs a unique knowledge base. For us, evaluation theory is that knowledge base. (p. 1)

Similarly, in the introduction to *Evaluation Theory, Methods, Models, and Applications*, Stufflebeam and Coryn (2014) assert one theme of their book is anchored in their belief that

> the evaluation discipline should be grounded in sound theory—that is, a coherent set of conceptual, hypothetical, pragmatic, and ethical principles forming a general framework to guide the study and practice of evaluation. (p. xxix)

Donaldson and Lipsey (2006) argue that evaluation theory has become a

> central thread in the social fabric of the evaluation profession; . . . [it] can facilitate community amongst evaluators practicing across the globe, . . . and [can] help evaluators become better ambassadors for the profession of evaluations and educators of potential clients. (p. 61)

In Part I of her Voices From the Field interview, Christina Christie reinforces all of these assertions as she argues that evaluation theory is important to both enhancing our understanding of evaluation's role and improving its practice.

Voices From the Field

Christina Christie: Evaluation Theory! Why Should We Care?

We should care about evaluation theory for several reasons. Evaluation theory provides a framework to think and talk about what it means to do evaluations within a particular context. It gives us a language to speak about things, and it provides the evaluation community with a shared understanding of concepts such as stakeholders, users, and program participants. When we think about evaluation as a practice, we must think about the complexities that evaluators encounter. Evaluation theory helps us to understand some of those complexities and how to best conduct an evaluation study and engage the complexities that might arise in the context of any given evaluation. Evaluation is a different activity than research. Evaluation is intended to inform some decision and/or inform potential program improvements or modifications. Evaluation theory also helps us to understand how standards related to rigor and credibility shift and fit within the contextual constraints of the programs and projects that we study.

Christina Christie is a professor and chair of the Department of Education in the School of Education and Information Studies at the University of California, Los Angeles. She has served on the Board of the AEA and is the former chair of the Theories of Evaluation Division and the Research on Evaluation Division of the AEA. Veronica Thomas interviewed her in the winter of 2020.

While evaluation, as a discipline, has been criticized for being atheoretical and methods-driven, over the past 25 years there has been increasing recognition of the important role that evaluation theory can and should play in the field. Evaluation theories seek to answer the question of how to do evaluations in the most adequate and efficient way. They also often prescribe what is desirable for the evaluator to do.

Distinguishing Evaluation Theories, Models, and Approaches

Making a clear distinction among evaluation theories, evaluation models, and evaluation approaches is, indeed, a daunting task in the field. The term *theory* is conventionally used in evaluation literature; however, Alkin (2004b) argues that it would be more appropriate to use the term *approach* or *model*. Stufflebeam and Shinkfield (2007) utilize the terms *evaluation approach* and *evaluation model* interchangeably for ease of communication, more often using the former.

The inconsistency in usage can be problematic for those scholars truly interested in understanding real distinction among the concepts. For example, some scholars refer to a particular paradigm, such as empowerment, as a model, but others might refer to that same paradigm as an approach. Although it has not resolved the ambiguity in the field, N. L. Smith (2010, p. 384) offered the following distinction for consideration:

- *Evaluation theories* are explanations of underlying fundamental issues such as the nature of evaluation's purpose, valuing, evidence, and use; they reflect thinking about how and why we engage in evaluation.

- *Evaluation models* are those more or less coherent resolutions that provide a compatible set of prescriptions for how to conduct an evaluation; they are conceptual frameworks that incorporate positions (stated either explicitly or implicitly) on various underlying theories about fundamental issues.

- *Evaluation approaches* are those broader conceptual collections, often representing groupings or classifications of models sharing similar principles; classification serves to categorize related ways of thinking about and conducting evaluation (e.g., consumer-oriented approaches and participatory/collaborative are examples of such a grouping of models).

In this chapter, we choose to use the term *evaluation theory* to encompass both evaluation theories and evaluation models and the term *evaluation approach* to include grouping or classification of various theories and models.

Classifying Evaluation Approaches and Theories

Two classifications of evaluation theories have received considerable attention in the field. These include Stufflebeam and Shinkfield's (2007) five-category framework and the evaluation tree (Alkin & Christie, 2004; Christie & Alkin, 2013; Christie & Alkin, 2008; Mertens & Wilson, 2019). We briefly discuss these classifications in this section. However, readers are encouraged to read some of the sources cited to gain more detailed information on these two classifications of evaluation theories.

Five-Category Classification

In terms of evaluation theories (or approaches), Stufflebeam and Shinkfield (2007) classified them into five categories. A detailed description of each theory within the five categories is provided in Stufflebeam and Coryn (2014). In determining their categories, Stufflebeam and Shinkfield (2007) reported that they considered prior assessments of program evaluation such as Stake's (1974) analysis of nine program evaluation approaches; Hastings's (1976) review of the growth of evaluation theory and practice; Guba's (1990) book, *The Paradigm Dialog*, and his 1977 presentation and assessment of six major philosophies in evaluation, House's (1983) analysis of evaluation approaches; Scriven's (1991, 1994) writings on the transdisciplinary nature of evaluation; and a host of previous inventories and analyses of evaluation models found in the literature.

Table 4.2 includes a summary of one classification system put forth by Stufflebeam and Coryn (2014) and Stufflebeam and Shinkfield (2007) for evaluation approaches and theories. The first classification, "pseudo-evaluations," is included because the authors argue that to cover the state of the art in the field, it is necessary to include bad and questionable practices as well as best efforts in their classification scheme.

Table 4.2 Stufflebeam and Colleagues' Classification of Evaluation Approaches and Theories

Classification of Various Theories and Approaches	Description
Pseudo-evaluations	These are evaluations that fail to produce valid assessments and often are motivated by political objectives or profit motives; that promote a positive or negative view regardless of what might be the program's actual value; or that seek to misrepresent value interpretations about some project, program, or object. Examples include pandering evaluations, evaluations by pretext, and politically controlled studies.
Quasi-evaluation studies	Question-oriented approaches focus on a set of narrowly defined questions that might be derived from a program's behavioral or operational objectives, a funding agency accountability requirement, or an expert's preferred set of evaluative criteria (e.g., objectives-based studies, performance testing), and methods-oriented approaches focus on use of a particular method (e.g., experimental studies, cost-benefit analysis); they are grouped together as quasi-evaluation studies because both tend to narrow an evaluation's scope and often deliver less than a full assessment of merit and worth. Examples include objectives-based studies, outcome evaluation as value-added assessment, benefit and cost analysis, and experimental studies.
Improvement- and accountability-oriented evaluation theories and approaches	These approaches stress the need to fully assess a program's value and seek comprehensiveness in considering the full range of questions and criteria needed to assess program merit, worth, importance, probity, feasibility, safety, or equity. Examples include consumer-oriented studies and accreditation and certification studies.
Social agenda and advocacy	These approaches aimed at increasing social justice through program evaluation are strongly oriented toward democratic principles of equity and fairness and utilize practical procedures for involving the full range of stakeholders. Examples include responsive evaluation or client-centered studies, constructivist evaluation, and deliberative democratic evaluation.
Eclectic	These are approaches that have made no commitment to any particular evaluation philosophy, methodological approach, or social mission; evaluations within this category are designed to accommodate needs and preferences of a wide range of evaluation clients with the aim of seeking a program's merit and worth unconstrained by the parameters of a single model or approach. Examples include utilization-focused evaluation.

Sources: Stufflebeam, D. L., & Coryn, C. L. S. (2014). *Evaluation theory, models, and applications* (2nd ed.). San Francisco, CA: Jossey-Bass; Stufflebeam, D. L., & Shinkfield, A. J. (2007). *Evaluation theory, models, and applications*. San Francisco, CA: Jossey-Bass.

In the activity that follows, readers also have an opportunity to review evaluation studies that reflect these approaches.

Activity
Categorizing Evaluation Studies

Using the listing of evaluation-related journals found in Chapter 3 (p. 104), locate an evaluation study that takes one of these approaches. Indicate why you feel the study fits into this category. Also describe the evaluation's stated objectives, methods, and key results.

The Evaluation Tree

Alkin (2004b) stressed that when examining various evaluation prescriptive theories comparatively, it is helpful to have a framework showing how they are related and one highlighting features that distinguish theoretical perspectives. Thus, Alkin and Christie's (2004) evaluation tree and later elaborations of this tree (e.g., Alkin, 2013; Christie & Alkin, 2008, 2013) were put forth to describe the purpose and uses of various evaluation models and approaches. Their evaluation tree consists of three roots representing the foundation for evaluation work and supporting the development of the field in different ways. The three roots include (a) *social accountability*—stemming from evaluations designed to improve programs and society and the need for accounting, actions, or resources; (b) *social inquiry*—stemming from a concern for employing a systematic and justifiable set of methods for determining accountability; and (c) *epistemology*—addressing arguments about the nature of knowledge, often drawing from three major paradigms: postpositivism, constructivism, or pragmatism (Christie & Alkin, 2013).

The evaluation tree also includes three major branches that classify different evaluation theories by their primary focus on one of three essential elements of evaluation methods, values, and use. The evaluation theories and theorists aligned with the three tree branches include the following:

- *Methods theories* are guided by and emphasize research methodology. Theorists include Ralph Tyler, Peter H. Rossi, and Donald T. Campbell.

- *Values-based theories* maintain that placing value on the subject of the evaluation is central to the process; this branch is split into two fundamental perspectives, the objectivist influenced and subjectivist influenced. Theorists include Michael Scriven, Ernest House, Egon Guba, and Yvonna S. Lincoln.

- *Use theories* focus on the way in which evaluation information will be used and originally focused on the role of evaluation and those who will use the information. Theorists include Hallie Preskill, David M. Fetterman, and Michael Quinn Patton.

It is noteworthy to point out that Alkin and Christie did not view the theories on the three branches as mutually exclusive. A theory's placement on a particular branch of the evaluation tree was a function of its relative emphasis. Alkin and colleagues (e.g., Alkin, 2013; Christie & Alkin, 2008, 2013) have reexamined the original evaluation tree and made several modifications from its original presentation, including a repositioning of some of the theorists, the addition of other theorists, and a reconceptualization of the valuing branch.

Christina Christie indicates in Part II of her Voices From the Field interview what she sees as exciting evolving areas in evaluation theory related to the use, methods, and values branch of the evaluation tree. In particular, she discusses promising areas addressing program complexity, broadening methodological perspectives, and recognizing evaluator values and positionality.

Voices From the Field

Christina Christie: Evaluation Theory! Where Are We Going?

In terms of where evaluation theory is going, I consider some developments in the areas related to the three branches—use, methods, and valuing—of the evaluation theory tree. As for the use branch, the field is really pushing on understanding systems and trying to determine how we gather and share evaluation information for the purpose of learning in large complex systems. In terms of the methods branch, work is continuing to evolve, challenging the long-held belief that the experimental design is the gold standard and that quasi-experimental evaluation is subpar. Research on evaluation is expanding our understanding of how well good quasi-experimental designs approximate experimentally designed evaluations, with some concluding that strong quasi-experimental designs are equally as valid and rigorous as experimental designs. So much theory development is happening now around the valuing branch with emphasis on equity, diversity, and inclusion. While theories on the use and methods branches are where we get our procedures and prescriptions for practice, theories on the valuing branch provide positionality (or stance) an evaluator takes and the extent to which those values become part of practice. Culturally responsive evaluation, for example, takes program evaluation to another level. Thinking about what it means to be culturally responsive is a way for evaluators to think about their own values.

Students want to understand how they will know where they might fall on the evaluation theory tree and how evaluation theory will inform their practice. And, students who plan to be not an evaluator, but maybe an administrator or policymaker, want to know how evaluation theory can inform the work that they want to see get done. As such, evaluation theorists need to talk more about evaluation theory and the "So what?" question for practice.

Christina Christie is a professor and chair of the Department of Education in the School of Education and Information Studies at the University of California, Los Angeles. She has served on the Board of the AEA and is the former chair of the Theories of Evaluation Division and the Research on Evaluation Division of the AEA. Veronica Thomas interviewed her in the winter of 2020.

Mertens and Wilson's Four-Branch Tree of Evaluation Approaches

Mertens and Wilson (2019) point out that while Alkin's evaluation tree has some usefulness, it is

> limited in that it primarily reflects the work of white Western theorists and is not inclusive of evaluation theorists who are feminist, people of color, persons with disabilities, members of the lesbian/gay/bisexual/transgender/queer or questioning (LGBTQ) community, communities in economically poor countries, or members of Indigenous groups. (p. 40)

To redress with oversight as well as expand the evaluation tree, Mertens and Wilson mapped out three branches (or essential elements) of the evaluation tree—use, methods, and valuing—to three major research paradigms (discussed earlier in this chapter) used in the evaluation field. They concluded that the use branch maps onto the pragmatic paradigm, the methods branch maps onto the postpositivist paradigm, and the valuing branch maps onto the constructivist paradigm. See Table 4.3 for more of this mapping along with an explanation.

Table 4.3 Mertens and Wilson's (2019) Mapping of Major Paradigms to Christie and Alkin's (2013) Evaluation Tree

Christie & Alkin's (2013) Evaluation Tree Branches	Mertens & Wilson's (2019) Paradigms Mapping Onto the Evaluation Tree Branches	Examples of Theorists and/or Theories	Explanation
Use	Pragmatic	David M. Fetterman/Empowerment Evaluation J. Bradley Cousins, Jean A. King/Participatory Evaluation Michael Quinn Patton/Utilization-Focused Evaluation Hallie Preskill/Organizational Learning Daniel L. Stufflebeam/Context, Input, Process, Product (CIPP) Model	Theories/theorists place emphasis on evaluation approaches that facilitate use of evaluation findings.
Methods	Postpositivist	Donald T. Campbell Huey-tsyh Chen Thomas D. Cook Gary T. Henry Melvin M. Mark Peter H. Rossi Ralph W. Tyler	Theories/theorists focus on the methods mostly in the tradition of randomized controlled trials.
Valuing	Constructivist	Elliot W. Eisner Jennifer C. Greene Egon Guba Ernest House Yvonna S. Lincoln Michael Scriven Robert E. Stake	Theories/theorists place emphasis on the manner in which evaluation data are judged and valued, by whom, and the underlying issues considered to accomplish this valuing.

Mertens and Wilson (2019) expanded the evaluation tree to include a fourth branch—social justice—that is mapped onto the transformative paradigm (see Figure 4.1).

The social justice branch encompasses theoretical frameworks that have a primarily emphasis on advancing social justice. This branch includes frameworks such

Figure 4.1 Mertens and Wilson's Four-Branch Tree of Evaluation Approaches and Theories

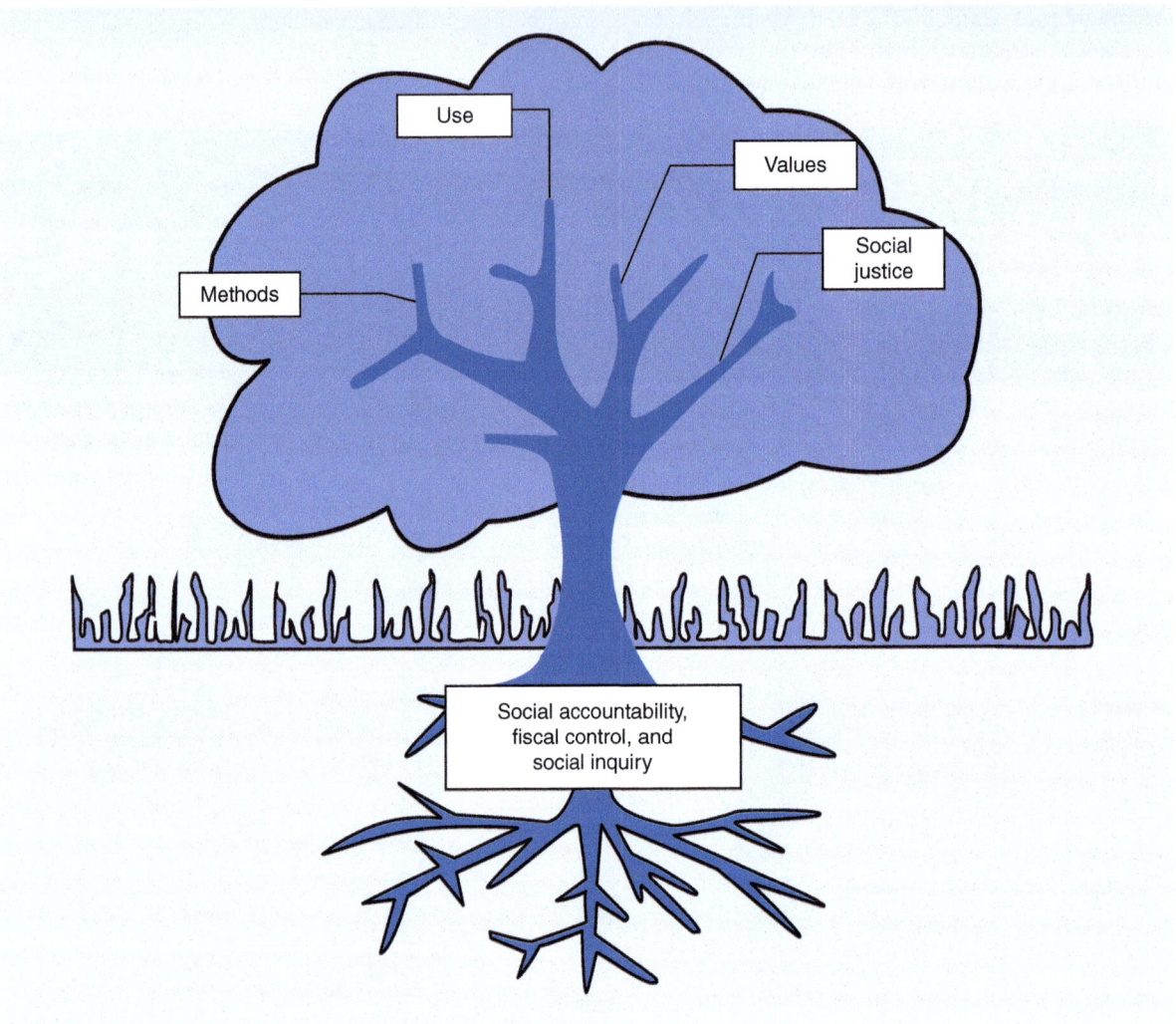

Source: Mertens, D.M. & Wilson, A. T. (2019). (2nd.) Program evaluation theory and practice: A comprehensive guide. NY: Guildford Press. Reprinted with permission of Guilford Press.

as cultural responsiveness, human rights, feminist, disability rights, Indigenous, and queer theories. Some theories and theorists that Mertens and Wilson placed on the social justice branch include (a) deliberative democratic evaluation (e.g., Barry MacDonald, Saville Kushner, Jennifer C. Greene), (b) feminist (e.g., Sharon Brisolara, Denise Seigart, Sharlene Hesse-Biber), (c) disability/deaf rights (e.g., Donna M. Mertens, Martin Sullivan, Carol J. Gill), (d) Indigenous (e.g., Fiona Cram, Linda T. Smith, Joan LaFrance), and (e) African American/critical race theory (e.g., Stafford Hood, Rodney Hopson, Asa Hilliard, Henry T. Frierson, Veronica G. Thomas).

Mertens and Wilson (2019) noted that, similar to Christie and Alkin (2013), they do not view the branches on the evaluation tree as mutually exclusive; instead, placement of the theories and theorists on the tree is primarily a function of relative emphasis within the various models.

Evaluation Theories Within a Cultural Context

Social programs and evaluations of those programs are entrenched in theories, including social science theories, theories of change, program theories, and evaluation theories. These theories derive from various sources including expert opinion, scientific research, and practical experience. As discussed in Chapter 1, our understandings of the world are shaped, in large part, by our understandings of culture—our cultural values and perspectives. Clearly, theories are not neutral inasmuch as they reflect implicit and explicit assumptions and biases about how people behave and how things work. A such, it is essential to interrogate theories for culturally embedded (and biased) perspectives regarding the definitions of social problems, the programs developed to address them, and the intended beneficiaries of these programs.

Cultural competence is not automatically present or absent in a particular evaluation theory. It exists, or fails to exist, as a function of how the researcher uses the theory in his or her work. The postpositivist paradigm, for example, suggests that by using the right tools we can capture and understand reality. This postpositivist position revised earlier positivist assumptions that reality exists independent of the observer and can be apprehended accurately by objective processes (Guba & Lincoln, 1998). As covered in other chapters, contemporary researchers and evaluators acknowledge that objectivity is a goal that can never be attained because research is influenced by the theories and biases of researchers. Culturally competent approaches that are consistent with postpositivism concede the difficulty of doing this work without the influence of our own cultural expectations and biases (Green, 1995).

An interpretivist/constructivist lens argues that cultural competence cannot be based on the acquisition of knowledge about past ways of life or undiluted cultural experiences in other contexts, but instead must be attained by focusing on immersion in the current lived experience of culture as it has adapted and developed to meet contemporary challenges; therefore, cultural competence requires readiness to engage with alternative, distinctive accounts of what is significant and necessary to gain an accurate understanding of the world (C. Williams, 2006).

Morgan (2014) argues that there has been a strong fit between pragmatism and social justice advocacy on issues of equity, fairness, freedom from oppression, and the need to build just institutions. Research embedded in pragmatism seeks to advance social justice through a problem-solving, action oriented process of inquiry based on democratic values and commitment to progress (Biesta, 2010; Greene & Hall, 2010; Johnson & Onwuegbuzie, 2004).

Using a critical paradigm, the evaluator draws connections between the problem under consideration and the oppressive, social, political, and economic arrangements that created and sustained the problem. The critical paradigm is squarely focused on issues of social justice through research that engages "with the historical, political, and economic structures that have contributed to formulations of ethnic identity, group status, and opportunities for individuals" (Williams, 2006, p. 213).

There are efforts toward more cultural competence in evaluation approaches and theories. For example, the AEA (2011) put forth a *Public Statement on Cultural*

Competence. In this statement, it stresses that culturally competent use of theory requires all of the following:

- Thoughtful consideration of alternative theoretical perspectives
- Fitting theory to the cultural context of evaluation practice
- Developing culturally specific theory where appropriate
- Balanced consideration of both strengths and limitations of cultural practices when theorizing
- Vigilance to avoid equating cultural variables with problems or deficits
- Embracing complex explanations attentive to how power works within systems (p. 6)

Evaluation Approaches and Theories: A Summary Description of Selected Examples

In Table 4.4, we summarize several of the extensively relied-on and emerging evaluation approaches and theories in the field, providing an overview of the approach or theory, its major proponents, and a description of its primary emphasis.

Table 4.4 Selected Evaluation Approaches and Theoretical Frameworks

Evaluation Theory/Approach	Theorists/Proponents	Major Emphasis/Description[1]
CIPP Model	Daniel L. Stufflebeam	Includes discussion of four complementary sets of evaluation focusing on project context, input, process, and product or outcome (e.g., Stufflebeam, 1971, 2004; Stufflebeam & Zhang, 2017)
Culturally Responsive Evaluation	Katrina Bledsoe Henry T. Frierson Melvin Hall Stafford Hood Rodney Hopson Hazel Symonette Veronica G. Thomas	Honors the cultural context in which an evaluation takes place by bringing needed, shared life experience and understandings to the evaluation tasks at hand (e.g., Frierson, Hood, Hughes, & Thomas, 2010; Hood, Hopson, & Frierson, 2015; Hood, Hopson, & Kirkhart, 2010; Madison, 1992; Samuels & Ryan, 2011; Symonette, 2004; Thomas, 2004; Thompson-Robinson, Hopson, & SenGupta, 2004)
Culturally Responsive Indigenous Evaluation	Nicole Bowman Joan LaFrance Richard Nichols American Indian Higher Education Consortium	Provides theoretical, methodological, and practical evaluation design and strategies for carrying out a culturally responsive evaluation of services and programs provided for and/or designed by Indigenous Peoples (Bowman, 2006; Bowman, Dodge-Francis, & Tyndall, 2015; LaFrance, 2004; LaFrance & Nichols, 2010; Waapalaneexkweew [Bowman-Farrell] (2018); Waapalaneexkweew [Bowman] & Dodge-Francis, 2018)

Developmental Evaluation	Michael Quinn Patton	Focuses on understanding the activities of a program operating in dynamic, novel environments with complex interactions; emphasizes innovation and strategic learning rather than standard outcomes and is focused on thinking about programs in context; particularly suited to innovation, radical program redesign, replication, complex issues, and crises (e.g., Patton, 2011)
Empowerment Evaluation	David M. Fetterman	Fosters program improvement through empowerment and self-determination; evaluator engages a diverse range of program stakeholders and acts as a "critical friend" or "coach" while guiding them through the evaluation process; seeks to increase the probability of program success by providing stakeholders with the tools and skills to self-evaluate a mainstream evaluation within their organization (e.g., Fetterman, 1994, 2001, 2015; Fetterman & Wandersman, 2007)
Kirkpatrick's Four-Level Model of Evaluation	Donald L. Kirkpatrick James D. Kirkpatrick Wendy K. Kirkpatrick	Aims toward offering systematic approach of analyzing and evaluating the results of training and educational programs; probably the best-known model for evaluation of training across four levels: (a) reaction, (b) learning, (c) behavior, and (d) results (e.g., D. Kirkpatrick, 1994; J. Kirkpatrick & Kirkpatrick, 2016)
Realist Evaluation	Ray Pawson Nick Tilley	Centers on finding not only what outcomes are produced from interventions but also how they are produced and what is significant about the varying conditions in which the interventions take place; seeks to answer the question, What works for whom, in what circumstances, and why? (Pawson & Tilley, 1997)
Systems-Oriented Evaluation	Beverly Parsons Patricia Jessup Margaret Hargreaves	Argues that program theories and evaluations are generally too linear in nature and that social interventions or programs must be viewed as part of a complicated or complex system; focuses on evaluating systems and not simply programs (Parsons, 2010, 2013; Parsons, Jessup, & Moore, 2016; Reynolds, 2007)
Transformative Evaluation	Donna M. Mertens	Challenges the old-school approaches that focused on problems and deficiencies and asserts that all social groups and communities have strength and assets and that people are experts in their own situations and contexts (Mertens, 2009, Mertens, Sullivan, Bledsoe, & Wilson, 2010; Mertens & Zimmerman, 2015)
Utilization-Focused Evaluation	Michael Quinn Patton	Stresses that evaluations should be judged by their utility and actual use with focus on intended use by primary intended users (e.g., Patton, 1997, 2008)
Values-Engaged Evaluation Theory	Jennifer C. Greene Jori N. Hall Ayesha S. Boyce	Espouses a democratic approach to evaluation that is highly responsive to context and emphasizes stakeholder values; seeks to provide contextualized understandings of social programs that have particular promise for underserved and underrepresented populations (Greene, Boyce, & Ahn, 2011; Greene, DeStefano, Burgon, & Hall, 2006)

Note: The publications cited are meant to be selective and not a comprehensive representation of the particular theory/approach.

SUMMARY

This chapter examined major paradigms, theories, and models that have informed the evaluation field. These include scientific paradigms, social science theories, program theories, and evaluation models, theories, and approaches. There are clearly too many theories and models to extensively cover in this chapter. Therefore, we focused our attention on those we felt have had a major presence in the field.

The chapter indicated how theories are capable of contextualizing and explaining the consequences of policies, programs, and evaluators' actions, including their impact on society and behavior and the role of social and institutional domains when doing evaluations. Social programs are generally conceptualized and implemented around a theory of how the desired change will or should occur. Social science theories can assist the evaluator in multiple ways. In particular, they can help evaluators assess the likelihood that programs will be able to accomplish certain objectives, guide evaluation measurement and design decisions, and provide a context for interpreting evaluation findings.

Another important theory in evaluation is program theory. This explains why the program does what it does and provides the rationale for expecting that doing so will achieve the desired results. Program theory includes a sequence of sets or logical chain of if–then relationships that link investments to activities to results. Essentially, it is the thinking behind how a particular program or intervention will bring about results.

Program theories, like social science theories, can be biased to the extent that they focus exclusively on the assumptions and goals of policymakers who operate from a dominant paradigm, and thus, they fail to pay attention to issues of equity and social justice. However, there are growing numbers of scholars in the evaluation community calling for program theories that accommodate the perspectives of culturally diverse and marginalized communities.

Evaluation theories, primarily prescriptive in nature, are conceptual positions or arguments posing a resolution to some fundamental question about evaluation practice. They provide guidance in determining the purpose for evaluation and define what is acceptable evidence for decision making. The evaluation field should care about evaluation theory, and evaluation theory should do more to connect evaluation theory with practice.

It is our hope that the discussion and activities in this chapter exposed readers to the diversity of theoretical frameworks in the field in terms of major assumptions, values, and methodological emphasis. We continue to encourage readers to critically think about and interrogate programs, theories, and models with a view toward their ability to exclude or include perspectives of individuals from nondominant groups.

SUPPLEMENTAL RESOURCES

Theory of Change: A Practical Tool for Action, Results, and Learning

www.aecf.org/resources/theory-of-change/

This manual, created for the Annie E. Casey Foundation's Making Connections initiative, defines theory of change using Casey's impact, influence, and leverage platform and shows community advocates how to create their own theory of change by showing the relationships between outcomes, assumptions, strategies, and results. The manual will assist users in

- learning how to create a theory of change with multiple community partners;
- understanding how a theory of change helps define and prioritize strategies needed to achieve results; and
- knowing different ways a theory of change can be used—evaluation, strategic planning, and fundraising, for example.

It also provides various examples of community change initiative theories of action, which are different from theories of change.

Using Theory of Change to Design and Evaluate Public Health Interventions: A Systematic Review

Breuer, E., Lee, L., De Silva, M., & Lund, C. (2015). *Implementation Science, 11*(63).

https://implementationscience.biomedcentral.com/articles/10.1186/s13012-016-0422-6

Despite the increasing popularity of the theory of change approach, little is known about the extent to which the theory of change has been used in the design and evaluation of public health interventions. This review aims to determine how theories of change have been developed and used in the development and evaluation of public health interventions globally.

Theory of Change

www.betterevaluation.org/en/resources/guide/theory_of_change

This guide, written by Patricia Rogers for UNICEF, looks at the use of theory of change in an impact evaluation. It demonstrates how it can be useful for identifying the data that needs to be collected and how it should be analyzed. It also highlights its use as a framework for reporting.

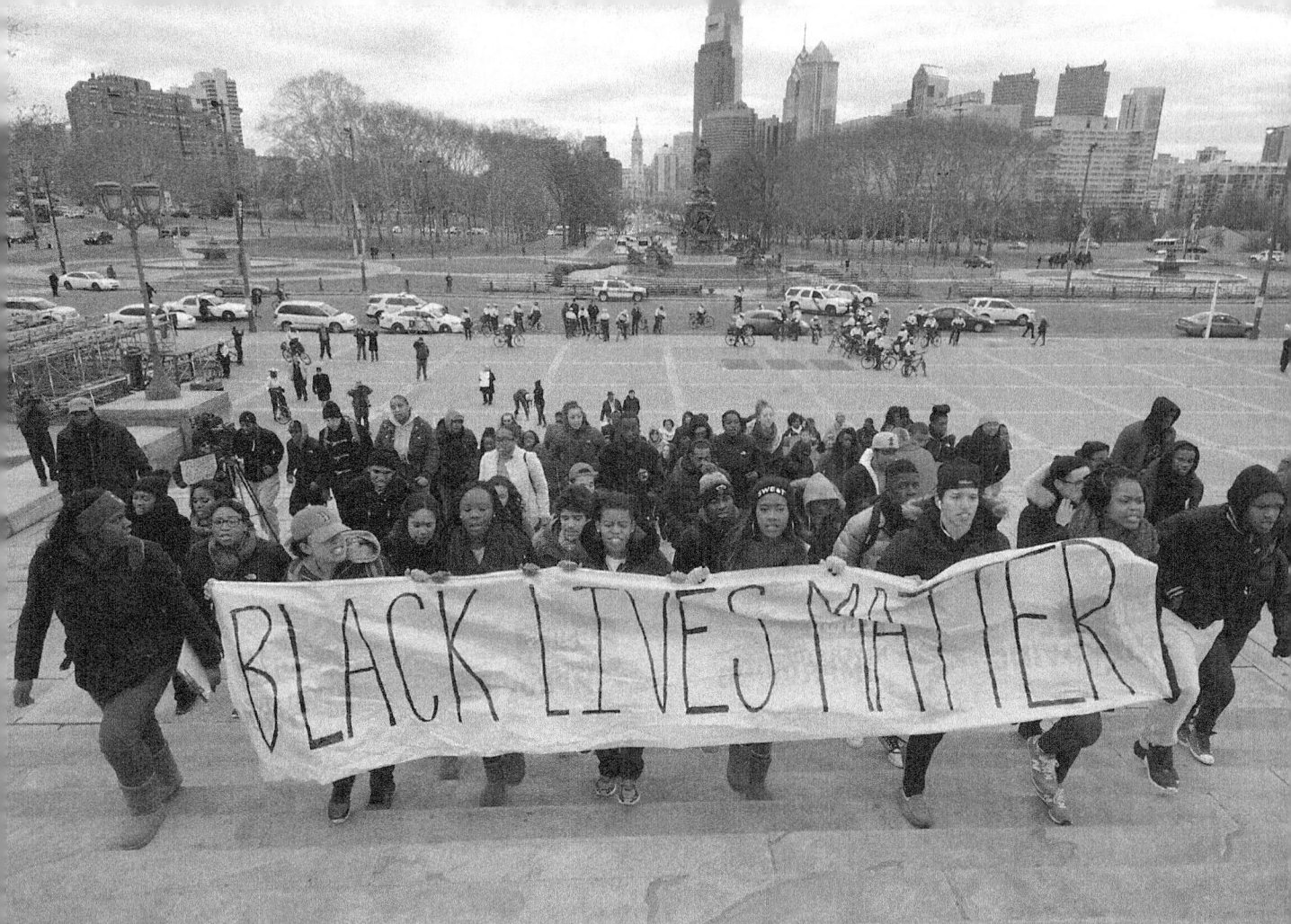
istock/Bastiaan Slabbers

There is growing demand for social justice in society and in evaluation and for moving past reliance on traditional paradigms toward perspectives that seek to address fairness, intersectionality, and racialized and other systemic oppressions.

CHAPTER 5

Social Justice and Evaluation
Theories, Challenges, Frameworks, and Paradigms

For evaluation to be in service to society, it must acknowledge society's diversities and attend to goals of societal improvement. To do this, evaluations, including their frameworks, assumptions, models, and methods, need to move beyond dominant paradigms (introduced in Chapter 1) to ensure that voices are heard, values and cultures are respected and included, and definitions of *expert* and *expertise* are expanded.

After reading this chapter and participating in the activities, readers will be able to meet the following learning objectives:

- Explain how stereotypes and behaviors tied to social justice ills such as racism, sexism, ableism, and homophobia can impact evaluation

- Discuss what it means to be a culturally competent evaluator

- List ways cultural competence should be a part of all evaluation designs and implementations

- Explain how critical race theory, feminist theory, queer theory, and changing models of disability provide a context for social justice models of evaluation

- Describe some similarities and differences among the following social justice–oriented evaluation paradigms and frameworks:
    - Transformational
    - Empowerment
    - Feminist
    - Participatory
    - Deliberative democratic
    - Collaborative
    - Equity-focused

Introduction

A major goal for this chapter is to present the need for social justice in society and in evaluation and discuss some social justice–based theories. A second goal is to help the reader understand the roles that evaluation has and hasn't played in social justice efforts and present evaluation paradigms and frameworks that have social justice at their core. We begin the chapter with an overview of social justice, including different definitions of social justice followed by a discussion of marginalized groups and the impact of a lack of social justice on people in those groups. We cover the concept of intersectionality (first defined in Chapter 1) and discuss its importance to evaluators, summarize theories that provide context for social justice evaluation, and discuss race, racism, and evaluation. Finally, we provide an overview of seven social justice–oriented evaluation frameworks and paradigms.

After completing the chapter and the activities, readers will be able to discuss the roles that evaluation has and can play in social justice areas and understand ways that stereotypes and privilege can impact evaluation. We expect readers to have an understanding of contemporary social justice–oriented evaluation frameworks and how theories such as critical race theory provide context to these frameworks.

Social Justice

Over the past several decades, there has been a growing body of literature tying social justice to evaluation practice. Barry MacDonald (1976) and Ernest House

(1980) were among the first scholars to explicitly couple social justice interests and evaluation. MacDonald advocated the use of democratic evaluation as a mechanism to depict the multiple realities of a program with justice and truth. He argued for democratizing evaluation knowledge and broadening the interests served beyond decision makers and experts to also encompass the interests of citizens, at large. House (1990) viewed social justice as "one of the most important values that the field should aspire to fulfill with evaluation being an institution for democratizing public decision making by making programs, policies, and decisions open to public scrutiny and deliberation" (quoted in Thomas & Madison, 2010, p. 571).

Definitions of Social Justice

As can be seen in Table 5.1, there are many different definitions of social justice.

Table 5.1 Different Definitions of Social Justice

Social justice is "a broad term for action intended to create genuine equality, fairness and respect among people" (University of New Hampshire, 2020).

"Social justice means the rights of all people in our community are considered in a fair and equitable manner. Social justice specifically targets the marginalised and disadvantaged groups in our society" (Workforce Council, 2015, p. 3).

"Social justice is a concept of fair and just relations between the individual and society, as measured by the distribution of wealth, opportunities for personal activity, and social privileges" (Wikipedia, 2020a, para. 1).

"Social justice is justice that follows the principle that all individuals and groups are entitle[d] to fair and impartial treatment. Social justice attempts to prevent human rights abuses. Social justice is based on notions of equality and equal opportunity in society. It focuses on the full and equal participation of all citizens in economic, social and political aspects of the nation" (USLegal, 2019, para. 1).

Social justice is the "fair and proper administration of laws conforming to the natural law that all persons, irrespective of ethnic origin, gender, possessions, race, religion, etc., are to be treated equally and without prejudice" (BusinessDictionary, n.d., para. 1).

"Social justice is the virtue which guides us in creating those organized human interactions we call institutions. In turn, social institutions, when justly organized, provide us with access to what is good for the person, both individually and in our associations with others. Social justice also imposes on each of us a personal responsibility to collaborate with others, at whatever level of the 'Common Good' in which we participate, to design and continually perfect our institutions as tools for personal and social development" (Center for Economic and Social Justice, 2020, para. 7).

"Social justice is really the capacity to organize with others to accomplish ends that benefit the whole community" (Novak, 2009, para. 1).

Different definitions highlight different themes. For example, some definitions such as that from BusinessDictionary (n.d.) focus on social justice as equal treatment, while others such as those from Novak (2009) and the Center for Economic and Social Justice (2020) emphasize the whole community and the common good. The word cloud in Figure 5.1, developed from the definitions in Table 5.1, illustrates, as would be expected, that *social* and *justice* are the two most prominently appearing words, with the next most prominent word being *fair*. As Eric Jolly points out, "fair is not always equal and equal is not always fair":

> You are working with two children, one of whom is seriously overweight. The other is seriously underweight. Your goal is to bring them both to good health. Is it fair to treat them equally? Will you achieve your goal if you do so? Of course not. Fair is not always equal and equal is not always fair. (quoted in Campbell-Kibler and Campbell, 2007, para. 8)

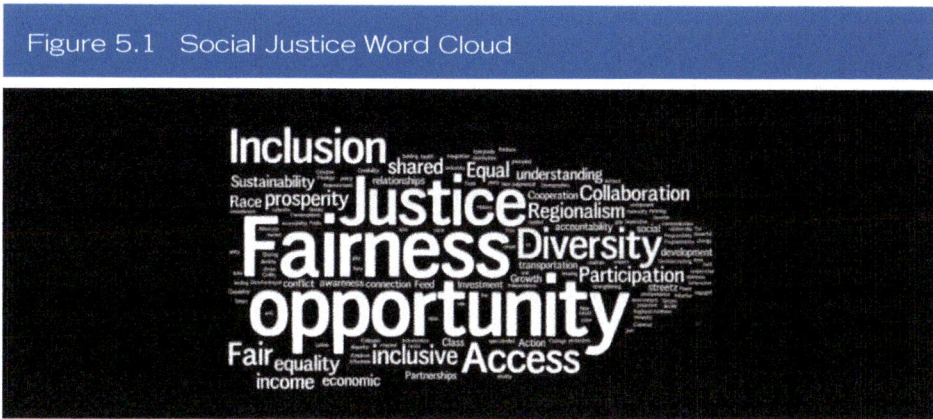

Figure 5.1 Social Justice Word Cloud

In the following activity, readers have an opportunity to reflect on and determine what is important to include in their own definitions of social justice.

Reflect and Discuss
Defining Social Justice

In small groups, discuss what you think should be included in a definition of social justice and why you made the choices you did.

Marginalized Groups

Issues of social justice tend to center on groups who are marginalized in society and thus have unequal access to opportunities and outcomes. The European Institute for Gender Equality (2020) defines **marginalization** as "different groups of people within a given culture, context and history at risk of being subjected to multiple discrimination due to the interplay of different personal characteristics or grounds, such as sex, gender, age, ethnicity, religion or belief, health status, disability, sexual orientation, gender identity, education or income, or living in various geographic localities" (para. 1). As well as groups who are marginalized, there are groups who are dominant in a society. As covered in Chapter 1, in the United States, the dominant groups are white, generally of European origin, and of middle to high income. Within those dominant groups, men who are cisgender—that is, men whose sense of personal identity and gender corresponds with their birth sex—are more dominant than others.

Being a part of a dominant group gives one many advantages, such as access to better schooling (Cook, 2015), better health care (Nelson, 2002), better housing and neighborhoods (Rice, 2019), and higher-paying jobs (Salsberg & Kastanis, 2018). These advantages are part of what is often described, as we discussed in Chapter 1, as privilege.

Impacts of Marginalization

The impact of being a member of one or more marginalized groups is substantial and needs to be considered when social programs are being evaluated. For example:

- "Although the longstanding achievement gap in the [United States] between [B]lack and [W]hite children remains, it has declined over the past 50 years in both mathematics and reading. The national *income* achievement gap, however, has grown over the past 50 years and is now larger than the [B]lack–[W]hite achievement gap" (Jank & Owens, n.d., p. 12).

- "In 2017, [B]lacks represented 12% of the U.S. adult population but 33% of the sentenced prison population. whites accounted for 64% of adults but 30% of prisoners. And while Hispanics represented 16% of the adult population, they accounted for 23% of inmates" (Gramlich, 2019, para. 5).

- The unemployment rate for Black workers generally hovers at approximately twice the unemployment rate for white workers. This pattern remains relatively stable over time even in the midst of high unemployment for whites (J. Jones, 2018).

- "Persons with disabilities [at all age levels] have lower employment rates than persons without disabilities" (National Center for Educational Statistics, 2017, para. 1).

- "Just 9% of students from the lowest income group finish college as compared to 54% from the highest income group." Over time, graduation rates are increasing at a much higher rate for students from the highest-income group than for students from the lowest-income group (Jank & Owens, n.d., p. 14).

- Americans with lower incomes tend to have poorer health compared to those with higher incomes (Chetty et al., 2016).

- Lesbian, gay, and bisexual youth make up 12.2% of youth in correctional facilities, while best estimates show that only 6% to 8% of youth in the general population identify as lesbian, gay, or bisexual. Almost 60% of incarcerated girls are **sexual minorities**. Data were not reported for youth who are transgender or in transition (Wilson et al., 2017).

- Gay and bisexual boys, in custody, were nearly 11 times more likely than heterosexual cisgender boys to report having experienced sexual violence by peers (Wilson et al., 2017).

Fixing the Group vs. Fixing the System

In social policy and social programming, the response to disparities such as those described earlier is often to "fix" the people rather than to fix the system that is behind the disparities. The belief has been, and too often remains, that disparities are the "fault" of marginalized individuals and groups. For example, people were told that the problems women face were "the result of our inferiority, weakness, madness, hysteria, having our periods, being pregnant or 'all in our heads'" (Schweitzer, 2017, p. 331). A basic tenet of **second-wave feminism**—that the personal is political—is an acknowledgement that many of the problems women face are the result of real inequities that hamper women as individuals and as a group from achieving their full potential (Hanisch, 1969).

A similar belief—that racial disparities are the fault of individuals of color—was part of the reason that African American Studies programs were established. One of the goals of African American Studies is to move society to an acknowledgement that while "race is not real . . . racism shapes life opportunities" (D. White, 2017, p. 4) and that "no American institution has been unaffected by racism, racist policy, or racial discrimination" (D. White, 2017, p. 3).

The reports of disparities and attempts to remedy them tend to focus on one or another marginalized group and do not acknowledge that individuals belong to a number of different groups, each of which has different amounts of privilege. Table 5.2 provides a visual representation of the variety of areas where there is privilege and where there is oppression.

In the following activity, readers look within themselves to define characteristics that provide them more and less privilege.

Activity
Finding My Privilege and Oppression

Look at Table 5.2 on the following page on privilege and oppression, and find demographic characteristics that may cause you to have privilege and other characteristics that are more likely to cause you to be oppressed. Write down one or two specific benefits you receive from being a member of a more privileged group and one or two disadvantages or challenges you have as a result of your membership in a more oppressed group.

Table 5.2 Privilege and Oppression

Privilege	Oppression
Able-bodied	Person With a Disability
European Heritage	Non-European Heritage
Gentile, Not Jewish	Jewish
Heterosexual	LGBTQ
Light Skinned	Dark Skinned
Literate	Non-Literate
Male	Female
Native English Speaker	Non-Native English Speaker
Traditional Gendered	Gender Fluid
Upper Middle Class	Working Class, Poor
White	Person of Color
Young	Old

Source: Morgan, K. P. (1996). Describing the emperor's new clothes: Three myths of educational (in) equity. In *The Gender Question in Education: Theory, Pedagogy, & Politics* (pp. 105–122). Boulder, CO: Westview Press.

As the earlier activity made clear, each of us fits into more than one group, and we all are a combination of privilege and oppression. For example, even the most privileged of us grow old and, thus, can become subjected to ageism. Membership in more than one marginalized group is, as was introduced in Chapter 1, called intersectionality. Crenshaw (1989) introduced the idea that when it comes to thinking about how inequalities persist, categories like sex, gender, race, and class are best understood as overlapping rather than distinct. The complexity of individuals' lived experiences can't be fully explained or understood by focusing on a single social category such as race or ethnicity. All of these characteristics interact. Using Black women as an example, Crenshaw explains how intersectionality helps us understand context and the complexities of discrimination and inequalities:

> The most common linguistic manifestation of this analytical dilemma is represented in the conventional usage of the term "Blacks and women." Although it may be true that some people mean to include Black women in either "Blacks" or "women," the context in which the term is used actually suggests that often Black women are not considered. . . . [T]his single-axis framework erases Black women in the conceptualization, identification and remediation of race and sex discrimination by limiting inquiry to the experiences

of otherwise-privileged members of the group. . . . This focus on the most privileged group members marginalizes those who are multiply-burdened and obscures claims that cannot be understood as resulting from discrete sources of discrimination. (pp. 139–140)

Intersectionality is of great importance to evaluators and evaluations. As is covered in detail in Chapter 13, intersectionality is directly related to the disaggregation of data, or the breaking of data into different subgroups to explore "what works for whom in what context." It also helps us understand, as Campbell and Jolly (n.d.e, para. 1) point out, that "as individuals we have many demographic characteristics including our race, gender, ethnicity, age, geographic location, education, income, disability status, [and] veteran status. . . . Rather than focusing on only one demographic category, high quality evaluations need to determine which categories are integral to the evaluation and focus on them."

Theories Providing Context for Social Justice Evaluations

As was introduced in Chapter 1 and is covered in detail in other chapters, theories and models based on the dominant paradigm may leave out the experiences and perspectives of those from marginalized groups and even contribute to the "fix the individual vs. fix the system" framework. A number of theories have gone beyond the dominant paradigm to bring to the forefront the lives and experiences of marginalized people and to develop different sets of assumptions about what research is done and how. As will be covered later in the chapter, these theories have influenced the development of evaluation frameworks that have a social justice perspective at their core. The following are short descriptions of theories tied to race, gender, gender identity, and disability. While the theories are different, there is overlap across them. For example, as Kosofsky Sedgwick (1990) points out, "In twentieth-century Western culture gender and sexuality represent two analytic axes that may productively be imagined as being as distinct from one another as, say, gender and class, or class and race. Distinct, that is to say, no more than minimally, but nonetheless usefully" (p. 30). Reflecting Crenshaw (1989), she also speaks about the need for closer attention to "the multiple, unstable ways in which people may be like or different from each other" (Kosofsky Sedgwick, 1990, p. 23).

Critical Race Theory

Along with pioneering the concept of intersectionality, Crenshaw (2011) was instrumental in the development of critical race theory and included intersectionality as an essential component of critical race theory. She and other legal scholars, including Derrick Bell, Patricia Williams, and Camara Phyllis Jones, popularized the notion of critical race theory within the subfield of critical legal studies in the 1980s. The assumptions and concepts behind critical race theory were then adapted for use in other groups. At the core of critical race theory is the acknowledgement that "racism is engrained in the fabric and system of the American society . . . [and] institutional racism is pervasive in the dominant culture. . . . [Critical race theory] identifies that these power structures are based on [W]hite privilege and [W]hite supremacy, which perpetuates the marginalization of people of color" (UCLA School of Public Affairs, 2009, para. 2). In 2015, Bonilla-Silva described the following tenets of critical race theory:

- Racism is "embedded in the structure of society."
- Racism has a "material foundation."
- Racism changes and develops over different times.
- Racism is often ascribed a degree of rationality.
- Racism has a contemporary basis. (p. 74)

Drawing on the first tenet of racism as embedded in the structure of society, Crenshaw (2011) points out the potential for normalization of racism where racial inequality can be seen as normal or natural rather than the result of a "racialized social system." This normalization can have a strong negative impact on the development and evaluations of social programs. If evaluations do not attend to how systems, at a variety of levels, may be perpetuating the discrimination and inequities that programs seek to ameliorate, evaluation results will be at best unhelpful.

In 2002, Solórzano and Yosso introduced five components of critical race theory. These components, summarized and further discussed by Thomas (2009, p. 62), included the following:

- Placing race and its intersectionality with other forms of subordination at the center of research
- Using race in research to challenge the dominant scientific norms of objectivity and neutrality
- Having the research connected with social justice concerns and potential praxis with ongoing efforts in communities
- Making experiential knowledge central to the study and linking this knowledge to other critical research and interpretive perspectives on race and racism
- Emphasizing the importance of transdisciplinary perspectives that are based in other fields (for example, ethnic studies, women's studies, African American Studies, studies on Chicanos and Chicanas and on Latinos and Latinas, history, and sociology) for enhancing an understanding of the effects of racism and other forms of discrimination on persons of color

From a research and evaluation perspective, critical race theory provides a framework for challenging established knowledge, analyzing racial inequalities, and exposing oppressive social and power structures.

Feminist Research and Theory

In the late 1960s, as part of the second wave of feminism, critical analysis was directed toward research, including social science research, and how it was being done. Research was criticized in terms of who was studied (generally men), what was studied (generally issues of interest to men), and how things were interpreted (generally from a male perspective) (Campbell, 1989; Harding & O'Barr, 1987). For example, women in their menstruating years were systematically excluded from clinical research even when diseases that affect women and men were being studied (Freeman et al., 2017). When women were included in studies, the results were often skewed. For example, investigations of sex differences were more likely to use the term *superiority* when the differences were in men's favor than when they favored women (Mastroianni, Faden, & Federman, 1994; Parlee, 1975). From these and other critiques came a focus on nonsexist research methods (Harding & O'Barr, 1987) and guidelines on reducing bias in research from organizations such as the American Educational Research Association (Shakeshaft et al., 1985) and the American Psychological Association (McHugh, Koeske, & Frieze, 1986).

In 1987, Harding argued against "just adding women" to studies as a model of nonsexist research. Rather, she argued for a focus on women's experience. Harding stresses that a "goal of social science research should be to provide explanations of social phenomena that women want and need rather than providing for welfare departments, manufacturers, advertisers, psychiatrists, the medical establishment or the judicial system with answers to questions that they have" (p. 8). She also argued for "locating the researcher in the same critical plane as the overt subject matter" (p. 8) to "avoid the 'objectivist' stance that attempts to make the researcher's cultural beliefs and practices invisible while simultaneously skewering the research's objects, beliefs and practices to the display board . . . the beliefs and behaviors of the researcher are part of the empirical evidence for (or against) the claims advanced in the results of the research" (p. 9).

Crossman's (2019) definition of feminist theory owes much to Harding's (1987) earlier work. She defines **feminist theory** as a theory that "shifts its assumptions, analytic lens, and topical focus away from the male viewpoint and experience and toward that of women. In doing so, feminist theory shines a light on social problems, trends, and issues that are otherwise overlooked or misidentified by the historically dominant male perspective within social theory" (Crossman, 2020, paras. 1–2).

A related feminist theory is **feminist standpoint theory**. Merriam-Webster (2020d, para. 1) defines *standpoint* as "a position from which objects or principles are viewed and according to which they are compared and judged." In feminist standpoint theory, social science research and evaluation are practiced from the standpoint of women or particular groups of women. Feminist standpoint theory draws on three important claims:

> (1) Knowledge is socially situated. (2) Marginalized groups are socially situated in ways that make it more possible for them to be aware of things and ask questions than it is for the non-marginalized. (3) Research, particularly that focused on power relations, should begin with the lives of the marginalized. (Bowell, n.d., para. 1)

Critical race theory and feminist theory have implications for evaluators and evaluations including highlighting the importance of looking not just at the individual but also at the context and the overall systems in which the individuals and the programs being evaluated are operating. They also address the "myth of evaluator objectivity" that Melvin Hall raises in his Voices From the Field interview in Chapter 1 and include an emphasis on the lived experiences of members of marginalized communities, which is covered in other areas in more detail in other chapters.

The following case study shows, making experiential knowledge a part of the evaluation can make a difference.

> ### Case Study
> #### Being Heard
>
> In an evaluation of a program for students defined as being at risk of school failure, the evaluator was in a conversation with two students who were helping with the evaluation. As part of the conversation, one student said, "I would like to get better grades, but if I do, they will kick me out of the program." The other student responded: "You can get good grades and still stay in the program; you just have to have a bad attitude." Further data collection and analysis found that fear of having to leave the program was negatively affecting student behavior, something that program staff did not know.
>
> *Source:* P. B. Campbell, unpublished evaluation study.

Jori Hall (2020) argues that in addition to addressing methodological issues, evaluators need to look at themselves and their profession and examine their own privilege. She points out the importance of "raising the collective consciousness of privileged communities or, in this case, the evaluation profession" (p. 29) and suggests that studying the liberation efforts of oppressed groups, such as Black Lives Matter, can help evaluators critically examine privilege.

Queer Theory

One of the key concepts in queer theory is the idea of "heteronormativity," which pertains to "the institutions, structures of understanding, and practical orientations that make heterosexuality seem not only coherent—that is, organized as a sexuality—but also privileged. . . . Heteronormativity is a worldview that promotes heterosexuality as the normal and/or preferred sexual orientation, and is reinforced in society through the institutions of marriage, taxes, employment, and adoption rights, among many others. Heteronormativity is a form of power and control that applies pressure to both straight and gay individuals, through institutional arrangements and accepted social norms. (University of Illinois Library, 2020, para. 5)

Queer theory "emerged in the late 80s and early 90s, deliberately appropriating the term of abuse usually hurled at gay people ('queer') in order to challenge its offensive meaning. It draws on French philosopher Michael Foucault's writings on sexuality and his notion that bodies are given meaning by discourse and social structures of knowledge and power. The binary oppositions (man/woman, gay/straight) on which discourse, and thus subjectivity, are founded are revealed to be not fixed, but fluid, fictional—and can, therefore, be destabilised" (Hanman, 2013, para. 4). For queer theorists, "sexuality is a complex array of social codes and forces, forms of individual activity and institutional power, which interact to shape the ideas of what is normative and what is deviant at any particular moment, and which then operate under the rubric of what is 'natural,' 'essential,' 'biological,' or 'God-given'" (Klages, 2006, p. 117).

For evaluators, keeping queer theory in mind when designing and implementing evaluations can mean that, regardless of the evaluation model, attention is being paid to participants who may be lesbian, gay, bisexual, transgender, or queer (LGBTQ) and to possible issues and conflicts. Being aware of the fluidity of gender, sexuality, and sex means having an awareness that what used to be considered stable demographic categories, such as gender and sex, can change and thus need to be questioned at each data collection point in longitudinal evaluations. Too, as covered in more detail in Chapter 12, it means that much like race, standard categories are no longer enough, and it is important for participants to be given an opportunity to self-identify their gender, sex, and sexuality.

Sexual minorities are likely to be present in many evaluation populations; however, evaluators may be unaware of their inclusion because of the stigma attached to participants "outing" themselves (Mertens & Wilson, 2019). Further, Mertens and Wilson (2019) stress that because of the sensitivity of issues surrounding LGBTQ status, evaluators need to be aware of and engage in safe ways to protect such individuals' identities and ensure that discriminatory practices are brought to light in order to bring about a more just society.

Disability Theory

In the 1960s, the civil rights movement began to take shape, and disability advocates saw the opportunity to join forces alongside other minority groups to demand equal treatment, equal access, and equal opportunity for people with disabilities. The struggle for disability rights has followed a similar pattern to many other civil rights movements—challenging negative attitudes and stereotypes, rallying for political and institutional change, and lobbying for the self-determination of a minority community (Anti-Defamation League, 2018).

The passage of the Americans with Disabilities Act (ADA) in 1990, and its 2008 update, was a major step forward. The ADA prohibits discrimination against individuals with disabilities in all areas of public life, including jobs, schools, transportation, and all public and private places that are open to the general public. It also guarantees equal opportunity for individuals with disabilities in public accommodations, employment, transportation, state and local government services, and telecommunications (ADA National Network, 2019).

A major effort of the disability rights movement has been to change the underlying models that impact how people with disabilities are viewed and treated and how programs that serve them are designed and evaluated. For evaluators, it is important to be aware of the different models, how they may be used in program development, and what implications their use may have for program definitions of success.

The **Medical Model of Disability** is one that is familiar to the general public. It assumes disability is an individual problem caused by disease, trauma, or another health condition. The "problem" requires sustained medical care with the goal of a "cure" or an individual's adjustment and behavioral change that would lead to an "almost-cure" (Disabled World, 2019).

A variation of this model, the **Empowering Model**, focuses on having individuals with disabilities and their families, rather than the medical community, decide the course of their treatment and what services they wish to benefit from, thus turning the professional into a service provider whose role is to offer guidance and carry out clients' decisions. Under both of these models, the problems that are associated with disability are individual problems, and society has no underlying responsibility to make a "place" for these individuals (Disabled World, 2019; D. Kaplan, n.d.; Retief & Letšosa, 2018).

A model of disability that is particularly damaging and is fortunately less prevalent today is the **Moral Model of Disability**, which holds people morally responsible for their own disabilities. Some cultures still associate disability with sin and shame for both the person with a disability and his or her family, which often leads to guilt, isolation, and ostracism. Another model that has been good for raising money but not helpful for self-determination is the **Tragedy and/or Charity Model** where people with disabilities are seen as victims of circumstance, deserving of pity (D. Kaplan, n.d.; Retief & Letšosa, 2018). The following case study describes one of the better-known examples of an application of the Tragedy and/or Charity Model.

Case Study
The Jerry Lewis Muscular Dystrophy Telethon

Every Labor Day weekend for almost 24 hours, from 1966 to 2010, the Jerry Lewis MDA Labor Day Telethon raised billions of dollars for the Muscular Dystrophy Association. While Lewis and other popular stars of the day were raising money, they were also fostering stereotypes and presenting people with disabilities as pitiable (Andrews, 2017).

In his 1991 critique of the telethon, which went on for another nine years, Ben Mattlin wrote that speaking of "the dystrophic child's plight," or calling disability a "curse" reinforces the offensive stereotype that we are victims. . . . Similarly, phrases like "dealt a bad hand" and "got in the wrong line" are unfair. Disability is not "bad" or "wrong." . . . There is no shame in needing others, no loss of dignity. Our needs are more personal and continuing than other people's—nothing to be ashamed of." (para. 14)

The work of the disability rights movement has led to a model of disability that promotes social justice. The **Social Model of Disability or the Disability Model** (Oliver, 1996) views "disability" as a socially created problem; that is, what makes people disabled is not their medical condition, but the attitudes and structures of society. In other words, this model argues that it is society that disables people. In this model, social discrimination is the most significant problem experienced by persons with disabilities and is the cause of many of the problems that are regarded as intrinsic to the disability under the other models (Retief & Letšosa, 2018).

Proponents of the Social Model of Disability make a sharp distinction between "impairment" and "disability." The point of emphasizing this distinction is to show how much and sometimes all of what is disabling for individuals who have impaired bodies has to do with physical and/or social arrangements and institutional norms that are themselves alterable (stairs vs. ramps, presentation of data using only auditory means vs. universal design for communication, restrictive definitions of job requirements vs. expansive accommodations for different modes of performing work, etc.) (Goering, 2015). In this model, impairment is understood as a state of the body that is nonstandard, defined as "lacking part of or all of a limb, or having a defective limb, organ or mechanism of the body" (Oliver, 1996, p. 22). Oliver (1996) argues that impairment is nothing less (or more) than a description of the physical body. Disability, by contrast, is the "disadvantage or restriction of activity caused by a contemporary social organization which takes no or little account of people who have physical impairments and thus excludes them from participation in the mainstream of social activities" (Oliver, 1996, p. 22). An illustration of the social model of disability in practice would show the design of a community with wheelchairs in mind, with no stairs or escalators. Here, the argument is that if our built environment was constructed in such a manner, then wheelchair users would be able to be as independent as everyone else in the community.

As indicated in the following activity, there has been discussion as to whether or not disability should be viewed primarily as a condition and whether or not people with disabilities should be viewed primarily as members of minority groups.

> ### Reflect and Discuss
> #### Medical Condition or Culture or Both
>
> Read the following two paragraphs and, in small groups, discuss your responses to them.
>
> Within the deaf community there are those who see deafness as a disability and those who view deafness as a culture and identify as members of cultural and linguistic minorities. While members of both groups may support the Social Model of Disability, those who see deafness as a disability may also see deafness in terms of the Medical Model, where through the use of such medical devices as cochlear implants, deafness can be "fixed." Those with the cultural view don't necessarily reject medical aid, but embrace the identity of being deaf (Berke, 2019).
>
> It is important in social justice evaluations not just to respect deaf culture and sign language throughout the evaluation process but also to review the goals and objectives of the project to be evaluated and the degree to which those goals and objectives reflect the concerns and values of the deaf communities involved (Mertens & Wilson, 2019).

As will be discussed later in the chapter, evaluation paradigms and frameworks, with social justice at their core, incorporate aspects of these theories in their work. For example, one of the goals of **empowerment evaluation** is to foster self-determination (Fetterman, 1994), while the **transformative evaluation** paradigm focuses on increasing social justice and engaging members of culturally diverse groups (Mertens, 2005, 2007, 2009).

In her 2019 Voices From the Field interview (see page 164), Ayesha S. Boyce speaks about the roles that these theories play in her evaluation decision making. "I think of myself as a critical scholar," she says. "For example, I inform myself by staying current with critical race theory and related research areas such as microaggression, microvalidation, and intersectionality research [which can have implications for evaluation]. I attempt to remain informed about these theories. It is important for evaluators to be aware of these theories and to read more than just evaluation literature."

Race, Racism, and Evaluation

Race and racism have major implications for evaluation as well as for society in general. As House (2017, p. 168) pointed out, "a critical task for evaluators in any evaluation is to identify potential biases that might impede their conduct of honest, accurate, and fair evaluations." He went on to specify three suppositions tied to racism and evaluation:

1. If a society sees itself as democratic, and in many ways is democratic, and yet is racist and does not recognize the extent or nature of that racism, the society will promulgate programs and policies that purport to help the affected minorities; many programs and policies will actually damage these minorities significantly.

2. Racism in America is not a simple vestige of the past. Rather, American racism is created and recreated in the present. Several identifiable social entities, mechanisms, processes, and structures currently generate racist beliefs and behaviors.

3. Evaluation plays an important role in these processes. Evaluation is not a cause of the racism, but for racist processes to have their effects, the evaluation function must be distorted, co-opted, or corrupted. (p. 180)

Referring to Ralph Ellison's 1952 novel, *Invisible Man*, Porter (2018) writes about how within the dominant culture, there can be invisible others:

> This form of invisibility comes into play when, as an evaluator, you work in a context and glimpse something that you cannot fully appreciate or you cannot even see a phenomenon. A social asset in a community that enables resilience is ignored, an organizational practice that puts children in harm's way is misrepresented. People are left behind because our frames of reference mean they cannot be seen, even when they are in front of you. This seems to require more than hiring evaluators who know a context. Not being able to see something is also rooted [in] underlying prejudices, which require personal evolution to confront. (para. 10)

House (2017) provides guidance to evaluators as to what they can do to reduce the impact of racism on evaluation:

> As evaluators, we should check our own predispositions. No white person growing up in this country can be entirely free of racial framing, and racist attitudes and activities are likely to be invisible and taken for granted. We should also check the work of our colleagues for such dispositions. And we should work together; we need help from peers on this issue, given the pernicious nature of racism. (p. 169)

One way to do this is to use a racialized perspective or lens, which, as was discussed in Chapter 1, is what we are doing in this book.

> Using a racialized lens should compel evaluators to reflect on their own thinking about race and to consider how this informs the manner in which they conceptualize, implement, and disseminate their evaluations. Doing so can provide invaluable insights in areas that might not seem relevant without this frame. (Thomas, Madison, Rockcliffe, DeLaine, & Lowe, 2018, p. 521)

As we said in Chapter 1, examining one's own biases and racial attitudes and stereotypes is easier said than done. Powerful, yet often invisible, predispositions are a part of an evaluator's implicit bias and racial framing. People are all influenced by implicit bias or attitudes or stereotypes that affect their understanding, actions, and decisions in an unconscious manner (Staats, Capatosto, Tenney, & Mamo, 2017).

Challenges to Social Justice and Evaluation

Traditional Definitions of Rigor

As will be discussed in greater detail in Chapter 11, often the quality of an evaluation is measured by the methodological rigor of the methods used in the evaluation, with rigor traditionally being defined as controlling for as many extraneous, or unrelated, variables as possible, which because of the complexities and real-life contexts of evaluations can rarely be done in evaluation. An overemphasis on rigor can cause some voices not to be heard equally, or at all, and can allow important differences in cultural context to be left out, making an evaluation less strong. To provide findings that can impact practice and policy, evaluations need to use designs that can answer complex evaluation questions and don't harm program participants (Johnson, Kirkhart, Madison, Noley, & Solano-Flores, 2008; Parker, 2004).

Deficit Models

As referred to earlier in the chapter, underlying many of the social programs that are developed in a wide range of areas including education, health, criminal justice, and broadening participation is an underlying assumption that program participants are deficient in some way and need to be fixed. The **deficit model** is based on the premise that deficiencies in a culture are the cause of differences between minority group members and members of the dominant group. "Evaluators must be wary of deficit models that, essentially, blame individuals for social problems, rather than consider how institutional practices or societal responses to the certain individuals or cultural groups place them at increased risk for negative outcomes" (Thomas & Madison, 2010, p. 571).

For example, deficit models assert that racial/ethnic minority groups do not achieve as well as their white peers in school and life because their family culture is dysfunctional and does not reflect characteristics that are considered important to the white American culture (Salkind, 2008). In this model, children of color are seen as lacking in some ways, as needing to be fixed and needing to develop skills valued by the dominant culture (Gerstein, 2016). A consequence of applying this model is that few studies of lower achievement in mathematics among African American students situate that performance into the larger context of mathematics teaching and learning in schools in the United States (Ladson-Billings, 1997). Too, Campbell (1995) points out in her aptly titled book chapter, "Redefining the 'Girl Problem' in Mathematics," that as long as the emphasis is placed on girls and their "deficits" rather than the environments and contexts, including the messages girls and boys receive about who is and isn't good in mathematics, things will not change.

When programs are designed to fix individuals' weaknesses as defined by the dominant culture, without looking at the context or the broader environment or the individuals' strengths, they are, by definition, not moving social justice forward.

Neither are evaluators of such programs who don't question the use of the deficit model. There are alternatives. As Parker (2004) points out, there can be an

> anti-deficit model where in education, for example, evaluators look at the resources available for students of color vs others, look at systemic factors and look at subjects from a strength perspective which values the capacity, skill, knowledge connections and potential in individuals and communities while not ignoring the challenges or spinning struggles into strengths. (pp. 89–90)

Cultural Conflict of Interest

Another challenge to social justice and evaluation is the presence of cultural conflicts of interest. As was covered in more detail in Chapter 2, we define a cultural conflict of interest as occurring when an individual's cultural mores (social or cultural rules) are seen as the norm, the right way, or even the only way. For example, in our dominant culture, individual success is privileged. We tend to see a successful person as one who does well financially or has the potential to do so. This limited view colors our definitions of what success is when we are looking to judge the success of programs, colleges, majors, and individuals. An evaluator's inability to recognize other views could mean, for example, that a job training program for Indigenous People would be found to be successful if participants found good jobs outside of the reservation, without considering the impact of their leaving on the community. Policies made based on these types of conclusions can decrease rather than increase equity and reinforce the dominant culture (Thomas & Campbell, 2017).

Efforts to Reduce the Impact of Racism on Evaluation

Illuminating ways to minimize the impact of racism on evaluation is a professional responsibility as well as an individual one, and the field in general—and the American Evaluation Association (AEA) in particular—has been taking greater responsibility in this area. For example, the Joint Committee on Standards for Educational Evaluation's *Program Evaluation Standards*, which were described in more detail in Chapter 2, include a charge to be fair in addressing stakeholder needs and purposes and to be responsive to stakeholders and their communities. Further, the AEA's *Evaluators' Ethical Guiding Principles*, which were also described in greater detail in Chapter 2, urge evaluators to assess and make explicit the stakeholders', clients', and evaluators' values, perspectives, and interests concerning the conduct and outcome of the evaluation. The AEA has also, as covered in Chapter 2, done extensive work on cultural competence in evaluation including, in 2011, releasing a *Public Statement on Cultural Competence in Evaluation* that was approved by the full membership and is available on its website (www.eval.org/ccstatement).

In 2017, with support from the W. K. Kellogg Foundation, AEA hosted a series of regional Dialogues on Race and Class in America to discuss how attention to issues of race and class must be a significant part of the evaluator's frame of reference and an explicit part of the evaluation's scope of work. The moderator, Melvin Hall, has two very significant takeaways from the project. The first is the need for evaluators to be more involved where important policy decisions are made because too often decisions are made without the benefit of evidence collected in a systematic and purposeful way. The second takeaway, which is of particular importance for this book, "is a concern that the training evaluators receive may not provide the skillset necessary to efficaciously handle the thorny issues of race and class when they emerge through an evaluation process" (M. Hall, 2018b, para. 3).

Cultural Competence and Cultural Responsiveness

As we pointed out in Chapter 1, all evaluators need to have cultural competence to be competent evaluators. They need to have the ability to understand, communicate with, and effectively interact with people across cultures in evaluation, and to understand and deal with issues of objectivity and bias (Campbell & Jolly, n.d.f; Make It Our Business, 2017).

SenGupta, Hopson, and Thompson-Robinson (2004) go beyond the relatively simple definition of cultural competence presented earlier to describe it as a

> systematic, responsive inquiry that is actively cognizant, understanding, and appreciative of the cultural context in which the evaluation takes place; that frames and articulates the epistemology of the evaluative endeavor; that employs culturally and contextually appropriate methodology; and that uses stakeholder-generated, interpretive means to arrive at the results and further use of the findings.
>
> Cultural competence in evaluation takes place through continuing an open-ended series of substantive, ethical, and methodological insertions and adaptations that aligns the inquiry process with the characteristics of the groups/contexts being examined. (p. 13)

Cultural competence is not mastery of a particular set of knowledge and skills. Neither is it a state that one achieves, but instead it is a process of learning, unlearning, and relearning; it is a stance where the evaluator is prepared to engage with diverse segments of communities to include cultural and contextual dimensions important to the evaluation (AEA, 2011). Culturally competent evaluators not only respect the cultures represented in the evaluation but recognize their own culturally based assumptions, take into account the differing worldviews of evaluation stakeholders and target communities, and select culturally appropriate evaluation options and strategies (AEA, 2011; SenGupta et al., 2004).

With the increasing emphasis on recognizing cultural diversity and its importance for ethical and high-quality evaluation practice, cultural competence is viewed as an ethical imperative that represents the intentional effort of the evaluation team to produce work that is valid, honest, respectful of stakeholders, and considerate of the general public welfare or common good. The *Public Statement on Cultural Competence in Evaluation*, described earlier, stresses that culturally competent evaluations emerge from an ethical commitment to fairness and equity for stakeholders and that sufficient attention to culture in evaluation may compromise group and individual self-determination, due process, and fair, just, and equitable treatment of all persons and interests (AEA, 2011).

As pointed out in Chapter 1, it is not enough for evaluators to be culturally competent; they must be culturally responsive and apply their competence to their work. An evaluation is culturally responsive if it fully takes into account the culture of the program that is being evaluated, where "the evaluation is based on an examination of impacts through lenses in which the culture of the participants is considered an important factor, thus rejecting the notion that assessments must be objective and culture free, if they are to be unbiased" (Frierson, Hood, & Hughes, 2002, p. 63). Frierson et al. (2002) explain that "culturally responsive evaluators honor the cultural context in which an evaluation takes place by bringing needed, shared life experience and understandings to the evaluation tasks at hand" (p. 63). Joined by Thomas in 2010, they added that "in order to accomplish this task [of conducting a culturally responsive evaluation], the evaluator must have a keen awareness of the context in which the project is taking place and an understanding of how this context might influence the behavior of individuals in the project" (Frierson, Hood, Hughes, & Thomas, 2010, p. 75). Chapters 8–14 of this book cover the "how to" or practical aspects of doing a culturally responsive evaluation.

> There can be consequences for evaluators not being culturally competent and responsive. Evaluators often interpret data and draw conclusions in isolation and without attention to bias. This results in a hierarchy of experts who "know more and know better" than those who are experiencing the work directly, or than those who bring a different cultural and historical orientation to knowledge and data. Additionally, interpreting and drawing conclusions from data without the participation of those engaged in and affected by the work inequitably takes ownership of knowledge and decision making power out of their hands." (Center for Evaluation Innovation, Institute for Foundation and Donor Learning, Dorothy A. Johnson Center for Philanthropy, & Luminare Group, 2017, p. 4)

The following activity provides readers with an opportunity to review a vignette of an actual event related to cultural competence in evaluation and reflect on how they would respond.

Reflect and Discuss
What Would You Do?

For a project on the role of cultural relevance and cultural competence in working with communities, an organization hired, without community input, an experienced white evaluator who had previously worked with the white director of the organization. The evaluator had no experience working with people of color as supervisors or equal partners although the evaluator had collected data from people of color.

People of color from communities involved in the project leadership questioned the evaluator's philosophy of evaluation and asked about the evaluator's experience and comfort with working with people of color. The director and other white senior project staff said the questions were rude to the evaluator. The evaluator suggested she, on project funds, would go to each of the four sites and learn from them about their culture and community and begin to build trust.

One of the community project leaders pointed out that, yet again, people of color would be asked to train a white professional about their culture and community to help the evaluator begin to gain experience with communities of color so that, because she is white, she would be more likely to be hired for similar evaluations than more experienced evaluators of color.

What do you think the evaluator should do? Why?

Evaluation Models and Social Justice

Regardless of the evaluation model or methods used, for an evaluation to be high quality, an evaluator, or the evaluation team, must be culturally competent—knowledgeable about the cultures involved in the program and project—and they must apply that knowledge to the evaluation. Any evaluation model can have a social justice aim, and findings can move social justice forward; however, this is different from being a social justice–oriented evaluation model.

We define a social justice–oriented model of evaluation as one that depends on a culturally competent framework and a social justice aim, but goes further. It includes a strength-based perspective that focuses on uncovering assets and strengths of communities, particularly marginalized communities, rather than simply uncovering problems. A social justice–oriented evaluation includes basic assumptions and methods that help to ensure that the evaluation will have social justice implications regardless of the topic. It plans for a process of learning and not simply judging and infuses the cultures of the target individuals, program implementers, groups, and communities throughout the evaluation inquiry process. Social justice evaluations situate the evaluand within its sociocultural, historical, political, and organizational context to better understand the antecedents and links between interventions and outcomes.

Earlier in this chapter and in Chapter 1, there has been discussion of the concept of intersectionality. As will be covered in more detail in Chapter 13, intersectionality is a key component in the development of any analysis plan that is part of an evaluation focusing on social justice. Many, if not most, social justice programs have as goals the improvement of opportunities and quality of life for individuals and their communities. Such programs may have differential impacts by gender, class, ability, ethnicity, and race and by combinations of those demographics. Without evaluations that are sensitive to these issues and intersectionality, evaluators may inadvertently support or recommend programs for continuation where the group as a whole gains, but those who are advantaged gain more than other groups (Hall, 2018a).

An additional component to social justice–oriented evaluation is **equitable evaluation**.

> Although equitable evaluation (EE) and culturally responsive evaluation (CRE) are heavily intertwined, and address tenets of one another, they start from different perspectives. CRE puts culture and context at the center of the evaluation while in EE, equity is at the center of the evaluation. Critical questions start with a historical perspective as related to equity, the design is intended to advance equity, and self-determination of the evaluation is key. (Bledsoe, n.d., para. 5)

There are three principles to equitable evaluation, as outlined by the Equitable Evaluation Initiative (2020):

1. Evaluation and evaluative work should be in service of equity.
   - Production, consumption, and management of evaluation and evaluative work should hold at its core a responsibility to advance progress towards equity.

2. Evaluative work can should answer critical questions about the:
   - Ways in which historical and structural decisions have contributed to the condition to be addressed
   - Effect of a strategy on different populations
   - Effect of a strategy on the underlying systemic drivers of inequity
   - Ways in which cultural context is tangled up in both the structural conditions and the change initiative itself
3. Evaluative work should be designed and implemented commensurate with the values underlying equity work:
   - Multi-culturally valid
   - Oriented toward participant ownership (para. 3)

Examining power and who has it and exercises it is key to social justice–oriented evaluation. As Mertens (2005) points out, in social justice–oriented evaluation, the inclusion of stakeholders with less power "is not only for accurate representation of their viewpoints, but also to empower the less advantaged in terms of being able to take an active agent role in social change" (p. 87).

Social Justice–Oriented Evaluation Frameworks and Paradigms

As was covered in Chapter 4, there are a wide variety of evaluation paradigms and frameworks. In Table 5.3 we highlight some paradigms and frameworks that have an explicit social justice focus. We have chosen not to include culturally responsive evaluation and the underlying cultural competence of evaluators as a separate social justice evaluation framework because we see it as an essential part of any high-quality evaluation. As discussed in this and earlier chapters, the application of cultural competence to make evaluations culturally responsive is an ethical imperative. And as will be discussed in later chapters, not being culturally responsive in an evaluation can negatively impact what questions are asked, what data are collected and how, what analysis is done, and what conclusions are drawn.

Table 5.3 Social Justice-Oriented Evaluation Frameworks and Paradigms

Transformative Evaluation	A metaphysical framework that "directly engages the complexity encountered by researchers and evaluators in culturally diverse communities when their work is focused on increasing social justice" (Mertens, 2009, p. 10).
Empowerment Evaluation	A framework that uses evaluation concepts, techniques, and findings to foster improvement and self-determination (Fetterman, 1994)
Feminist Evaluation	A framework that emphasizes participatory, empowering, and social justice agendas with gender inequities that lead to social injustice as a central focus (Sielbeck-Bowen, Brisolara, Deigart, Tischler, & Whitmore, 2002)

Participatory Evaluation	A process that recognizes the importance of the evaluator's role as knowledgeable insider rather than neutral outsider and facilitates development of trust between assessor and those being assessed (Shapiro, 1988)
Deliberative Democratic Evaluation	The use of democratic processes "to construct valid conclusions where there are conflicting views" (House & Howe, 2000b, para. 1)
Collaborative Evaluation	A process that "systematically invites and engages stakeholders in program evaluation planning and implementation" (O'Sullivan, 2012, p. 518)
Equity-Focused Evaluation	"A judgment made of the relevance, effectiveness, efficiency, impact and sustainability—and, in humanitarian settings, coverage, connectedness and coherence—of policies, programmes and projects concerned with achieving equitable development results" (Bamberger & Segone, 2011, p. 9)

These frameworks and paradigms do not include specific methods, designs, or measures. Mertens and Wilson (2019) point out that no single methodology is associated with the transformative paradigm. This holds true for these other frameworks and paradigms as well. The models can be applied with a variety of evaluation methods and designs that are covered in Chapters 11 and 12. Some of these frameworks can be used in conjunction with others. For example, a social justice–oriented evaluation could be done using both the collaborative and empowerment frameworks. The equity-focused framework could also be used in conjunction with any of the others.

It should be noted that there are times when, for example, participatory, collaborative, or deliberative democratic evaluations may be done in ways that do not qualify as social justice–oriented evaluation. Based on our definition of social justice–oriented evaluation, that could mean, for example, that the evaluation didn't have a social justice aim.

Transformational Evaluation

In 2001, Donna M. Mertens wrote that the development of an inclusive/transformative model of evaluation was driven by the following factors: "(1) a shift in population demographics; (2) the pervasiveness and intransigence of social problems; (3) the social consciousness that has undergirded the leaders in the field of evaluation since its inception; and (4) efforts to increase international cooperation among evaluators world-wide" (p. 368). Later, she explained how the "transformative paradigm emerged in response to individuals who have been pushed to the societal margins throughout history and who finally have a means to bring their voices into the world of research" (Mertens, 2009, p. 3) As indicated in Table 5.3, Mertens (2009) describes transformational evaluation as a metaphysical framework. By including the term *metaphysical*, Mertens ties the transformative paradigm to "the fundamental nature of reality and being" (p. 86), and she poses such questions as "How is reality defined? By whom? Whose reality is given privilege?" (Mertens, 2007, p. 216).

In her 2019 Voices From the Field interview, Donna M. Mertens describes what led her to develop the transformative paradigm.

Voices From the Field

Donna M. Mertens: Developing the Transformative Paradigm

Upon joining the faculty at Gallaudet University, I knew I could learn the language and the culture [of people who are deaf and hard of hearing]. I gathered my students together and asked them to have conversations with me about how research could be relevant to them. I give credit to the Deaf community for their willingness to be honest with me. Their impression of research was that it was done on them for oppressive reasons that characterized them as less than whole and as not capable. As a member of the research community I had to process the harsh reality that they were putting in front of me and ask some very serious questions as to how do we flip the script on methodology so that it becomes something that is a tool for liberation and transformation.

I looked for methodological literature that would talk about transformation. The literature didn't bear out that intersectionality was being taken seriously. We needed to find something that brought together what the feminists were saying, what the Deaf community was saying, antiracism work, and the variety of critiques of research. Not finding any framework that provided an umbrella for all the dimensions of diversity that are used as a basis for discrimination, I created the transformative paradigm.

Donna M. Mertens is a professor emeritus who taught research and evaluation at Gallaudet University for 31 years, and she is a past president of the AEA. She was interviewed by coauthor Patricia B. Campbell in the fall of 2019.

The transformative paradigm provides "a framework of belief systems that directly engages members of culturally diverse groups with a focus on increased social justice" (Mertens, 2010, p. 470). Along with "extending the meaning of traditional ethical concepts to more directly reflect ethical considerations in culturally complex communities," it attends to "power issues in terms of determining the evaluation focus, planning, and implementation" (Mertens, 2005, pp. 86–87). Others have slightly different interpretations. For example, for Greene (2008, quoted in Mertens, 2012, p. 804), the transformative paradigm "focuses on the tensions that arise when unequal power relationships permeate a research context that addresses intransigent social problems" while K. Jackson et al. (2018, p. 11) describe the transformative paradigm as "a research framework that centers the experiences of marginalized communities, includes analysis of power differentials that have led to marginalization, and links research findings to actions intended to mitigate disparities."

The following activity provides an example of a transformative study for readers to reflect on and discuss.

Reflect and Discuss
Applying a Transformational Paradigm

In 2013, a collaborative project was funded to better understand factors that influence partnerships between science institutions and community-based organizations when implementing informal science programs in

> underserved communities. The study included a group of 13 community advisors who represented historically underrepresented or marginalized communities. Their role was to reflect on and inform the implementation research. However, as the advisors explain as follows, that role changed:
>
>> In the fall of 2015, frustrated with results that did not seem to represent the realities in our communities, we asked to lead an autonomous strand of research framed from our point of view shaped by our community experiences. We believe that dominant-culture research focused on understanding diverse communities yields inaccurate results because the research questions, data collection, and interpretation of results lack the "unfiltered" worldviews of our communities. In addition, we feel that cultural norms, neighborhood characteristics, and unspoken considerations, tensions, and fears in each of our communities are difficult to address unless community perspectives are an integral part of the research. It is important to note that we conducted this research essentially on our own time, as funds for the research were not included in the original grant. (Purcell et al., personal communication, June 2018)
>
> In small groups, discuss the ways you feel this work was or was not transformative.

Empowerment Evaluation

In his 1993 presidential address to the AEA, David Fetterman introduced the concept of empowerment evaluation. He describes it as "the use of evaluation concepts, techniques and findings to foster improvement and self-determination" (Fetterman, 2004, p. 4). More colloquially, he explains that "in essence empowerment evaluation is the 'give someone a fish, you feed her for a day; teach her to fish, and she will feed herself for the rest of her life' concept as applied to evaluation. The primary difference is that in empowerment evaluation the evaluator and the individuals benefiting from the evaluation are typically on an even plane, learning from each other" (Fetterman & Kaftarian, 1996, p.11). Empowerment evaluation is designed to help people help themselves and improve their programs using a form of self-evaluation and reflection. Participants conduct their own evaluations often with the help of an outside evaluator who serves as a coach or facilitator. In empowerment evaluation, program participants learn to continually assess their progress toward self-determined goals and to reshape their plans and strategies according to this assessment (Fetterman, 1994).

Fetterman and Wandersman (2007) proposed the following guiding principles for empowerment evaluation, which they reiterated in 2017: "(1) improvement, (2) community ownership, (3) inclusion, (4) democratic participation, (5) social justice, (6) community knowledge, (7) evidence-based strategies, (8) capacity building, (9) organizational learning, and (10) accountability" (p. 134). With empowerment evaluation, they "are educating others to manage their own affairs in areas they know (or should know) better than we do. At the same time, we are creating new roles for evaluators to help others help themselves" (Fetterman & Wandersman, 2017, p. 133). The following case studies describe the wide variety of areas in which empowerment evaluation has been applied.

> ## Case Studies
> ### Empowerment Evaluation Around the World
>
> In their 2017 celebration of the 21st anniversary of empowerment evaluation, David Fetterman and Abraham Wandersman listed ways empowerment evaluation has been used, including
>
> - by educators to improve schools in academic distress in rural Arkansas;
> - by teachers evaluating their own impact within the internationally practiced Visible Learning model;
> - by faculty, students, and administrators preparing for accreditation review in the School of Medicine at Stanford University;
> - by Peruvian women to build small businesses and become more economically self-sufficient; and
> - by fourth- and fifth-grade students to make their school more inclusive and inviting.
>
> Empowerment evaluation has also been used in teen pregnancy prevention and substance abuse prevention programs, to help bridge the digital divide in communities of color and in minority tobacco prevention initiatives. Empowerment evaluation has been used in remote Amazonian regions and squatter settlements in South Africa, as well as high-tech settings like Google and Hewlett-Packard in Silicon Valley. (Fetterman & Wandersman, 2017, p. 134)

Feminist Evaluation

Feminist evaluation emphasizes participation, empowerment, and social justice. Like the other social justice–oriented frameworks, it does not advocate a precise approach, but may be defined as a way of thinking about evaluation (Seigart & Brisolara, 2002). There are six basic tenets to feminist evaluation, as Sielbeck-Bowen, Brisolara, Seigart, Tischler, and Whitmore (2002) have described:

1. Feminist evaluation has as a central focus the gender inequities that lead to social injustice.

2. Discrimination or inequality based on gender is systemic and structural.

3. Evaluation is a political activity; the contexts in which evaluation operates are politicized; and the personal experiences, perspectives, and characteristics evaluators bring to evaluations (and with which we interact) lead to a particular political stance. A feminist evaluation encourages an evaluator to view her- or himself as an activist.

4. Knowledge is a powerful resource that serves an explicit or implicit purpose.

5. Knowledge should be a resource of and for the people who create, hold, and share it. Consequently, the evaluation or research process can lead to significant negative or positive effects on the people involved in the evaluation/research. Knowledge and values are culturally, socially, and temporally contingent. Knowledge is also filtered through the knower.

6. There are multiple ways of knowing; some ways are privileged over others.

Based on their experiences with feminist evaluation, Sielbeck-Mathes and Selove (2014) suggest that

> in order to gain attention and respect for the adoption of feminist frameworks, principles, and values for conducting program evaluation, it is imperative that we frame our conversations to connect rather than compete, align rather than malign and foster acceptance rather than objection from those we need to communicate to and with. This requires an understanding of [others'] position on issues that follow from the language or lens of their value and belief systems. (para. 3)

They go on to argue that

> key tasks associated with feminist evaluation include 1) understanding the problem from the perspective of the women the program is designed to serve, 2) studying the interior and external context of the program to understand the realities and lived experiences of women, and 3) identifying the invisible structures that can undermine even the most diverse, gender-responsive, trauma informed program. (Sielbeck-Mathes & Selove, 2014, para. 5)

Participatory Evaluation

In participatory evaluation, Shapiro (1988) calls for program evaluators to assume the role of both independent outsider and knowledgeable insider. Here, the evaluator and the participants can better examine and expose the intended and unintended consequences and benefits of the programs. As she explains, "an evaluator who is a participant in a sense of the member of the group, or has familiarity and trust with that group, is in a better position to ask the right questions to illuminate the complexity of the issue under investigation" (Shapiro, 1988, p. 88). It is a process that recognizes the importance of the evaluator's role as knowledgeable insider rather than neutral outsider and facilitates development of trust between assessor and those being assessed (Shapiro, 1988). While participatory evaluation didn't grow out of feminist theory, Shapiro feels that participatory evaluation is compatible with feminist theory and practice.

In 2002, the Partnership for Public Health published a guide to participatory evaluation, where the authors compared participatory evaluation to conventional evaluation. The primary difference they reported was that in participatory evaluation, project staff, members of the community, and/or other stakeholders drive the evaluation and, with the evaluator, determine the indicators of program progress and are responsible for data collection, analysis, and preparation of the final report. In conventional evaluation, it's the funders and program leaders who drive the evaluation and the professional evaluators and outside experts who determine the indicators and implement the evaluation including writing up the final report. In participatory evaluation the evaluator is seen more as a facilitator and a critical friend, while in conventional evaluations the evaluator is the expert (Zukoski & Luluquisen, 2002). Because of their emphasis on local knowledge, participatory evaluations are most appropriately used when

- there are questions about program implementation difficulties;
- there are questions about program effects on beneficiaries; [and]
- information is wanted on a stakeholder's knowledge of a program or views of progress. (Zukoski & Luluquisen, 2002, p. 3)

Conventional evaluations, it is felt, are better used when

- there is a need for independent judgment;
- specialized information is needed that only experts can provide; [and]
- program indicators are standardized, rather than particular to a program. (Zukoski & Luluquisen, 2002, p. 3)

The following case study provides an example of a participatory evaluation process.

Case Study
Students as Evaluators

In the mid-1980s, I began working with students as evaluators in New York City and continue to do so. In the student evaluator model, working with an experienced evaluator/facilitator, young people design and carry out evaluations of specific programs in which they are involved. They are Shapiro's (1988) "knowledgeable insiders." Students participating as student evaluators include middle school students, students who have been classified as "at risk," students in gifted and talented programs, and returning dropouts. Each group of student evaluators either is participating in a specific program or has participated in the program in the recent past. Along with being a part of the process to determine the questions to be answered by the evaluation and designing the evaluation, they present their data-based conclusions and recommendations to the program directors, who have made a commitment either to implement the students' recommendations or to explain why they won't or can't do so.

The student evaluator model is a powerful tool that allows young people to assess their own effectiveness and impact of their programs through a carefully guided process. The information that the students gather would not otherwise be known to program coordinators and administrators.

Source: Adapted from Campbell, P.B,, Edgar, S. & Halsted, A.L. (1994). Students as evaluators: A model for program evaluation. *Phi Delta Kappan.*, 76, 160–164.

Deliberative Democratic Evaluation

Deliberative democratic evaluation has as its goal "to construct valid conclusions where there are conflicting views. The approach extends impartiality by including relevant interests, values, and views so that conclusions can be unbiased in value as well as factual aspects" (House & Howe, 2000b, para. 1). House and Howe (2003) explain their view this way:

> In our opinion, no one has formulated better ways of reconciling conflicting perspectives, values, and interests than through democratic processes, imperfect though such processes might be. When evaluators encounter differing perspectives, they would do well to incorporate procedures that have served other democratic institutions. In our judgment, the conclusions of the evaluation will be more valid, the study will be perceived as more legitimate, and the ensuing public discussion will be more productive. (p. 80)

As with the other social justice–oriented frameworks, this approach employs traditional data collection and analysis techniques but, unlike participatory evaluation, relies heavily on the expertise of the evaluator. Like participatory evaluation, stakeholder perspectives are collected, processed, and analyzed "in a systematic, unbiased fashion, making those perspectives part of the process of arriving at evaluative conclusions" (House & Howe, 2003, p. 79). However, "in the deliberative democratic approach the evaluator is still in charge of the evaluation study and responsible for the findings, but stakeholder perspectives, values, and interests become an integral part of the study" (House & Howe, 2003, p. 79).

Howe and Ashcraft (2005) point out that

> the deliberative democratic approach to evaluation is grounded in deliberative democratic theory, which adopts a relatively strong stance toward stakeholder participation. Deliberate democratic theory emphasizes developing political practices and institutions that mitigate power imbalances among citizens so as to permit their free and equal participation. A necessary feature of practices and institutions that satisfy this ideal is that the procedures are designed to engage participants in genuine deliberation, motivated by the goal of fostering the common good, rather than engaging them in strategic bargaining, motivated by the goal of maximizing their perceived self-interest. (pp. 2275–2276)

In 2005, Howe and Ashcraft described the application of a deliberative democratic approach to the evaluation of school choice policy in the Boulder (Colorado) Valley School District. They found in their application of the model that "deliberative democratic evaluation cannot be a democratic practice unto itself. Rather, it must be seen as contributing to deliberations carried out by other democratic bodies, a school board, in this case" (p. 2295). In spite of the difficulties, they concluded that "it does not follow that evaluations should simply gather the information sought by the powers that be and feed it into democratic bodies" (pp. 2295–2296) and explained that evaluations must observe the principles of deliberative democratic evaluation if they are to provide the grist for genuine democratic deliberation. Deliberative democratic evaluation has three basic principles—inclusion, dialogue, and deliberation—that are listed as follows with accompanying questions reflecting each.

1. Inclusion
    a. Whose interests are represented in the evaluation?
    b. Are all major stakeholders represented?
    c. Should some stakeholders be excluded?
2. Dialogue
    a. Do power imbalances distort or impede dialogue and deliberation?
    b. Are there procedures to control power imbalances?
    c. In what ways do stakeholders participate?
    d. How authentic is the participation?
    e. How involved is the interaction?

3. Deliberation
   a. Is there reflective deliberation?
   b. How extensive is the deliberation?
   c. How well considered is the deliberation? (House & Howe, 2000b, pp. 2–3)

Collaborative Evaluation

"*Collaborative evaluation* is a term widely used in evaluation, [and] its meaning varies considerably. Often used interchangeably with *participatory* and/or *empowerment evaluation*, the terms can be used to mean different things, which can be confusing" (O'Sullivan, 2012, p. 518, italics added). We are using O'Sullivan and D'Agostino's (2002) definition of collaborative evaluation as an approach that engages program stakeholders actively in the evaluation process. When stakeholders collaborate with evaluators, their understanding increases, and the utility of the evaluation is often enhanced. Like participatory evaluation, in collaborative evaluation, stakeholders share responsibility for the evaluation; evaluation questions are developed together; evaluation expertise grows among board members, parents, teachers, service providers, and other key stakeholders; and evaluation evidence is used for program improvement (O'Sullivan & D'Agostino, 2002). "It systematically invites and engages stakeholders in program evaluation planning and implementation" (O'Sullivan, 2012, p. 518).

Collaborative evaluation distinguishes itself from other evaluation frameworks that include an emphasis on participation and collaboration, in that it uses a sliding scale for levels of collaboration. This means that different program evaluations will experience different levels of collaborative activity. Table 5.4 provides an overview of the opportunities and challenges of using a collaborative approach to evaluation based on the experiences of a group of evaluators from South Africa and the United States. While they were focusing on collaborations with nongovernmental organizations (NGOs), their conclusions hold for collaborations with a variety of organizations.

Table 5.4 Opportunities and Challenges of Applying a Collaborative Approach to Evaluation

Opportunities

- Hands-on learning by doing
- NGOs know their programmes and contexts
- Demystification of the evaluation process for NGO staff
- Co-ownership of the evaluation
- Human capacity building in monitoring and evaluation skills
- Evaluation is manageable and meaningful
- Evaluation reports are "user-friendly"
- Shared decision making and responsibility

Challenges

- Converging diverse skills and experiences
- Collaboration takes time
- NGOs have high staff turnover
- Unrealistic expectations
- Reactions to results
- Cost implications

Source: Diamini et al. (1997, pp. 26–31).

Equity-Focused Evaluation

Bamberger and Segone (2011, p. 9) describe **equity-focused evaluation** as

> a judgment made of the relevance, effectiveness, efficiency, impact and sustainability—and, in humanitarian settings, coverage, connectedness and coherence—of policies, programmes and projects concerned with achieving equitable development results.
>
> The goal of equity-focused evaluation, which is most frequently used in international work, is to provide "assessments of what works and what does not work to reduce inequity, and it highlights intended and unintended results for worst-off groups as well as the gaps between best-off, average and worst-off groups. It provides strategic lessons to guide decision-makers and to inform stakeholders" (Bamberger & Segone, 2011, p. 9).
>
> Equity-focused evaluations provide evidence-based information that is credible, reliable and useful, enabling the timely incorporation of findings, recommendations and lessons into the decision-making process. (Bamberger & Segone, 2011, p. 9)

In many ways that reflects social justice–oriented evaluation models in general. However, Bamberger and Segone (2011) also say equity-focused evaluation "involves a rigorous, systematic and objective process in the design, analysis and interpretation of information in order to answer specific questions, including those of concern to worst-off groups" (p. 9). Their use of an "objective process" can be problematic from a social justice perspective. As discussed in Chapter 1, we are not objective, and too often that which is seen as objective is that which reflects the dominant paradigm, including the values and beliefs held by those who are most powerful or dominant in a society. Similarly, the use of "rigor" in this definition can also be problematic from a social justice perspective. As we indicated earlier and will describe in more detail in Chapter 11, traditional definitions of rigor target having as much control over the environment as possible so only one variable can be examined. In the messiness and complexity of social justice programs or in programs in general, an emphasis on control can be problematic. The following case studies provide some examples of equity-focused evaluation.

> ## Case Study
> ### Equity-Focused Evaluation Case Studies
>
> These case studies illustrate different ways in which equity-focused evaluations have been designed and used by UNICEF and its partners.
>
> Evaluation of the UNICEF Education Programme in Timor-L'Este 2003–2009. "This case illustrates how equity issues can be addressed in a context where there is only limited access to quantitative data, and the evaluation must mainly rely on a mixed-method approach" (Bamberger & Segone, 2011, p. 98).
>
> Evaluating the equity outcomes of the Cambodia Community Led Total Sanitation Project. "One of the central objectives of the project was to develop methodologies to ensure the participation of all sectors of the population, including the poorest and most vulnerable. A central goal of the evaluation was to assess the equity outcomes of the project" (Bamberger & Segone, 2011, p. 98).

Bamberger and Segone (2011) point out that, reflecting empowerment evaluation, "equity-focused evaluation processes should be used to empower worst-off groups to the maximum extent possible, as well as to ensure that evaluation questions are relevant to the situation of these groups" (p. 12). Also, reflecting the basics of cultural competence, equity-focused evaluators "should be culturally sensitive and pay high attention to ethics . . . [and] sensitive to local beliefs, manners and customs and act with integrity and honesty in their relationships with all stakeholders, including worst-off groups" (p. 12). In her 2019 Voices From the Field interview, Ayesha S. Boyce speaks about some practical ways that evaluators can infuse social justice into all of their evaluations.

Voices From the Field

Ayesha S. Boyce: Applying Social Justice Perspectives to My Evaluations

Social justice is often an add-on to evaluations. To include it takes more work and more time, usually for the same amount of money, but it is important to do. I bring up equity, diversity, and inclusion (EDI) at two different levels in evaluations—informal and formal. Informally, I bring up issues of EDI in conversations, in meetings, and in emails. It allows me to ask if there are any diversity efforts tied to the program to be evaluated and, if so, what they are. It also allows me to have conversations with people about the culture and the climate of the program and those who are being served. These are not things that often show up in an evaluation plan but are the result of conversations that are important to have informally.

Formally, [a social justice perspective] shows up when you are looking at criteria that determine program quality and effectiveness, and include criteria that are tied to climate, diversity, inclusion, and equity. It is important to have evaluation questions related to equity regardless of whether a program is about broadening participation or is a diversity initiative. I add equity and diversity to the evaluation questions and include diversity and equity in the criteria for quality. As part of the questions about program effectiveness, I examine for whom the program is working well and for whom it is not, and as part of the process of assessing program climate, I ask participants how they feel about their inclusion in the program.

Ayesha S. Boyce, an assistant professor at the University of North Carolina–Greensboro is an evaluation teacher, scholar, and practitioner. She is the co-director of the UNCG Office of Assessment, Evaluation, and Research Services. She was interviewed by coauthor Patricia B. Campbell in the fall of 2019.

SUMMARY

A major focus of this chapter was to provide the reader with an overview of the need for social justice in society and in evaluation. We examined some prevailing social justice theories and provided an overview to help the reader understand the roles that evaluation has and hasn't played in social justice efforts. Along with the overview, the chapter presented evaluation paradigms and frameworks that have social justice at their core. Readers should now have an understanding of contemporary social justice–oriented evaluation frameworks and the commonalities among those frameworks, such as

- acknowledging one's own perspectives and biases;
- incorporating the pervasive influences of gender, race/ethnicity, disability, and poverty in the work;
- empowering those who are part of that which is being evaluated; and
- avoiding the separation of research from action and advocacy.

SUPPLEMENTAL RESOURCES

Resources for Culturally Responsive Evaluation

www.informalscience.org/evaluation/developing-evaluation-plan/resources-culturally-responsive-evaluation

This website provides a list of resources for understanding and performing culturally responsible evaluations including the Centers for Disease Control and Prevention's (CDC) "Practical Strategies for Culturally Competent Evaluation."

EvalIndigenous

www.evalpartners.org/evalindigenous/about

This project works "to inform individuals engaged in evaluation with Indigenous communities through a) documenting the evaluation and research protocols developed by Indigenous communities and organizations; b) facilitating learning and sharing of experiences[;] c) promoting innovation in approaches and methods used in Indigenous evaluation[;] and d) disseminating information regarding 'lessons learned.'"

BetterEvaluation

www.betterevaluation.org

This is the site of "an international collaboration to improve evaluation practice and theory by sharing and generating information about options (methods or processes) and approaches."

Social Justice Theory Resources

Critical Race Theory

Delgado, R., & Stefancic, J. (2017). *Critical race theory: An introduction* (3rd ed.). New York: New York University Press.

Dixson, A., & Rousseau, C. K., & Donnor, J. K. (Eds.). (2017). *Critical race theory in education:*

All god's children got a song. New York, NY: Routledge.

Feminist Theory

Harding, S., & O'Barr, J. F. (Eds.). (1987). Sex and scientific inquiry. Chicago, IL: University of Chicago Press.

Nielsen, J. M. (Ed.). (1990). *Feminist research methods.* Boulder, CO: Westview Press.

Queer Theory

Butler, J. (1999). *Gender trouble* (10th anniversary ed.). London, England: Routledge.

Kosofsky Sedgwick, E. (1990). Epistemology of the closet. Berkeley: University of California Press.

Disability Theory

Rousso, H. (2013). *Don't call me inspirational: A disabled feminist talks back.* Philadelphia, PA: Temple University Press.

Siebers, T. (2008). *Disability theory.* Ann Arbor: University of Michigan Press.

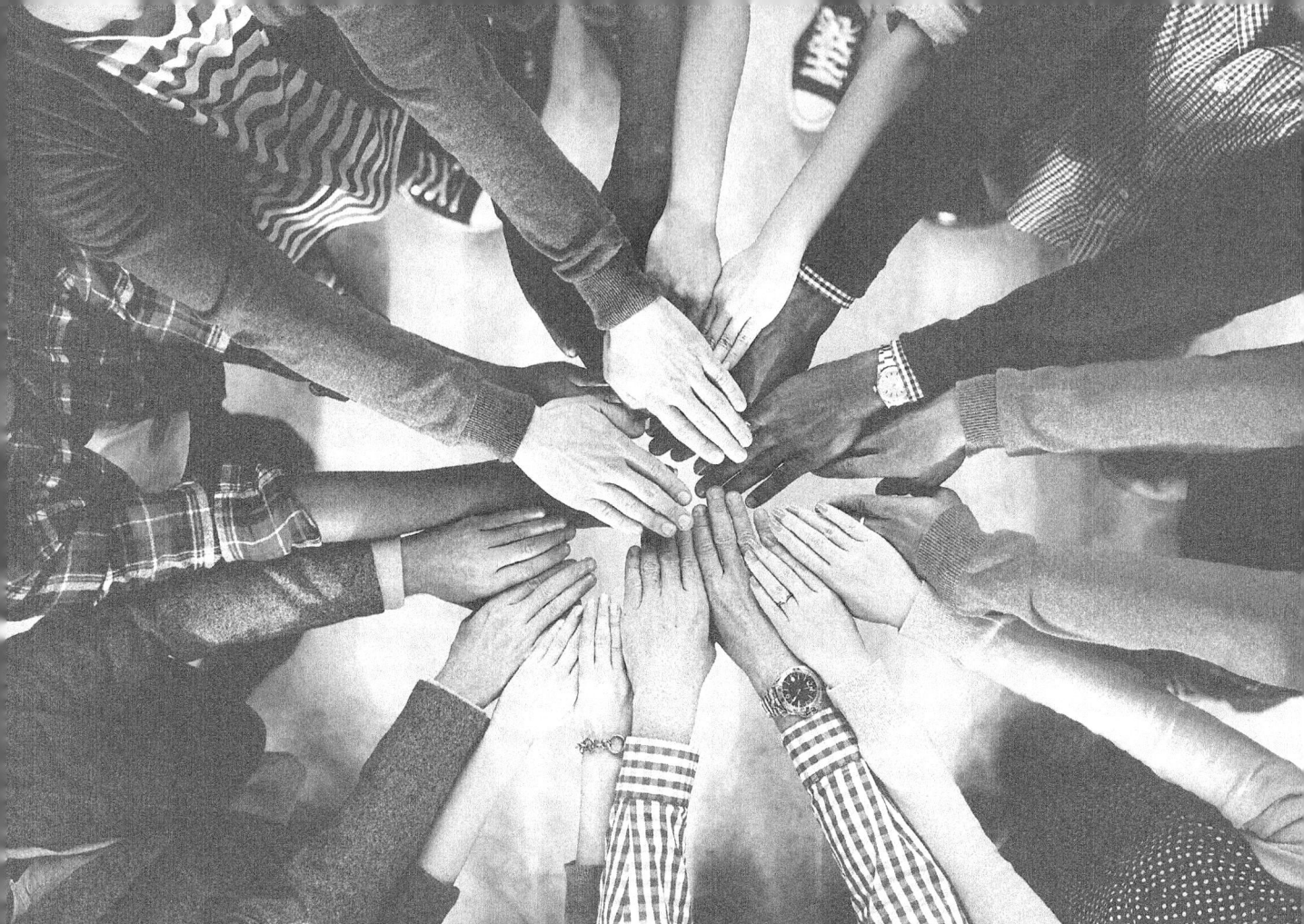
Shutterstock/Rawpixel.com

Different types of evaluations can either hide or illuminate issues related to inclusion, culture, and social justice depending on how evaluators plan and implement those evaluations as well as how findings from such evaluations are disseminated.

CHAPTER 6

Evaluation Types With a Cultural and Racial Equity Lens

Members of the school board and the superintendent are interested in uncovering the success (or lack thereof) of a five-year initiative to improve teaching and learning in their large urban school district. Program planners in a southern rural county want to learn about the needs of family caregivers of aging parents with mild cognitive impairment in order to provide programs that more effectively meet the needs of the area's diverse residents. The funder of a multisite state economic development training grant in the northeastern part of the country is interested in finding out what the project looks like at each site, to what extent the project staff at each site are administering the project in accordance with the written curriculum, and if site supervisors are adequately trained to oversee the project and work with the diverse clientele. These are just some of the myriad issues that different types of evaluations can address within their own unique cultural context.

After reading this chapter and participating in the activities, readers will be able to meet the following learning objectives:

- Explain the major categories and types of evaluations
- Describe when and why various types of evaluations are used
- Discuss the power and privilege evaluators have in conducting various types of evaluations
- Integrate issues of inclusion, cultural competence, and racial equity when considering various types of evaluation

Introduction

The field of evaluation has grown substantially over the past several decades. With this growth, evaluation has become an increasingly complex and multifaceted endeavor with varying philosophical perspectives around its purpose, values, methods, and roles for evaluators. Rather than the one-size-fits-all (or nearly all) approaches of past decades, today's evaluators have a variety of strategies (e.g., methods-driven vs. theory-driven), conceptual lenses (e.g., social justice, feminist), and approaches (e.g., culturally responsive, empowerment, appreciative inquiry, participatory, system-oriented), as well as reporting and data visualization tools, to select from when engaging in their work. These approaches are not mutually exclusive. For example, a system-oriented approach to evaluation can also be culturally responsive (Thomas & Parsons, 2017). Also, some approaches have similar features and, as such, are easier to couple together in practice. Evaluation approaches, for instance, that place emphasis on collaboration, community participation, and capacity building, such as participatory, democratic, transformative, and empowerment approaches, which were covered in more detail in Chapter 5, can readily support a culturally responsive evaluation approach if they have a deliberate emphasis on the integration of culture and social justice.

This chapter examines the major categories and types of evaluation, including their purpose, major strengths, when they are typically utilized, and their primary audiences. No one particular category/type of evaluation is inherently good or bad, but instead, its value is a function of its ability to meet the information needs at a particular point in time. Addressing culture and racial equity is relevant when considering all evaluation types. Depending on how evaluators plan and implement the various types of evaluations discussed in this chapter, they can either hide or illuminate issues related to inclusion, culture, and social justice.

Regardless of the type of evaluation conducted, it is the evaluator's responsibility to have a good understanding of the evaluand, be knowledgeable about the history and background of the target population and the surrounding community, and implement the evaluation in a manner that is methodical as well as respectful and responsive to the culture under study. As discussed in other chapters of the book, this can be difficult given the dominant positionality of many evaluators. As a result, evaluators from the dominant group (e.g., white) oftentimes have difficulty even seeing how they are failing to be inclusive and culturally responsive in their practice.

Classifying Evaluations

Scriven (1993) described evaluation as a transdiscipline—that is, a discipline that supplies essential tools, scholarship, and practice for other disciplines (e.g., statistics, measurement), while retaining unique characteristics (e.g., common logic, theory), an autonomous structure, and research efforts of its own. As a transdiscipline, the field includes many types of evaluations that have been used across multiple disciplines (e.g., public health, education, criminal justice, business) and applied areas (e.g., workforce development, youth development, health promotion). However, the type of evaluation selected for use is not area or discipline dependent, per se, but depends on other factors, such as

- the primary purpose of the evaluation;
- who will use the evaluation information and in what ways;
- the stage of the program (i.e., before, beginning, middle, end); and
- what questions the information users want to answer.

While evaluation can take place at any point during the life of a program, evaluation of a program during its early stages will be classified as distinctly different from an evaluation of a mature, well-established program. Further, an evaluation done for the purpose of gathering information to provide feedback to the program for making improvements is classified differently than an accountability-oriented assessment aimed at judging if the program works as intended. Improvement-oriented evaluations might point to problems that need to be corrected to make the program operate more smoothly, while accountability-oriented evaluations are critical for fulfilling responsibilities to external audiences.

A single program is likely, and it is even advisable, to have more than one type of evaluation over the life of the project. For example, an evaluation of a workforce development program during its early stages (e.g., first 6–12 months) might focus on the program's rationale, implementation, and ability to attract, recruit, and retain low-income, ethnically diverse populations; however, evaluation of the workforce development program in its established or mature stage is likely to focus on the program's success in terms of the employment outcomes of diverse program participants. The primary users of early program evaluation are generally program administrators or other internal audiences seeking information to guide program improvement and mid-course corrections. Primary users of mature program evaluations are oftentimes external audiences (e.g., funders, policymakers) in addition to internal audiences, both of whom want information on program effectiveness or the extent to which the program achieved its desired outcomes. From a social justice perspective, however, the results from evaluations should also be of use to participants, the community, and other stakeholders.

An Overview of Formative and Summative Classification

There have long been efforts to classify evaluations by their ultimate purpose and the timing of their implementation. Probably the most long-standing distinction of evaluation types is Scriven's (1967) formative and summative classification. This classification continues to be used in many evaluations. Despite discussions around the limitations of the formative–summative classification (H. Chen, 1996; Patton, 1996), this classic distinction is still used in the field and is sometimes even required by various government funders in evaluations of their programs. Further, many evaluators continue to communicate their evaluation plans and results using a formative–summative framework. Both types of evaluations are valuable within the appropriate set of circumstances, and one is no more important than the other.

One of the most comprehensive definitions of **formative evaluation** that we favor was put forth by Stufflebeam and Shinkfield (2007):

> Formative evaluation assesses and assists with the formulation of goals and priorities; provides direction for planning by assessing alternative courses of actions and draft plans; and guides program management by assessing implementation of plans and interim results. (p. 702)

Formative evaluations are generally collected to provide feedback to the program staff, and their results typically remain in-house. To be most useful, formative evaluations must provide feedback to program administrators in a timely manner so that programs can make corrections or modifications early while the program is in progress rather than waiting until the end.

Generally, formative evaluations are conducted during the early to midway stages of a project's implementation. For relatively new programs, in particular, there is often a concern about fidelity or the extent to which delivery of an intervention adheres to the protocols and program model originally developed. Formative evaluations can determine if (appropriate) staff/service providers have been hired; offices have been opened; services are being provided (as intended); and target participants have been reached, enrolled, and maintained in the program. Formative evaluation can assess fidelity, and these results can guide program implementation over time to improve the overall performance. However, there are occasions when formative evaluations are done to monitor the fidelity of more established programs to determine whether program activities are continuing to be delivered as intended or as revised. In addition to focusing on quality of implementation or program processes, formative evaluation is used to assess other areas such as stakeholder attitudes (including satisfaction with services) and pilot testing of evaluation measurement instruments.

Additional uses of formative evaluations exist beyond early to mid-stage project monitoring. Some evaluators point to the value of incorporating formative evaluation practices throughout the entire life of a program rather than simply as a procedural checkpoint after the program has been designed (e.g., Hall, Freeman, & Roulston, 2014). Gary Henry and colleagues (Henry, Smith, Kershaw, & Zulli, 2013) stress that under certain circumstances (e.g., combining existing, longitudinal, administrative data sets and a progression of analytical models) formative evaluations can be done to estimate preliminary program outcomes and identify promising program components based on their effectiveness during implementation. Data obtained from a formative evaluation have also been used as baseline data for subsequent monitoring of the project indicators.

Formative evaluations are very learning-focused, and they aim to help administrators and other decision makers obtain the real-time feedback they need to make better strategic decisions. Formative feedback to administrators can occur formally, through the submission of quarterly, biannual, or annual written reports on progress and process, or informally, through regular (e.g., monthly or bimonthly) check-in calls to update administrators on what has been gleaned as evaluators observe the program in action or talk with key stakeholders. Formative evaluations have the potential to stimulate a nuanced understanding and awareness of how contextual and cultural dimensions interact with the program design, implementation, and operations. Formative evaluations conducted through culturally responsive and social justice approaches include particular attention to things such as the target community's demographics; stakeholders' norms; values, needs, and interests across the diverse groups represented in the program; and program reach (or lack thereof) across diverse targeted groups. Equitable access of services is often an issue addressed in culturally responsive and social justice–oriented formative evaluation.

Summative evaluations, on the other hand, are conducted not for the primary purpose of guiding improvement, but instead for accountability or making judgment of a program's worth—that is, whether the project achieved intended objectives.

Summative evaluation reports are typically submitted at the end of the project. Sometimes, however, summative evaluation reporting is done at the end of a predetermined operating cycle or at a time deemed appropriate to measure outcomes (i.e., after the program has stabilized, after changes have been made and sufficient time has passed for results to be realized). With their primary audiences being program sponsors (funders) and other decision makers, summative evaluations are useful in accountability efforts that need to determine success and failure. Summative evaluations seek to answer questions such as *How have the target individuals and/or communities changed as a result of this program?* and *To what extent were the program's overall goals achieved?* The following activity provides an opportunity for readers to discuss different contexts that may be more suited to a formative versus a summative evaluation.

> ### Reflect and Discuss
> #### Optimal Circumstances for a Formative vs. Summative Evaluation
>
> In small groups, discuss, from your observations or personal experiences (e.g., work, community, or academic setting), a circumstance where a formative evaluation is needed and could provide timely and useful information.
>
> Now, using this same reflective process, identify a current situation where a summative evaluation is needed and could provide timely and useful information.
>
> Give your rationale for the examples provided.

Data collected in summative evaluations can be individual-, community-, and/or institutional-level outcomes. Summative evaluation data collected at the individual level include assessing changes in program participants' knowledge, attitudes, skills, behaviors, expectations, emotional status, or life circumstances as a result of the intervention provided. For example, (a) a summative evaluation of a mathematics enrichment program might assess the extent to which participating students improve logical reasoning processes required to solve advanced mathematics problems; (b) a summative evaluation of a health promotion program might assess the extent to which participating adults engage in lifestyle changes such as increased physical activity and improved stress management; and (c) a summative evaluation of a juvenile drug court program might assess the extent to which the program reduces participating youth recidivism and improves their social functioning. Summative evaluation can focus on institutional changes, such as modification in policies or procedures as a result of a particular program. Evaluation of a district-wide teacher professional development program, for instance, might document school-level policy changes in terms of scheduled time for teacher collaboration that emerged after the program ended.

Summative evaluations are generally implemented for some external audiences or decision makers (funders or potential future funders) to justify the continuation (or discontinuation), expansion (or shrinkage), or modification of the program. The results from a summative evaluation can also provide information that enables project administrators to make decisions regarding the specific services and the future direction of the program that could not have been made during the early or middle stages of the program cycle. A summative evaluation of a diabetes maintenance and prevention program, for example, might indicate that the program demonstrated positive results for its female participants but did not result in positive changes for male participants. Based on these findings, the program administrators may determine that they need to implement a different type of diabetes maintenance and prevention curriculum for men focusing on their unique needs and concerns.

Summative evaluations with a culturally responsive and social justice orientation address diversity and equity issues. Such evaluations might seek to address questions such as *Who benefited from the program?* and *Who is not receiving equitable benefits and may even be further marginalized by the project?* Chapter 10 has more examples of questions for different types of evaluations.

Distinguishing and Coupling Formative and Summative Evaluations

Scriven (1991) noted that the best illustration of the distinction between formative and summative evaluations was Robert Stake's analogy as depicted here:

> When the cook tastes the soup, that's formative.
>
> When the guests taste the soup, that's summative.
>
> —Robert Stake

Source of soup bowl photo: https://pixabay.com/vectors/soup-bowl-food-steam-pot-steaming-297736/

Using this analogy, when the cook tastes the soup while it is cooking, that is a metaphor for formative evaluation. It is formative because if after tasting the soup it is not to the cook's liking or taste preferences, the cook can explore strategies to make it taste better or fix the problem, such as adding more salt, pepper, or other seasoning to enhance the flavor. Subsequently, the cook can collect more formative data by retasting the soup. In this example, tasting occurred during the cooking process for the purpose of improving the soup before it had finished cooking. When the guests taste the soup after it has finished cooking and it is served, this is a metaphor for summative evaluation. At this point, the guests can offer a conclusive opinion or evaluative judgment of "goodness" of the soup.

With only the implementation of a summative evaluation, the evaluator is unable to capture important cultural information that might provide useful insight on the process of change. For example, a summative evaluation of students' mathematics competency, based solely on test scores, might simply conclude that Black students, in comparison to their white counterparts, fare significantly poorer on the state's mathematics examination. In this instance, evaluation users have no additional data available to make sense of this outcome. However, a formative evaluation might uncover a variety of characteristics that influence the learning outcomes (e.g., lower teacher quality and fewer mathematics learning resources in minority-dominant schools in comparison to schools that include mostly white and Asian students). These data give insight to structural and other inequities that may be greatly influencing the differences in test scores. The formative results also point to certain steps (e.g., improved teacher quality) that can be undertaken to close this achievement gap.

The emphasis on formative versus summative evaluation will change over the life cycle of the program. Whereas formative evaluations will likely be more prominent during the program's early stages, summative evaluations are dominant as the program matures and is completed. A summative evaluation can indicate what works (or did not work) while a formative evaluation is a useful complement to the summative evaluation by providing information that might help one understand why something worked (or did not work) and illuminating positive or negative factors (e.g., power dynamics, policies) operating during the life of the program that may have influenced participants' outcomes.

Other Evaluation Classifications

In addition to the classic formative–summative distinction, there are other evaluation classifications found in the literature that, in many ways, build on the formative–summative classification. In *Designing Evaluations*, a publication of the U.S. Government Accountability Office (GAO, 2012), evaluations are classified as process or implementation evaluations, outcome evaluations, and net impact evaluations. Process or implementation evaluations are studies designed to address the quality or efficiency of program operations or their fidelity to program design. Outcome evaluations assess the extent to which a program achieves its outcome-oriented objectives or other important outcomes. Net impact evaluation is a form of outcome evaluation that assesses the net effects of a program (or its true effectiveness) by comparing the observed outcomes to an estimate of what would have happened in the absence of the program. Since a program's desired outcomes are known to be influenced by factors (e.g., economic and labor market trends, political constraints) outside the program, the outcomes that are actually observed represent a combination of both program effects and the effects of those external factors. In net impact studies, questions about program effectiveness must be more sophisticated, and the evaluation design should attempt to identify the extent to which the program caused or contributed to those observed changes by ruling out extraneous threats to validity, as will be covered in more detail in Chapter 11. The Centers for Disease Control and Prevention (CDC) similarly classifies evaluations in terms of formative evaluation, process/implementation evaluation, outcome/effectiveness evaluation, and impact evaluation.

The U.S. Department of State classifies evaluations in two categories: performance evaluations and impact evaluations. Performance evaluations examine the inputs, outputs, outcomes, and performance of an intervention while impact evaluations focus on measuring the change attributable to a given intervention.

Chelimsky (1997) proposes three general perspectives as a way of classifying evaluations by their intended purpose:

- *Evaluations for accountability* include those conducted to yield measurement of results or efficiency suited to the information needs of auditors and government sponsors of evaluation.

- *Evaluations for development* are those done for the provision of evaluative help to strengthen institutions suited to the information needs of government reformers, public managers, and capacity builders.

- *Evaluations for knowledge* are those done for the acquisition of a more profound understanding of factors underlying public problems, of the fit between these factors and policy and program solutions proposed, and of the theory and logic (or lack thereof) that lie behind the intervention particularly suited to the information needs of researchers, program designers, and others.

Although Chelimsky argues that these different types of evaluation represent notable differences on a variety of dimensions and purposes, she does not view these as exhaustive or mutually exclusive with regard to method.

Different Types of Evaluations

In this section, we shift from discussion of broad classifications of evaluation to discussion of specific types of evaluations. Many of these evaluation types fit into one of the broad classifications presented earlier. Regardless of the type of evaluation undertaken, there can and should be attention to issues of culture, social justice, and inclusion. In his 2019 Voices From the Field interview, Henry T. Frierson argues that while some evaluation types can more readily lend themselves to culturally responsive and social justice approaches, every evaluator, despite the type of evaluation being implemented, should use a culturally responsive lens. This better ensures that the evaluators are less likely to miss critical nuances reflected within the project's cultural context that could affect the meaning of the results and interpretations.

Voices From the Field

Henry T. Frierson: Culturally Responsive Evaluation Across Different Evaluation Types

My focus has long been on culturally responsive evaluation as a practice that should be operating for all types of evaluations. Every evaluator should use, or try to use, a culturally responsive evaluation (CRE) approach. Some evaluation types, such as participatory evaluation as advocated by David M. Fetterman, more readily lend themselves to a CRE perspective. Despite the type of evaluation conducted, evaluation outcomes and results should be put into the context of the culture in which the project is based to ensure that what is observed and reported is indeed true or accurate. The evaluator should have a sense of the evaluation results within the specific cultural context. Truthfulness in reporting and interpreting data regardless of whether the data are qualitative or quantitative is essential. Often, stakeholders, particularly those involved in running or even participating in a project, have serious questions or concerns with what is being presented in a report regarding the project and their community. For example, the evaluation team may have missed critical nuances reflected within the project's cultural context. Those missed nuances could more accurately help inform the meanings and implications of the findings. Using a CRE lens across different evaluation types will better ensure that evaluation outcomes and results are agreed on as being true, even if not totally accepted, by various stakeholders because cultural nuances were taken into consideration when collecting the data and interpreting the results. This can mitigate potential arguments with stakeholders over the meaning of the outcomes. When we are talking about the evaluation of a program that can make a difference in the lives of people, if the reported findings are not accurately portrayed, it can have a negative effect not only on the project but on the people served or participating as well. Hence, evaluators should be humble and accept the fact that they may not be familiar with, or may even be clueless about, the cultural context of the project they are evaluating. In such instances, they should look for published and other resources to help them develop skills to provide a more accurate picture of what they are seeing or the data they are collecting.

Henry T. Frierson is associate vice president, dean of the Graduate School, and professor of research and evaluation methodology at the University of Florida. Veronica G. Thomas interviewed him in the fall of 2019.

Table 6.1 provides a summary of the various types of evaluations. In this summary, we classify evaluation as generally formative or summative in nature. We say "generally formative" or "generally summative" because of our recognition, as well as that of

Table 6.1 Summary of Evaluation Categories by Type

Category I: Formative or implementation evaluations assess and assist with the formulation of goals and priorities; provide direction for planning by assessing alternative courses of action and draft plans; and guide program management by assessing implementation of plans and interim results (Stufflebeam & Shinkfield, 2007).

Conducting formative or implementation evaluations using an *inclusion, social justice, and racial equity lens* can promote equity and inclusion by considering whether community conditions; power dynamics; or cultural, racial, or equity issues affect project process and implementation by gaining valuable perspectives from people and communities who are oftentimes silenced, ignored, or misunderstood, and by understanding more fully the reach and who is being served (e.g., disparities by different racial and ethnic groups).

Evaluation Categories/Types	Program Stage When Conducted	Primary Audience(s)	Major Purpose	Sample Question Answered1
Needs Assessment	Conducted before program is developed and/or during operation of existing program at appropriate interval	Program staff	Gather information to determine who needs the program, how great the need is, and what might work to meet the need	What community resources are currently available to address the need under consideration?
Evaluability Assessment	Conducted immediately following program design to identify weaknesses and just prior to deciding when to evaluate a program	Program staff	Gather information to determine whether an evaluation is feasible at present time	To what extent are program goals and objectives clearly defined and agreed on?
Process or Implementation Evaluation	Conducted early and during various phases of implementation	Program staff	Gather information to understand program's inner workings and what it is actually doing	How well is the program reaching hard-to-reach target populations?
Progress Evaluation	Conducted at various times in life of project but most useful when done at targeted periods	Program staff	Gather information to assess extent to which program is progressing in meeting its goals or benchmarks	To what extent are participants positively moving toward the intended outcomes?

Category II: Summative or outcome and impact evaluations render a summary judgment on certain critical aspects of a program's performance, for instance, to determine if specific goals and objectives were met (Rossi, Lipsey, & Henry, 2019).

Conducting summative or outcome and impact evaluations using an *inclusion, social justice, and racial equity lens* can promote equity and inclusion by disaggregating summative or outcome data to determine whether burdens and benefits of the project were distributed across different racial/ethnic groups and by considering the extent to which there were unintended changes due to cultural and racial issues/context.

Evaluation Categories/Types	Program Stage When Conducted/Primary Audience	Primary Audience(s)	Major Purpose	Sample Question Answered
Outcomes	Conducted at end of program, during operation of existing program, or at selected interval(s) when immediate or intermediate outcomes are expected to have occurred	Policymakers, external funders	Gather information to determine extent to which program achieved intended outcomes, usually focusing on short- and medium-term changes in participants resulting directly from program	To what extent were intended outcomes similarly achieved by diverse groups of participants?

(Continued)

Table 6.1 (Continued)

Evaluation Categories/Types	Program Stage When Conducted/Primary Audience	Primary Audience(s)	Major Purpose	Sample Question Answered
Impact	Conducted sometime after the program ends or during operation of existing program at selected interval(s) when impacts are expected to have occurred	Policymakers, external funders	Gather information to determine broader, long-term net effects of program (e.g., effect on entire school, community, organization, society, or environment)	Has the program resulted in new community partnerships, coalitions, or other efforts to improve residents' well-being?
Cost Benefit and Cost Effectiveness	Conducted at end of program or during operation of selected interval(s) when cost benefits are expected to be realized	Policymakers, external funders	Gather information to determine efficiency by standardizing outcomes in terms of their dollar costs and values	Is the cost of program services reasonable in relation to the benefits?

Category III: Other evaluation types include evaluations that do not neatly fit into the formative–summative paradigm because of their major purpose and the timing of the evaluation.

Conducting other types of evaluation using an *inclusion, social justice, and racial equity lens* can promote equity and inclusion by adapting the evaluation process to the cultural and racial nuances of the target community as the context warrants.

Evaluation Categories/Types	Program Stage When Conducted/Primary Audience	Primary Audience(s)	Major Purpose	Sample Question Answered
Developmental Evaluation	Conducted at any time and as an alternative to the formative–summative paradigm	Program managers, policymakers, external funders	Gather evaluative data for a developing or emerging initiative in dynamic environments where participants, conditions, interventions, and context are turbulent and pathways for achieving desired outcomes are uncertain	How can the initiative be more dynamic and adapt to the context in ways that are within the control of the project?
Rapid Evaluation	Conducted over a short period of time during early to middle stages of program implementation	Program managers, policymakers, external funders	Gather information to provide timely and actionable evidence on precise, shorter-term questions mostly focusing on program operations and services but sometimes also focusing on outcomes	What is the most effective outreach strategy for reaching high-risk male youth of color?
Metaevaluation	Conducted generally after the evaluation is completed but, in some instances, done formatively or before an evaluation to review the evaluation plan or concurrently alongside the evaluation	Policymakers, external funders	Gather information to perform a systematic evaluation of an evaluation and its subcomponents or to compare two or more evaluations	To what extent was the evaluation done well and does the evaluation meet professional standards and practices?

[1] More detailed questions by evaluation type are discussed in Chapter 10.

others, that the formative–summative distinctions do not always oppose each other, nor must they be mutually exclusive categories. Also, depending on the context, some evaluations can serve formative and summative purposes (H. Chen, 1996; Stufflebeam & Shinkfield, 2007; Wholey, 1996). One example is the Government Performance and Results Act (GPRA) of 1993 (PL 103-62) that sought to improve congressional decision making, service delivery, and program effectiveness as well as provide public accountability (Wholey, 1996). Since we recognize that there are other types of evaluation (e.g., developmental evaluations, metaevaluations) that do not neatly fit into the boundaries of the formative–summative distinction, we have included such a category in the table.

We also describe, in Table 6.1, the different types of evaluation by (a) program stage when they are generally conducted; (b) primary audience, or individuals/groups that will use the evaluation information to make decisions; (c) major purpose; and (d) sample questions answered. The table also highlights how issues of inclusion, social justice, and a racial equity lens can be incorporated in each evaluation category. Following the table, there is more detailed discussion of these various types of evaluations as utilized in practice.

Formative and Implementation Evaluations

These evaluations provide a rich opportunity to consider cultural, inclusion, and racial equity factors by focusing on and uncovering community conditions; power dynamics; and cultural, racial, or equity issues that affect project process and implementation and by more fully understanding project reach including the extent to which certain members of the community (e.g., low-income groups, people of color) were not served although they were the intended project beneficiaries.

Needs Assessments

By gathering critical information prior to program design, the evaluation can yield information that provides a better understanding of the problem under consideration and what services are most appropriate to meet that need for particular cultural and racial/ethnic groups or communities. Low-income and other marginalized groups often have unmet needs that must be uncovered and understood. **Needs assessments** can be invaluable in providing insights into the most pressing needs for unserved groups and how to address them. Such assessments have been conducted or commissioned by a variety of organizations including health care institutions and agencies; educational institutions; and federal, state, local, and municipal agencies for the purpose of determining priorities, making organizational improvement, and/or allocating resources.

Rossi, Lipsey, and Henry (2019) define a needs assessment as an evaluative study that answers questions about the social conditions a program is intended to address, the nature of the need for a program, and the appropriate target population. Needs assessments are essential for accurately identifying actual and potential unmet needs of diverse populations and allowing for program services to be tailored in a manner that is effective for addressing those needs. The essential task for the evaluator as needs assessor is to describe the situation that concerns major stakeholders in a manner that is as careful, objective, and meaningful to all groups as possible and to help draw out the implications of that diagnosis for structuring effective intervention.

By needs, we are referring to "the measurable gap between two conditions—'what is' (the current status or state) and 'what should be' (the desired status or state)" (Altschuld & Kumar, 2010, p. 3). A need can occur as a result of the desire to correct a deficiency or to improve a current state. Needs assessments are based on the assumption that certain populations and/or communities have needs that are not being met at all or are being insufficiently addressed. Prior to designing a program to address an unmet need or gap, it is important to understand the problem under consideration that the target population faces and the key factors that contribute to the problem. The following case study provides an example needs assessment.

Case Study
Example of a Needs Assessment Statement of Purpose

Verité Healthcare Consulting, LLC, based in Alexandria, Virginia, conducted a community needs assessment (CNA) of the New York State (NYS) Delivery System Reform Incentive Program (DSRIP), the primary means by which the state implemented its Medicaid Redesign Team Waiver Amendment. The CNA results were reported to Advocate Community Providers (ACP)/ New York Community Preferred Providers (NYCPP), a physician-led emerging Performing Provider System (PPS) and a lead organization under the DSRIP in NYS.

Delivery System Reform Incentive Program Brief Description

The purpose of the DSRIP is to restructure and transform the safety net care delivery system for Medicaid recipients and to attain a 25% reduction in avoidable hospital use by the Medicaid population and uninsured individuals over a five-year period. The DSRIP is structured as an incentive payment program in which networks of providers, called PPS, work together in a coordinated fashion to implement projects that affect system transformation, achieve clinical improvements, and address population-level health goals in part through prevention activities.

Purpose of Needs Assessment

The purpose of the CNA is to analyze and document priority health and health service challenges for the Medicaid and uninsured population in the community and to inform DSRIP project selection and design. The ACP CNA documents the demographics and health care needs of the population to be served and the health care and community-based service resources currently available in the service area. The CNA presents and analyzes a wide range of demographic, health, and health care delivery system indicators, including but not limited to domain metrics, as well as information from key informant interviews, Medicaid focus groups, and a survey of health care, behavioral health, and social services providers.

Source: Health Consulting, LLC. (2014, December 15). Excerpted from Community Needs Assessment for New York State DSRIP Project Plan Application.

In the conceptualization and design of programs, it is essential to consider the cultural context of the environment and population that will be served by the program. Communities have their own particular cultures, histories, webs of relationships, and social structures that influence both their needs and their assets. A needs assessment that is conducted ahead of program implementation can document important cultural considerations, as well as the nature and scope of the need, who needs the program, and what might work to close the gap or meet the need in the target population. Needs assessments can yield information that provides a good understanding of the nature and scope of a problem in that particular context *prior to* implementing a program to reduce or eliminate that problem, in context, and to address the unmet needs. For example, a needs assessment of long-term medical and psychosocial care needs and services for Hispanic female rape survivors might focus on the extent to which there are adequate and culturally appropriate services for this population (rape counselors, translators, legal support, etc.), which, in turn, could inform the program planning for expanding and/or enhancing existing support services in this area. Results from a needs assessment of African American cancer patients found that the participants perceived a lack of culturally specific support services located within their neighborhoods; other needs participants identified included a lack of social support, a lack of resources related to appearance, a lack of resources for continued care, and a lack of support services for children of survivors (Mosavel & Sanders, 2011). Here, culturally responsive needs assessment data could prove invaluable when designing support programs for this population. Failure to gather cultural and contextually relevant information during the needs assessment prior to program design could lead to faulty and misdirected program initiatives.

A needs assessment can help program planners and other decision makers prioritize those identified needs as well as determine (a) what groups to target for services, (b) the best way to publicize or market services, (c) estimates of the number of persons who could benefit from the program or services, (d) the geographical distribution and sociodemographic characteristics of potential clients, and (e) barriers that might be encountered by clients (or potential clients) (Royse, Thyer, & Padgett, 2010). As seen in the following steps, a significant amount of planning, buy-in, and collaboration is required for a successful needs assessment to take place.

Step 1: Clarify the purpose and determine the focus and scope of the needs assessment.

Step 2: Determine the data required to identify needs and gaps in order to make informed and justifiable decisions.

Step 3: Identify relevant partners for the needs assessment; this generally involves building a needs assessment team or committee.

Step 4: Determine data sources to inform the needs assessment.

Step 5: Collect new information and/or gather existing information relevant to the target population(s), community, and issue(s) under consideration.

Step 6: Analyze and interpret information to draw conclusions such as identifying trends, gaps and strengths, and where improvements are needed.

Step 7: Use or encourage use of results to determine short- and long-term goals.

After the needs assessment is complete and reported back to its intended audiences, program planners and other key decision makers can take action through prioritizing the identified needs, appraising the options for meeting those needs, and implementing an action plan including allocation of resources. Actions taken as a result of a needs assessment clearly must be monitored and evaluated to determine if the changes implemented are having the desired effect of meeting the needs of the target population/community.

Evaluability Assessments

Sometimes during the formative evaluation stage, an evaluator might detect that a program is not ready for a formal evaluation. In such instances, it is advisable to conduct an **evaluability assessment**. The evaluability assessment, generally qualitative in nature, is an approach initially introduced by Joseph Wholey (1977, 1979) as a pre-evaluation activity to ensure that programs were properly implemented and ready for summative evaluation. More recently, Wholey (2015) argued that a program is ready for evaluation when it meets four criteria:

- Program goals are agreed on and realistic.
- Information needs are well defined.
- Evaluation data are obtainable.
- Intended users are willing and able to use evaluation information.

If a program meets these criteria, the evaluation is thought to be justified, feasible, and likely to yield useful information that contributes to improved program management and performance. Programs with unrealistic or ill-defined goals (such as changing an entire city over a six-month period) or where key stakeholders disagree on the objectives are not likely to succeed, and thus evaluation becomes a waste of valuable and limited resources.

Evaluability assessments are formative in nature and most valuable when they are conducted at two points in the program life cycle: (a) immediately following program design to identify any weaknesses and (b) just prior to deciding whether to evaluate the program. During the latter, the evaluability assessment can help determine whether, at this particular time, an evaluation is worthwhile in terms of its likely benefits, consequences, and costs. The evaluability assessment can also indicate whether the program is able to provide the information required for a process evaluation or outcome evaluation. Many evaluators ask evaluability-assessment-type questions prior to implementing a process or implementation evaluation without formally referring to their work as an evaluability assessment.

While Wholey's (1979) initial conceptualization of an evaluability assessment was primarily focused on assessing program readiness for impact evaluation and meeting the information needs of program managers and policymakers, the purposes of evaluability assessments have been expanded to include use in program change and improvement. Wholey views evaluability assessment as one of several exploratory evaluation approaches. Sometimes evaluability assessments are performed by a program staff member, but they are generally perceived as more credible when conducted by a professional evaluator because of this individual's more likely strong knowledge of program evaluation. In a review of the state of practice of evaluability assessment as represented in the published literature over two decades, Trevisan (2007) found that evaluability assessments were done in a wide variety of programs, disciplines, and settings with the most common rationale for conducting an evaluability assessment being to determine program readiness for impact assessment, program development, and formative evaluation. Regardless of the discipline and setting, the kinds of questions answered in evaluability assessments include the following:

- Is the program rationale and justification realistic?
- Are the intervention's intended outcomes clearly identified, realistic, and commonly understood by relevant stakeholders?

- Does the intervention have in place or have the capacity to develop procedures to generate the data required for the evaluation?
- Are there external factors (e.g., cultural, political, financial) that would hamper the evaluation?

Wholey (2015) continues to argue for use of evaluability assessments, particularly as a management tool, even though some evaluators (e.g., M. Smith, 2005) point to a decline in their use and appeal since the 1970s and 1980s. The following activity summarizes the six-step process put forth by Wholey for conducting an evaluability assessment.

Reflect and Discuss
Six-Step Process for Conducting an Evaluability Assessment

In the *Handbook of Practical Program Evaluation*, Joseph Wholey (2015, pp. 92–96) discusses a six-step process for evaluability assessment, as abbreviated here. After reviewing and reflecting on this information, answer the questions at the end of the process description.

Step 1: Involve intended users and other key stakeholders by meeting with policymakers, managers, and other stakeholders closely involved in the evaluability assessment.

Step 2: Clarify the program design by exploring perspectives on program design, results to date, results expected in the next year or two, problems that inhibit effective performance, and uses and intended uses of information that is available or desired.

Step 3: Explore program reality by comparing the intended program with the actual program, relying on existing information (e.g., project reports), and conducting site visits or interviews and discussions with knowledgeable persons.

Step 4: Assess the plausibility of the program by utilizing what has been learned in Steps 1–3 and making a rough estimate of the likelihood that the intended services will be delivered to the intended recipients and the likelihood that intended outcomes will occur.

Step 5: Reach agreement on any needed changes in program design or in the program itself through exploring what has been learned and determine what steps should be taken.

Step 6: Reach agreement on the focus and intended use of any further evaluation by offering a set of evaluation options and having stakeholders agree on one or more of these evaluation options.

Questions for Discussion

1. What particular challenges do you see as possible at each stage of the evaluability process?
2. How might the evaluator overcome some or all of the identified challenges?

Process Evaluations

A process (or implementation) evaluation can take place once or several times throughout the life of the project. Multiple aspects of the program can be examined by a process evaluation including program implementation, context, and research process.

At the most basic level and probably most frequently done, a process evaluation can examine some or all of the following aspects of project implementation:

- **Fidelity**, or the extent to which the project is being implemented as originally intended
- **Dosage**, or how much of the intended intervention is being delivered
- **Uptake**, or how much of the intervention is actually being received by participants and by different types of participants
- **Program reach**, or the proportion of the intended priority audience that participates in the intervention
- **Participant responsiveness**, or the participants' level of engagement in and receptivity to the program activities
- **Staff competency**, or staff members' qualifications including their cultural competency to work with the target population
- **Culture** and **context**, or aspects of the environment (e.g., culture, context, infrastructure issues) that may influence intervention implementation or study outcomes

Some process evaluations even examine evaluation methods and design processes to consider the influence of such factors as randomization, program contamination, or the extent to which the control group was exposed to the program.

The following case study illustrates what might be the foci of a process evaluation of a teen pregnancy and parenting program.

Case Study
Process Evaluation of Teen Pregnancy and Parenting Program

Damamli, an African term meaning "beautiful vision," is a program dedicated to supporting pregnant and parenting teen mothers in Maryland, placing emphasis on educating young mothers to be able to thrive independently. The program provides a three-phase support system to ensure that teen mothers are equipped with the skills they need to become independent and self-sufficient young women and mothers. In particular, the teen mothers receive training in the following functional areas: pregnancy prevention, developmental stages, anger management, discipline, communication, money management, household management, health, hygiene, employment preparedness, and community resources (Hearts & Homes for Youth, 2020).

A process evaluation of this particular teen pregnancy and parenting program might examine the following issues:

- Type, quality, and quantity of services delivered
- Demographic characteristics of the beneficiaries of project services
- Resources used to deliver the services, plus the barriers and facilitators to program delivery
- How implementation problems were resolved
- Recruitment and retention procedures, particularly sustaining the involvement of hard-to-reach participants

In the early and middle stages of a project, results from process evaluations can assist stakeholders to determine what the project is actually doing and how it is operating. The process evaluation can yield information that will tell administrators if there is a need for changes or midcourse corrections. For example, results from a process evaluation might point to the need to refine or modify participant recruitment strategies because certain marginalized target populations are not being reached, successfully recruited, or maintained in the project. After the project ends, a process evaluation, through its comprehensive picture of how the project functions, can yield important insights into why and how the outcomes or results were achieved (or not achieved). In other words, process evaluations can help explain both success and failure. If outcomes of the summative evaluation are not favorable, a process evaluation can help evaluators discern the extent to which failure may be the result of implementation failure or theory failure.

Implementation failure, introduced in Chapter 4, is the lack of expected results due to poor implementation of the intervention's services and activities. Stame (2010) identified two main issues that contribute to implementation failure: (a) the implementers' attitudes, beliefs, and behaviors and (b) the context, seen not simply as the geographical or institutional location into which programs and projects are embedded, but also as the prior set of social rules, norms, values, and interrelationships gathered in these places). An example of implementation failure would be no improvements in diabetic clients' health outcomes because the service providers were unable to schedule clients, as proposed, to meet with their doctor on a regular basis throughout the intervention. It might not be the service providers' fault that this occurred inasmuch as it could be due to unusually hazardous weather and other environmental conditions affecting the community that made it impossible to keep the clients' doctor visits on track.

Theory failure, also introduced in Chapter 4, occurs when project activities are implemented to the standards of the design strategy but the expected outcomes are not found, suggesting that the theory that linked the activities to the expected outcomes is incorrect. While program theory often assumes that a program's activities relate to outcomes in a simple and straightforward way—that is, the program (independent variable) produces a change in the target population (dependent variable)—this is often not the case (see Chapter 13 for more detail on independent and dependent variables). Stame (2010) notes that program theories hypothesizing linear causality from program input to program output and outcome may be too simplistic and even incorrect. In reality, there are complex factors that exist but are often absent in the program theory of change. In such instances, program theory failure may occur.

Progress Evaluations

This type of formative evaluation assesses a program's progress in achieving its intended goals. The goals serve as benchmarks for measuring progress. During a **progress evaluation**, the evaluator collects data to determine whether or not the benchmarks (or interim outcomes) were attained at particular points in time. A progress evaluation can also uncover unexpected developments that might point to the need for modifications of the program. In a behavioral modification program, for example, a progress evaluation might assess changes in participants' attitudes midway through a multiyear program, providing both feedback on what seems to be working and evidence of outcomes early on in the life of the program. While implementing a progress evaluation can be done throughout the life of a project, it is most useful during the program's early stages when activities are piloted and their individual effectiveness or articulation with other program components is unknown (Frechtling, 2010). Similar to information from a process or implementation evaluation, findings from a progress evaluation can later be used in a summative evaluation as baseline data.

In the following activity, readers plan a formative evaluation.

Activity
Planning a Formative Evaluation

Discuss the different types of formative evaluations examined in this chapter.

Now, as a team, imagine that your group was asked to plan a formative evaluation for your academic department, a university program, or your job's department or division. Briefly describe the evaluand you chose to consider, including an identification of the unit's mission and goals and its key stakeholders.

Then, in small groups, discuss how you would proceed.

Questions for Discussion

- What type of formative evaluation would you plan?
- What would be the rationale for your selection?
- What kinds of recommendations would you hope to be able to provide to the unit's administrator(s) (department or division chief, department chairperson, dean of the college, etc.)?

Summative, Outcome, and Impact Evaluation Types

Evaluations discussed in this section are those done primarily for the purpose of providing insights into program outcomes (intended and unintended) for the target population, communities, and/or systems. These types of evaluations are conducted during operations of mature programs at predetermined interval(s) when outcomes and impacts are expected to have occurred or at the end of the program (often in conjunction with baseline data collection prior to or at the beginning of project implementation). Results from summative or outcome and impact evaluations can help program administrators, funders, and other decision makers discern whether a program is meeting its objectives and having other unintended results.

When looking at outcomes and impacts, it is important that evaluators and others (e.g., funders) specifically attend to marginalized populations (e.g., low-income groups, people of color, people with disabilities) and the historical tendency to define "successful" outcomes and impacts from the perspective of the dominant group. Evaluators need to be in an ongoing mode of asking questions such as (a) Who is benefiting? (b) Who is not receiving equitable benefits? and (c) Who might even be further marginalized by the program being evaluated?

Outcome Evaluations

Outcome evaluations, sometimes referred to as effectiveness evaluations, are summative evaluations that assess the extent to which a program is producing the intended changes (and unintended changes). An outcome evaluation is the type of evaluation most people think about when they hear the term *evaluation*. It focuses on determining whether a program improves one or more targeted outcomes for those served. Outcome evaluations often are interested in ascertaining data on changes in participants' knowledge, attitudes, skills, behaviors, expectations, emotional status, or life circumstances as a result of their participation in the intervention. For example, an outcome evaluation of a smoking cessation program might ask:

- Did the program help participants stop smoking?
- Did certain types of people (e.g., male vs. female; middle age vs. young adult) have more positive outcomes than did others?

An outcome evaluation of a juvenile justice program might ask whether participation in the program led to changes in young people's skills, knowledge, attitudes, or behaviors and if those changes were associated with reduced juvenile justice system involvement. In an outcome evaluation, changes are generally expressed in numeric or quantitative format, and it, ideally, requires that targeted participants are compared to a control (or comparison) group of participants who are similar to the targeted participants in relevant ways except for the fact that they are not exposed to the program. Control and comparison groups are discussed in detail in Chapter 11.

In the following activity, readers reflect on and discuss a formative outcome evaluation of the previously presented teen parenting and pregnancy prevention project.

Reflect and Discuss
Outcome Evaluation of Teen Pregnancy and Parenting Program

The case study on page 184 illustrated some of the issues a process evaluation of a teen pregnancy and parenting program might examine:

- Type, quality, and quantity of services delivered
- Demographic characteristics of the beneficiaries of project services
- Resources used to deliver the services, plus the barriers and facilitators to program delivery
- How implementation problems were resolved
- Recruitment and retention procedures, particularly sustaining the involvement of hard-to-reach participants

Reflect on these process issues and then identify factors that an outcome evaluation of this same program might be interested in pursuing.

Compare and contrast the issues you identified with those identified by others.

Outcome evaluations are generally more expensive and time-consuming to conduct—that is, compared to process and implementation evaluations—and they require the involvement of experts with a track record of documenting their knowledge of and experience with evaluation research and statistics. Funders and certain other stakeholders (e.g., community members) may prioritize an outcome evaluation over a process evaluation for providing information about a program's effects on participants, while program managers and staff may prioritize the process evaluation because it can provide information useful to determine areas for program improvement. In an ideal situation, the process evaluation is just the first step, and it sets the stage for an outcome evaluation.

Outcomes can be looked at in terms of short-term results, intermediate (or medium-term) results, and long-term results. **Short-term outcomes** are assessed at the end of the intervention or shortly afterward. These are the immediate benefits or changes as a result of the intervention, often occurring within a year of program completion. **Long-term outcomes**, generally assessed in impact evaluation (as discussed in the next section), are more distant benefits or changes that are expected as a result of the intervention. Oftentimes, long-term results are referred to as impacts to convey the notion that they have broader and more durable significance than short-term results. These might include changes in conditions, policies, or organizational structure. **Intermediate outcomes** represent the layer of outcomes between short-term and long-term results. These medium-term results include a specified intermediate state that results from and follows short-term results and contributes to the desired long-term outcome. For example, an intermediate result might be actions taken by participants based on what they learned in the program. Short-term, intermediate, and long-term outcomes are related and build on each other, as demonstrated in the following case study.

A comprehensive evaluation will document process as well as outcomes since reporting process or outcomes in isolation provides an incomplete picture. For example, a process evaluation indicating a high attendance rate of teachers attending the district-wide professional development (PD) workshop does not reveal anything about teacher outcomes (e.g., new knowledge and skills, use of skills acquired in the classroom) as a result of attending the PD workshop. On the other hand, an outcome evaluation, alone, indicating that some teachers reported using skills acquired during the PD in their classroom while others did not will not provide sufficient contextual information to better understand the circumstances that might have facilitated or prevented teachers' use of skills gained in the classroom.

Case Study
Strong Through Every Mile Program Examples of Short-Term, Intermediate, and Long-Term Results

In an article published in *BMC Public Health*, Dayna Maniccia and Janel Leone (2019) presented the theoretical framework and protocol for the evaluation of Strong Through Every Mile (STEM), a 10-week structured running (exercise) program designed to increase psychological, social, and physical well-being among survivors of intimate partner violence. The authors reported STEM to be (to their knowledge) the only community-based structured running program designed to improve the quality of life of survivors of intimate partner violence. Maniccia and Leone provided the illustration shown in Figure 6.1 to indicate the short-term, intermediate (medium-term), and long-term outcomes expected from this project.

Figure 6.1 STEM Program Model

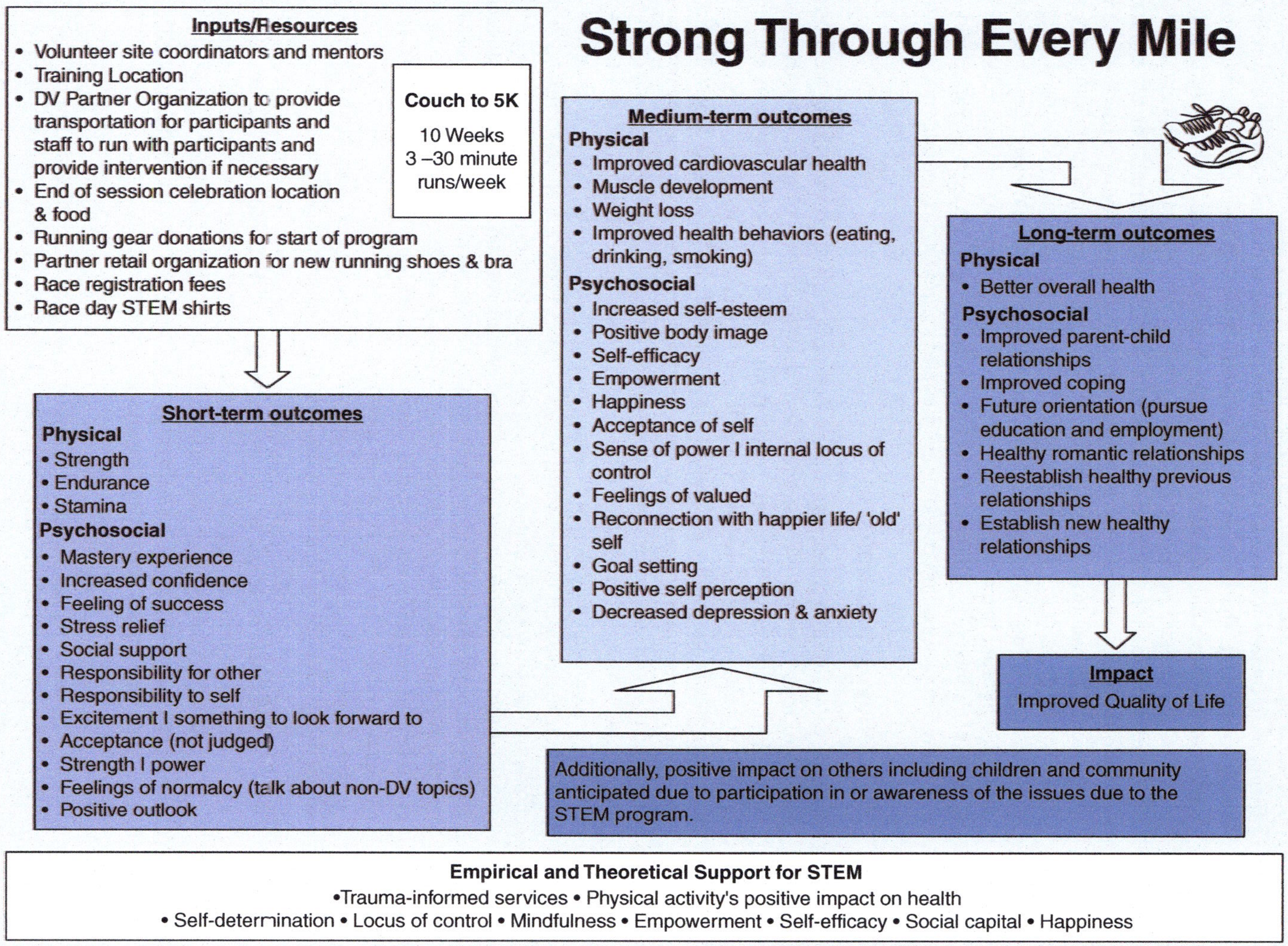

Strong Through Every Mile

Inputs/Resources
- Volunteer site coordinators and mentors
- Training Location
- DV Partner Organization to provide transportation for participants and staff to run with participants and provide intervention if necessary
- End of session celebration location & food
- Running gear donations for start of program
- Partner retail organization for new running shoes & bra
- Race registration fees
- Race day STEM shirts

Couch to 5K
10 Weeks
3–30 minute runs/week

Short-term outcomes

Physical
- Strength
- Endurance
- Stamina

Psychosocial
- Mastery experience
- Increased confidence
- Feeling of success
- Stress relief
- Social support
- Responsibility for other
- Responsibility to self
- Excitement I something to look forward to
- Acceptance (not judged)
- Strength I power
- Feelings of normalcy (talk about non-DV topics)
- Positive outlook

Medium-term outcomes

Physical
- Improved cardiovascular health
- Muscle development
- Weight loss
- Improved health behaviors (eating, drinking, smoking)

Psychosocial
- Increased self-esteem
- Positive body image
- Self-efficacy
- Empowerment
- Happiness
- Acceptance of self
- Sense of power I internal locus of control
- Feelings of valued
- Reconnection with happier life/ 'old' self
- Goal setting
- Positive self perception
- Decreased depression & anxiety

Long-term outcomes

Physical
- Better overall health

Psychosocial
- Improved parent-child relationships
- Improved coping
- Future orientation (pursue education and employment)
- Healthy romantic relationships
- Reestablish healthy previous relationships
- Establish new healthy relationships

Impact
Improved Quality of Life

Additionally, positive impact on others including children and community anticipated due to participation in or awareness of the issues due to the STEM program.

Empirical and Theoretical Support for STEM
- Trauma-informed services • Physical activity's positive impact on health
- Self-determination • Locus of control • Mindfulness • Empowerment • Self-efficacy • Social capital • Happiness

Source: Maniccia, D.M., & Lecne, J.M. (2019). Theoretical framework and protocol for the evaluation of Strong Through Every Mile (STEM), a structured running program for survivors of intimate partner violence. BMC Public Health 19, 692.

Impact Evaluations

Similar to outcome evaluation, the impact type of summative evaluation generally takes place after a program has ended. While outcomes are thought to be finite and measurable changes that occur shortly after the program ends, impact is the much broader longer-term effect. Therefore, in contrast to an outcome evaluation, an impact evaluation assesses any broader, longer-term changes that have occurred as a result of the program, intended and unintended, positive and negative, direct and indirect. These impacts seek to uncover net effects of the program on, for example, the entire community, school, organization, environment, or society.

Impact evaluations seek to reconstruct the counterfactual, or an estimate of what would have happened in the absence of the intervention. Focused on the long-term results, impact evaluations are useful for measuring sustained changes brought about by the program or making policy changes or modifications to the program. In some instances, impact evaluations are undertaken 5–10 years after the intervention has ended in order to examine its long-term effects. Unfortunately, because of feasibility considerations (e.g., limitations of time, monies, staff), many program evaluations are limited to process and outcome studies and are unable to conduct impact studies.

Efficiency Evaluations

If there were unlimited resources for social programs such that the achievement of goals and objectives were considered desirable, regardless of cost, then there would be no need to conduct efficiency evaluations. These types of evaluations are needed, however, because cost is always a consideration relative to what the program is doing and the value of its results. A detailed discussion of all the various types of efficiency evaluations is beyond the scope of the chapter. However, for a brief overview of the different types of efficiency evaluations, their history, and a brief glossary of terms and analyses, the reader is referred to Brian Yates's (2009) introduction to a special issue of *Evaluation and Program Planning* focusing on cost-inclusive evaluation.

Efficiency evaluations answer questions about project costs in comparison to the monetary value of its benefits or its effectiveness for bringing about changes in the social conditions it addresses. The concern with program effectiveness will logically precede an emphasis on program efficiency. There is no point in carrying out an ineffective program efficiently (Drummond, O'Brien, Stoddart, & Torrance, 1987). However, after the desired levels of results are achieved and/or maintained, an evaluation of a program's efficiency becomes a major concern.

Rossi and colleagues (2019, p. 238) provided some useful examples of efficiency issues that frequently arise in decision making about social programs:

- Policymakers decide to allocate funding to a basic literacy program for new immigrants that has shown positive effects in an impact evaluation. An important consideration is the extent to which the program's benefits (positive outcomes, both direct and indirect) exceed its costs (direct and indirect inputs required to produce the intervention).

- A government agency is reviewing national disease control programs currently in operation. If additional funds are to be allocated to disease control, the administrations want to know which program would show the biggest payoff per dollar of expenditure.

- Evaluations in criminal justice have established the effectiveness of various alternative programs for reducing recidivism. The most effective program is also the costliest. The question for the decision makers is whether the greater effectiveness of that program justified its highest cost.

- Board members of a private foundation are debating whether to support a program of low-interest loans for home purchases or a program to provide work skills training for married women to increase family income. They want to know which will produce the greatest economic benefits for low-income families.

These examples address cost and other resource allocation issues that decision makers must face at some point in their decisions regarding whether to fund, de-fund, expand, or reduce a program. Once administrators and other decision makers know how effective and efficient their programs are, they can then make an informed decision whether its results are worth the costs. A successful intervention that requires substantial resources to implement may not be a good choice to further invest in if similar outcomes can be obtained with markedly fewer resources.

Two of the major types of efficiency evaluations include cost-benefit and cost-effectiveness evaluations. Both are summative-type evaluations that examine the impacts of a program relative to its costs. The desirable outcome from both cost-benefit and cost-effectiveness evaluations is to be able to conclude whether the intervention is worthwhile to the extent that the achieved benefits (positive outcomes) exceed the incurred costs (inputs required to produce the results and/or opportunities presently foregone).

Cost-benefit evaluations examine the relationship between the value of resources used by a program and the value of resources produced by the program. Here, value is measured as the same, typically in monetary terms, for both the costs and the benefits. The question this type of evaluation seeks to answer is whether the program produces sufficient benefits in relation to its costs. During the mid-1970s, there was significant use of cost-benefit analyses, especially in evaluating the extent to which mental health services reduced unnecessary use of health services (e.g., Cummings & Follette, 1976). Consider the following example stressing the importance of determining the value of an intervention in view of its costs. Discuss responses to the questions raised.

Reflect and Discuss
Importance of Detecting Cost Benefits

In his edited volume, Robert Brent (2003) makes a cogent case for the value of cost-benefit evaluation. In the chapter "Introduction to Health Care Evaluation" (p. 4), he provides the following real-world example.

The Cost of Saving Lives: An Example

The American Cancer Society endorsed the protocol of having six sequential stool tests for detecting cancer of the bowel. Five sequential tests were previously the standard practice. However, it was found that for every extra case that was detected by the sixth test, the cost was $47 million. "Hey," you can imagine doctors saying, "one can never be too careful when it comes to matters of health." One may not know exactly what is the value of detecting the one case of colon cancer. But one can suspect that it is not as high as $47 million, given that for that same amount society can feed over 12,000 people for a year (at $10 a day). Only by subjecting health care expenditures to an economic evaluation can we uncover the bases for making worthwhile decisions.

(Continued)

> (Continued)
>
> *Source:* Excerpted from Brent, R. J. (2003). Introduction to health care evaluation. In R. J. Brent (Ed.), *Cost-benefit analysis and health care evaluation* (pp. 3–4). Northampton, MA: Edward Elgar.
>
> **Question for Discussion**
>
> When considering the case from the perspectives of various key stakeholders (identified as follows), what might be the major factors for determining the overall value or worth of the new protocol?
>
> - Doctors
> - Cancer patients and their families
> - Funders
> - Policymakers
> - Broader societal members
>
> Provide a rationale for your answer.

In a cost-benefit analysis, some main methodological issues include identifying benefits, measuring benefits, and determining cost (present and future). This, of course, will vary depending on the nature of the intervention or the social condition it seeks to remedy. Hauck, Smith, and Goddard (2004), for instance, point out that in a medical intervention, the most obvious benefit is the improved health of individuals. They further acknowledge that such an intervention may also generate wider societal benefits including benefits to third parties such as relatives (e.g., reduction in time spent caring for the patient), the wider community (e.g., reduction in infection risk), or the economy in general (e.g., effects on the labor market). Some studies also include indirect morbidity benefits (e.g., patients whose treatments result in their ability to work productively generate an economic benefit to society) in their analyses (Hauck et al., 2004). Once the relevant benefits are identified, they have to be measured in monetary terms (Hauck et al., 2004).

Cost-effectiveness evaluation is sometimes viewed as an alternative to cost-benefit evaluation. A cost-effectiveness evaluation compares an intervention to another intervention (or the status quo) by estimating how much it costs to gain a unit of a desired outcome, such as one year of life gained or death prevented. This is considered by some to be a more pragmatic approach to efficiency evaluations because it does not use monetary measures of benefits (Hauck et al., 2004) but instead considers the relationship between the value of resources used in program implementation and nonmonetary outcomes produced by the program. A common constraint in conducting a cost-benefit analysis is the inability to monetize benefits (Better Evaluation, n.d.b). In such cases, a cost effectiveness analysis is useful. In health care, for example, it is difficult to put a value on outcomes (e.g., lives saved); however, the outcomes themselves can be counted and compared (e.g., the number of lives saved). Examples of cost-effectiveness evaluations from the CDC are described in the following case study feature.

Case Study
CDC Cost-Effectiveness Evaluations

Intervention Is More Effective and Less Costly

In the example below, we compare the childhood vaccination program to the status quo of no vaccination program. We can see that the costs of implementing the program are less than the medical and productivity costs averted. Because the intervention is cost saving, the results are not presented as a cost-effectiveness ratio. Instead, they are presented as net cost savings.

Childhood Vaccination Program Example

Costs of implementation	$ 7.5 billion
Cost averted (medical costs & productivity losses)	−$76.4 billion
Net costs (negative value means cost savings)	−$68.9 billion

Intervention Is More Effective and More Costly

The example below presents the results from a cost-effectiveness analysis of a screening intervention for preventing chlamydia infections among high risk women (compared to the status quo of no screening). The results are presented as a cost-effectiveness ratio. This cost-effectiveness ratio can be compared to another intervention to determine which is more cost-effective.

Sexually Transmitted Diseases Treatment Example

Calculate Net Cost

Costs of implementation (cost of testing and treatment)	$23,844
Cost averted (cost of treating pelvic inflammatory disease [PID])	$13,033
Net costs (positive value means money spent)	$10,811
Identify Change in Health Outcomes	In this case, 10.6 PID cases averted
Calculate Cost-Effectiveness Ratio	
Net costs/change in health outcome = $10,811/10.6 =	$1020 per PID case averted

Note: This analysis modeled the intervention as applied to 10,000 women.

Source: Centers for Disease Control and Prevention, Office of the Associate Director for Policy and Strategy. (2019). *Polaris Economic Evaluation: Cost-effectiveness analysis.* Retrieved https://www.cdc.gov/policy/polaris/economics/cost-effectiveness.html

---

Over 40 years ago, Levin (1975) argued that the vast majority of evaluations fail to consider the cost component. This neglect, he believed, was due to the fact that the methodological basis for much evaluation research derived from the experimental sciences focusing on whether there were statistically significant differences between intervention and control/comparison groups with little emphasis on whether these differences were also socially significant with accompanying cost analyses of such differences. With more accountability and limited resources to allocate among competing programs (e.g., in areas such as public health), considerably more emphasis is being placed on evaluating costs and benefits.

Some policymakers and other stakeholder groups are concerned about the equity impacts of social investments on social inequalities. However, standard methods of economic evaluation such as cost-benefit analysis and cost-effectiveness analysis generally only provide information about the efficiency impacts of social investments on total costs and benefits. Since ideals of equity, fairness, or justice are complex, context-dependent, and value-laden, and they mean different things to different people, it can be difficult (although not impossible) to operationalize the impact of programs in equity terms (Sen, 2011).

Perhaps the greatest value of an efficiency evaluation is that it forces us to think in a disciplined fashion about both program costs and benefits (Rossi et al., 2019). Efficiency evaluations provide useful information particularly to funders who wish to see the return on their investment or the benefits of their money to the program beneficiaries. The outcome of these evaluations can have important consequences for future spending priorities, decisions about the direction of initiatives, and the level of accountability available for publicly funded initiatives (Marsh, 2010).

Alternative Types of Evaluations

As discussed earlier in this chapter, some types of evaluations do not neatly fit into the formative or summative classification by crossing the formative–summative boundaries (e.g., representing both or neither type).

Rapid Evaluations

In some instances, evaluations are allotted as little as a few weeks to be carried out, from start to finish. Despite the limited time frame, such evaluations are expected to be accurate, detailed, and insightful so that important program-related decisions, such as whether to continue, scale up, or discontinue, can be made with confidence. Rapid feedback evaluation, an idea originally conceptualized by Joseph Wholey and colleagues as an extension of evaluability assessment, grew out of their experiences working with federal program managers and their awareness of clients' needs for the timely delivery of findings to inform key programming decisions (Bellavita, Wholey, & Abramson, 1986; Wholey, 1983). Rapid feedback evaluations involve a quick assessment of program performance in terms of agreed-on objectives and indicators. This approach represents a process for testing changes to program operations and services to quickly know whether and for whom the change caused its intended improvement. Rapid evaluation reflects the notion that rough approximations delivered at the right time are better than precise results delivered too late for decision makers to act on them (McNall & Foster-Fishman, 2007).

Rapid evaluation, which can be formative or summative in nature, was created to provide program managers with quick answers to support program decisions. It can be used as an exploratory or formative evaluation technique yielding information that help clarify program goals, improve program quality, and clarify evaluation criteria for the design of a more intensive full-scale evaluation. Yet, in other cases, it may be summative in nature when the intended users (e.g., policymakers) conclude that they have enough information from the rapid evaluation that an intensive full-scale evaluation is not necessary. This is more likely to be the case with rapid evaluations that use a rigorous, scientific approach to provide decision makers with timely and actionable evidence of whether operational changes improve program outcomes.

Rapid evaluation methods came out of "a need for a quick, accurate, and economical method of evaluation of facilities and client satisfaction" (Anker, Guidotti, Orzeszyna, Sapirie, & Thuriax, 1993, p. 15) and concerns about the practicality and cost-effectiveness of surveys. Over the past 30 years, several methods of rapid evaluations have been conducted under various names such as real-time evaluation, rapid assessment, rapid feedback evaluation, and rapid cycle evaluation. Rapid evaluations seek to provide trustworthy, actionable information to decision makers at critical points in time.

Two major advantages of rapid evaluation are speed and cost-effectiveness, both important qualities in the real world of social programming where both time and money are in limited supply. This approach is invaluable for program staff under pressure from funders and other stakeholders to demonstrate some program performance on a specific issue or emerging problem beyond what is usually presented in quarterly and annual reports. Rapid evaluations are undertaken with the recognition that while longer-term evaluations might yield important information, the results might come too late to be of use. Although rapid evaluation takes much less time to conduct than traditional evaluations, it does not mean it is a rushed evaluation. The amount of preparation work done beforehand can be quite significant and comparable to preparing for a traditional evaluation. Two examples of rapid evaluation from Mathematica are provided in the following case study feature.

Case Study
Rapid Evaluations

On its website, Mathematica describes several cases of rapid evaluation done within the context of its work. Two examples are summarized as follows.

Rapid Evaluation Example I

Determining the most effective outreach strategies for increasing program engagement and uptake of employment services resources. A variety of government, private, and nonprofit organizations across the country offer reemployment services to veterans. In partnership with the U.S. Department of Labor and local agencies, Mathematica designed and tested a series of personalized emails, informed by insights from behavioral science, to encourage stronger job-seeker engagement with reemployment services. Through a quick-turnaround study, Mathematica measured statistically significant increases in service take-up and program completion as a result.

Rapid Evaluation Example II

Examining whether a new messaging approach, including proactive reminders, improves TANF participants' timely submission of work activity participation hours. Many local Temporary Assistance for Needy Families (TANF) and other public assistance programs struggle with on-time and accurate submissions of required participation documentation. In Colorado, Mathematica is partnering with a county workforce center to try out different nudges—email and postcard reminders—in an effort to improve the rate of timely reporting by participants.

Source: Mathematica. (2020). *Rapid-cycle evaluation.* Retrieved from https://www.mathematica-mpr.com/our-capabilities/rapid-cycle-evaluation

Rapid evaluations have been used extensively worldwide to study various public health initiatives to include study of (a) the HIV/AIDS crisis in racial and ethnic minority communities in three U.S. cities (Needle et al., 2003); (b) sexually transmitted infections (STIs) in St. Petersburg, Russia (Aral, St. Lawrence, Dyatlov, & Kozlov, 2005); (c) HIV and STIs in a gold mining town in Tanzania (Desmond et al., 2005); (d) drug use in South Africa (Vincent, Allsop, & Shoobridge, 2000); and (e) tuberculosis control in KaNgwane, South Africa (Lee & Price, 1985) (all cited in McNall & Foster-Fishman, 2007). The evaluation of ongoing responses to humanitarian emergencies presents an extreme example of an urgent need for evaluation findings in real time (McNall & Foster-Fishman, 2007). In response to the unfolding crisis in Kosovo in 1998 to 1999,[1] the Danish International Development Agency (DANIDA) conducted what is believed to be the first real-time evaluation (RTE) of a humanitarian emergency response (McNall & Foster-Fishman, 2007). Since then, the Evaluation and Policy Analysis Unit of the United Nations High Commissioner for Refugees (UNHCR) has used RTE to assess responses to humanitarian crises in various places including Sudan-Eritrea, Angola, Pakistan, Afghanistan-Iran, and Chad (Bartsch & Belgacem, 2004; Sandison, 2003).

Rapid evaluations can be conducted during any stage in the program life cycle. Prior to program initiation, a rapid evaluation can be used to determine what issues need to be addressed by a program. Rapid evaluation collected prior to program implementation can also yield baseline data for measuring program performance as well as provide valuable contextual information about local cultures and beliefs, norms, assets, and risk behaviors that can be integrated into the program design. At a program's midway, a rapid evaluation can be used to identify and fix problems as they occur. Lastly, at a program's end, a rapid evaluation can be used to assess successes, weaknesses, and potential for replication and/or scale-up.

The following activity provides readers an opportunity to identify where, within their person or professional context, rapid evaluations might be useful.

Activity
Rapid Evaluation and You

Think of instances in your life (at school, at work, or in another professional or personal setting) where a rapid evaluation could be useful.

Organize into small groups. Describe the situation to your group members, indicating

- the rationale for a rapid evaluation; and
- the value of a rapid evaluation, in contrast to a traditional evaluation, in the situation.

Metaevaluations

In 1969 in the *Educational Products Report*, Michael Scriven introduced metaevaluation to the field as a methodology to describe his evaluation of a plan to evaluate educational products. In this report, Scriven defined metaevaluation as any evaluation of an evaluation, evaluation system, or evaluation device. This is essentially a systematic and formal evaluation of evaluations to determine the quality of their processes and findings—or, more simply put, an evaluation of evaluations. Metaevaluation has

---

[1] In 1998 and 1999, the United States and its NATO allies attempted to put an end to escalating violence between ethnic Albanian guerrillas and Yugoslav forces in the Federal Republic of Yugoslavia's Kosovo region. During 1998, open conflict between Serbian military and police forces and Kosovar Albanian forces resulted in the deaths of over 1,500 Kosovar Albanians and forced 400,000 people from their homes. The international community became gravely concerned about the escalating conflict, its humanitarian consequences, and the risk of it spreading to other countries.

been expanded to include the process of delineating, obtaining, and applying descriptive information and judgmental information about an evaluation's utility, feasibility, propriety, and accuracy and its systematic nature, competence, integrity/honesty, respectfulness, and social responsibility to guide the evaluation and publicly report its strengths and weaknesses (Stufflebeam, 2001; Stufflebeam & Shinkfield, 2007).

Metaevaluations have great value in ensuring the quality of the evaluation, earning and maintaining credibility for the evaluation from both clients and other evaluators, and providing direction for improving evaluation plans, operations, draft reports, and means of communicating findings (Stufflebeam & Shinkfield, 2007). In the third edition of the Joint Committee on Standards and Educational Evaluation's *Program Evaluation Standards* (Yarbrough, Shulha, Hopson, & Caruthers, 2011), evaluation accountability was added as a new attribute calling for rigorous documentation of evaluations and their internal and external metaevaluation for formative and summative purposes.

Many scholars view metaevaluations as essential and a part of the professional obligation of evaluators although they note there are various ways metaevaluations can be undertaken. For example, Scriven (1991) believes that metaevaluation should first be done by evaluators on their own work. He acknowledges, however, that this approach has little credibility because the results of self-evaluation are notoriously unreliable. Therefore, whenever possible, Scriven advises using an independent evaluator for the metaevaluation. This is an individual who has no other roles and responsibilities relative to the program, the evaluation, or the organizations and institutions that staff those programs and evaluations. Further, when the stakes are high and the program evaluation quality should be unimpeachable, more complex and better-resourced metaevaluations are warranted (Yarbrough et al., 2011).

Metaevaluations can be conducted by making an assessment of evaluations through reports and other relevant sources such as information and judgments from various stakeholders such as the evaluator, client, program staff, program beneficiaries, and others. In other instances, metaevaluations might necessitate the additional monitoring and collection of data to address evaluation quality over longer periods of time, as well as long-term impact and utility (Yarbrough et al., 2011).

A metaevaluation often utilizes qualitative procedures such as content analysis or criteria checking that seeks to answer questions such as these:

- Did the report clearly describe the program?
- Were the techniques of data analysis explicit?
- Were the instruments for data collection valid?
- Did the report clearly justify the recommendations made?

Patton (1997, 2011) suggests three broad questions to focus the metaevaluation: (a) Was the evaluation done well? (b) Is the evaluation worth using? and (c) Did the evaluation meet professional standards and principles? In addition to Patton's three questions, we add another broad question to focus the metaevaluation: Did the evaluation pay close attention to issues of culture and context?

Metaevaluation has been considered a hallmark of good evaluation for over four decades (e.g., House, 1987; Scriven, 1969; Stufflebeam, 2001; Yarborough et al., 2011). Based on research reported by Cooksy and Caracelli (2009), however, there is not convincing evidence to indicate that metaevaluations have become a standard in the practice for individual evaluations, except perhaps in the form of the kind of management quality control reviews that occur at government agencies such as the U.S. GAO or large consulting firms.

Developmental Evaluations: Another Alternative to Formative–Summative

While the formative–summative approach to evaluation has an important role, it is not typically structured to support adaptive learning in complex and emerging initiatives or new developments where next steps are unknown (Patton, 2006, 2011). **Developmental evaluation** was conceptualized by Michael Quinn Patton in the early 1990s and expanded later (e.g., Patton, 2006, 2011) as an alternative to the traditional formative–summative paradigm and as a way to address innovation and complexity. Developmental evaluation, Patton contends, supports adapting and changing an innovation for ongoing development, whereas formative evaluation supports improving a program and helping it get ready for the summative evaluation. In a July 2010 *AEA365* post, Michael Q. Patton makes a distinction between innovations and standard projects and programs and the types of evaluations needed as follows:

> Innovations are different from standard projects and programs. Innovators are often different from people implementing typical programs. Innovators are in a hurry, value rapid, real time feedback, have a high tolerance for ambiguity, embrace uncertainty, learn quickly, and adapt rapidly to changed conditions. They're not always sure where they're heading, so they resist being boxed in by concrete, pre-set targets. They're propelled into action more by vision than by clear, specific and measurable outcomes. They want an evaluation approach attuned to their fast pace and innovative spirit. They are at home in complex dynamic systems. Such systems characterize the world in which they live and work. Thus, they want an evaluation approach [development evaluations] attuned to complexity. (quoted in Kistler, 2010, para. 2)

Patton also describes how developmental evaluation is distinct from monitoring. He argues that monitoring serves best to track progress against implementation plans when a detailed implementation plan has been funded for a model-based project. Developmental evaluation is best used with innovations, which often lack detailed implementation plans and predetermined monitoring indicators because they are occurring in complex dynamic systems and both the work and the indicators are emergent, developmental, and changing. In their practical guide to developmental evaluation, Dozois, Langois, and Blanchet-Cohen (2010, p. 14) summarized the important ways developmental evaluation differs from traditional evaluation:

- The primary focus is on adaptive learning rather than accountability to an external authority.
- The purpose is to provide real-time feedback and generate learning to inform development.

- The evaluator is embedded in the initiative as a member of the team.
- The [evaluator] role extends well beyond data collection and analysis; the evaluator actively intervenes to shape the course of development, helping to inform decision-making and facilitate learning.
- The evaluation is designed to capture system dynamics and surface innovative strategies and ideas.
- The approach is flexible, with new measures and monitoring mechanisms evolving as understanding of the situation deepens and the initiative's goals emerge (adapted from Westley, Zimmerman, & Patton, 2006).

Patton (2011) points to a developmental evaluation as appropriate for evaluating innovations or developing and emerging initiatives in dynamic environments where participants, conditions, interventions, and context are turbulent, pathways for achieving desired outcomes are uncertain, and conflicts about what to do are high. He also argues that this type of evaluation could be particularly useful in complex situations where the knowledge base is not well established. Complex and dynamic social and environmental change initiatives call for equally dynamic and nimble approaches to evaluation rather than more traditional approaches where an implicit assumption is that the progression of the problem to a solution can be laid out in a relatively clear sequence of steps (Gamble, 2006). Rather than try to reduce complexity, developmental evaluation seeks to create structured feedback mechanisms that provide the guidance to programs seeking to evolve, adapt, and thrive in complex conditions. See the following case study of a developmental evaluation reported by Patton (2011).

Case Study
Developmental Evaluation of Leadership Program

Michael Patton (2011) describes a developmental evaluation with a community leadership program where the evaluation team was asked to bring evaluative thinking and data to bear as the team conceptualized, developed, and tried out new approaches for new groups including immigrants, Indigenous Peoples, people from distressed rural communities, elected officials, and young people. The program developed new approaches in light of new federal and state policies affecting rural communities.

The developmental relationship lasted over 6 years and involved different evaluation designs each year including participant observation, several different surveys, field observations, telephone interviews, face-to-face interviews, focus groups, case studies of individuals and communities, cost analyses, theory-of-change conceptualizations, futuring exercises, and training participants to do their own community-based evaluations. Each year the program changed in significant ways and new evaluation questions emerged. Program goals and strategies evolved. No summative evaluation was ever conducted, no final report was ever written. The program continues to evolve and continues to rely on developmental evaluation.

Source: Excerpted from Patton (2011, p. 3).

The developmental evaluator's role focuses on helping innovators embed evaluative thinking into their decision-making processes as part of their ongoing design and implementation initiatives. As described in Chapter 1, evaluative thinking is "critical thinking applied in the context of evaluation, motivated by an attitude of inquisitiveness and a belief in the value of evidence, that involves identifying assumptions, posing thoughtful questions, pursuing deeper understanding through reflection and perspective taking, and informing decisions in preparation for action" (Buckley, Archibald, Hargraves, & Trochim, 2015, p. 378).

Developmental evaluation is not prescriptive, and it has the opportunity to be responsive to culture, inclusion, and the local context. It seeks to support and accommodate emergent, innovative, and transformative processes that often define the social change initiative; to nurture learning; and to provide rapid, real-time feedback. The developmental evaluator is integrally involved as a project team member, questioner, observer, and facilitator. This type of evaluation is grounded in a genuine and conscious commitment to learning and openness to change (Preskill & Beer, 2012). Examples of questions that can help guide a developmental evaluation include the following:

- What has been developed to date, or is developing and emerging, as the initiative takes shape?
- How can the initiative be more dynamic and adapt to the context in ways that are within the control of the project?
- What are the implications of what has been developed?

Developmental evaluation is particularly suited to situations that are (a) highly emergent and volatile where the environment is constantly changing (e.g., response to a natural disaster); (b) difficult to plan for or predict because the variables are interdependent and nonlinear (e.g., a financial meltdown); (c) socially complex, requiring collaboration among stakeholders from different organizations, systems, or sectors; and (d) innovative, requiring real-time learning and development (Dozois et al., 2010; Gamble, 2006; Patton, 2008; Preskill & Beer, 2012). It is optimal when there is buy-in from the project staff for such an approach, the project/organization has a culture that supports learning, there is a willingness to adapt the project's structure and procedures to accommodate new ways of doing things and a willingness to allocate resources to support innovation, and the process is participatory in nature from the leadership to support staff.

Developmental evaluation is not the solution for every project, issue, or situation inasmuch as a traditional evaluation often fulfills the intended purpose of judging whether a particular model, intervention, program, or policy is working or not (Cunningham & Elmi, 2015). However, when contexts are overly complex, uncertain, and dynamic, then developmental evaluation is a potential option.

The first step in the developmental evaluation process is determining the scope of the work. The evaluator needs to determine what things those leading the initiative are hoping to do and what contributions they think developmental evaluation can contribute to their efforts. Given the dynamic context of innovation, it is helpful for the developmental evaluator to anticipate how the scope of a developmental evaluation process might evolve and plan to periodically revisit the scope (Patton, 2011). In a developmental evaluation, questioning and learning take place simultaneously with action. Developmental evaluation is characterized by short cycles of design, data collection, feedback, and evaluative synthesis and reflection. This type of evaluation is typically a much more embedded process than traditional evaluation, and, as such, evaluators must be willing to invest in building relationships at the beginning of the process. Further, developmental evaluators, like all other evaluators, need to be attuned to manifestations of power dynamics and inequities operating within the innovations.

Putting It All Together

The following activity provides an opportunity for readers to reflect on all the various types of evaluations discussed in this chapter and to determine which type would be the best option for the scenarios provided.

Activity
Putting It All Together: What Would You Do?

Organize into small groups and discuss the six hypothetical project scenarios presented as follows. Then, reflect back on the different types of evaluations discussed in this chapter and indicate what type of evaluation you would recommend and why.

Scenario 1: The county executive is interested in obtaining information in order to understand the concerns and problems residents have and to ultimately identify and prioritize issues for action.

Scenario 2: The project director of a teen pregnancy and parenting program for low-income youth of color want to know the extent to which the project is successfully reaching its intended population.

Scenario 3: The funder of a science, technology, engineering, and mathematics (STEM) project is interested in finding out the extent to which the project is resulting in any significant changes in the participating girls' attitudes toward pursuing STEM majors in their postsecondary education.

Scenario 4: Funders of a community-based health program are unsure whether the funded program, although in operation for 18 months, is ready for a formal evaluation; however, they require some systematic data to help them determine the program's readiness.

Scenario 5: Organization X wants the evaluator to be a facilitator and learning coach who brings evaluative thinking to the table that informs ongoing change and innovation that is supportive of the organization's goals.

Scenario 6: A program director of a youth literacy program is interested in determining if the program has actually had an effect on the participating students.

Now, the groups can construct their own scenarios that would call for various types of evaluations discussed in this chapter.

SUMMARY

This chapter intended to provide readers with a good understanding of the different types of evaluations that fall within the mostly formative and summative dimensions as well as those that cross the boundaries of established categories or represent something quite different, such as developmental evaluations. A key emphasis in this chapter has been to consider evaluation types in terms of their major purpose, primary intended audience, and program stage. In planning and implementing the various types of evaluations discussed in this chapter, evaluators have a responsibility to obtain a good understanding of the evaluand, be knowledgeable about the history and background of the target population and the surrounding community, and implement the evaluation in a manner that is respectful and responsive to the intended users of the evaluation. While this can be difficult for some evaluators given their dominant positionality and difficulty in even seeing how they are failing to be inclusive and culturally responsive in their practice, it can be overcome with ongoing awareness of issues of power and privilege and deliberate steps to ensure that social justice, inclusion, and equity are prominent in its planning, implementation, and dissemination.

SUPPLEMENTAL RESOURCES

W. K. Kellogg Foundation Step-by-Step Guide to Evaluation: How to Become Savvy Evaluation Consumers

www.wkkf.org/resource-directory/resource/2017/11/wk-kellogg-foundation-step-by-step-guide-to-evaluation

This document supersedes the original 2008 and 2014 *Evaluation Handbook* and is designed to provide guidance to people with little or no experience with formal evaluation. It covers evaluation basics such as (a) determining which methodologies and approaches to use and when, (b) the importance of community engagement and racial equity in the evaluation process, and (c) communicating your findings.

Evaluability Assessment Checklist

www.gov.uk/government/uploads/system/uploads/attachment_data/file/248656/wp40-planning-eval-assessments.pdf

See pages 20–23 of the report, *Planning Evaluability Assessments: A Synthesis of the Literature With Recommendations* (Davies, 2013), for a checklist of things to consider in an evaluability assessment in (a) project design, (b) information availability, and (c) institutional context.

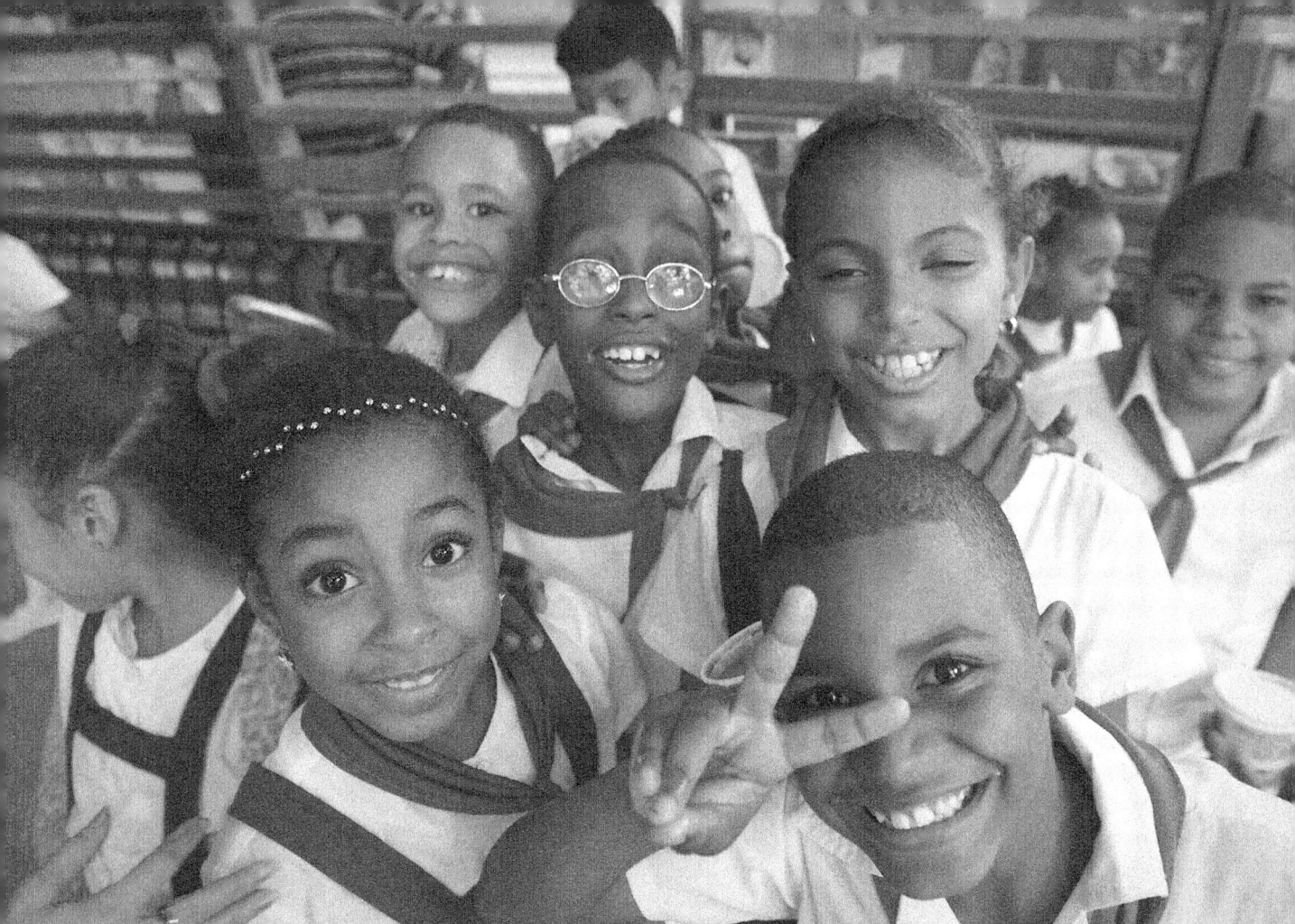
Istock/Joel Carillet

A keener understanding of the complex nature of social problems, how they are identified and the, oftentimes, racialized assumptions underlying social programming can provide evaluators with a broader conceptual lens for helping programs better work toward more socially just outcomes.

CHAPTER 7

Social Programming, Social Justice, and Evaluation

Evaluators must forge an evaluation practice that serves broad democratic ideals of diverse participation, social justice, and equity. They do this by meaningfully engaging, understanding, and uncovering the quality of the social programming experience for diverse participants, as well as the appropriateness and contextual fit of the program's design and the outcomes for people in programs within the context of their oftentimes racialized environments. Before this can be realized, it is essential that the evaluator understand the oftentimes racialized nature of social problems and social programming in a diverse society such as the United States.

After reading this chapter and participating in the activities, readers will be able to meet the following learning objectives:

- Explain how social problems and social programs get identified, politicized, and sometimes framed through a racialized lens

- Know why it is important for evaluators to have a broader understanding of social problems and social programming

- Understand "wicked problems" and be able to explain how they contribute to the marginalization of certain people and how they reflect the intersectionality of different social problems that social programming attempts to address

- Assist program administrators and others to clearly articulate the key components of a program, including writing good SMART objectives

- Develop logic models that depict the program's story, connecting its various components to their intended outcomes, as well as how contextual factors can be woven into such models

- Know the value of traditional, as well as nontraditional, depictions of logic models to describe a program's story

Introduction

This chapter will discuss social problems and social programming through a social justice lens. As evaluators speak for others through the work that they do, it is important that they have a keen understanding, as House and Howe (2000a) point out, of the reality that evaluations of social programs exist within some authority structure or some particular social system; that evaluations do not stand alone as simply logic or a methodology, free of time and space; and that evaluations are certainly not free of values or interests. Better understanding how social problems are identified and the assumptions underlying social programming designed to ameliorate these problems can provide evaluators with a broader conceptual lens for explaining the experiences and outcomes of individuals and communities impacted by these programs and for helping programs better work toward more socially just outcomes.

The chapter will describe the various components of a social program that should be clearly articulated before planning and implementing the evaluation, as well as the evaluator's potential role in assisting in clarifying these components. The last section of the chapter introduces the logic model and discusses how this visual representational aid assists in clarifying the theory of change for the social program under examination and planning the evaluation. Both traditional (linear and causal pathways) and nontraditional, nonlinear (e.g., circular, Afrocentric, Indigenous) logic model formats with their corresponding strengths and limitations are discussed. In particular, ways for depicting cultural and contextual factors that might influence the program are presented.

Understanding Social Problems and Social Programs Through a Social Justice Lens

Wicked Problems

To the extent that evaluators have a keen understanding of the nature of social problems in a diverse country such as the United States, they are better able to understand the appropriateness and fit of the social program within the target community. Evaluators work with programs designed to ameliorate wicked problems that threaten the physical and psychological well-being of children, families, communities, and entire populations. Wicked problems involve multiple and diverse stakeholders and are socially and politically complex. As such, issues of trust, respect, and equity often are, implicitly or explicitly, embedded in discussions toward resolution of the problem.

Design theorists Rittel and Webber (1973) first introduced the term *wicked problem* to draw attention to the complexities and challenges of planning and social policy problems. They described wicked problems as a class of social system problems that are socially complex, highly resistant to resolution, multicausal, and ill formulated and where there are many clients and decision makers with conflicting values. Table 7.1 illustrates the 10 characteristics of wicked problems as put forth by Rittel and Webber.

Wicked problems are difficult or almost impossible to solve because of the interconnected nature of these problems with other problems; incomplete, contradictory knowledge (no clear solution); the number of people and opinions involved; and the large economic burden (Rittel & Webber, 1973). As introduced by Rittel and Webber (1973), wicked problems referred to social planning problems, but the term has since been applied in multiple contexts where Indigenous and other minority groups experience injustice and inequities (Hopson & Cram, 2018). Many of today's most urgent social challenges are widely viewed to be wicked problems—that is, complex, largely intractable, contested issues. Examples of wicked problems coupled with social injustices include racial disparities in educational outcomes, mass incarceration, racial and gendered discrimination, unfair housing policies and practices, poverty, gun violence, food insecurity, inequitable health care and access, and domestic violence. Decades of efforts to eliminate problems such as poverty, economic underdevelopment, inequality, and crime may have lessened the problems but certainly have not solved them by any meaningful standard. Particularly troublesome is that some wicked problems, such as income inequality, have actually worsened since the 1970s (Congressional Budget Office, 2018; Stone, Trisi, Sherman, & Taylor, 2018).

Table 7.1 10 Characteristics of Wicked Problems

Wicked Problems Characteristics	Brief Description
There is no definitive formulation of the problem.	Different people describe the problem differently.
There is no stopping rule.	There is no solution that is final; it is difficult to determine success with wicked problems because they bleed into one another (e.g., poverty and food insecurity).
Solutions are not true/false or clearly right or wrong.	There is likely a matter of finding acceptable solutions, compromises, or good enough options.
There is no immediate and no ultimate test of a solution.	There is no immediate determination or test of how good a solution attempt has been.
Every solution is a "one-shot" operation.	There is no real opportunity to learn by trial and error; every attempt counts and has significant impacts.
There is no set number of exhaustive desirable solutions.	There is a range of possible solutions to the problem, with the acceptability or desirability depending on perspective of the various stakeholders.
The problem is essentially unique.	Despite similarities between a current problem and a previous one, there might be an additional distinguishing property that is of overriding importance.
It is a symptom of another problem.	Every problem is multicausal, and there are many interdependencies.
Multiple explanations exist.	Explanations of wicked problems vary greatly depending on the individual perspective, and the choice of explanation determines the nature of the problem's solution.
Planners (policymakers) have no right to be wrong.	Planners attempting to solve a wicked problem must be fully responsible for their actions.

Source: Adapted from Rittel, H. W. J. & Webber, M. M. (1973). Dilemmas in the general theory of planning. Policy Sciences, 4, 155–169.

Wicked problems contribute to the marginalization of individuals based on their race/ethnicity, gender, sexual orientation, age, religion, and other points and intersections of difference from a cisgender, white, male, able-bodied norm; further, wicked problems are intensely political because ameliorating a wicked problem is often about the redistribution of goods and services to those who may be seen as "less deserving" in the common sense of the wider society (Hopson & Cram, 2018). Social problems, like those mentioned earlier, that are identified as wicked problems are especially challenging to solve because they involve a number of different stakeholders with different views. For example, if we were to ask 10 individuals about mass incarceration, we would be likely to obtain 10 different responses as to what are the main contributors to mass incarceration and an even greater number of ideas as to the best ways of resolving mass incarceration. The responses are likely to be informed by respondents' worldview, including their personal values and circumstances, as well as their own situated knowledge of the issue. As noted by Domenico, Hospes, and Ross (2012), wicked problems have cause–effect relationships that are difficult or impossible to define, and they cannot be framed without creating controversies among stakeholders. Solutions require collective action among societal groups with strongly held, conflicting beliefs and values. The following case study describes global food insecurity as a wicked problem.

> ## Case Study
> ### Global Food Insecurity as a Wicked Problem
>
> According to the United Nations, food security exists when all people at all times have physical, social, and economic access to sufficient, safe, and nutritious (FAO, IFAD, UNICEF, WFP, & WHO, 2019). People experiencing moderate food insecurity face uncertainties about their ability to obtain food and are forced to reduce, at times during the year, the quality and/or quantity of food they consume due to lack of money or other resources. This situation diminishes dietary quality, disrupts normal eating patterns, and can have negative consequences for nutrition, health, and well-being. Individuals facing severe food insecurity experience hunger, have likely run out of food, and, at the most extreme, go for days without eating, putting their health and well-being at grave risk.
>
> A myriad of socioeconomic problems are linked to food insecurity. These include issues such as poverty, social inequality, poor health resources, poor working conditions, and inadequate education. These, in turn, result in a lack of access to the resources needed to produce or purchase food. In addition to socioeconomic factors, environmental degradation, loss of biodiversity, and unsustainable land-use practices contribute significantly to the problem of global food security.

The following activity asks readers to identify and think about wicked problems in their community.

> ## Activity
> ### Wicked Problems You See
>
> Identify an issue within your (broader or immediate) context that you would characterize as a wicked problem.
>
> Identify the various key stakeholders, including people/groups/organizations who are affected by and can affect the problem. For the stakeholders that you identified, provide a brief written description of how each stakeholder group is likely to frame the problem (e.g., causes, consequences) and potential solution(s).
>
> Now, go back to Table 7.1 and delineate the characteristics of the problem that are commensurate with Rittel and Webber's (1973) 10 characteristics of wicked problems.

Hopson and Cram (2018) expand discussion of wicked problems to include "complex ecologies of evaluation" spanning government, nongovernment, philanthropic, tribal, and community settings. They describe ecology as representing "the diverse natural, physical, and organizational realities and settings of projects, programs, and policies" (p. 7). Further, they argue that evaluators have the potential to add immense value to unpacking, understanding, and responding to wicked problems where and when they confront them around the world, particularly if the field moves away from its too-often-narrow focus on methods, tools, and theories. Hopson and Cram eloquently state that

> evaluators are encouraged to lift their heads up from decisions about method to look about and think about place and space, to contemplate the land on which they stand and the cultural contexts in which they work. (pp. 7–8)

Many social programs that evaluators are tasked with evaluating focus on wicked social problems that are intimately interconnected with other problems. For example, poverty is tied to poor and inadequate housing; children who live in poor housing often attend underresourced neighborhood schools and receive lower-quality education than their more affluent counterparts; low-quality education is related to poor life outcomes (few employment opportunities, lower lifetime income levels, etc.). Evaluators should be cognizant of these connections even if they are not a stated focus of the social program under study. Furthermore, attention to the power dynamics and causes of particular social problems under consideration can help evaluators employ both a micro-analysis (focusing on the individual) and a macro-analysis (focusing on larger structures of society such as political, legal, and economic systems) to capture the meanings of the processes and outcomes they see during the evaluation.

Social Problems: Definition, Description, and Theoretical Underpinnings

Whereas private problems are matters for the individual to resolve, social problems are public issues that generally engender a public response to solve. Behaviors or conditions are identified as social problems only when they (a) have negative consequences for large numbers of people, (b) are recognized as conditions or behaviors that need to be addressed, and/or (c) have a significant number of people mobilize to eliminate the behavior or condition (Heiner, 2016). Once a behavior or condition is identified as a social problem, some data about it become vital to the development of policies and practices to remedy the problem. Typically, policymakers seek data on the size of the problem, its location in the social structure, and its trajectory or trends in particular environments. Evaluators are often called on to conduct a needs assessment (discussed in detail in Chapter 6), which can answer questions around the nature, magnitude, and distribution of a problem that a social program is intended to address.

Objective Element of Social Problems

Sociologists tend to put forth definitions and descriptions of social problems that entail both an objective and a subjective component and vary across societies, among individuals and groups within a society, and across historical time periods (Barkan, 2012). The objective element of a social problem is that to be identified as such the condition or behavior must be a real, objective condition; must be a phenomenon that induces material and/or psyche suffering for certain segments of the population; and must be able to be measured, explained, and solved. There is an objective reality to the social problem even though there may be different perspectives to its measurement, explanation, consequences, and solution. Individuals become aware of social problems through their own life experiences, the media, and education. For example, while there is debate about the objective consequences of climate change, this condition is generally established by a substantial body of data accumulated from work by academic researchers, government agencies, and other sources.

Subjective Element of Social Problems

The subjective element is that there must be a perception that a condition or behavior needs to be addressed for it to be considered a social problem. As discussed in Chapter 4, this reflects a social constructivist viewpoint (Rubington & Weinberg,

2010), whereby conditions become social problems through a collective process of definition and interpretation influenced by individuals' beliefs, values, and life experiences. From a social constructivist perspective, while various types of negative conditions and behaviors currently exist, they may not be considered sufficiently negative to acquire the status of a social problem. Many negative conditions or behaviors only become social problems if citizens (often from the dominant group), policymakers, or other parties call attention to the condition or behavior. Not all undesirable societal conditions are elevated to the status of social problems that engender public concern because, in large part, there is no public outcry about these conditions and only a small proportion of the country's population has pushed for something to be done about them. Examples include negative behaviors and conditions such as political and corporate corruption, limited energy supply, and resource depletion, all of which are real threats in the United States, yet there is no widespread outcry to ameliorate these conditions.

Critical constructivism, a synthesis of conflict theory and symbolic interactionism, seeks to explain why some seemingly harmful phenomena (e.g., corporate corruption) get little public attention and are not deemed social problems by emphasizing the role of elite interests in the process of social problem identification. This approach overlaps the critical lens of conflict theory to understand power relationships and inequality with the constructivist lens of symbolic interactionism to unpack the process of meaning-making and interpretation of the social environment (Heiner, 2013). Critical constructivism argues that the manner in which social problems are identified, constructed, and presented to the public often reflects the interests of society's elite more than those of the general public—oftentimes at the expense of those with the least power (Blau, 2014; Heiner, 2013). Hence, to the extent that social problems are constructions, even conditions that hurt people need not be deemed social problems. For example, segregated facilities such as restaurants, hotels, schools, and toilets in the South persisted for over 100 years without being considered a problem by the members of the dominant culture in this country. Similarly, the impoverishment and massacre of a high proportion of the Indigenous population was not a problem while it was happening, but only deemed a problem long after its occurrence and negative consequences. According to Heiner (2013), those without power accept the existence of certain social problems because they believe the messaging and accept the cultural norms, beliefs, and values. Further, members of the dominant and powerful group enforce their social order on vulnerable groups through policies, laws, media, and social institutions to promote the status quo, which ultimately maintains their privileged status (Anderson & Taylor, 2013). As Murray Edelman (1987) aptly points out,

> problems come into discourse and therefore into existence as reinforcements of ideologies, not simply because they are there or because they are important for well-being. They signify who is virtuous and useful and who is dangerous and inadequate, which action will be rewarded and which penalized. . . . They construct areas of immunity from concern because those areas are not seen as problems. (p. 8)

Unfortunately, in this 24/7 media-driven society, there is also a competition for attention among the problems that are publicly discussed; as some problems come to dominate social and political news and discussion, others fade from the scene.

Almost 50 years ago—and even more applicable today—Anthony Downs (1972) wrote about "issue-attention cycles" to put forth the notion that after a period of time an issue begins to bore the public and is replaced with something else, even if the original issue has not been resolved. As an example, he points out that ghetto riots were headline news from the 1965 Watts riots in Los Angeles until about 1970, when they were reduced to minor items, even though the ghettos continued to erupt in violent protest through at least the early '70s. Downs argued that the logic that explains official, public, and media attention to political problems turns not on their severity but rather on their dramatic appeals. Generally, three qualities (at varying degrees) characterize social problems that often go through this issue-attention cycle:

- The majority of persons from the dominant group in society are not suffering from the problem (e.g., poverty, crime, unemployment) nearly as much as some minority group(s).

- The sufferings caused by the problem are generated by social arrangements that provide significant benefits to a majority or a powerful minority of the population.

- The problem has no intrinsically exciting qualities or no longer has them; for example, when urban city racial riots were being shown nightly on the nation's television screens, public attention naturally focused upon their causes and consequences. But when they ceased (or at least the media stopped reporting them so intensively), public interest in the problems related to them declined sharply. (Downs, 1972, pp. 41–42)

To the extent that evaluators gain a broader conceptual and theoretical lens for deconstructing how social problems exist and are dealt with through power, policy, and social programming, they will be in a better position to develop and implement more useful evaluations of programs and projects designed to address various social problems.

Sources of Social Problems

Factors that cause and/or help perpetuate social problems occur at multiple levels of social life. Some consider the locus of social problems to be at the individual level, and the system bears no blame. Here, it is believed that "maladjusted" individuals engaging in bad behaviors or those with bad attitudes, values, and beliefs cause social problems in society (W. Ryan, 1976). This perspective is rooted in **Social Darwinism**, or the belief in the "survival of the fittest"—the idea that certain people become powerful in society because they are innately better. Social Darwinism has historically been used to justify imperialism, racism, eugenics, and social inequality. A person-blame perspective, or deficit model as discussed in Chapter 5, would argue, for example, that one reason for the racial achievement gap is that African American parents, especially those from low-income groups, do not care about their children's learning, fail to teach them good study habits, and do not encourage them to take school seriously. This perspective would also argue that poor people are poor because they are lazy and do not want to work. The person-blame perspective reinforces negative stereotypes, and unfortunately, this perception can negatively influence the ways that policies are defined, and programs are designed, to "help" poor or other marginalized individuals.

Then, there is the belief that the source of social problems is at the societal or system level. This perspective argues that societal conditions are the major sources of social problems. Here, dealing with such social problems is thought to, first, involve understanding the distribution of power within our society. This includes recognition of the government, economy, system of (in)justice, and political, educational, and other institutional frameworks that constrain opportunities for certain groups of people. In other words, instead of simply blaming poor people for being poor, systems perspectives argue that attention must be given to elements (e.g., housing costs, health care, unfair wages, segregated schools) of society that keep poor people in poverty. A systems perspective calls for changing structures and power inequities that generate and facilitate social problems. Social problems can also be manifested as a result of the interactions of individual- and systems-level factors.

Social Problems' Fluid Nature

Behaviors and circumstances deemed social problems are created with a complex grid of shared cultural understandings communicated through rituals, books, customs, institutional rules and policies, news media, and entertainment (Heiner, 2013). Social problems come into discourse and therefore into existence as reinforcement of ideologies oftentimes signifying who is (or is not) virtuous and useful, who is dangerous or inadequate, and which actions are to be rewarded or penalized (Edelman, 1987).

Social problems are not fixed; instead, they change over time in size, demographic patterning, and nature. Conditions defined as social problems at any given time are not facts, but social constructions that reflect and reinforce established beliefs about the self, the other, and the social settings in which we live, and, among other uses, they rationalize inequities based on race, class, and gender (Edelman, 1987). Definitions of social problems differ by both audience and time. For example, prior to the 19th century, domestic violence was not viewed as a social problem inasmuch as a husband had a legal right and "marital obligation" to exert discipline and control over his wife through the use of physical force. Today, of course, domestic violence, or use of physical force in relationships, is regarded as a social problem rather than a marital right. Poverty, unemployment, and discrimination against women and minority groups are generally accepted, at the present time, as social problems, but throughout much of human history they were regarded as part of the natural order (Edelman, 1987). In the early 1980s, homelessness was primarily a problem affecting very poor single men, but by the early 1990s, single parents and their children comprised almost one-half of the country's homeless population, and thus it was deemed a major social problem within U.S. society. Even today, some individuals and groups in this country view the availability of abortion as a social problem, while others view restrictions on abortion as a social problem. Changing dynamics have a profound effect on what social problems are recognized and what social programs are funded.

The following activity provides an opportunity for readers to identify and discuss major social problems in their community.

> # Reflect and Discuss
> ## Major Social Problems in Your Community
>
> - What do you see as a major social problem in your community?
> - Who is most negatively affected by this social problem, and how?
> - What actions, if any, do you see being undertaken to ameliorate these problems?

Social Programs Through a Social Justice and Transformative Lens

To produce evaluations that are useful and have potential for impact across diverse stakeholder groups and constituencies, it is critical that evaluators understand the nature of social programming (or interventions) designed to ameliorate social problems, through a social justice and **transformative lens**, prior to undertaking the evaluation. Social justice– and transformative-oriented perspectives examine the holistic nature of social problems by seeking to understand the interdependency among individuals, communities, and societies using a more judicious democratic process in generating knowledge about social problems and social interventions and using this knowledge to both advance and transform social progress. It should be stressed that this orientation is not embraced by all evaluators; yet, it has a nascent presence in evaluation theory and practice. As was discussed in Chapter 5, advocates of social justice and transformative perspectives look at social programming from the beginning with the moral perspective that respect for the rights of others includes respect for diverse worldviews and lived experiences, and the right to disagree and to learn from disagreement.

We assert that social justice and transformative perspectives should be included in seeking understanding of social problems and subsequently in evaluating social programs. This is particularly the case when examining programs targeting people of color and other marginalized groups, such as persons with disabilities, since these groups often do not get to define the nature of their own problems and have genuine and meaningful input into the solutions (**social programs**) to address the problem. Kushner (2009) summarized five outcomes as the argument for a social justice orientation in evaluation. These outcomes include (a) providing an open exchange of ideas across stakeholder groups, (b) making the evaluation process a space where power inequalities can be (procedurally) neutralized (i.e., equal treatment for all), (c) promoting independence and impartiality of the evaluator whose obligation is to address everyone's dilemma, (d) promoting free and open publication of evaluation reports, and (e) increasing recognition of collective responsibility for enhancing public information. Consideration of these outcomes provides a useful starting point for evaluators to begin their own reflection about the place of social justice in their own learning and evaluation practice. The following activity provides an opportunity for readers to think about, reflect on, and discuss how they might approach understanding program context through a social justice and transformative lens.

> ## Reflect and Discuss
> ### Social Programming and Evaluation Through a Social Justice and Transformative Lens
>
> Imagine that you were asked to evaluate a housing program within one of the most depressed areas of Detroit, Michigan.
>
> From social justice and transformative perspectives, what might be some contextual issues on which you would gather information to better understand the program's outcomes once received?
>
> What are some things that you, as the evaluator, might do? Might look for? Might ask about? Whom might you seek to talk with, and why?
>
> Organize into small groups and discuss your reflections with others in your group.

Considering the nature of social problems and social programs through a social justice lens can promote evaluative thinking aimed at better understanding the link between the intervention (or social program) and outcomes by explicitly situating the intervention, and its stakeholders, within its sociocultural, historical, political, and organizational context (Thomas & Parsons, 2017). Such critical thinking applied to the evaluation context can serve as the foundation for planning, implementing, and disseminating evaluation findings that serves broad democratic ideals of diverse participation, social justice, and equity. Individuals who evaluate programs serving minority and other marginalized populations (e.g., low-income groups, persons with disabilities), in particular, should take notice of the extent to which the policies, activities, and theories of change that serve as the basis for these interventions may, implicitly or explicitly, reinforce negative biases, **racial framing** (House, 2017), or framing based on other demographic characteristics of particular groups. For the evaluator, the task of program evaluation is not an objective and detached examination into the inert, static, external realities of social programs; instead, it looks at the fluid, subjective world of people's lives, as experienced, interpreted, recalled, and mediated by them, and the oftentimes-racialized systemic contexts in which social programs, communities, and individuals are embedded (Thomas, Madison, Rockcliffe, DeLaine, & Lowe, 2018).

In her Voices From the Field interview, Dominica McBride points out that the evaluator's mindset is critical to embracing a social cultural equity lens for examining social programs, valuing the community and its strengths, and providing evaluative data that can be a resource for community members as they advocate for social programs to ameliorate certain social problems.

Voices From the Field

Dominica McBride: Reflective Action, Social Programming, and Evaluation

The evaluator's mindset is critical. The social cultural equity lens influences how evaluators look at things, how we analyze data, and what happens afterwards. There is a self-reflective piece where we must question our own assumptions, decisions, and actions given our training and the broader context. Our mindset needs to be one of valuing the skills and talents of the community and including them in evaluation decision making such as having a say in evaluation questions and tools. The evaluator must have cultural humility that involves showing respect to members of the community and behaving in a way that says that I can and want to learn from persons different from my own group. As agents of social change, evaluators must have a core commitment to seeing this change take place and engaging in actionable steps to make it happen. The evaluator can be an agent of social change through an activist/advocate lens by speaking truth to power.

Evaluators should also consider what collective action within the community is needed to move things in a different, more equitable direction. The evaluator must work in collaboration with other people who are doing this social programming work. Community partnership/engagement is a priority, and evaluation is seen as an opportunity to provide leadership and build the capacity of the community. Because of the partnership an evaluator has with the community, more valid data can be collected; partnerships can too be rehabilitative by providing data for program improvement and data to meet needs and support community empowerment. Evaluative data can drive a broader focus on the issue by serving as a resource for the community to advocate and use data to make the just change they want to see in their community. For example, in response to a community-based youth violence prevention project in Illinois where the government cut funding, evaluators worked with the program staff to help them use data to demonstrate the need and to show why their funding should be reinstated. While the evaluator competencies are a great foundation for people who want to be evaluators, we also need people who are proficient in how we make social change happen—effective advocacy, community organizing, and mobilizing people to take collective action.

Dominica McBride is CEO of BECOME, a Center for Community Engagement and Social Change, in Chicago, Illinois. Veronica G. Thomas interviewed her in the fall of 2019.

Power, Political, and Economic Nature of Social Problems

Social problems are often defined by those in power. However, acceptance of definitions of social problems only from the point of view of the "powerful" individuals within a society can be problematic. The powerful can define social reality in a manner that manipulates public opinion (Eitzen, Baca-Zinn, & Smith, 2013). Political elites promote one understanding of an issue over another to advance a particular policy position. Through emphasizing certain features of an issue, downplaying others, and assembling those features into a coherent narrative with clear implications for policy actions, they are able to frame public perception, either favorably or unfavorably, regarding the problem (Winter, 2008).

As discussed earlier in this chapter, political perspectives and ideologies help to frame social problems within the United States. They single out which conditions of behaviors are identified as social problems, how they are defined, and how the problem should be solved. The manner in which a social problem is articulated has a dramatic effect on the kinds of social programming that are proposed for ameliorating the problem. For example, liberal Democrats often view poverty as a condition resulting from circumstances beyond an individual's control such as lack of opportunity and structural factors (e.g., racism) within institutions and systems (Cato Institute, 2019). They feel that it is an injustice that poor people are poor. As a result, their solutions call for systemic changes aimed at expanding opportunities for disenfranchised individuals and communities. Liberals generally push for increased federal support and safety net programs for individuals and families to protect them from poverty. Conservative Republicans tend to view poverty as at the individual level resulting from a lack of motivation, limited intelligence, inability to delay gratification, and other personal characteristics of poor people. They view poverty as a social problem due mostly to poor people's behavior (Cato Institute, 2019). Conservatives tend to defend the existing system and are less supportive of using the federal government to help people out of poverty. They often advocate for more personal responsibility and argue that if poor people tried a little harder, or were not so lazy, they would not be poor anymore.

There is also an economic side to social problems. The economic burden, of course, rests on those groups (e.g., poor people) who experience the social problem or condition. However, there can be a benefit to other individuals and groups. This benefit generally serves to bolster the influence and economic outcomes of the privileged individuals and groups. In his book, *The Poverty Industry: The Exploitation of America's Most Vulnerable Citizens*, Hatcher (2016) argues that there is a vast scale of disadvantaged people being exploited for profit. He used the concept of the "poverty industry" to describe how state governments and their private industry partners are profiting from the social safety net, turning America's most vulnerable populations into sources of revenue. The poverty industry, according to Hatcher's analysis, is stealing billions in federal aid and other funds from impoverished families, abused and neglected children, and the disabled and elderly poor.

Readers are encouraged to complete the activity that follows to draw a sharp comparison between the benefits for one group and the suffering for another group as a result of the same social problem.

Activity
Research the Literature: Who Suffers and Who Benefits

Conduct a review of the literature in one of two areas: financing and organization of U.S. schools and the educational system, or U.S. health care delivery.

Based on your literature review, media coverage, and your own situational knowledge of the issue, explain how and why some groups of people suffer from current status in the area, and who they are, while others, simultaneously, benefit. Draw some conclusions from your analysis.

Eitzen and colleagues (2013) stress that conventional social problem identification focuses on the symptoms of social ills and the people who deviate from the norm, rather than the sources of the problem. As examples, they noted (and we add) that, as a society, we are more apt to

- study the person who commits a crime instead of the law or the prison system that exacerbates negative individual outcomes;
- scrutinize persons with cognitive and mental disabilities rather than the social institutions, social conditions, and quality of life that may facilitate or perpetuate cognitive and mental decline;
- explore the culture of the poor (from a deficit perspective) rather than how the characteristics of the rich fuel income inequalities;

- investigate the pathologies of students and their families rather than the inadequacies of education; and
- study the characteristics and consequences of poverty rather than the social structure that allows conditions like poverty to exist.

There is a special role that evaluators can play in helping relevant stakeholders to think through alternative or broader social problem definitions and solutions. In particular, evaluators can facilitate discussions surrounding the fit between popular conceptions of the problem, often found in newspapers and other sources, and the implicit or explicit definitions included in legislative or administrative remedies (Rossi & Berk, 1990).

Equity-Based Social Programming

Many of our social problems are caused by or result in disparities and inequities between minority and majority groups. At the international level, in particular, momentum has been growing for a stronger focus on equity in human development. Therefore, inherent in the goal of many internationally based social programs is the explicit emphasis on disparities and inequities. **Equity-focused interventions** seek to reduce disparities between the most and least disadvantaged groups within a population. These programs aim at ensuring that services and benefits reach the most hard-to-reach segments of the population and avoid intervention-generated inequities (Segone, 2012). The major aim of this type of social programming is the elimination of the unfair and avoidable circumstances that deprive individuals of their rights and basic resources that are available to other groups.

Bamberger and Segone (2011) stress that the focus on equity in social programs poses important challenges and opportunities to the evaluation function, and they raise several questions in this matter, including

> [a] What are the methodological implications in designing, conducting, managing, and using equity-focused evaluations? [b] What are the questions an equity-focused evaluation should address? and [c] What are the potential challenges in managing equity-focused evaluations? (p. 8)

Equity-focused evaluations, discussed in Chapter 5, explicitly focus on examining the equity dimensions of interventions, going beyond conventional quantitative data to the analysis of behavioral change, complex social processes and attitudes, and collecting information on difficult-to-reach socially marginalized groups (Bamberger & Segone, 2011). Evaluations of equity-focused programs involve analysis and interpretation of information to answer specific questions, including those of concern to worst-off groups, such as what works and what does not work to reduce inequity, and the gap between best-off and worst-off groups (Segone, 2012).

Structural Racism, Social Programming, and Evaluation

Special consideration of **structural racism** (or race-based inequalities) in relation to social problems and social programming is warranted because of the insidious nature of the relationships among them. Many would agree that when thinking about the prominent social problems in U.S. society (e.g., poverty, crime, education gaps, health disparities), race is always a factor in the equation. Yet, in the conceptualization of social programs designed to address these societal problems, there is often failure to take into account how policies and institutions that affect opportunities often reinforce a system that racializes outcomes through underlying and hidden structures that shape biases and create disparate results, even in the absence of racist actors or racist intentions (Powell, Heller, & Bundalli, 2011).

Numerous social programs have been implemented to address issues such as the racial achievement gap, income inequality, and health disparities. However, these problems rarely address structural racism and the race-based inequalities in the social, economic, and political systems that contribute to these outcomes (Thomas et al., 2018). Structural racism has been described as

> the many systemic factors that work to produce and maintain racial inequities in America today. These are aspects of our history and culture that allow the privileges associated with "[W]hiteness" and the disadvantages associated with "color" to remain deeply embedded within the political economy. Public policies, institutional practices and cultural representations contribute to structural racism by reproducing outcomes that are racially inequitable. (Aspen Institute Roundtable on Community Change, n.d., p. 1)

Structural racism is the normalization and legitimization of an array of dynamics—historical, cultural, institutional, and interpersonal—that routinely advantage whites while producing cumulative and chronic adverse outcomes for people of color (K. Lawrence & Keleher, 2004). Evaluators are often asked to examine the effectiveness of programs that are designed to yield a quick "magic bullet" fix to problems derived from years of structural racism and oppression. While evaluators alone cannot solve the racism problem, they certainly can at least elevate this harsh reality in the discourse on the eradication of social problems that derive from a national legacy of structural racism, exploitation, and bigotry. Evaluations that ignore these factors obscure the impact of social forces on social problems.

Social programs that purport to address racial disparities may be resisted by the community to the extent that the programs are viewed as promoting further marginalization and stereotyping of community members. For example, school officials who initially support sharing of school achievement data with programs, and evaluations of those programs, may withdraw access to that information when it is viewed that these data will be used for comparison purposes and ultimately become an instrument that will further marginalize the low-income urban students of color reflected in the district data. Therefore, social programming should include strategies anticipating, identifying, and addressing resistance in the community that will not only improve the work's overall effectiveness, but also allow the evaluation to include these strategies in its assessment (Center for Assessment and Policy Development, 2013).

Integrating Program Planning and Evaluation Planning

Conventional wisdom is that the planning for the evaluation should take place early in the social program planning process. Program planning and evaluation planning are essentially two perspectives on the same project, and, ideally, a close relationship should exist between the two efforts. There are multiple benefits to early integration of the program planning and evaluation planning. This creates, from the beginning of the program, a transparent evaluation process whereby all relevant stakeholders know the purpose of the evaluation, its methodology (i.e., what data will be collected, how, and when), and how the results intend to be utilized for program improvement and decision making. This can also help build consensus and trust around the evaluation process and product. Good social program planning continuously keeps the evaluation in mind; and likewise, good evaluation planning is grounded in sound social program planning.

Social Program Evaluations vs. Social Project Evaluations: Distinctions and Implications

Many evaluators and others use the terms *program* and *project* and *program evaluation* and *project evaluation* interchangeably, although others make a clear distinction. In this text, we tend to use the terms *program* and *project* fairly synonymously. However, it is worth pointing out a distinction made in some of the literature. The National Science Foundation (NSF), for example, in its *User-Friendly Handbook for Project Evaluation* (Frechtling, 2010), distinguishes between the terms by describing a **program** as a coordinated approach to exploration in a specific area. Here, a program consists of a collection of related projects, subprograms, and/or activities managed in a coordinated way to obtain benefits not available from managing them individually. The multiple projects within the program are complementary to one another. On the other hand, the NSF describes a **project** as a singular investigative or developmental activity funded by a particular program. Projects, unlike programs, have a defined start and end point and specific objectives that they intend to achieve. Projects may also have various components. For example, an after-school enrichment project (which may be part of a larger school reform program) could have multiple components including a tutoring component, a counseling component, and a parental involvement component. See Figure 7.1.

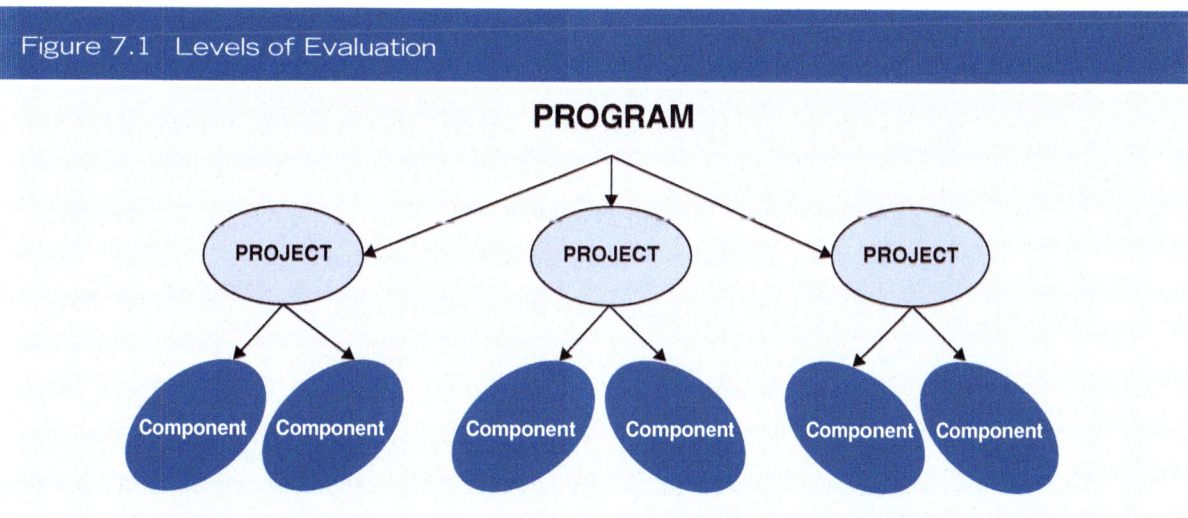

Figure 7.1 Levels of Evaluation

Source: National Science Foundation.

With this distinction in mind, the NSF recognizes two basic levels of evaluation: program and project. Hence, program evaluation is an effort that determines the processes and outcomes of the multiple projects within the program. In contrast, a **project evaluation** focuses on examining processes and outcomes of a specific, individual project funded under the umbrella program. As illustrated in Figure 7.1, projects have specific components, which also may be the focus of an evaluation.

Key Program/Project Components Every Evaluator Must Understand

Evaluators should have clarity and a good understanding of the components of a program or project to successfully assist clients during the conceptualization phase of program design, to determine if a project is ready for a formal evaluation, and to be able to write a reasonable **evaluation plan**. Each program or project (herein referred to as program in this section) has five major components: a mission, goals, objectives, activities, and resources. Before an evaluation begins, at a minimum, the program's mission, goals, and objectives must be clear to all involved in the effort. During the planning and proposal stage of program design, an evaluator may be consulted for assistance in clarifying the proposed program's statement of mission, goals, and objectives. These key program components, which should be clearly articulated and widely known among the program's key audiences, are discussed in the following section. Examples of each component are provided.

Program Mission

The program's **mission** is a statement that describes its overall reason for existence. This statement defines the program's purpose and direction. A good mission statement should be free of jargon and accomplished in a brief statement or short paragraph at most. In developing a mission statement, answers to several questions should be kept in mind:

- What social problem or condition does the project exist to eliminate or reduce?
- What needs does the program exist to meet?
- What population is being served by the program?
- What geographic area does the program serve?
- What philosophy underlies the program development and implementation?

Mission statements are broad and do not go into much detail, but they do provide some insight into what the program intends to do to eliminate or decrease the problem under consideration.

Program Goals

Once a clear mission statement is articulated, there should be specification of the program's goals. The goals should derive from the program's mission, and include broad statements of what the program needs to accomplish to achieve the desired results. Program goals help provide focus for the program. In developing program goals, the following questions should be kept in mind:

- What changes (e.g., knowledge, attitudes, behaviors/skills) does the program desire to bring about in its participants?
- What broader impact does the program desire to have on the individuals and/or communities being served?
- What contributions does the program hope to make to the field?

Program Objectives

After the program's mission and goals are established, the objectives should be articulated. The goals serve as the foundation for developing the program's objectives, which are precise and measurable statements of what the program intends to accomplish during a specific period of time to achieve each goal. Objectives are the building blocks or steps taken toward achieving the goals. Translating broad objectives into measurable outcomes is not always a simple task since it involves setting practical limitations on the quantifiable outcomes that express the goals.

Good objectives provide a way to measure success and, thereby, become an important part of evaluation planning. Useful objectives are SMART, meaning they are

specific—that is, the objectives are well defined in indicating what is to be done and how one will know that it is done;

measurable—that is, the objectives are quantifiable or include a metric with a target that indicates success;

achievable—that is, the objectives can be attained by the program given the proposed capacity and time frame;

relevant (and realistic)—that is, the objectives are consistent with the program's mission and goals and realistic within the available people, resources, and time constraints and other supports needed to accomplish the intended outcomes; and

timely—that is, the objectives are stated in a manner that includes a specific time when they will be accomplished (Centers for Disease Control and Prevention [CDC], 2018).

Objectives that are stated in a broad or vague manner must be reformulated to be made SMART, as illustrated in Table 7.2.

Table 7.2 Example Objectives From Non-SMART to SMART

Non-SMART Objective	Why Non-SMART	Reformulated to SMART Objective
Teachers will be trained on the selected scientifically based health education curriculum.	It is not specific, measurable, or timely.	By year two of the project, staff will have trained 75% of health education teachers in the school district on the selected scientifically based health education curriculum.
Ninety percent (90%) of youth participants will participate in lessons on assertive communication skills.	It is not specific or timely.	By the end of the school year, district health educators will have delivered lessons on assertive communication skills to 90% of youth participants in the middle school HIV-prevention curriculum.

Source: Adapted from CDC (2018). (Also see supplemental resources at end of chapter.)

Readers have an opportunity to make somewhat vague and broader objectives into SMART objectives by completing the following activity.

Activity
Making Objectives SMART

What follows are several general and vague program objectives. Reformulate these objectives, making them SMART, by using the criteria discussed in this chapter.

- Increase student reading achievement
- Increase midlife adults' engagement in physical exercise
- Enhance student motivation
- Reduce bullying behavior
- Reduce school truancy

While goals are broad and abstract, objectives are narrow and concrete. Further, objectives should be feasible given the program's resources (time, money, personnel, etc.). There are different ways objectives can be classified. A simple classification for objectives is outcomes-oriented versus process-oriented objectives. *Outcomes-oriented objectives*, sometimes referred to as results-oriented objectives, focus on the results or changes in the target population (individual-level outcomes such as increased job skills) and/or community-level changes (e.g., reduction in crime) as a result of the program. For example:

> There will be a 50% increase in the percentage of participating students who meet or exceed the standards on the state mathematics examination by the end of the next school year.

Process-oriented objectives, on the other hand, focus on the activities to be completed within a specific period of time. For example:

> Of all program attendees, 85% will complete at least 15 math activities by the end of the school year.

Another way to classify objectives is to organize them in terms of behavioral, performance, process, and product objectives. Behavioral objectives focus on results or changes in human action (e.g., increase parenting skills). Performance objectives focus on a specific time frame within which a behavior will occur at an expected proficiency level (e.g., increase the percentage of students scoring at the advanced level on a district-wide subject-matter exam). Process objectives focus on the activities to be completed within a specific period of time (e.g., conduct 12 educational fairs over the next 24 months). Product objectives focus on tangible item results (e.g., produce three educational brochures).

Program Activities

Once the program's mission, goals, and objectives are clear, the next step is to identify the program's **activities**. These include the services and tasks undertaken by the program that contribute to the achievement of the mission, goals, and objectives. In essence, the activities are the specific interventions that the program offers to the target population.

Program Resources

The program's **resources** are the things and people needed to support the program's activities. Typical program resources include money (grant funding, donations), staff, volunteers, partnerships, and collaborations.

Putting It All Together: Program Mission, Goals, Objectives, Activities, and Resources

Once evaluators have a good understanding of a program or project's major components (i.e., its mission, goals, objectives, activities, and resources), as well as the program's cultural and contextual characteristics, they are able to better think about the things that could be examined in an evaluation of the program. The following case study presents the components of a hypothetical project adapted from an actual project worked on by the first author.

Case Study
The Components of a Sample Project

What follows is a summary description of a project designed to address the issue of school underachievement. school students who are at risk for academic failure residing in Urban City, USA.

Mission Statement

The Talent Development Project's mission is to address the problem of underachievement among middle

Goal Statements

The goals of the Talent Development Project are threefold, including

(Continued)

(Continued)

- to improve the intellectual skills of students;
- to elevate the affective skills of students; and
- to enhance the social skills of students.

SMART Objective Statements

Twelve months after participating in the Talent Development Project, 80% of all the participating students will show statistically significant increases in

- mathematics achievement test scores;
- academic self-efficacy;
- emphatic behaviors; and
- personal mastery.

Activities

The activities of the Talent Development Project include

- an after-school program;
- an in-school tutorial program;
- professional development for teachers and other school staff;
- service enhancement activities;
- family–school–community partnerships;
- school-based assessments; and
- follow-up activities.

Resources

The Talent Development Project's resources include

- program staff;
- volunteers;
- grant funding;
- local donations;
- equipment and facilities; and
- collaborative partners.

By completing the activity that follows, readers can create their own hypothetical project to include a description of the major components of a program.

Activity
Design Your Own Project

Organize into small groups. Develop a hypothetical project in a selected area of your choice (e.g., education, health, criminal justice). In your hypothetical program, you are to do each of the following:

- Give your hypothetical program a name
- Write a clear and concise mission statement
- Write three program goals
- Write six SMART objectives (two per goal)
- Give a list of program activities
- Give a list of program resources

Clearly, for an evaluator to accurately plan and implement an evaluation to examine the effort and fidelity of program activities, as well as effectiveness, it is essential that there be a clear understanding of the mission, goals, and objectives. Furthermore, the evaluator should pay close attention to the expected link between the program's activities and expected outcomes. There are tools available that can assist evaluators to discern the intended linkage between/among program components. One of the most important, and probably most widely used, tools available is the logic model.

Logic Models: Linking Program Components

The logic model is a graphic representation or picture of how a particular project or initiative is supposed to work. Knowlton and Phillips (2013) describe a logic model as simply a visual display of pathways of actions to results. This is intended to communicate the intended relationship among the program's various components. Logic models should not simply depict the status quo (what is), but instead should depict what the program will do—how the program will improve a particular condition or outcome as a result of the implementation of articulated activities and strategies. Descriptions and examples of the use of logic models abound in the literature across various disciplines and can be found in, for example, publications by Coffman (1999), Frechtling (2007), S. Kaplan and Garrett (2005), Knowlton and Phillips (2013), Funnell and Rogers (2011), McLaughlin and Jordan (2015), and the W. K. Kellogg Foundation (2004, 2017).

A question can arise for new evaluators as to who is responsible for designing the program logic model. It certainly should not be the responsibility of a single person, such as a program director, evaluator, or some outside consultant, who comes in and spends a few hours studying the program, then leaves. Only through co-construction via key stakeholders working together can a logic model be created that is meaningful and effective for its intended purpose. These stakeholders can include program planners, program staff, evaluators, program participants, individuals knowledgeable about the target group, individuals from the target group or community, experts who are knowledgeable of the relevant research, and other stakeholders from the community. (Chapter 8 discusses stakeholders in detail.)

Benefits of Logic Models for Program Planning

A logic model is an invaluable tool for program managers and staff in conceptualizing, planning, and communicating with others (e.g., policymakers, potential funders, community members). It can help build a unified vision and common understanding of the program by requiring stakeholders to come to consensus about the various components of the program. Good logic models also result in more precise communication about the various aspects of the program and how they fit together to achieve the intended outcomes. Co-construction of the logic model can be a tool to engage diverse stakeholders, enhance teamwork and collaboration, and build ownership of the program among those involved in developing the logic model.

A logic model makes assumptions about the program explicit, and it increases coherence when trying to explain the complexity of the program's design and intended results. It maps how the program intends to achieve its goals. An important feature of the logic model is that it helps stakeholders distinguish between what a program does (activities) and what results (outcomes) it expects to achieve. It can also increase internal and external buy-in about what the program is, how it works, and what it's trying to achieve, thus inspiring different stakeholder groups to communicate about the program in the same manner.

As a powerful communication tool, the logic model can be used to demonstrate to potential funders that the program is sound and well thought out, and it can streamline the grant application by succinctly describing the program. Of course, the benefits of a logic model can only be realized if it is a good model. Based on a review of the literature on logic models, we suggest the following questions be asked to determine if the logic model is a good one.

- Does the logic model make sense?
- Is the information in the logic model meaningful?
- Is the logic model culturally appropriate (in terms of how it is graphically represented as well as the narrative information)?
- Are the strategies and activities, as depicted in the logic model, doable?
- Can the information, such as the intended outcomes, be verified?
- Is the information in the model easy to follow and understand?
- Is the logic model depiction visually appealing and user-friendly?

A logic model should be, essentially, a "living" document that is responsive to program changes; that is, logic models should be carefully designed but not fixed or too rigid that they ultimately stifle innovative thinking and change. Programs can (and should) change over time in response to refinements made by the implementers, formative feedback from evaluators, political realties impacting the program change, changes in stakeholder interests and beliefs, and external influences (e.g., demographic changes in the community). Therefore, logic models should be flexible and dynamic such that when significant changes are made to a program, those modifications are reflected in an updated logic model. This will only occur to the extent that logic models are regularly reviewed and updated to reflect innovation and current conceptions of the program.

Limitations of Logic Models

Before diving into a deeper discussion of logic models, we want to alert readers to a few precautions. As Knowlton and Phillips (2013) noted,

> the proper reference, "logic model," is no guarantee of logic. . . . There is some danger in seeing a graphic display on paper and considering it true. . . . Typically models do not take unintended consequences into account although every program has side effects. (p. 11)

Another caution is that although use of logic models has increased substantially over the past few decades, readers may be disappointed to learn that there is no strict standardization in the content, format, and visual look. This is not a necessarily a bad thing, but it does mean that logic models can vary in their complexity and take many different forms, including flowcharts, tables, pictures, and diagrams, and can include different components. However, most (certainly not all) logic models are limited to a single page, have some fundamental components (discussed in the next section), and provide a simplified visual representation of the relationship among components of a program depicted in a linear, causal pathway (from left to right) from program activities to an aspirational set of outcomes. Having said this, a potential concern with logic models is that they can be too reductionistic and linear.

Logic models clearly aim for simplicity rather than accurately capturing every detail of an intervention. A challenge here is finding the right balance of providing sufficient depth and breadth to understanding the program and its context, without being so complicated that it loses its appeal and ability for users to quickly grasp the program being described. Programs and their services, provided in the real world, are undoubtedly influenced by a range of factors beyond those often highlighted in logic models. All programs, particularly those serving marginalized groups, are often complex and messy, not simple and linear.

These noted cautions about logic models should be acknowledged and not taken lightly. Considering these potential pitfalls, the goal for program planners, evaluators, and others involved in logic model development should be to develop a useful logic model that balances brevity and complexity while simultaneously distilling an intervention to its key components and relationships without oversimplifying connections. While logic models cannot definitively represent the real world of uncertain causal relationships, they do have great value in social program planning and evaluation, as discussed in the following sections.

Logic Models and Evaluation Planning

The cornerstone of an effective evaluation is an intimate understanding of the program (project) under consideration. Hence, logic models can be very useful in evaluation planning since they provide the evaluator with a visual depiction of how the program is supposed to work. Logic models can help evaluators better match the evaluation to the program by helping them focus on critical components of the program. As an advance organizer, the logic model aids the evaluator to focus on the important elements of the program and to identify what evaluation questions should be asked and why, as well as what measures of performance are key (McLaughlin & Jordan, 2015). If a particular result is included in the logic model, then it generally should be included in the evaluation as a factor to track and measure.

The logic model can help the evaluator prioritize where to spend the limited resources allocated to the evaluation. It helps the evaluator focus more specifically on what information stakeholders really need to know about the program. If a logic model does not exist when the evaluator is hired, it will be extremely useful if the evaluator, in collaboration with various stakeholders, works to create one. Table 7.3 summarizes the major benefits of logic models for evaluation planning.

Components of Logic Models

As stated earlier, there is no single way to depict a logic model. However, for the most simplified format of logic model typically used in the field, there are four basic components that appear: inputs, activities, outputs, and outcomes.

Table 7.3 Benefits of Logic Models for Evaluation Planning

Provide Focus	Help the evaluator determine what to evaluate by providing focus on the most important activities and outcomes to examine
Determine Questions	Help identify the questions the evaluation will ask
Identify Indicators	Help determine what key metrics and data to collect to provide evidence to answer the evaluation questions
Aid Data Collection	Help determine appropriate data sources, methods, instruments, and samples
Determine Timing	Help plan for timing of data collection efforts
Facilitate Learning	Help evaluator and others develop a good understanding of the program
Maximize Use of Resources	Facilitate more efficient use of evaluation resources by providing greater focus to the evaluation

Inputs are resources (human and financial) and contributions that are required to support the program. These are the things that are invested to make the program operate. Inputs might include staff, volunteers, funding, program infrastructure, materials, and facilities.

Activities, as described earlier in this chapter, are the strategies, services, and tasks undertaken by the program to bring about the desired change. Activities answer the question, *What did they do in the program?* The activities are the program's interventions. In the earlier example of the Talent Development Project (see the case study on page 223), the activities included an in-school tutorial program, professional development of teachers and other school staff, service enhancement activities, and some family, school, and community partnerships.

Outputs are the products, goods, and services generated by the project from the program activities. Sample outputs for the Talent Development Project described earlier include the number of students served, the number of workshops provided to parents, and curriculum developed. It should be noted that many evaluators do not separate out activities and outputs in their models; however, McLaughlin and Jordan (2015) made a distinction by pointing out that activities represent what the program does whereas outputs are what the program produces. Outputs answer questions about "how many" and should not be confused with outcomes.

Outcomes are the actual changes, benefits, and/or impacts in individuals, communities, organizations, and systems that occur as a result of exposure to the program's activities (interventions) and outputs. The outcomes answer the question, *So, what difference did the program make?* In thinking about outcomes, there should be clarity on who will experience the changes. Results or changes can occur at the individual or participant level, family level, community level, organization level, or system level. Example individual-level outcomes might be new participant knowledge gained, increased participant skill level, and changes in participants' attitudes and values. Family-level changes might include an increase in family cohesion and engagement. Community-level changes might include increases in public safety. Organization- or system-level changes might include an increase in collaboration or communication among partners within a system (e.g., families, schools, and communities).

Some logic models include only an outcomes column, whereas others break the outcomes down into short-term outcomes, intermediate (or medium-term) outcomes, and longer-term outcomes. As described in Chapter 6, short-term outcomes are those early, most immediate changes and benefits most closely associated with the direct and immediate results of the program and are generally achievable within weeks, months, or one year. Examples of short-term outcomes include changes in individuals' knowledge, attitudes, or motivations about a particular issue as a result of participating in the program. The intermediate (or medium-term) outcomes are those expected to result from or follow the short-term outcomes—that is, what results should occur next. Longer-term outcomes, sometimes referred to as impacts, are more distant in time and may take years or decades to occur. These are the things that are desired to occur over time, resulting from the achievement of the short-term and intermediate outcomes. Longer-term outcomes are more difficult to measure and are attributed to the program's actions.

Because programs do not exist in a vacuum, some logic models include additional components such as assumptions and/or environmental conditions. Including these additional features in the logic model allows it to capture more cultural and context-specific information. The assumptions are things the program developers argue are underlying beliefs or ideas about why the strategies and activities implemented by the program will lead to the desired outcomes. Environmental conditions include other circumstances and influences on program results that are beyond the program's control but can influence the success (or lack thereof) of the program. These might include political, social (e.g., community), and economic conditions. These factors might evolve over time and require a change in program strategies and activities.

Types and Looks of Logic Models

There is no one correct standard or format for the look of a program logic model. While the typical logic model is designed to be read from left to right in a linear fashion, others might be vertically represented to be read from bottom to top as a way of expressing the sequencing and relationship of program components. A typical program-level logic model is depicted in tabular format that simply itemizes the program inputs, activities, outputs, and outcomes as illustrated in Figure 7.2.

Figure 7.2 Example of Simple Logic Model

Project: Intervention on Healthy Eating

Inputs (What is invested)	Activities (What is done)	Outputs (What products, goods, and services are generated)	Outcomes (What results)
• Staff • Volunteers • Grant funding • Donations • Collaborations	• Workshops • Outreach	• Number of new curricula developed • Number of workshops offered • Number of completed participants	• Increased participant knowledge of healthy eating • Changes in participant attitudes on portion sizes

Source: Author created.

Instead of just columns, some logic models use arrows to show detailed progression of program logic—that is, to illustrate what leads to what (see Figure 7.3). Some also add other components such as reach, assumptions, and contextual or environmental factors. **Reach** illustrates the targets (e.g., middle school students, parents) of the project. Assumptions are the beliefs of stakeholders about how the program will work. The assumptions are generally based on the theoretical and empirical literature, best practices, and past experience with the current or similar programs. Contextual or environmental factors are those that the program may have little to no control over, but include external factors (e.g., cultural norms, job market, political climate) that might interact with and influence the program or intervention. Contextual factors can include things such as political constraints that impede program implementation, socioeconomic conditions impacting the target population, and competing initiatives sponsored by other agencies.

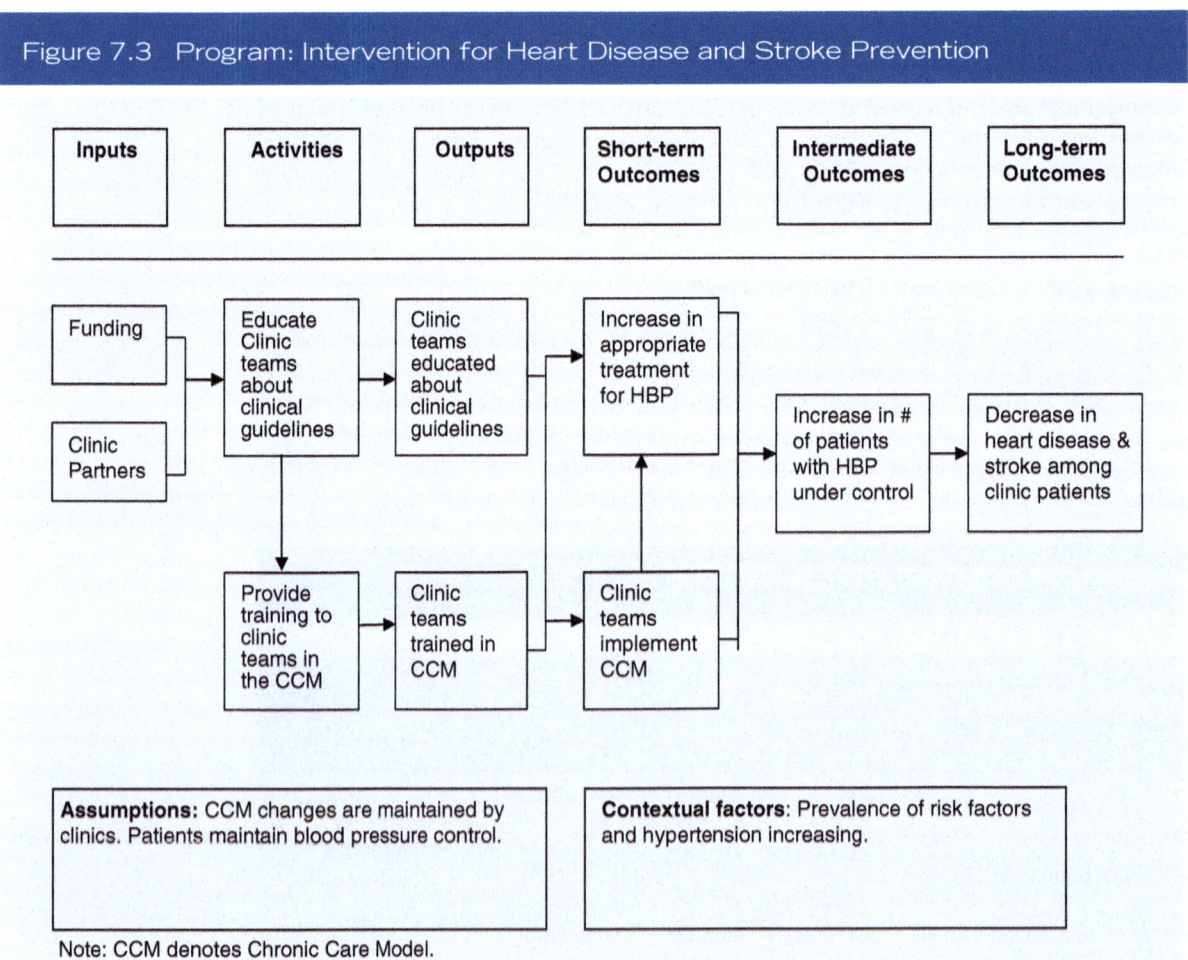

Figure 7.3 Program: Intervention for Heart Disease and Stroke Prevention

Note: CCM denotes Chronic Care Model.

Note: CCM denotes Chronic Care Model.

Source: Centers for Disease Control and Prevention.

Nested Logic Models

A single logic model may focus on an entire program or project or only a few components of a program or project. However, there are instances where logic models can be nested. When the development of a program logic model becomes too complex, **nested logic models** that capture varying levels of detail about the program might be needed. Nesting refers to the process of creating one or more detailed logic models that fit within a larger model (Kirby, 2004). Nested models can be used to describe and explain complex systems or initiatives and are often used to manage descriptions of larger, more complex programs. These nested logic models depict the hierarchy of various levels and how they connect within a single system with each logic model depicted built with reference to the level above (or below) and in relation to the organization's or program's overall mission (Hernandez, 2000; Wauchope, 2001).

Using a nested logic model example from Abdi and Mensah (n.d.), as illustrated in Figure 7.4, one can see essentially three different logic models for the physical activity program targeting children and adolescents: organization level, program level, and project level. Here, it provides a high-level overview of the programs underlying theory, which may be of interest to program funders and community partners (organization-level model). Then it depicts additional information on the specifics of the program of interest. Here, there are three logic models, all providing related but different information.

Figure 7.4 Example of Nested Logic Model

Organization Level

Inputs	Activities	Audience	Outputs	Short-term Outcomes	Long-term Outcomes
• Funding • Partnerships with other organizations • Coordination and oversight	• Policies/procedures and standards • Identificaion of physical activity best practices • Evidence-informed framework and evidence generaton	• Departments and units of the organization	• Number of policies/procedures and guidelines developed and implemented • A physical activity best practices guideline • A framework on evidence generation and use	• Increased awareness of available resources to support capacity building in program areas	• Improved skill set among program staff • A coordinated capacity building approach at the orgainzation level

Program Level

Inputs	Activities	Audience	Outputs	Short-term Outcomes	Long-term Outcomes
• Capacity building sevices and resources for staff • Scientific and technical experts	• Training workshops • Consultations • Webinars	• Internal staff working on physical activity related projects	• Number of workshops • Number of consultations • Number of webinars	• Increased staff knowledge on planning and evaluation	• Increased capacity among staff to deliver evidence-informed physical activity programs

(Continued)

Figure 7.4 (Continued)

Project Level					
Inputs	**Activities**	**Audience**	**Outputs**	**Short-term Outcomes**	**Long-term Outcomes**
• Staff • Time • Supplies for program materials • Equipment for activiites • Volunteers • Community centre facilities	• Bi-monthly community sports activity event at local community centre	• Adolescents aged 12 to 17 years old	• Number of bi-monthly community sports activities	• Increased awareness of the importance of physical acivity • Increased awareness of physical acivitiy community programming • Increased participant attendance of community programs	• Reduction in the prevalence of overweight and obesity

Source: Ontario Agency for Health Protection and Promotion (Public Health Ontario), Abdi S, Mensah G. Focus On: Logic models-a planning and evaluation tool. Toronto, ON: Queen's Printer for Ontario; 2016. Reprinted (or adapted) with the permission of Public Health Ontario.

The advantage of traditional, linear logic models is that they are not difficult to create, although they can be depicted in various ways. The only consistency generally found in terms of the look of a logic model is that it is presented on a single page. Traditional, linear logic models can be created fairly easily in either a Microsoft Word table or a Microsoft Excel worksheet.

In the following activity, readers have an opportunity to practice developing their own logic model.

Activity
Develop Your Own Draft Logic Model

Either using the project description that follows or the description of the hypothetical project developed earlier in the Design Your Own Project activity (page 224), you are to develop your own project logic model. This activity should be completed in small groups so that input can be gleaned from a variety of individuals. Imagine, as the evaluator, you were asked to prepare and present this draft logic model to program staff for comment and feedback.

Hypothetical Project

West Coast University X has a partnership with a local school district to implement a program where approximately 1,200 middle school students in grades 7–9, from underresourced schools, spend a full day on the university campus to broaden their understanding of and interest in college life.

> *Goals and Objectives:* The goal of this project is to provide these students with a greater understanding of the academic and social life of college students. Specific objectives (not yet SMART) include (a) increasing the middle school students' interest in postsecondary education, (2) elevating their knowledge of academic requirements for postsecondary education, and (3) expanding their understanding of the day-to-day lived experiences of college students.
>
> *Activities:* During the campus visit, students attend workshops, visit classes and laboratories, have one-on-one discussions with students and administrators, and visit campus facilities such as the student center, libraries, and bookstore.

Beyond Traditional Linear Logic Models

Fuzzy Logic Models

Some evaluators, particularly those who embrace more complexity and systems thinking, argue that the traditional, linear focused logic model should be transformed. They contend that life is messy, and that programs rarely unfold over time as they were originally intended to in the logic model. Traditional logic models, in their opinion, are static, simple, and predictable, while real life is dynamic, complicated, and somewhat unpredictable (Hutchinson, 2015). Hence, the fuzzy logic model concept evolved out of the desire to make the traditional logic model dynamic, nonlinear, and stakeholder friendly. Fuzzy logic models aim to embrace fluid and approximate reasoning and varied context to improve the capacity of logic models to navigate nonlinearity, feedback loops, and other concepts of complexity integral to the environmental programs and policies. It considers the dynamic nature of the systems surrounding a program. It gives a visual image of the complexities that can affect processes and outcomes.

Keene and Metzner (2011) argue that "fuzzifying" a traditional logic model with graphic design and data visualization creates new opportunities to account for complexity and expands access and use of the evaluation process to a greater diversity of stakeholders over a longer period of time.

The fuzzy logic model, in name, did not catch on much in the evaluation field. This may be due, in part, to the long history of the traditional logic model and its demonstrated benefits. However, there is increasing acceptance of the shortcomings of traditional, linear logic models and efforts to offer alternatives.

Circular Logic Models

Not all logic models are depicted as linear, casual pathways. While linear models are better at guiding discussions of cause and effect and how far down the chain of effects a particular program was effective, a circular model is more effective at depicting the interdependence of various program components to produce the intended effects (Community Toolbox, n.d.). An example of a circular and dynamic logic model is illustrated, on the next page, in Figure 7.5.

Culturally Relevant Logic Models

There have been efforts in the field to ensure that logic models are culturally appropriate and engaging for diverse populations. In the sections that follow, we discuss approaches to logic models designed with African American and Indigenous populations in mind.

Figure 7.5 Example of a Circular Logic Model for a School-Based Health Promotion Intervention

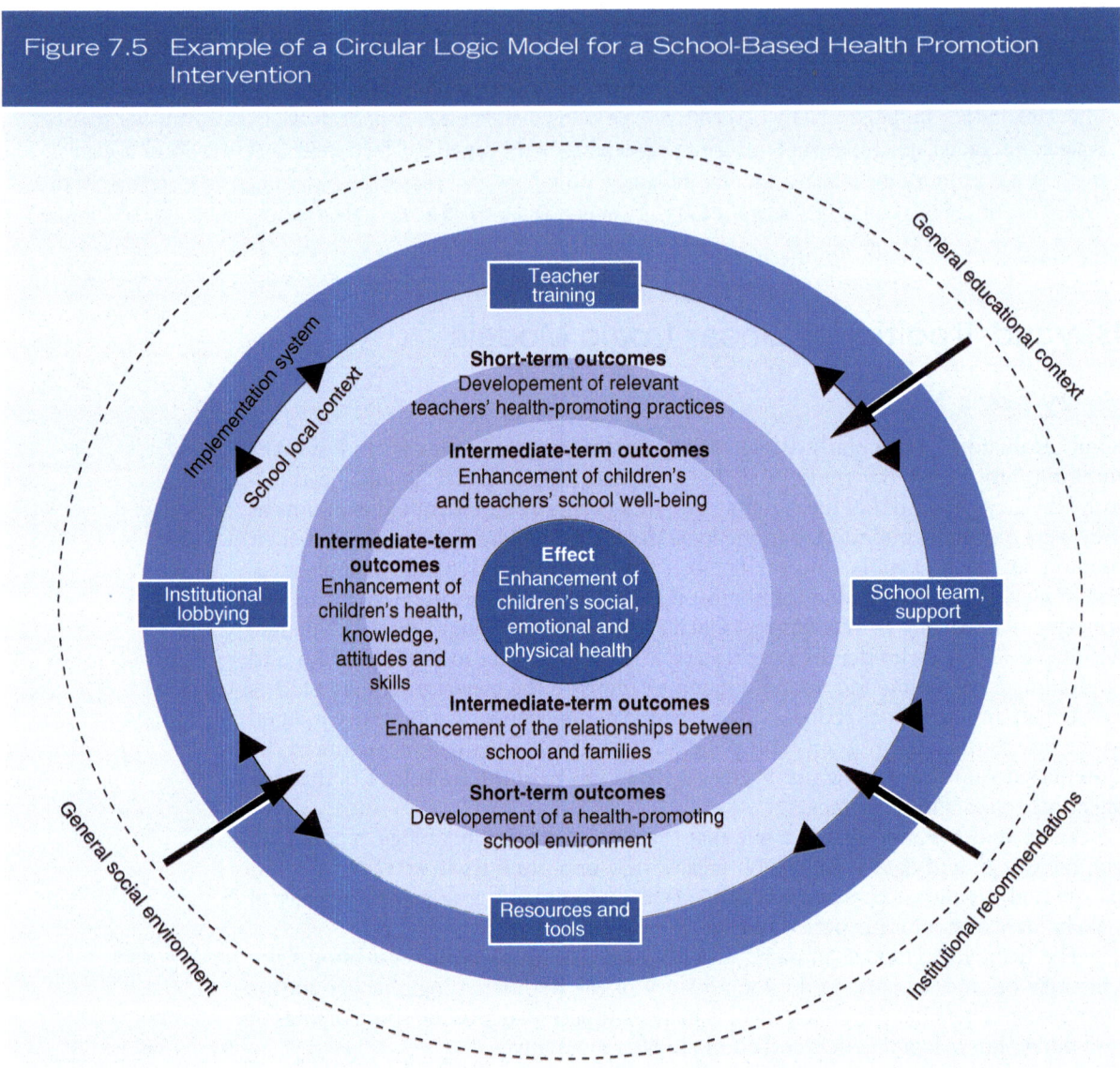

Source: Reproduced from Vivian Barnekow, Bjarne Bruun Jensen, Candace Currie, Alan Dyson, Naomi Eisenstadt and Edward Melhuish (Eds.). Improving the lives of children and young people: case studies from Europe Volume 3. School. (p. 51) ©2013. http://www.euro.who.int/__data/assets/pdf_file/0017/232505/e96926.pdf. May 4th, 2020.

Afrocentric-Centered Logic Model Approaches

As a leading voice in the national conversation on responsible fatherhood, the Center for Urban Families in Baltimore, Maryland, implements the Baltimore Responsible Fatherhood Project (BRFP). The project's goals are to increase fathers' emotional and financial support of their children and families. The BRFP assists fathers with parenting skills and issues involving child support. The project's theory of change is based on social-cognitive theory (discussed in Chapter 4) infused with Nguzo Saba (Swahili) principles of collective work and responsibility. An underlying premise of the project is that interventions that draw on **Afrocentric** values are likely to be more effective with this population, most of whom are African American men (Klempin & Mincy, 2009).

The logic model for the BRFP is depicted in Figure 7.6. This model was designed in a manner to be both meaningful and engaging to the population being served. In this model, inputs include case management, funding, and partnership. The model uses nontraditional language (i.e., learning areas) to characterize shorter-term outcomes, including healthy relationships, parenting skills, job readiness, and child support management.

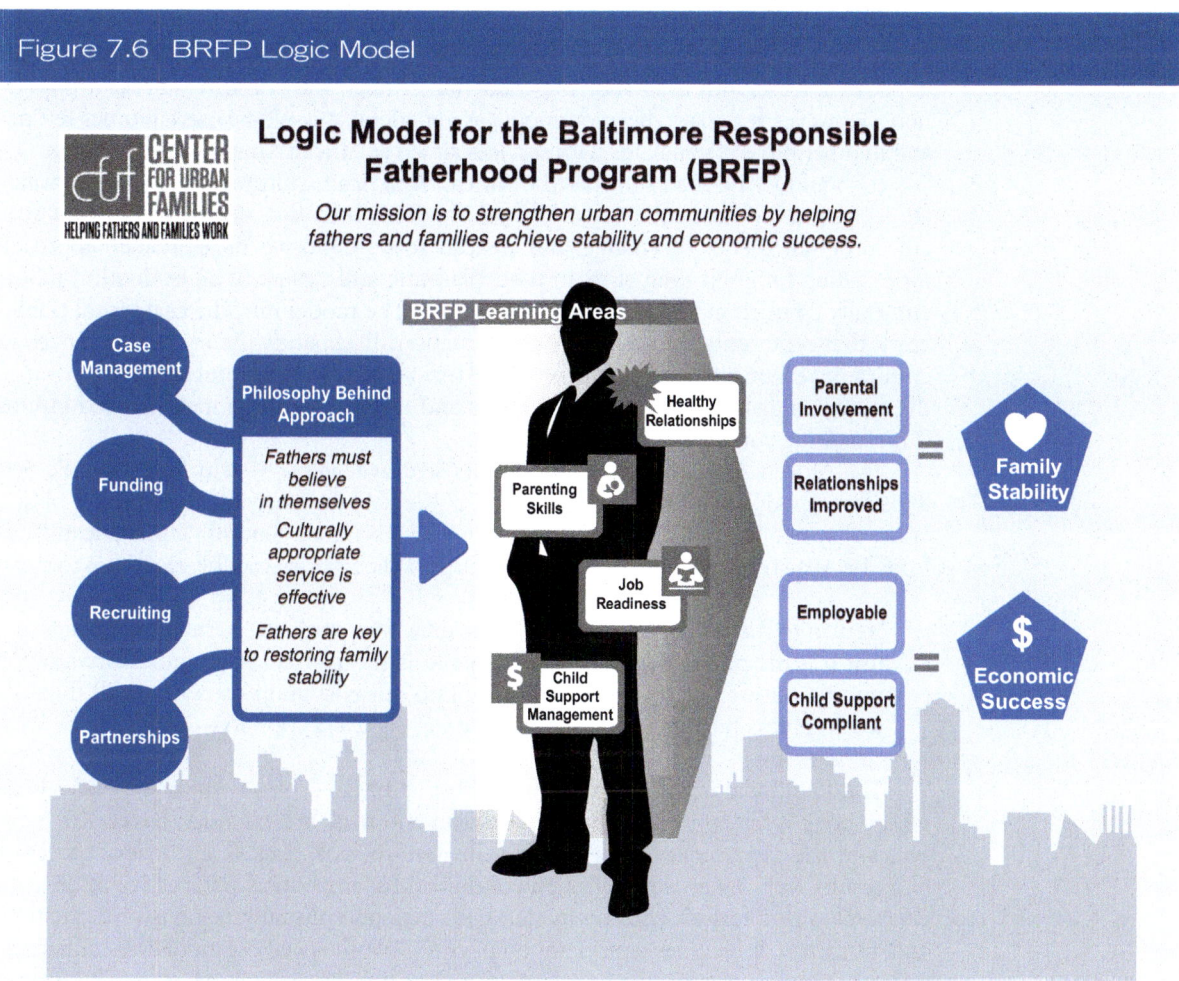

Figure 7.6 BRFP Logic Model

Source: Center for Urban Families. (n.d.). *Logic model for the Baltimore Responsible Fatherhood Program (BRFP)*. Retrieved from http://bmafunders.org/wp-content/uploads/2014/01/under-construction-logic-model-cfuf.pdf

Frazier-Anderson, Hood, and Hopson (2012) developed the African American Culturally Responsive Evaluation System for Academic Settings. They characterize this as

> an adaptation of a logic model for use in African American communities. To date, there has not been a systematic set of procedures to guide evaluators in

their efforts to conduct culturally responsive evaluations with African American populations for use in African American communities. We believe that the [African American Culturally Responsive Evaluation System for Academic Settings] is a first step in this process. (p. 360)

They viewed this as an alternative to the traditional, linear model. Instead, the African American Culturally Responsive Evaluation System for Academic Settings model was seen as one that provided a visual depiction of culturally responsive evaluation recognizing that the African way of thinking is not necessarily linear; it also provides a visual of symbolic significance for the African American community. The model was originally designed and intended for use with evaluations in academic settings with African American populations. However, it has also been promoted as a model that could be used in other settings and in other professional fields with services aimed at African American populations.

It should be pointed out that the African American Culturally Responsive Evaluation System for Academic Settings logic model is intended not to represent a specific program theory of change, but instead to be inclusive of a broader approach for assisting program evaluators in their planning and design of an evaluation that is culturally competent and culturally responsive. The model introduces a visual framework that represents the stages in an evaluation. It expands theory and practices in culturally responsive evaluation within African American communities to advance the equitable distribution of opportunities and resources among marginalized groups (Frazier-Anderson et al., 2012).

The African American Culturally Responsive Evaluation System for Academic Settings logic model, as illustrated in Figure 7.7, depicts the image of the Sankofa bird, a visual of symbolic significance entrenched in African culture. **Sankofa** is an African word from the Akan tribe in Ghana, which, according to Elleni Tedla, roughly translates to mean

> "return to the source and fetch." The source is our culture, heritage and identity. It is the power that is within us. Sankofa means that as we move forward into the future, we need to reach back into our past and take with us all that works and is positive. (Frazier-Anderson et al., 2012, pp. 361–362)

The traditional image of the Sankofa bird is that of a bird with an egg in its beak whose body is facing forward but whose head and neck are extended backward. Symbolically, this represents the need for evaluators to look back (e.g., review processes and results with stakeholders) from a cultural and sociopolitical perspective in order to effectively move forward. In the model, CRE denotes culturally responsive evaluation, and, as shown, it includes consideration of cultural influences, sociopolitical influences, and contextual analyses at various levels (community, district, school, etc.). The African American Culturally Responsive Evaluation System for Academic Settings model has been regularly used by Rodney K. Hopson and Karen E. Kirkhart in their Foundations of Culturally Responsive Evaluation workshops at the annual meetings of the American Evaluation Association (AEA) and the Center for Culturally Responsive Evaluation and Assessment (CREA) (Hopson, personal communication, February 16, 2020).

Logic Models From an Indigenous Framework

Over the past decade, increasing numbers of indigenous evaluators have been redefining evaluation practices in a manner to be responsive to the values of **Indigenous** communities and their ways of knowing (e.g., Bowman, Dodge Francis, & Tyndall,

Figure 7.7 American Culturally Responsive Evaluation System for Academic Setting Logic Model

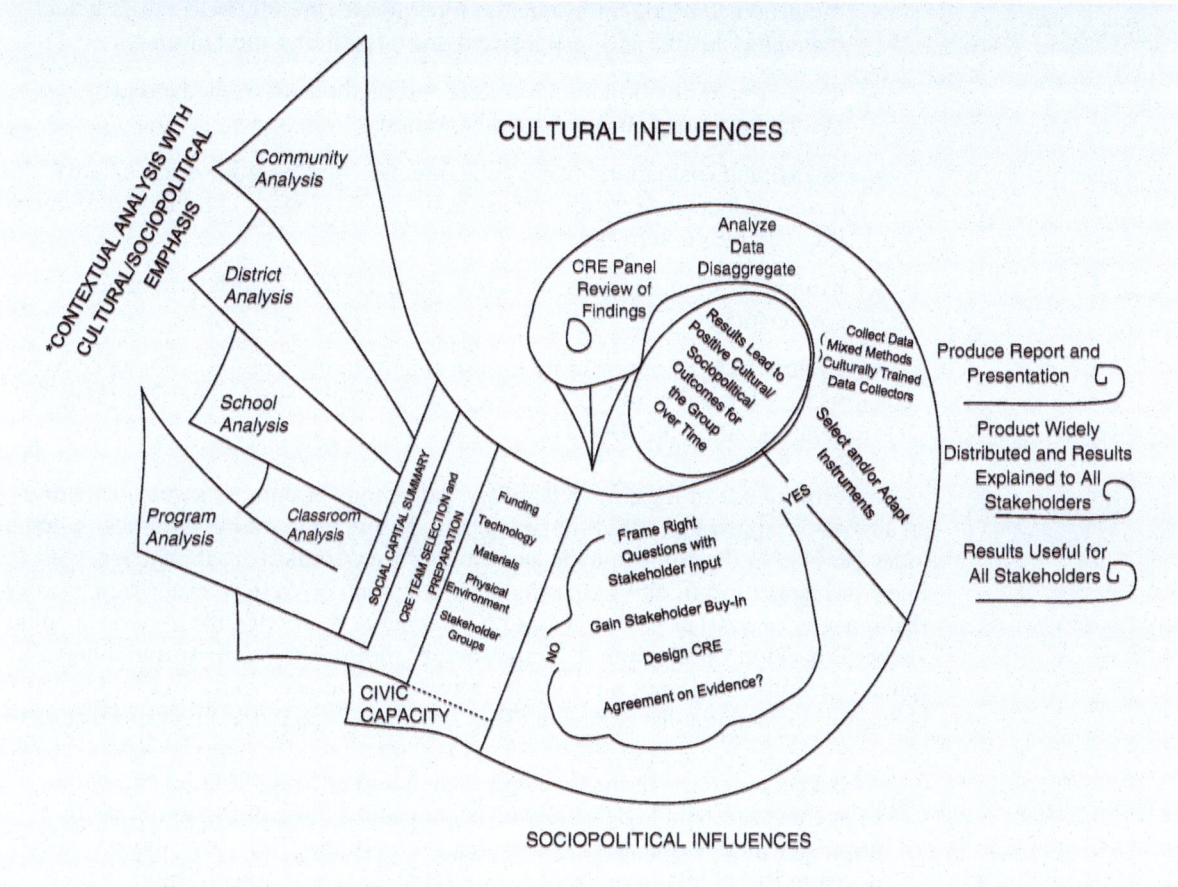

Source: Frazier-Anderson, Hood, and Hopson (2012).

Note: *Cultural/sociopolitical factors are emphasized throughout the evaluation.

2015; LaFrance & Nichols, 2009, 2010; LaFrance, Nichols, & Kirkhart, 2012; Martinez, Running Wolf, Big Foot, Randal, & Villegas, 2018). Here, the term *Indigenous* includes members of American Indian tribes, Native Hawaiians, Alaska Natives, First Nations peoples, and Aboriginal peoples of Canada and the Pacific Islands (LaFrance & Nichols, 2009).

Before discussing how logic models are developed and depicted from an Indigenous framework, it is first necessary to provide more information on the Indigenous framework in order for readers to have a context to think about logic models within this contextual framework. The **Indigenous evaluation** is not just a matter of accommodating or adapting majority perspectives to Indigenous Peoples contexts. Rather, it requires a total reconceptualization and rethinking. It involves a shift in worldview (LaFrance & Nichols, 2010; LaFrance et al., 2012; Martinez et al., 2018). In the development of an Indigenous framework for evaluation, the American Indian Higher Education Consortium was guided by the following principles:

- American Indian tribes have ways of assessing merit or worth based on traditional values and cultural expressions. This knowledge should inform how evaluation is conducted and used in our communities.
- Indigenous framing for evaluation incorporates broadly held values while remaining flexible and responsive to local traditions and cultures.
- Responsive evaluation uses practices and methods from the field of evaluation that fit our needs and conditions.
- By defining evaluation, its meaning, practice, and usefulness in our own terms, we take ownership. We are not merely responding to the requirements imposed by Western practices.
- Evaluation should respect and serve tribal goals for self-determination and sovereignty.
- Evaluation is an opportunity for learning from our programs and effectively using information to create strong, viable tribal communities. (LaFrance & Nichols, 2009, pp. 4–5)

In terms of use of logic models, many Indigenous evaluators argue for the use of an alternative approach to traditional logic models when working with these communities because "Indigenous knowledge values holistic thinking that contrasts with the linear or hierarchical thinking that characterizes much of Western evaluation practice" (LaFrance et al., 2012, p. 62). Working in collaboration with the American Indian Higher Education Consortium, LaFrance and Nichols (2009) demonstrated how utilization of culturally relevant metaphors (common in Indigenous ways of knowing) can be used in logic model development. They developed evaluation processes that were

> robust enough to accommodate and value different "ways of knowing" within Indigenous epistemologies, build ownership and a sense of community within groups of Indian educators and evaluators, and effectively contribute to the development of high-quality and sustainable science and mathematics education programs. (LaFrance & Nichols, 2010, p. 14)

Further, LaFrance and Nichols (2009) argue that a model incorporating symbols reflective of cultural knowledge and worldviews is a better indicator of logic models for Indigenous populations than a traditional linear and narrative-driven logic model. The sequential ordering of logic models, LaFrance and Nichols point out, does not fit Indigenous communities. Instead, evaluations for Indigenous communities mostly involve "telling their stories."

Describing a program's logic through **storytelling** is a primary feature of the Indigenous evaluation framework with a graphic or drawing used to describe the story as best determined within its own context. In this sense, creating the story and identifying assumptions, from an Indigenous perspective, is similar to the Western evaluation practice of developing program theory. LaFrance and Nichols (2009) point out that there is no one specific way to approach story creation, but the key is to take time to list all the elements and their relationships. This, from their perspective, differs from simply listing goals, objectives, and activities. The goal of story creation is similar to the logic model in that it considers how activities relate to proposed outcomes.

However, instead of a traditional logic model, Indigenous frameworks encourage story modeling as a more creative alternative.

The drawing of the story creation model communicates the program story using cultural representations in a manner that is understandable in the community (LaFrance & Nichols, 2009). The model can be a canoe, medicine wheel, tree, or fishing net—whatever fits within the cultural context (see Figure 7.8). It links activities to outcomes, but it may, or may not, include immediate and long-term outcomes. It may also illustrate how program participants engage in the program such as pullers of a canoe, or harvesters of a fishing net, or the roots, trunks, or branches on a tree (Joan LaFrance, personal communication, April 3, 2020). In using a culturally appropriate logic model, evaluators enable Indigenous groups practice evaluation in ways that reflect their own values and ways of knowing while respecting cultural differences. Indigenous evaluators encourage careful use of language, avoiding terms such as *logic modeling* and *theory of change*, instead focusing on the more familiar and straightforward explanation such as creating and telling a story.

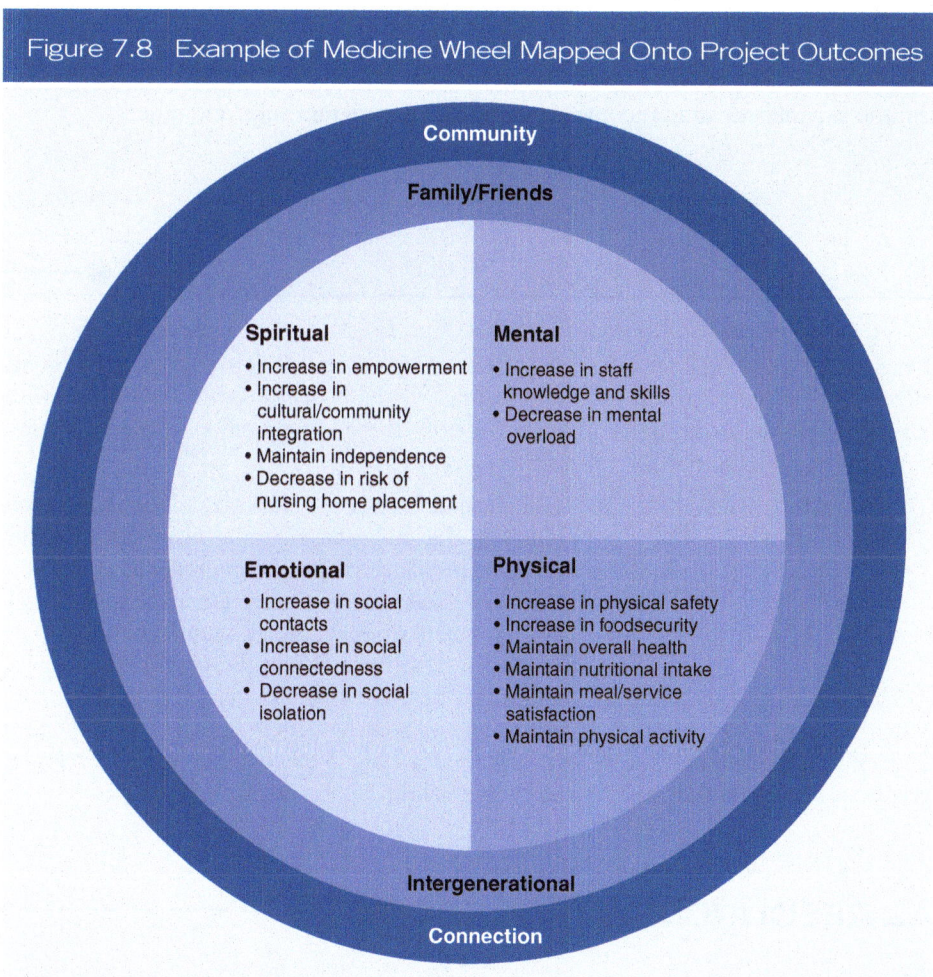

Figure 7.8 Example of Medicine Wheel Mapped Onto Project Outcomes

Source: Jenkins, S., Robinson, K., & Davis, R. (2015). *Adapting the medicine wheel model to extend the applicability of the traditional logic model in evaluation research.* Proceedings of the 2015 Federal Committee on Statistical Methodology (FCSM) Research Conference (p. 7). Retrieved from https://nces.ed.gov/fcsm/pdf/F2_Jenkins_2015FCSM.pdf

Additionally, Jenkins, Robinson, and Davis (2015) argued that traditional, linear logic models may not represent all of the elements critical to efforts in Indigenous communities. In an effort to ensure inclusion of important cultural concepts (e.g., spiritual well-being) and to operationalize measurement of those concepts in planning outcome evaluations of programs that provided nutrition and supportive services for Indigenous People (American Indians, Alaska Natives, and Native Hawaiians), Jenkins et al. mapped the traditional logic model to the *medicine wheel*. The medicine wheel is the universal symbol of a circle, which represents perfection, as well as infinites, since the circle has no beginning or end and is divided into four quadrants (Oxendine, 2014). Among different Indigenous traditions, the medicine wheel has been interpreted as a tool of healing and inner understanding (e.g., Hengen, 2013). In their work, Jenkins et al. created a medicine wheel to orient the expected project outcomes across the traditional quadrants of Indigenous practice: spiritual, mental, emotional, and physical. Figure 7.8 illustrates this medicine wheel. They stress that by employing a *participatory evaluation* approach, coupled with the use of the medicine wheel as a logical framework, evaluators are in a better position to obtain buy-in for the evaluation from stakeholders, including tribal leaders, line staff, and service recipients, and that research questions are more likely to make sense to participants and the findings will more accurately represent the experiences and outcomes of tribal elders, program staff, and others.

SUMMARY

This chapter provided a discussion of social problems, particularly wicked problems, and social programming designed to ameliorate those problems through a racialized and social justice lens. We sought to make clear, through illustrative examples and cogent arguments, why it is important for evaluators to have a fundamental understanding of this perspective in order to be more effective in their practice, especially when working with programs serving diverse and marginalized communities.

Additionally, the chapter examined the key components of a social program that need to be clearly articulated before planning and implementing the evaluation. While it is expected that program staff and administrators have already articulated these components, the evaluator may need to collaborate with them to clarify these components before evaluation planning begins.

The logic model can be a useful visual tool to assist stakeholders in depicting the program theory and to assist evaluators in evaluation planning. The benefits and limitations of logic models were presented. Additionally, both traditional (linear) and nontraditional (nonlinear) formats are described. While the nontraditional logic models may be more difficult to create, they present an opportunity for stakeholders to visually depict the program's story in a manner that is more culturally relevant and contextualized for the target audience(s).

SUPPLEMENTAL RESOURCES

Writing SMART Objectives

www.cdc.gov/healthyyouth/evaluation/pdf/brief3b.pdf

This brief, published by the CDC, is about writing SMART objectives. It includes an overview of SMART objectives, how to write SMART objectives, a SMART objectives checklist, and examples of SMART objectives.

Readings on Wicked Problems

Peters, P. G. (2017). What is so wicked about wicked problems: A conceptual analysis and a research problem. *Policy and Society*, 36(3), 385–396.

Weber, E. P., & Khademian, A. M. (2008). Wicked problems, knowledge challenges, and collaborative capacity builders in network settings. *Public Administration Review*, 68(2), 334–349.

LOGIC MODEL RESOURCES

Enhancing Program Performance With Logic Models

https://lmcourse.ces.uwex.edu/

This is a link to an online course from the University of Wisconsin–Extension that helps program practitioners use and apply logic models. Individuals will learn what a logic model is and how to use one for planning, implementation, evaluation, or communicating about their program.

CDC Evaluation Documents, Workbooks, and Tools: Logic Models Series

www.cdc.gov/eval/tools/index.htm

This links to numerous CDC materials and resources developed to assist their staff and grantees with evaluation. The materials and resources cover topics such as evaluation development tools, logic models, evaluability assessments, indicators and performance measures, evaluation reporting, and economic evaluations and tools.

Developing a Logic Model or Theory of Change

https://ctb.ku.edu/en/table-of-contents/overview/models-for-community-health-and-development/logic-model-development/example

This link is to examples of logic models that other people have found effective.

Logic Models: Templates, Examples, and Bibliography

https://fyi.extension.wisc.edu/programdevelopment/logic-models/bibliography/

This website has a variety of logic model resources and examples.

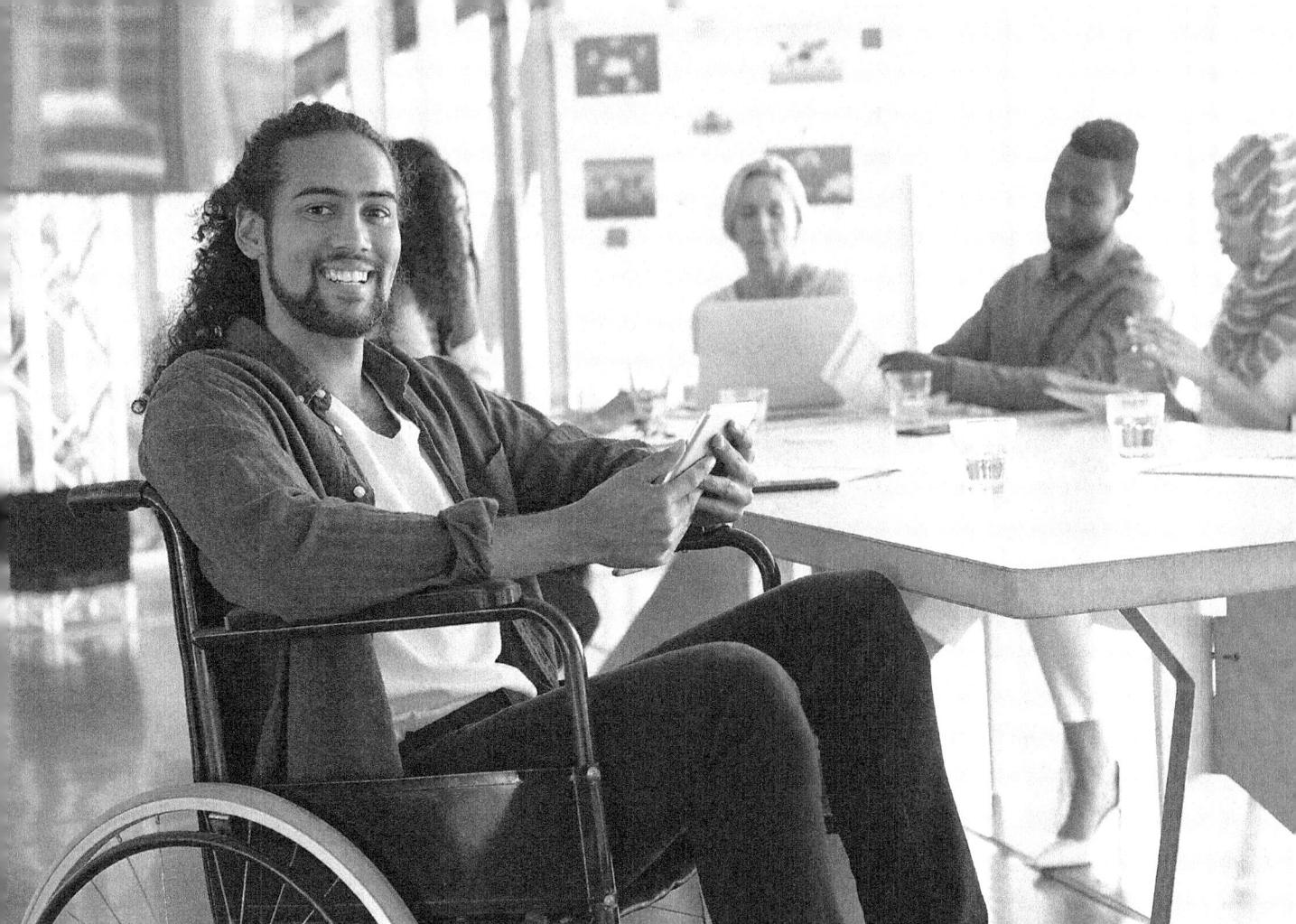
Shutterstock/wavebreakmedia

Engaging stakeholders representing diverse constituencies work best when there is ongoing dialogue between the evaluator and stakeholders and when all stakeholders are valued, respected, and treated as partners with something meaningful to contribute.

CHAPTER 8

Responsive Stakeholder Engagement and Democratization of the Evaluation Process

In the current sociopolitical climate as government and private businesses, as well as scientific enterprises, wrestle with decreasing levels of public confidence, stakeholder engagement has become an increasingly important avenue for fostering qualities of transparency, accountability, and trust. These qualities are crucial in any field-based work, including evaluation planning, implementation, and use of findings. While engaging stakeholders has been widely lauded as a key aspect of good evaluation, the scope and depth of engagement with stakeholders varies across different contexts.

After reading this chapter and completing the activities, readers will be able to meet the following learning objectives:

- Identify the right stakeholders to engage in a particular evaluation
- Delineate the benefits of responsive stakeholder engagement for both stakeholders and evaluators
- Explain the power of building relationships with diverse stakeholders for evaluation success and being responsive to their needs
- Describe a continuum of stakeholder engagement, ranging from monitoring and outreach to shared leadership and empowerment
- Prepare a communications plan for engaging stakeholders throughout the evaluation process
- Articulate strategies for overcoming challenges to stakeholder engagement

Introduction

As introduced in Chapter 1, in this era of "post-truth," "alternative facts," and "spin" where there is increasing resistance to knowledge and attacks on experts, stakeholder engagement is vital to promoting the credibility and legitimacy of the work of evaluators. This chapter focuses on stakeholder engagement—in particular, responsive stakeholder engagement—as a means of both democratizing the evaluation process and enhancing the validity and value of evaluation findings.

Who Are Stakeholders?

In the evaluation literature, **stakeholders** have been variously described. Bryk (1983) defined them as the people whose lives are affected by the program under evaluation and the people whose decisions will affect the future of the program. The U.S. Department of Health and Human Services Centers for Diseases Control and Prevention (U.S. DHHS CDC, 2011) describes stakeholders as people or organizations invested in the program, interested in the results of the evaluation, and/or having a stake in what will be done with the results of the evaluation. Rossi and colleagues (Rossi, Lipsey, & Freeman, 2004; Rossi, Lipsey, & Henry, 2019) defined stakeholders as individuals, groups, or organizations having a significant interest in how well a program functions. Stakeholders can take varied forms to include individuals (e.g., target participants, policymakers, project managers, project staff, public officials), institutions (e.g., universities, faith institutions, media), federal and nonfederal agencies and sponsors (e.g., foundations, funders), organized groups (e.g., citizens' groups, think tanks, research and evaluation organizations), and clients or other intended individuals/groups who would benefit from the project.

Different programs have different stakeholder groups. Table 8.1 provides a listing of typical stakeholders for educational, health, and criminal justice programs. While this listing might not be exhaustive or completely accurate within every context, it provides a starting point for evaluators to identify potential key stakeholder groups for the types of programs listed in the table.

Table 8.1 Typical Stakeholder Groups for Selected Program Type

Typical Stakeholders for Education Programs	Typical Stakeholders for Public Health Programs	Typical Stakeholders for Criminal Justice Programs
K–12 Education Programs • Students • Parents • School staff • District staff • School board • Taxpayers • Business community • Other community members *Higher Education Programs* • Students • Faculty • Administrators • Staff • Board of trustees • Taxpayers • Business community • Other community members	• Program managers and staff • Local, state, and regional coalitions interested in the public health issue • Local grantees of funds • Local and national advocacy partners • Other funding agencies, such as national and state governments • State or local health departments and health commissioners • State education agencies, schools, and other educational groups • Universities and educational institutions • Local government, state legislators, and state governors • Privately owned businesses and business associations • Health care systems and the medical community • Religious organizations • Community organizations • Private citizens • Program critics • Representatives of populations disproportionately affected by the problem • Federal, state, and local law enforcement representatives	• Federal, state, and local law enforcement • Juvenile justice authorities • Businesses • Families • Faith communities • Civic organizations • Health and social service agencies

Source: Centers for Disease Control and Prevention (2011).

Valuing Stakeholders and Diverse Stakeholder Engagement

Stakeholder engagement has been described as "involving all stakeholders (individuals and groups) that can affect or are affected by an evaluation process and/or its findings" (Bryson, Patton, & Bowman, 2011, p. 1). In the realities of fieldwork, stakeholder engagement often does not involve all individuals and groups (or representatives of such individuals and groups) who are affected or potentially could be affected by an evaluation process. Historically, marginalized groups (e.g., low income groups, persons with disabilities, people of color) have been left out of decision making and input related to program development, implementation, and evaluation. The evaluator may have to work through issues related to distrust, cultural differences, and power dynamics when seeking to engage these groups.

Stakeholders represent diverse constituencies in every evaluation context, and each constituency potentially has a unique and central perspective. An evaluator, however, might find it relatively easy or more efficient (e.g., save time) to simply ignore the perspective of certain stakeholders, particularly marginalized and difficult-to-work-with individuals and groups, when planning and implementing an evaluation. With increasing diversity among stakeholder groups and the evolving political context that evaluators are facing, evaluators must be very deliberate and reflective in determining how best to engage the full range of relevant stakeholders, from decision makers to community members, from those easy-to-work-with stakeholders to the more difficult stakeholders to engage with during the evaluation process.

The initial impetus for stakeholder engagement primarily grew out of the concern that evaluation results were not being used. One indicator of the success of an evaluation is the extent to which stakeholders utilize the knowledge gained from the evaluation for process and/or program improvement. Over three decades ago, Weiss (1983) argued that if stakeholders provided key input at the front end of the evaluation, they would take more pride of ownership, the results would gain credibility and authority, and utilization would increase. Thus, stakeholder engagement can result in a better-informed evaluation process as well as more useful results.

Engaging diverse stakeholder groups, across the entire evaluation process, can be especially challenging in instances where differential power relations and cultural conflicts between/among stakeholders and evaluators might actually discourage engagement. For example, the evaluator may come to learn that certain stakeholder groups were intentionally excluded from providing input or participating in the development and planning of the program. This may have occurred as a result of an elitist view or an authoritarian tendency of the program administrator and/or funding agency wherein the points of view of the poor, marginalized, and discriminated against (i.e., certain racial, religious, and political groups) were dismissed as irrelevant. Upon deeper discussion and reflection, the evaluator may learn that these individuals' viewpoints were ignored not because they were uninformed, ill informed, or irrelevant, but because their points of view were different from those of the program administrator and funder. Sometimes program administrators have fragile egos that prevent them from considering alternative perspectives, especially from marginalized or less powerful groups.

In engaging stakeholders, evaluators must also deal with the reality that not all stakeholder groups with a vested interest in the project will share the same concerns, opinions, or priorities. There may be multiple realities that are socially constructed by different stakeholders, and these realities can be in conflict. Different stakeholder groups prioritize different desires and interests from an evaluation. For example, in a school reform initiative, funders may prioritize learning about best practices that will improve their ability to make better funding decisions; policymakers may prioritize the evaluation producing sound and valid results that can provide convincing arguments to shape policy decisions; program administrators and staff (e.g., teachers) may prioritize the evaluation providing an inspirational story about the hard work they have done to move others to action; parents and students may want the evaluation to demonstrate that students' lives were improved and their learning outcomes were enhanced; and the larger community may prioritize the extent to which the evaluation was an empowering process that helped build capacity for the community members to better advocate for themselves and their children.

It is important that the evaluator provide an opportunity for representatives from all key stakeholder groups to express their varying perspectives and concerns. Undoubtedly, doing so will take more time (and resources) to gather and synthesize feedback, but it will provide rich and diverse information. Evaluators should engage these diverse stakeholders even if feasibility concerns (e.g., time constraints, financial resources) make it impossible to be fully responsive to or prioritize every stakeholder group's concerns in the evaluation. In almost all situations where all stakeholders' interests cannot be addressed simultaneously, or even at all, evaluators have the task of deciding which stakeholders' interests to focus on and in what sequence. This relates not only to issues of evaluation goals and objectives, but also to issues of fairness, ethics, and stakeholder prioritization—all topics discussed later in this chapter and/or elsewhere in this text.

Identifying and Classifying the Right Stakeholders

Stakeholder engagement, or the lack thereof, can help, or hinder, the evaluation before it begins, while it is being conducted, and/or after the results are collected and ready for use (U.S. DHHS CDC, 2011). The value of stakeholder engagement, in large part, is a function of engaging the *right* stakeholders. Identifying the right stakeholder group(s) is project context specific; that is, the right stakeholders in one context may not necessarily be the right stakeholders in another context. The evaluator cannot assume the key stakeholders identified by the funder and/or project administrator are automatically the only or right stakeholders to engage. Identifying the right stakeholders involves finding out who is involved in the local context of the evaluand, clarifying their roles and responsibilities, and determining whose interest and influence they represent. The right stakeholders can also be identified through consultation with knowledgeable members of the target community and soliciting specific recommendations to represent diverse groups and perspectives as well as insights gleaned from a review of the literature related to the particular topic and context. The quality of the evaluation will be enhanced with representation of diverse interests, especially by inclusion of traditionally marginalized groups who represent diverse perspectives and positions of power (Mertens & Wilson, 2019).

Stakeholder engagement is not something that is simply nice to do during the planning of the evaluation. Instead, it is an essential and mutually beneficial part of the entire evaluation process. Further, the extent to which stakeholders representing marginalized groups, particularly low-income communities of color, are engaged (or ignored) can have a major impact on the success or failure of evaluation and the credibility and utility of the results in these communities. During the planning stage, engaging the right stakeholders can create broader buy-in of what the evaluation is trying to accomplish and its potential value. Stakeholders can champion the evaluation effort beyond the typical reach of the evaluator by reaching others within their community and bringing in related communities. They can also inform the evaluation process with culturally and contextually relevant information, thus helping the evaluator better understand important issues that might have otherwise been missed. Stakeholders can work in partnership with the evaluator to ensure the evaluation focus, including its purpose and guiding questions, addresses the information needs of the relevant audiences, and they can offer insights on and from diverse target populations that can subsequently bolster access and participation. During the implementation phase, for example, engaging the right stakeholders can add value in the data collection efforts by collaborating with stakeholders as recruiters of potential participants and/or local data collectors. Engaging the right stakeholders during the dissemination and use of findings phase can, for instance, be beneficial in terms of yielding culturally and contextually competent insights into the meaning of various findings and ways for communicating those findings in diverse communities.

The evaluator must be sensitive to changing dynamics in the project context since new individuals, organizations, and groups may become stakeholders during the course of the evaluation that were not stakeholders during evaluation planning. Similarly, individuals, organizations, and groups that were stakeholders during evaluation planning may no longer be stakeholders at later points in the evaluation process. Contextual stakeholders, as described by Rossi et al. (2004), consist of individuals, organizations, groups, and other social units in the immediate environment of a project with interests in what the project is doing or what happens to the project. The evaluator must pay attention to all relevant contextual factors that influence who ultimately may have a stake or vested interest in the project and the resulting evaluation at the present time and potentially in the future. If new stakeholders are brought in during the middle of the evaluation, the evaluator should disclose and discuss their inclusion with the existing stakeholders. Likewise, the new stakeholders should be informed of current stakeholder representation on the project.

Stakeholder Classifications

Guba and Lincoln (1982) note that the concept of stake—that is, having a vital interest in a program or activity—is a very broad one, so one might expect the range of relevant stakeholders also to be very broad. As such, stakeholders have been broadly classified as a function of their relationship to the project under consideration. The CDC (U.S. DHHS CDC, 2011) classifies stakeholders in terms of three (non–mutually exclusive) groups of individuals to include:

- Those involved in the management of program operations (e.g., project administrators and management, program staff, partners, funding agencies)
- Those served or affected by the program (e.g., clients, patients, advocacy groups, community members, elected officials)
- Those who are intended users of the evaluation findings (e.g., persons in a position to make decisions about the program, such as partners, funding agencies, coalition members, and the general public or taxpayers) (p. 13)

There are also other ways stakeholders are categorized in efforts to help identify and prioritize stakeholder groups and to ultimately guide decisions on which stakeholders engage within a particular context. Table 8.2 illustrates common categorizations used for segmenting stakeholders. These include categorizing stakeholders as primary vs. secondary, direct vs. indirect, and internal vs. external. How stakeholders are classified is generally a function of determining each particular individual or group's position relative to the project (e.g., internal vs. external); the extent to which the individual or group is impacted, directly or indirectly, by the project's actions, decisions, or results; and whether the individual or group is directly or indirectly involved in the project's ongoing activities.

Table 8.2 Description of Different Stakeholder Classifications

Primary stakeholders: People or groups that are directly affected, either positively (beneficiaries or having something to gain as a result of the project's decisions, actions, or outcomes) or negatively (having something to lose as a result of the project's decisions, actions, or outcomes); examples of benefits might include increasing skills, goods, services, money, and/or social connections; losses might include less access to power and resources; primary stakeholders have a major interest in the success of the project since they are directly impacted by project outcomes.

Secondary stakeholders: People or groups that are indirectly affected, either positively or negatively, as a result of the project or decisions or actions of the project; secondary stakeholders can be influential even though they have an indirect interest in the project.

Direct stakeholders: People or groups that are involved with a visible role in the day-to-day activities of a project, including people who utilize the services of the project or are impacted by those services.

Indirect stakeholders: People or groups whose interests are enhanced or threatened by the project; those who are indirectly affected by the project; those with a representational stake in the project.

Internal stakeholders: People or groups from within the project, such as project managers, staff, and clients, with an interest in its success and failure.

External stakeholders: People and groups from outside the project, such as funders or investors, that are affected by or can affect the consequences and outcomes of the project.

The case study that follows describes a hypothetical project based on a real issue affecting many U.S. communities—opioid addiction. After readers review the case, they have an opportunity to identify, classify, and prioritize stakeholders for the project.

Case Study
Classifying Stakeholders

The following is a description of a hypothetical project based on a real issue affecting many U.S. communities. Review the project description and then complete the activities at the end of the description.

Real Context and Hypothetical Project Description

According to data reported by the National Institute on Drug Abuse (NIDA), in 2017 Ohio had the second-highest rate of drug overdose deaths involving opioids in the United States. There were 4,293 reported deaths—a rate of 39.2 deaths per 100,000 persons, compared to the average national rate of 14.6 deaths per 100,000 persons. In 2011, prescription opioids were the main underlying cause of overdose deaths in Ohio, with a total of 710 deaths reported that year. The number of deaths continued to grow, and by

2017, prescription drugs accounted for 947 reported deaths.

In response to this problem, Project End Zone, a community-based prevention program, was developed and implemented in Ohio. This federally funded project focuses on reducing overdoses almost exclusively related to abuse of prescription opioid pain relievers, including fentanyl, hydrocodone, methadone, and oxycodone. In addition to the evaluation, Project End Zone involves four integral components: community engagement, coalition building, prevention of overdoses, and training individuals to provide recovery services for opioid use disorders.

Activities

In small groups discuss the project and its context. First, identify who are the likely Project End Zone key stakeholders. Be sure to consider diverse individuals, groups, and organizations that deal with drug use and prevention, including leaders, advocates, and clients from the community. Take special care to promote the inclusion of underserved and/or underrepresented persons.

Second, go back and classify these stakeholders as primary vs. secondary, direct vs. indirect, and internal vs. external. Specify what might be their primary interest in the evaluation (build their own evaluation capacity, use the evaluation results to improve service delivery, etc.).

Third, extend your thinking about Project End Zone to prioritize who you believe are the "right stakeholders" for the evaluator to engage during planning, implementation, and dissemination of evaluation findings. Why did you select these particular stakeholders?

Key and Hidden Stakeholders

Evaluators must identify and engage key stakeholders who matter most, giving priority to those who

- are responsible for day-to-day implementation of the activities that are part of the project under consideration;
- can increase the credibility of the evaluation efforts;
- will advocate for or authorize changes to the project that the evaluation may recommend; and
- will or can fund or authorize the continuation (or discontinuation) or expansion of the project (U.S. DHHS CDC, 2011).

While in theory this description seems relatively straightforward, in practice it is not so obvious. Evaluators should not make the mistake of assuming that those individuals in leadership or decision-making positions are automatically the most important or only key stakeholders.

Visible stakeholders are often the most powerful individuals (e.g., project administrators, funders) and are relatively easy to manage. They are generally quite vocal and typically make their information needs explicit to the evaluator. In some evaluations, there are instances where important individuals or groups are out of sight—in essence, "hidden." Hidden stakeholders can be individuals or groups that are unknown or ignored by funders and project administrators. Unlike visible stakeholders, they often do not have a voice or a seat at the table. This omission can jeopardize both project implementation and evaluation of the project. Furthermore, hidden stakeholders, once disclosed, oftentimes do not voice their concerns either because they were not asked to do so or because they believe that their issues will be ignored, dismissed, or minimized. These individuals or groups are simply unidentified, ignored, and/or forgotten by the evaluation team. Often, these individuals and groups just may fit into the category of the "right stakeholders" to engage.

Hidden stakeholders can be significantly impacted by the project, be quite knowledgeable about the project's context, or have considerable influence on the project and/or the evaluation. For example, in developing and evaluating criminal justice reform initiatives, persons with physical and intellectual disabilities are generally ignored as key stakeholders, although national data from the U.S. Department of Justice (2015) and other reports (e.g., Vallas, 2016) indicate that people with disabilities are at a higher risk than people without disabilities of entering the justice system, and persons with disabilities already in the justice system face significant problems, including access to counsel, lack of accommodations, complex rules, systematic abuse, and solitary confinement. People with disabilities are among the most vulnerable in our society, yet they are routinely ignored, disregarded, and/or marginalized as key stakeholders in initiatives designed to ameliorate or improve a social problem.

Some key, but hidden, stakeholders may have been intentionally excluded from participating in the development of a project and its evaluation planning. This can occur as a result of elitist or prejudicial attitudes of persons in power (e.g., funders, program administrators) that cause them to ignore, for example, the perspective of the poor, peoples of color, or individuals with multiple-minority status. Engaging a narrow set of representatives from the key stakeholder groups is not only problematic in terms of equity, inclusion, and voice, but it can also backfire by alienating some individuals and groups that are critical to the success of the evaluation. The perspectives of hidden stakeholders who are invisible (or less visible) may, in reality, be important to better ensuring the validity and credibility of the evaluation.

Clearly, no stakeholders or stakeholder groups should be excluded because of demographic characteristics such as race/ethnicity, socioeconomic status, language, or disability. The following activity gives readers an opportunity to reflect on and discuss hidden stakeholders and answer a set of related questions.

Reflect and Discuss
Hidden Stakeholders Speak Out

In a task force report by the Clinical and Translational Science Awards (CTSA) Consortium Community Engagement Key Function Committee, Kimberly Horn and Geri Dino (2011, p. 119) described an actual case applicable to this chapter's discussion of hidden stakeholders:

> American Indian youth are one of the demographic groups at highest risk for smoking (Johnston et al., 2002; CDC, 2007) and yet there is little research regarding effective interventions for American Indian teens to prevent or quit smoking. Unfortunately, American Indians have a long history of negative experiences with research, ranging from being exploited by this research to being ignored by researchers. Specifically, they have been minimally involved in research on tobacco addiction and cessation in their own

> communities. The problem is compounded by the economic, spiritual, and cultural significance of tobacco in American Indian culture. In the late 1990s, the West Virginia University Prevention Research Center and its partners were conducting research on teen smoking cessation in North Carolina, largely among [W]hite teens. Members of the North Carolina American Indian community approached the researchers about addressing smoking among American Indian teens, focusing on state-recognized tribes.
>
> Based on the description from Horn and Gino (2011), answer the following questions:
>
> 1. Why do you believe that American Indian teens were "hidden stakeholders" in the teen smoking intervention and research (and evaluation) efforts in North Carolina?
> 2. What activities or action steps would you suggest for engaging this "hidden" population in the design and evaluation of smoking intervention programs?

The evaluator should look "outside of the box" for unidentified stakeholders who can provide a different perspective, invaluable insight, and feedback on the issues under consideration. For example, this could mean asking community members and/or participants about others who are or might be interested in the project or might find the results useful. Certain stakeholder groups may be relatively easy for funders, project administrators, and evaluators to overlook because such groups tend to maintain low visibility out of fear, distrust, or indifference to researchers and evaluators. The evaluator has a responsibility to seek these groups out to the extent that they have a major stake in the project under consideration and to determine what concerns they have in relation to the project. Equity and justice entail ensuring that all parties with a stake in the project have a voice in some aspect of the evaluation and assuring them that their concerns are being heard. While it may be impossible for the evaluator to fully meet the information needs of all stakeholder groups, all should be heard and, hopefully, all will see some value in the evaluation process and outcomes.

Democratizing the Evaluation Process With Stakeholders

Engaging the full range of stakeholders, including hidden stakeholders, is one way to better democratize the evaluation process early on. House and Howe's (2000a, 2000b) **deliberative democratic evaluation** approach, introduced in Chapter 5, stresses that the evaluation process must be based on the full and fair inclusion of all relevant stakeholders and represent the views of disadvantaged groups. They further add that the evaluator has a special responsibility to those stakeholders who might not normally be heard because they are relatively powerless, invisible, unorganized, or for some reason likely not to be included. Evaluators should not ignore imbalances of power, and doing so, House and Howe (2000a) argue, is to "endorse the existing social and power arrangements implicitly and to evade professional responsibility" (pp. 9–10). It is essential that the evaluator give voice to these hidden stakeholders.

Democratic evaluation is a way to "democratize" the evaluation process by explicitly addressing power relations through inclusion, dialogue, and deliberation (House & Howe, 2000b; K. Ryan, 2005). This approach seeks to include stakeholders' perspectives through ensuring that all key stakeholders, or their legitimate representatives (e.g., parents representing their children, minsters representing their faith community), are engaged in all aspects of the evaluation. This includes, for example, giving stakeholders a voice in determining key evaluation questions, identifying criteria for judging data quality, interpreting results, and formulating recommendations. Less powerful or hidden stakeholders should be engaged not as merely tokens or window dressing, but instead as partners and collaborators in the evaluation process. Having the full range of diverse stakeholders engaged in the evaluation process as partners and collaborators can better ensure that power imbalances do not inequitably set the evaluation agenda or inform conclusions. By engaging stakeholders from diverse groups (e.g., cultural, racial, ethnic, geographic, political, organizational, and linguistic) throughout the entire process, the evaluator can better determine if the evaluation goals and questions are relevant and meaningful to the full range of key stakeholders. Additionally, engaging a diverse range of stakeholders early on provides opportunities to question underlying project assumptions, explore competing explanations, and develop consensus around what the evaluation should address.

To better ensure that the right stakeholders are being engaged and to democratize the evaluation process, the evaluator must start with good understanding of the project, its history, underlying assumptions, and external forces impacting the project. Evaluators should ask themselves the following questions early on during evaluation planning while studying the project context:

- Who will be affected by the project?
- Who is at the table, and who is missing during key meetings?
- Which individuals/groups always seem to talk, and which individuals/groups never speak up?
- Which voices are marginalized and/or excluded but need to be included in this process?
- What is the history of this and other evaluation efforts in this particular community?
- Who are the individuals with deep content knowledge of the project and its community?
- Who can influence the process or outcomes of the project?
- Who are the individuals and/or groups that are the advocates of the project? The major detractors?
- Who could increase the credibility of the evaluation within the target community?
- Who should be consulted to plan and implement a culturally competent and ethical evaluation?
- Who are the people who are well respected by the community being served by the project under consideration?
- Who potentially stands to gain from the project and the evaluation, and who potentially stands to lose?

- Who might be important to consider for political reasons?
- Who will use the evaluation findings, and toward what ends?

Gregory Phillips and colleagues (2019) described how they explored new ways to engage multiple stakeholders in a process that was inclusive, democratic, and social justice oriented during a citywide evaluation of an HIV prevention program. As illustrated in the following case study, the evaluators' team members viewed themselves as "evaluation coaches" and guides.

Case Study of Inclusion, Democratic Participation, and Social Justice in Evaluation

In 2015, the Evaluation Center was funded by the City of Chicago to conduct a citywide evaluation of all HIV prevention programming. The authors (G. Phillips et al., 2019, p. 328) described their approach to ensure inclusion, democratic participation, and social justice. The text that follows is an excerpt from the report describing the strategies they employed.

Inclusion

The Evaluation Center worked hard to ensure both field-level staff and director-level staff were engaged in all evaluation activities by stressing the importance of having both types of individuals involved at the launch meeting. Field staff and program directors represent very different skill sets and experiences, so ensuring individuals from each level were included led to the development of quality, culturally relevant evaluation materials that could be integrated into the day-to-day activities of the program. By including field staff, who work most closely with the clients, data collection tools were tailored to the specific subpopulation(s) being served. By involving program directors, recommendations made based on findings were more likely to be implemented by the organization. In instances when there was staff turnover at a delegate agency, which was particularly common among field staff, a replacement was immediately identified, rather than relying on the project director as the sole contact.

Democratic Participation

The Evaluation Center avoided taking control of the decision-making and allowed the site to take the lead in identifying questions that were most important to them. While they finished the process with an extremely large questionnaire, their staff were happy and bought into the importance of collecting and sharing these data. Had the Evaluation Center made an executive decision to cut the instrument without including the site, the relationship could have been strained and the site likely would have felt less inclined to spend time collecting and sharing quality data. By remaining in an evaluation coaching role and guiding them in a particular direction, the Evaluation Center was able to be a part of the decision-making without discouraging their participation.

Social Justice

A key factor in the use of this evaluation approach was emphasizing inclusivity and ensuring broad access to an intervention, particularly by marginalized populations identified by the delegate agency teams. Through their role as an evaluation coach, the Evaluation Center team was able to have targeted discussions and host a webinar on how to improve and diversify recruitment to reach subgroups to increase the ability of the resulting evaluation to truly measure improvements among the population being served. By helping improve programming and increasing the ability of agency stakeholders to plan and implement programming in the future, the Evaluation Center played an active role in working toward social justice for marginalized populations and communities disproportionately affected by HIV. Specifically, this evaluation partnership serves primarily sexual and gender minority individuals, as well as Black and Latinx communities.

Relationships, Values, and Stakeholder Engagement

In many respects, success in one's personal and professional lives is enormously impacted by the relationships cultivated over time. So, too, in the evaluation process, building and cultivating relationships and engaging stakeholders are important. Stakeholder engagement has the potential to foster harmonious relationships and collaboration while simultaneously opening opportunities for stakeholders to be supporters and champions of the evaluation. Obviously, it is essential for evaluators to have technical expertise in engaging their craft. However, it is also important for them to develop good working relationships with project stakeholders. At a most basic level in developing such a relationship is a genuine belief in democratic values and that stakeholders are entitled to being treated fairly, respectfully, and honestly in the engagement process. As Jennifer C. Greene explains in her Voices From the Field interview, evaluation (and evaluators) always advances some values. Those values of equity, justice, inclusion, and voice are essential when engaging stakeholders. While engaging diverse stakeholders is not always easy, as Greene notes, respect, honesty, and trust must vividly be part of the evaluator–stakeholder process.

Voices From the Field

Jennifer C. Greene: Engaging Stakeholders With Respect, Honesty, and Trust

Evaluation is the social practice of valuing, and thereby evaluation always advances some values and not others. Values get advanced through which and whose evaluation questions get addressed, what kinds of data are used to inform answers to those questions, and especially what criteria are used to judge program quality. Evaluations should privilege values of equity, justice, inclusion, and voice, as these democratic ideals are the most defensible. Therefore, the evaluator has both the opportunity and the responsibility to advance these core democratic values as a primary basis for evaluative actions and judgments.

It is the evaluator's job to assertively, and always politely and respectfully, legitimize the core democratic evaluation principle that all stakeholders (or their designated representatives) should have the opportunity to inform, shape, and interpret the process and product of the evaluation. This responsibility requires not just talk, but also action. From establishing the key evaluation questions to reporting evaluation results, the evaluator is responsible for creating concrete avenues for meaningful participation by all stakeholders (or representatives thereof). These avenues can invoke other evaluator responsibilities, like arranging transportation for participating stakeholders, or the services of an interpreter, or child care, or meals for participants and families. That is, evaluators cannot just pronounce a stance of inclusion, but they must proactively enact concrete pathways for meaningful stakeholder voice and action.

Integral to this process of meaningful stakeholder participation in an evaluation study is the enactment of respect. Respect is integral to meaningful and consequential engagement of stakeholders in evaluation. For example, it is critically important to explicitly get permission from evaluation stakeholders to share their ideas and honor their commitments, while keeping their personal stories private. With respect, you are mindful that you are a visitor in others' spaces. With respect come trust, commitment, and caring. With respect also come meaningful evaluation data, conversations, and consequences.

Jennifer C. Greene is professor emerita in the Department of Educational Psychology at the University of Illinois at Urbana-Champaign. She served as 2011 president of the American Evaluation Association (AEA). She was interviewed by coauthor Veronica G. Thomas in the fall of 2019.

Responsive Stakeholder Engagement

In the 1970s, Robert Stake (1975, 1976) introduced the concept of **responsive evaluation** as one that "orients more directly to program activities than to program intents; responds to audience requirements for information; and [ensures] the different value-perspectives present are referred to in reporting the success and failure of the program" (Stake, 1975, p. 14). Responsive evaluation focuses on the concerns of the stakeholders, gathered through ongoing engagement with these individuals and groups during the evaluation. In responsive evaluation, the role of the evaluator is that of a full, subjective partner in the program, highly involved and interactive (Stake, 1975) and providing an avenue for continued communication and feedback throughout the evaluation process. Responsive evaluators seek to increase the usefulness of the evaluation to individuals in and around the program by responding to the audience requirements for information (Stake, 1975).

Central features of responsive evaluation include dialogue, openness, respect, inclusion, and engagement (Abma et al., 2001; Greene, 2001). Dialogue enhances the willingness of stakeholders to participate, to share power, and to change in the process (Abma et al., 2001).

Consistent with the notion of responsive evaluation, the preferred concept that we use to describe the engagement process is **responsive stakeholder engagement**. This refers to evaluators not simply engaging stakeholders but doing it in such a manner that stakeholders become active participants in the evaluation process and there are tangible and explicit outcomes from the evaluator–stakeholder engagement process. Responsive stakeholder engagement is an intentional and ongoing process of relationship building and connections with multiple and diverse stakeholders whereby the evaluator pays close attention to what stakeholders are signaling as their needs (and wants) and the evaluator, to the extent feasible and ethical, conducts the evaluation in a manner that directly responds to these needs and wants. Co-construction, a key feature of responsive stakeholder engagement, involves evaluators collaborating and forming genuine partnerships with key stakeholder groups to conceptualize, implement, and evaluate social interventions in a manner that is responsive to the project's context; it seeks to democratize the evaluation process by lessening the implicit and sometimes explicit power dynamics between evaluators and project stakeholders (Thomas, 2004).

Responsive stakeholder engagement involves understanding the program context, identifying diverse and relevant stakeholders, respecting and taking into consideration their varied perspectives, building trust, co-constructing, and sharing decision making. It honors the strong philosophical base of responsive evaluation whereby evaluators are expected to promote equality and fairness, help those with little power, thwart the misuse of power, reassure the insecure, and help people see things from alternative viewpoints. In responsive stakeholder engagement, evaluators are expected to continuously engage with and respond to (or at least recognize) the needs of the various key stakeholder groups.

In many instances, good evaluation can be as much about building relationships, communicating and visiting well, and creating rapport across varied constituent groups as it is about the technical side (e.g., crafting questions, developing evaluation designs and methods, analyzing data and hypothesis testing) of the process. Responsive stakeholder engagement is an intentional and ongoing process and focuses squarely on relationship building and connections with multiple and diverse stakeholders. In responsive stakeholder engagement, stakeholder knowledge, perspectives, and experiences are highly valued as a resource, and it is consistently integrated in the evaluation process.

Also, this type of stakeholder engagement is flexible enough to permit modifications to the project and/or the evaluation based on stakeholder feedback. For example, while conducting an evaluation of an adult literacy program, coauthor Patricia B. Campbell found, through stakeholder engagement, that literacy instructors wanted to perform their own evaluations and that the participant goals were different from those of the funder. As a result, the evaluation was modified so the outcome measures also included participants' literacy goals, and the evaluator collaborated with literacy instructors to develop materials for the instructors to be able to conduct their own formative evaluation. (See Chapter 4 for more information on formative evaluation.)

For stakeholder engagement to be responsive, it is important that the evaluator obtains a clear understanding of diverse stakeholders' interest, perceptions, and concerns related to both the project and the evaluation. In *Practical Use of Program Evaluation Among Sexually Transmitted Disease (STD) Programs*, Salabarría-Peña, Apt, and Walsh (2007) suggest asking the following questions to obtain this critical information:

- What do stakeholders perceive as the purpose of the program?
- What do they think about the program?
- What concerns, if any, do they have about the program?
- What have they heard about the proposed program evaluation?
- What areas do stakeholders think are important to address first in the evaluation?
- What do stakeholders hope to learn from the evaluation?
- What concerns, if any, do stakeholders have with the program evaluation?
- How available are stakeholders to participating in the evaluation process?
- What are the political implications of specific stakeholders' involvement?
- What are the program expectations of stakeholders' involvement in the evaluation?
- How can the evaluator meet stakeholders' evaluation and communication needs? (p. 18)

The following is a simple, yet important, tip for determining stakeholders' interests.

You don't have to—and in fact shouldn't—guess what stakeholder interests are. Ask them what's important to them. If there are stakeholders that aren't willing to be involved, try to talk to them anyway. If that isn't possible, try to find out their concerns from others who are likely to know. Most stakeholders will be more than willing to tell you how they feel about a potential or ongoing effort, what their concerns are, and what needs to be done or to change to address those concerns. (Community Tool Box, n.d.)

Adequately representing the needs and interests of stakeholders throughout the entire evaluation process, from conceptualization and design to dissemination of findings, is fundamental to good program evaluation. The relationships between stakeholders and evaluators can be either (or both) facilitators or barriers to a successful evaluation. As such, responsive stakeholder engagement must focus on both the process (e.g., quality) and outcomes (e.g., insights, actionable steps) of the engagement process. It should be tailored to the characteristics of the project, the community being served, and the needs of the stakeholders. The diversity and culture of stakeholders are acknowledged, supported, and respected. It is also essential that evaluators know and understand which stakeholders should be worked with, in what ways, and at which stages of the evaluation process to increase the chances that the evaluation will serve the intended purpose for its intended users (Bryson & Patton, 2015).

The Misuse of Responsive Stakeholder Engagement

Stakeholder engagement, particularly ongoing responsive stakeholder engagement throughout the entire evaluation process, is beneficial for a variety of reasons articulated throughout this chapter. However, there can be misuse of the stakeholder engagement process. Evaluators must be mindful not to engage stakeholders for their own self-serving ends. That is, identifying and prioritizing stakeholders to engage throughout the evaluation process should not be based on selecting individuals and groups that would be agreeable or would advocate for the evaluator's work under any circumstance. In instances when stakeholders who are engaged by the evaluator are viewed by others as biased and lacking independence from the evaluator, the value of stakeholder engagement diminishes considerably.

Additionally, certain stakeholders can also be guilty of domination and misuse of the engagement process to further their own interest. For example, some stakeholders (e.g., project administrators), through the engagement process with the evaluator, may try to restrict evaluator access to just "satisfied" or "happy" project participants or to those who have been prepped beforehand what to say to the evaluator (Perrin, 2019).

Evaluators should not be so focused on responding to the stakeholders' needs and preferences that they fail to act responsibly and ethically when some stakeholder interests run counter to professional ethics (Chapter 2 discussed ethics in detail) or sound technical practice. By engaging representatives from a diverse group of stakeholders, the evaluator is better positioned to achieve a more balanced perspective throughout the process.

Continuum of Stakeholder Engagement: From Nonresponsive to Responsive

Along with others (e.g., Bryson et al., 2011; International Association for Public Participation, n.d.), we believe that stakeholder engagement throughout the evaluation process can be viewed on a continuum from monitoring (i.e., nonresponsive) to empowerment (i.e., totally responsive). It can involve a variety of formal and nonformal activities between the evaluator and stakeholders. Table 8.3 illustrates a seven-level progression of the stakeholder engagement continuum from monitoring through empowerment. In the table, there is also an indication of the type of engagement strategies that can be employed as one moves from one level of stakeholder engagement to another, as well as what results are likely to emerge from the particular level(s) of stakeholder engagement. The further one progresses through the continuum of engagement, the greater the likelihood of involvement, impact, trust, and communication flow between the evaluator and stakeholders.

Table 8.3 Levels of Stakeholder Engagement: From Nonresponsiveness to Responsiveness

Level of Stakeholder Engagement	Nature of Engagement	Engagement Strategy Examples	To What End	Results for Evaluator
Monitor ⬇	No direct communication; the evaluator pays attention to stakeholders' attitudes and behaviors through indirect sources; engages with minimal effort	• Media scans • Internet searches • Conversations with other parties who have some knowledge of the relevant stakeholders' actions and attitudes	To understand community	Results may include nonresponsive to cultural nuances, stakeholders' needs and desires
Outreach ⬇	One-way communication; the evaluator keeps stakeholders informed of the status of the evaluation	• Fact sheets • Newsletters • Reports • Website updates • Mass email communications	To give feedback to stakeholders on evaluation progress and results	Results may include nonresponsive to cultural nuances, stakeholders' needs and desires
Consultation ⬇	Two-way communication between the evaluator and stakeholders; the evaluator informs, listens to, and solicits feedback from stakeholders	• Focus groups • Fishbowl technique • Town halls and other public meetings • Advisory boards and panels	To give and receive feedback;	Results may include the gathering of information on how to include stakeholder feedback in evaluation planning and implementation
Involve ⬇	Two-way communication between the evaluator and stakeholders; the evaluator solicits input and ensures stakeholders' concerns are directly reflected in the evaluation process; provides direct feedback to stakeholders on how their input influenced the evaluation process	• Focus groups • Town and other public meetings • Evaluation committees, advisory boards, and panels • Stakeholders as data collectors and context experts	To give and receive feedback	Results may include responsive to stakeholder feedback; sharing in evaluation processes, activities, and/or decision making
Collaborate ⬇	Two-way communication; the evaluator and stakeholders co-create (or co-construct) aspects of the evaluation	• Focus groups • Partnerships • Evaluation committees, advisory boards, and panels	To give and receive feedback	Results may include responsive to stakeholder feedback and cultural context; sharing in evaluation processes, activities, and/or decision making

Level of Stakeholder Engagement	Nature of Engagement	Engagement Strategy Examples	To What End	Results for Evaluator
Shared leadership ⬇	Two-way communication between the evaluator and stakeholders; bidirectional relationship between the evaluator and stakeholders; shared decision making between the evaluator and stakeholders	• Partnerships • Evaluation committees, advisory boards, and panels	To give and receive feedback	Results may include responsive to stakeholder feedback and cultural context; sharing in evaluation processes, activities, and/or decision making
Empower	Two-way communication; the evaluator uses evaluation to stakeholder evaluation capacity; gives stakeholders final decision making in aspects of the evaluation process by ensuring the evaluation serves and maximizes interests for stakeholders; the evaluator supports and facilitates stakeholder decision making	• Focus groups • Town and other public meetings • Evaluation committees, advisory boards, and panels	Responsive to stakeholders' decisions about the evaluation and implementing what they decide	Results may include providing options to inform stakeholder decisions; goal may be to build culturally appropriate capacity to engage in evaluative thinking and practice

Note: Adapted and expanded from various sources including Bryson and Patton (2015); Bryson, Patton, and Bowman (2011); CTSA Consortium Community Engagement Key Function Committee Task Force (2011); International Association for Public Participation (n.d.) at www.iap2.org.

The appropriate level of stakeholder engagement will depend on the evaluation context, including the nature of the stakeholder groups (e.g., their needs and desires) and their relationship to the community and the project under consideration in the evaluation process (e.g., stage of project, length of project). Different stakeholder groups might fall at different points on this engagement continuum for different purposes and at different phases of evaluation planning, implementation, and use of findings. Also, it is important that the evaluator focus on engagement with a few key stakeholder groups at a time since it is likely more effective to deeply engage with a smaller number of stakeholders than to have marginal or superficial engagement with lots of groups.

Barriers to Responsive Stakeholder Engagement

Understanding both the "how" and the "why" of responsive stakeholder engagement is key to developing a respectful and sustained engagement process. Stakeholders are often reluctant to engage with evaluators until they know that their input is wanted, valued, and influential. Responsive stakeholder engagement, being respectful and meeting stakeholders' needs, must be an ongoing process. However, throughout the evaluation process, a number of situations may impede stakeholder engagement. An important one includes a lack of trust between the evaluator and stakeholders. This lack of trust can exist for various reasons, including those stemming from issues related to diversity, power, and mismatched priorities between the evaluator and various stakeholder groups. This is less likely the case when there is only one primary stakeholder or a small number of stakeholders who know each other and have a history of working together. However, in larger, more complex projects and evaluations involving a number of different stakeholder constituencies with competing or even conflicting interests, power and status differences often emerge (Bryson & Patton, 2015).

It is not only important that evaluators make the commitment to engage stakeholders in the evaluation, but it is equally important for them to work proactively toward this end by shaping their approach to the stakeholders in ways that are culturally responsive, thus helping stakeholders feel comfortable (and wanted) in the co-construction of the evaluation. The learning curve for stakeholders can be longer than the learning curve for evaluators on most projects; for example, evaluators know more about project development than project directors typically know about evaluation (Brewington & Hall, 2018). Therefore, proactive, clear, and ongoing communication and education by the evaluator about the evaluation can reduce tension and democratize the process.

Since power dynamics can be complex and situational, it is important that evaluators keep a watchful eye on the dynamics that might be occurring between and/or among relevant stakeholders. First, the evaluator must be cognizant of these power dynamics, and second, the evaluator must be prepared to address them throughout the evaluation process using various avenues appropriate to the particular context (Brewington & Hall, 2018). The power and privilege of some stakeholders oftentimes drown other voices out, frustrating a democratic process (Leviton & Melichar, 2016). When diverse groups are involved, in many instances, some groups are overlooked or not heard. In communities with histories of power issues vis-à-vis the dominant society, the power issue needs to be consciously addressed by the evaluator (Nelson-Barber, LaFrance, Trumbull, & Aburto, 2005). This raises the issue of how to include all stakeholders in the evaluation process that empowers marginalized and often-forgotten groups yet at the same time is still engaging the dominant group(s). Care is needed in defining who is considered a marginalized group, to avoid stigmatization and exclusion of other groups that may have even less voice (Baur, Abma, & Widdershoven, 2010).

Additionally, because of varying interest in power dynamics among stakeholders, there may be tension or conflict between or among diverse stakeholder groups. For example, in a school reform project, there may be tension between project administrators and parents or between different groups of parents. The very worst course of action for the evaluator is to ignore the tensions (Leviton & Melichar, 2016). Instead, as Leviton and Melichar (2016) indicate, conflict should be anticipated and managed through careful inclusion of stakeholders and transparency about decisions including careful and, if necessary, repeated explanations and updates about the choices being made.

It is worth noting that conflict does not have to be destructive and, if handled well, can actually stimulate creativity and lead to innovations (Abma, 2006). Tineke Abma (2000) describes a situation where evaluators had to deal with conflict between two major stakeholder groups (i.e., management and therapists) during their evaluation of a vocational rehabilitation project. She stresses that evaluators can play an important role in making hidden conflicts visible. See the following case study for a summary of the stakeholder conflict case and the steps the evaluators took to manage this conflict and restore conditions for an ongoing process of social negotiation and assisting stakeholders to learn how to handle differences.

Case Study
Handling Stakeholder Conflict

Abma (2000) describes a case that deals with an evaluation of a vocational rehabilitation project for psychiatric patients. During this project, a conflict developed between management and the therapists who were involved in the evaluated program. Both stakeholder groups (management and therapists) felt misunderstood. Abma stresses that, as evaluators, they played a role in making hidden conflicts visible.

The Situation

During the project a conflict developed between the manager and therapists in the task force. There was discontent on both sides about the way the collaboration was proceeding and they blamed each other for the problems being experienced. The conflict threatened working relationships, took a lot of energy, generated feelings of powerlessness and frustration, and had negative consequences for the project as a whole.

As evaluators, we attempted to prevent the situation escalating further. Instead of searching for consensus, differences were articulated. This stimulated the parties in the conflict to consider the opposition between the manager and therapists not as a natural reality, but as the outcome of a social negotiation process. They began to see that the opposition was not a given, but a social construction and as such open for reconstruction. Reality again became negotiable. Instead of pointing towards each other, participants redefined the situation as a shared problem. All learned to understand the difference between delegation and involvement, and experienced that it is possible to work collaboratively towards results if everyone is willing to share power and take responsibility. (Abma, 2000, p. 202)

Power differentials do not go away by simply inviting diverse groups to the table. There must be concrete actions taken by the evaluator to mitigate distinctions among people of different project positions or statuses and cultural backgrounds. Evaluators have recommended engaging in actions such as training for stakeholders in the basics of evaluation, involving stakeholders through work in small groups that cross-cut the positions of stakeholders, cultivating openness and sensitivity to the expressed and unexpressed concerns of different groups, providing translators as needed, and integrating representatives of diverse stakeholder groups into planning and decision-making committees (Nelson-Barber et al., 2005).

In the following activity, readers will reflect on and discuss the potential for stakeholder conflict in the project described.

Activity
Identify Potential Stakeholder Conflict

In a journal article, Leviton and Schuh (1999) described the Rapid Early Action for Coronary Treatment (REACT) intervention.

REACT Description

In 1994, the National Heart, Lung, and Blood Institute (NHLBI) initiated the REACT study with the goal of evaluating a community intervention to reduce patient delay time, defined as the period from the onset of heart attack symptoms until a patient's contact with the medical care system. REACT was a four-year, randomized, multicenter collaborative community trial, with five academic study field centers, each affiliated with four communities. REACT used community organizations, community and media education, provider education, and patient education to convey the message about the importance of seeking help quickly when heart attack symptoms begin.

Organize into small groups. Discuss the intervention and potential conflict using the following questions as a guide:

1. Who are the key stakeholders in the REACT intervention?
2. What potential conflicts could emerge between/among the identified stakeholder groups?
3. What strategies could the evaluator use to minimize this tension?

Evaluators can reduce the level of mistrust between themselves and stakeholders by seeking to understand the stakeholders' perspectives and communicating with clarity and honesty. Being transparent and continuously delivering on promises goes a long way in strengthening trust between the evaluator and stakeholders. Relationships can also be strengthened by the evaluator asking the right questions at the right time to better understand varied perspectives. The attitude of the evaluator plays a major role in cultivating trust with stakeholders. The evaluator must "visit and listen" well. This means displaying an attitude of "working with," not simply working in, the community. The evaluator should display an attitude of humility and openness to learning and discovering together. While being interviewed for this book, Jennifer C. Greene (personal communication, November 14, 2019), pointed out that tensions can be reduced between the evaluator and stakeholders when the evaluator provides support to stakeholders such as stipends for transportation to meetings, interpreters for English language learners and persons with hearing impairment, child care, incentives, and other gestures of appreciation (food, gift cards, etc.).

Benefits of Responsive Stakeholder Engagement

Responsive stakeholder engagement, at its most basic level, involves engaging diverse individuals and groups that reflect the diversity of the community under consideration. Responsive stakeholder engagement can be a complex and labor-intensive task.

However, it adds value to the evaluation process, and can be mutually beneficial for stakeholders and evaluators. First, engagement of stakeholders throughout can help to both demystify and democratize the evaluation process. It can increase stakeholders' awareness, commitment, support of the evaluation while simultaneously reducing their distrust and fear of the evaluation. Engagement with stakeholders can create buy-in, foster collaboration, and better ensure transparency. Stakeholder engagement can enhance the evaluation knowledge and deep understanding of the project and its context. Table 8.4 depicts the value of engaging the "right" stakeholders during the three major phases of the evaluation process: planning, implementation, and dissemination and use of results.

Table 8.4 The Value of Responsive Engagement of the "Right" Stakeholders

During Evaluation Planning	→	During Evaluation Implementation	→	During Dissemination and Use of Evaluation Results
Right stakeholders can: • Provide culturally appropriate understanding of the program context including community history, strengths/assets, and past experiences with similar and other projects • Help build trust, reduce anxiety, and improve communications between the evaluator and the community • Give input on evaluation goals, objectives, questions, measures, and acceptable evidence • Help identify and prioritize the "right" stakeholders • Assist the evaluator in building support and understanding for the evaluation within the community • Identify potential challenges and provide guidance on overcoming such challenges		**Right stakeholders can:** • Provide insight on strategies for identifying and recruiting the target population • Advise on other sources of evidence beyond that originally conceptualized • Help "give voice" to data by examining findings and providing input into the meaning of observations, taking into consideration the cultural context in which data were gathered • Serve as sources of useful information		**Right stakeholders can:** • Review results to better ensure that the conclusions drawn reflect the community's cultural values and perspectives of the program's quality and effectiveness • Provide input into drawing conclusions in a balanced manner, taking into consideration the community's cultural context, relevance, and capacity • Give insights on dissemination strategies best suited to the context and needs for acting on findings and incorporating community strengths and capacities

An underlying assumption of responsive engagement is that diverse stakeholders are engaged in a manner that presents them with robust opportunities to increase learning about the project and to influence decision making throughout the evaluation process. Issues related to the identification and prioritization of relevant stakeholders, gaining access to and getting the cooperation of the different stakeholder groups, and implementing an appropriate methodology are evaluation challenges that can be meaningfully addressed through engaging with stakeholders (Thomas, 2004). The input and lessons learned through stakeholder engagement can yield more credible and useful evaluation. The more diverse the stakeholders involved in the engagement process, the more ideas generated and, thus, the more varied the perspectives for planning and implementing the evaluation. This will likely create more internal and external buy-in and support for the evaluation process.

Engaging diverse stakeholders can also enhance the objectivity of the evaluation and sharpen the quality of the results. Responsive stakeholder engagement can facilitate consensus building and ownership of findings, conclusions, and recommendations. This, in turn, will increase the likelihood that the evaluation results will be useful to a broad range of audiences. Another benefit to responsive stakeholder engagement is capacity building. In these instances, stakeholders have the opportunity to learn more about the evaluation process.

Responsive stakeholder engagement can significantly enhance communications between the evaluator and key individuals, groups, and communities impacted by the project under consideration. Such engagement provides stakeholders with an opportunity to have their issues heard and to provide input into the process of evaluation planning, implementation, and dissemination and use. Leviton and Lavizzo-Mourey (2013) point out, in the following case study based on a project to prevent Latino childhood obesity in the United States, that balancing stakeholder needs and engaging stakeholders from the very beginning, though messy, yields invaluable benefits when designing and evaluating a project to prevent Latino childhood obesity in the country.

Case Study
Salud America! The Messiness and Value of Stakeholder Engagement

Since 2007, the Robert Wood Johnson Foundation (RWJF) has supported *Salud America! The RWJF Research Network to Prevent Obesity Among Latino Children*. *Salud America!* is a research network to prevent Latino childhood obesity in the USA. It has developed essential scientific evidence, new researchers, communications, and a robust online national network of 2,000 experts, community leaders, and advocates aiming to reverse Latino childhood obesity.

The network started with input from hundreds of Latino community leaders from around the country, and now includes thousands. It was essential for Latino leaders to decide the priority topics for the network to study and evaluate. The ethical imperative was clear, given Latinos' often marginal position in American society. Relevance and evaluation quality were equally served, because so little prevention had focused on Latinos to date, yet prevention strategies clearly needed to be tailored to Latino cultures and life situations. The wisdom of communities about their own situation could be tapped through their leaders, who participated in a nominal group process. Community processes, when authentic, can be extremely messy. Yet this effort was orderly—more than feasible, because the infrastructure was in place to obtain stakeholder input.

Source: Excerpted from Leviton and Melichar (2016, p. 805).

Six-Step Process for Responsive Stakeholder Engagement

Depending on the nature of the project to be evaluated and its context, the stakeholder engagement progress can range from fairly simple and straightforward to labor intensive and complex. We present a six-step process for stakeholder engagement.

Step I: Prepare for Diverse Stakeholder Engagement. The best strategy to prepare for the process of responsive stakeholder engagement is to gain a thorough understanding of the project under consideration, including its history, the cultural context, and the environmental and political factors influencing project conceptualization, implementation, outcomes, and interpretation of those outcomes. This community scoping involves developing an in-depth understanding of the target community's social diversity, history, existing networks, and overall socioeconomic and cultural characteristics. In other words, evaluators should find out everything they can about the project and its context through collecting and scrutinizing written materials (e.g., project proposal, organizational chart, project logic model) and talking with key people involved with and/or knowledgeable about the project.

Step II: Identify The Full Range of Diverse Stakeholders. In accordance with the guidance provided in the Joint Committee on Standards for Educational Evaluation's Program Evaluation Standards (Yarbrough, Shulha, Hopson, & Caruthers, 2011), the evaluator should search out all relevant stakeholder groups (or their representatives). An essential part of the initial stage of stakeholder engagement is the identification of the full range of diverse stakeholders for the project under consideration. During this process, the evaluator should strive to be as inclusive as possible. This includes identifying the obvious and less obvious stakeholders. After identifying potential stakeholders, the evaluator should go back and reconsider this process to identify previously unidentified, or hidden, stakeholders. It should also be noted that project stakeholders may not remain static inasmuch as new issues evolve during the course of the evaluation, and new and/or different stakeholders may need to be identified. So, consideration of contextual stakeholders is important.

Stakeholder analysis can be conducted during the planning stage of an evaluation and revisited throughout the evaluation process as conditions change. This technique helps the evaluator identify and assess the importance of key people, groups of people, and institutions that may influence the success of the project and the evaluation. There are several stakeholder mapping tools and worksheet templates for stakeholder identification found in the literature (e.g., U.S. DHHS CDC, 2011). However, the stakeholder analysis can begin as a simple process of making a list of key stakeholders from brainstorming sessions with relevant individuals and groups. Guba and Lincoln (1989) proposed several practical strategies for identifying key stakeholders, starting with asking the individual who represents the evaluator's first contact with the project for nominations. Using this "ripple" or snowball technique whereby the evaluator asks stakeholders in already-identified groups about other, possibly overlooked groups or individuals that seem appropriate to include can be quite useful. Of course, a limitation of this approach occurs when there is potential bias in the identification of the project's first contact and that individual's subsequent recommendations. Adapting a template designed by the CDC, we developed Table 8.5, which can be used as a worksheet by evaluators for identifying stakeholders.

Table 8.5 Worksheet for Identifying Key Stakeholders

Questions for Identifying Potential Stakeholders	List of Stakeholders/Groups
Who has deep cultural, contextual, and content knowledge of the community being served by the project?	
Who are the individuals or groups that are well respected by the target community?	
Who is affected, directly and indirectly, by the program?	
Who is involved in program operations?	
Who is involved in program operations?	
Who is involved in program operations?	
Who will use evaluation results?	
Who are hidden, but potentially important, individuals or groups to engage?	
Who is providing support (e.g., financial) to the project?	

Using the list identified in the second column, determine which of these stakeholders can:			
Provide guidance (e.g., cultural, technical) to the evaluation	Enhance the credibility of the evaluation and its (agreed-on) purpose	Influence how evaluation results are used	Make decisions for initial funding, continuation, expansion, or reduced funding of the program

Step III: Identify and Prioritize Key Stakeholders. Evaluators should go back to the key questions presented earlier in this chapter to determine the breadth of their completeness in terms of stakeholder identification. With a wide range of diverse stakeholders for any given project under evaluation, it may not be feasible or advisable to engage all stakeholders with the same intensity at the same time. More realistically, different stakeholder groups can be engaged for different purposes and at different phases of the evaluation process.

Evaluators must be strategic and clear about whom they need to engage and when to engage across the full range of the evaluation process. In most evaluations, the evaluator will ultimately have to make decisions about which stakeholders can be reasonably included in the evaluation under consideration. Evaluators need to consider which stakeholders are a *must-have*—that is, individuals/groups essential to include—and which stakeholders would simply be *nice to have*, meaning they are still important but not essential. It is important that the evaluator does not allow cultural and other biases to affect consideration of which stakeholders are classified into the "must have" versus the "nice to have" categories. Prioritized stakeholders must include diverse groups with a myriad of perspectives, roles, and experiences relative to the project and the target community. And, most importantly, the evaluator must not (explicitly or implicitly) exclude certain stakeholders from the engagement process on the basis of characteristics such as race/ethnicity, socioeconomic status, gender, disability status, or language.

Preskill and Jones (2009) provide useful guidelines for prioritizing stakeholders. These guidelines suggest including stakeholders that (a) represent diverse perspectives and/or experiences and can raise questions and ideas that reflect all sides of the issue; (b) have deep expertise in the area being studied and can raise questions grounded in extensive research and practice; (c) are responsible for the program or initiative being evaluated and can use the evaluation findings to make improvements; (d) are in a position of influence and can raise questions relevant to politicians and other change agents; (e) are intensely interested in the issue and want to help the program or initiative reach its goals, and raise questions about possibilities and images of future success; and (f) are proponents of evaluation and build buy-in and support throughout the evaluation's design and implementation. Even after using these guidelines, it is still critical that the evaluator take a step back and reflect on whether there are additional individuals, groups, and/or organizations that are hidden or should be included that have not been identified. Furthermore, it is important that the evaluator not focus simply on groups that would promote the evaluator's own interest (e.g., make the evaluation easier to conduct) but instead bring different stakeholder groups to the table and prioritize them based on their potential contributions to the evaluation and the extent to which they represent an important stakeholder perspective to the project under evaluation.

Step IV: Determine Stakeholders' Values, Needs, Motivations, Interests, And Concerns. After identification and prioritization of key stakeholders, it is important to find out their values, needs, motivations, interests, and concerns. The evaluator must determine what they want and what motivates them to participate and remain engaged in the evaluation process. This information is often ascertained in preliminary evaluation planning through the use of various techniques such as key stakeholder interviews and stakeholder surveys.

Step V: Determine Where Key Stakeholders Fall on the Stakeholder Continuum. The evaluator must determine how stakeholders might be engaged at a particular point in time. This entails identifying the appropriate level and type of stakeholder engagement for a particular project or a particular stakeholder group at a particular time in the life cycle of the evaluation. A stakeholder analysis might indicate that certain stakeholder groups require a greater or lesser level of engagement than other groups depending on various factors (e.g., their buy-in or resistance to the project). Additionally, the level of engagement with particular stakeholder groups may need to be adjusted depending on changing contextual and political dynamics.

Step VI: Create a Process For Ongoing Stakeholder Engagement. The evaluator must develop a strategy for keeping key stakeholders engaged in the evaluation process. Stakeholder engagement is an ongoing process. It is dynamic, ever changing with the varying demands of the sociocultural political environment, the project, and the people affected by the project. As such, the evaluator must be prepared to make changes as necessary and create a process that keeps stakeholders interested and engaged. Stakeholder check-in is important. The evaluator should create open lines of communication with stakeholders that will allow them to address potential problems and collaboratively set up corrective actions. Transparency is key to ensure high levels of trust and confidence in the evaluator as well as the evaluation process. Evaluators should keep stakeholders in the loop on important decisions related to the evaluation.

This information should be communicated in a clear and concise manner. Evaluation efforts must be focused, and stakeholders must feel they are an important part of this process. Ultimately, treating stakeholders as partners is one of the most effective strategies for keeping them engaged.

Communicating With Stakeholders

At the heart of effectively engaging the right stakeholders at the right time is communicating with them. It is advisable for the evaluator to develop a communications plan early during the design phase although this plan will likely need to be revised. The communications plan should determine what information needs to be communicated, to whom, when, and how it should be communicated. The communications plan must demonstrate keen understanding of stakeholders' desires in the communication process. A template for designing a communication plan, provided in the following activity, for better engaging stakeholders includes (a) identifying the stakeholders to be communicated with during the process (the *who*), (b) determining what kind of communications each stakeholder group will receive (the *what*), (c) identifying how (e.g., in-person, reports, town meetings) stakeholders will be communicated with (the *how*), (d) specifying how often communications will flow between the evaluator and various stakeholder groups (the *when*), and (e) identifying who, from the evaluation or project team, has the primary responsibility for carrying out the communications with stakeholders.

This activity provides a communications plan template and invites readers to complete a communications plan using this template.

Activity
Developing a Stakeholder Engagement Communications Plan

Using the template provided, develop a stakeholder engagement communications plan for evaluation of the REACT intervention described in the activity on page 262 of this chapter.

Stakeholders (Who)	Message (What)	Medium (How)	Schedule (When)	Person/Group Responsible

Communication with stakeholders may be formal or informal. Some examples of formal communication include meetings, reports, presentations, conference calls, videos, social media (e.g., Facebook, Twitter), and media releases. This type of communication is usually planned and takes considerable time and effort for the evaluator to prepare. Informal communication is also important and can be a useful vehicle for relationship building. Such impromptu communications can include hallway conversations and other ad hoc discussions, informal meetings (e.g., over lunch), email, and voice mail. Whether the evaluator's communication with stakeholders is formal or informal, predictable and reliable communication is key. Clear communication with stakeholders will improve and better retain the engagement process across the life cycle of the evaluation. Chapter 14 covers modes of communicating with stakeholders in greater detail.

SUMMARY

As the evaluation field continues to explore ways to be more inclusive and increase use of evaluation findings for process improvement and other decision making, engagement of stakeholders across the entire evaluation process has gained prominence. Today, evaluators do not have the option of deciding whether or not they will engage stakeholders. Instead, evaluators must determine who, how, and when they will engage stakeholders across the entire evaluation process. Stakeholder engagement is an iterative, not linear, process in which there is much back-and-forth interaction between the evaluator and the stakeholders. There must be fair representation of all relevant stakeholders and not just the high-status (e.g., funder, project director) or agreeable ones. The stakeholder engagement process should not be haphazard or an afterthought. Instead, it must be responsive, practical, systematic, and deliberate.

Engaging the right stakeholders in a responsive and respectful manner has numerous benefits, including providing evaluators with more culturally and contextually relevant knowledge of the project and its surrounding community; diverse perspectives on information needs and what would be deemed credible evidence among various stakeholder groups; greater insights on the target population, ways to access this population, appropriate data collection strategies, and the meaning of the data collected; and more ideas and strategies for communicating evaluation results in ways to increase use. As evaluators think of who are the right stakeholders and how to practically engage throughout the evaluation process, there should be careful consideration of what each stakeholder group brings to the evaluation context. For example, some stakeholders bring community wisdom or technical expertise, while others bring important yet diverse perspectives on issues (e.g., substance abuse) the project seeks to remedy; and yet others bring influence and buy-in support. The evaluator must determine how important it is to have these varying qualities reflected throughout the process of evaluation planning, implementation, and dissemination and use of findings.

Responsive stakeholder engagement is no easy feat. However, it can be accomplished with careful planning and implementation. Overall, engaging stakeholders work best when there is ongoing dialogue between the evaluator and stakeholders and when stakeholders are respected and treated as partners with meaningful responsibilities. Evaluators respond to interpretations and definitions of evaluation contexts based on their own values, perceptions, and beliefs, which, in essence, shape the reality they construe from the evaluation of such contexts. Engaging with members of the community can impact the character and contours of these contexts, as perceived by the evaluator, and the subsequent evaluation knowledge generated (Abma, 2006).

In summary, we offer the following checklist of things for evaluators to work toward accomplishing in their efforts to ensure a respectful and responsive stakeholder engagement process:

- Gain an understanding of the project, including its cultural context
- Recognize and respect diverse stakeholders' wisdom about their own needs and assets
- Demonstrate, through actions, genuine respect for the diversity of stakeholders, including taking steps to minimize power differentials between evaluator and stakeholders and among different stakeholder groups
- Value the assets that diverse stakeholder groups can bring to the evaluation process
- Identify all relevant stakeholder groups, paying particular attention to those groups often hidden, left out, pushed out, or marginalized during project and evaluation planning and implementation
- Obtain input and consensus from representatives of key stakeholders (e.g., project staff, community members, funders) on both the process and outcome of stakeholder engagement—ensuring that the process has a clear and explicit purpose
- Prioritize the stakeholders that need to be engaged and clarify unique (and sometimes overlapping) roles and responsibilities throughout the evaluation process
- Solicit, in multiple ways, stakeholders' input (i.e., interests, perceptions, and concerns) on the project and the evaluation
- Involve stakeholders in key evaluation planning and implementation activities
- Develop ongoing and culturally appropriate ways of interacting and communicating with stakeholders
- Establish and implement procedures to monitor and maintain high levels of stakeholder engagement (e.g., routine check-ins to ensure that agreed-on stakeholders' interests and needs are being addressed, forming a stakeholder advisory group with representatives from the diverse stakeholder constituencies, and having regular meetings with such groups) as well as corrective practices for overcoming problems
- Communicate to stakeholders how their input affects decision making and evaluation actions
- Ensure that stakeholders are (and perceive themselves to be) valued, respected members of the evaluation process and their contributions are recognized monetarily and otherwise (e.g., awards)

Ultimately, diverse stakeholders bring an experiential knowledge of the project and its context that is oftentimes unknown to the evaluator. Bringing together, in strategic ways, individuals and groups who may be affected by the project and can influence decisions and actions impacting the project is vital. Meaningfully and authentically involving representatives from these diverse stakeholder groups will improve the likelihood that the evaluation will yield results that will be credible and relevant to local needs and realities.

SUPPLEMENTAL RESOURCES

Identifying and Analyzing Stakeholders and Their Interests

https://ctb.ku.edu/en/table-of-contents/participation/encouraging-involvement/identify-stakeholders/main

This webpage, posted by Community Tool Box, is a free, online resource for those working to build healthier communities and bring about social change, and it provides information on how to increase success by recruiting community members who have a vested interest in the effort both directly and indirectly.

The Value of Engaging Stakeholders in Planning and Implementing Evaluations

Gilliam, A., Davis, D., Barrington, T., Lacson, R., Uhl, G., & Phoenix, U. (2002). *AIDS Education and Prevention Journal, 14*(3, Suppl. A), 5–17.

This article describes the framework used by the CDC and provides examples of four studies that involved a participatory process with various stakeholders from health departments, community-based organizations, and community planning groups to national and regional organizations in designing and implementing evaluations that yielded results useful for program improvement.

The Role of Stakeholders in Educational Evaluation

Taut, S., & Alkin, M. (2010). In *International Encyclopedia of Education* (3rd ed., pp. 629–635). Oxford, UK: Elsevier.

This article discusses the evaluation literature regarding the role stakeholders play in educational program evaluation. The authors dichotomize stakeholder involvement into two categories that they refer to as deep and broad involvement.

Stakeholder Involvement in Evaluation: Three Decades of the *American Journal of Evaluation*

Rodríguez-Campos, L. (2012). *Journal of Multi Disciplinary Evaluation*, 8(17), 57–79.

This article focuses on the ways in which authors who published work in the *American Journal of Evaluation* have approached stakeholder involvement over the past three decades.

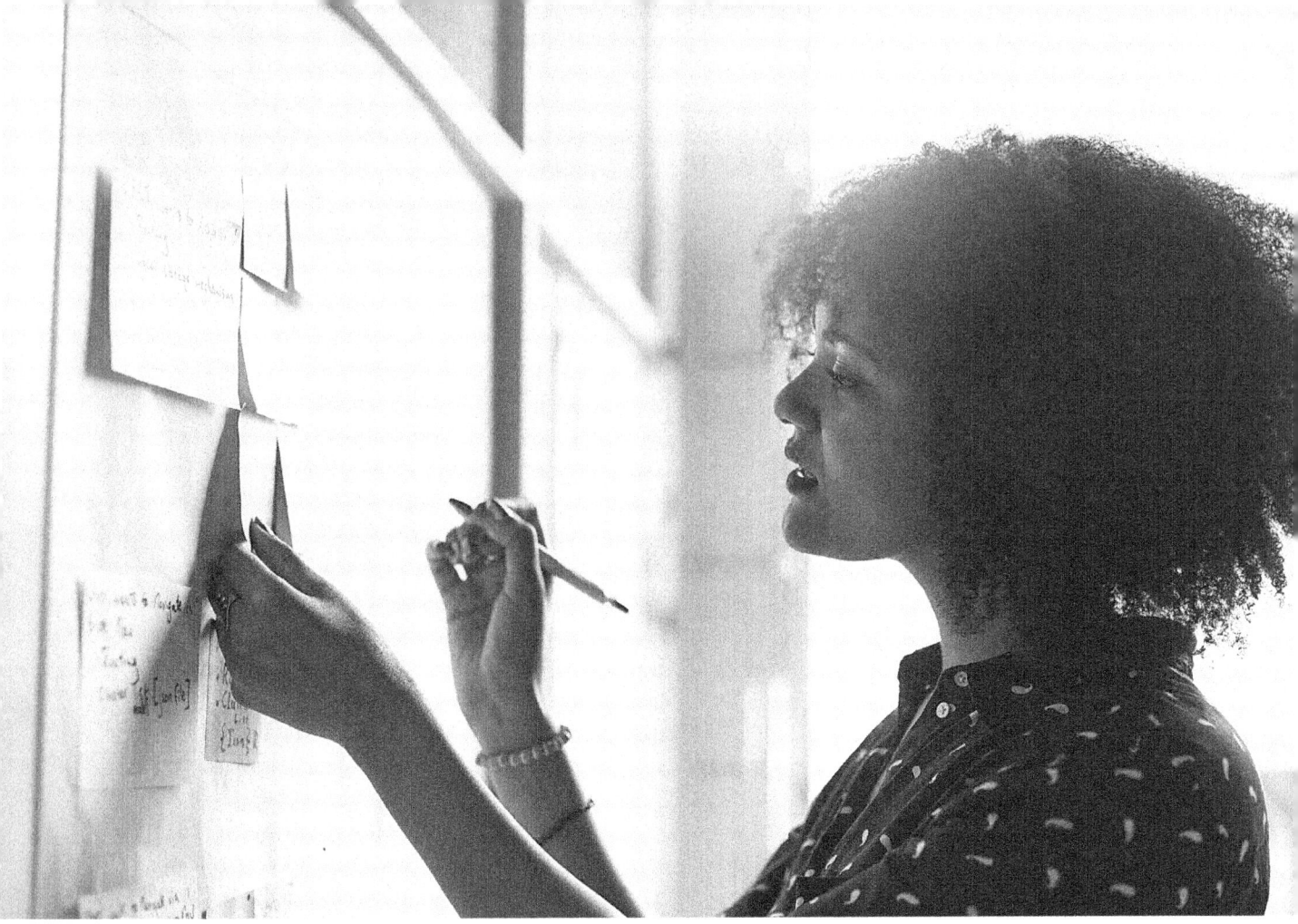
Istock/David Crespo

Evaluators should formulate a flexible evaluation plan that takes into account cultural and other contextual issues while simultaneously involving diverse stakeholders and attending to power imbalances that have the potential to impede the evaluation process.

CHAPTER 9

Planning the Evaluation

Depending on the evaluation context, its purpose, and the stakeholders' information needs, planning the evaluation can be either relatively straightforward or quite complex. In any case, however, good evaluation planning is essential because it gives the work focus, helps achieve objectives, and increases work efficiency.

After reading this chapter and participating in the activities, readers will be able to meet the following learning objectives:

- Explain activities in evaluation planning
- Describe the importance of stakeholder involvement throughout the evaluation planning process
- Take action to rebalance power differentials that can impede evaluation planning
- Perform an analysis of an evaluation context using specific guiding questions
- Put a process in place for gaining consensus on project and evaluation goals, priorities, and definitions of success
- Describe different types of indicators and know how to judge their usefulness in context
- Create evaluation planning and management tools
- Outline the components of a useful evaluation plan

Introduction

Arguably, evaluation planning is one of the most important steps in the evaluation process. Considerable time and effort must be invested in this early phase of the evaluation. Evaluation planning should not be rushed. It involves conceptualizing and formulating an overall evaluation strategy before implementing the evaluation. Evaluation planning is the anticipation and visualization of relevant issues, questions, methods, communications, and deliverables associated with the evaluation.

There is no single way to plan an evaluation. Each evaluation plan must be responsive and tailored to the unique characteristics of the program and its stakeholders, the information needs of evaluation users, the stage of the project, and available resources. Depending on the context, planning an evaluation can be either relatively straightforward or quite complex. In some initiatives, for example, stakeholders only want to determine if a single site project met its intended goals. Here, the evaluation may be planned around answering a single question, such as *Did students' reading comprehension increase after participating in the reading program*? In other instances, evaluation planning may be more complex given the intricacies of the project, including multiple sites and their varying contexts and the diverse information needs of end users. For example, in complex and evolving projects, such as integrated health care interventions or human services projects serving children and families, there may be ongoing adaptations of the intervention to local contexts and changing demographics of the target population. Preparing for evaluating such dynamic interventions is complex, often involving planning for assessing the many different facets of the program and determining how the synergy of multiple effects may lead to significant change.

Project planning, implementation, and evaluation work best when these activities are coordinated and synchronized. In an ideal situation, the evaluator is identified and in place prior to project implementation. This is most likely to occur when a grant application is being written and it requires an identified evaluator and the evaluation plan to be submitted along with the project proposal. Involving the evaluator during the grant application process has enormous advantages because the evaluator can gain a thorough understanding of the project's intent during its design and can establish a relationship with project administrators and other key stakeholders early in the process. Under these circumstances, the evaluator is better able to tailor the evaluation planning and implementation activities. Project staff can also benefit from the evaluator's expertise early on. For example, the evaluator can assist project staff with the development of their logic model, which was covered in Chapter 7; work with them to ensure that their project goals are clear and link to measureable objectives; and help them set milestones to determine if the project is progressing as intended. However, it is not unusual, for various reasons, that an evaluator is a late hire (e.g., after project implementation) and therefore tasked with planning an evaluation of a project already underway. Under these circumstances, the evaluator has ample "catch up" work to do to understand the existing project, its various parts, and different stakeholders.

This chapter will discuss activities involved in planning for an evaluation. While we will cover how to write an evaluation plan, the chapter is not simply about the written evaluation plan. Instead, it examines the myriad activities and steps an evaluator needs to do during comprehensive evaluation planning, particularly stressing the importance of broad and diverse stakeholder involvement. The chapter also introduces readers to some of the standard tools that can be customized for use in evaluation planning and management.

Dealing With Power Imbalances During Evaluation Planning

Evaluators need to pay attention to power imbalances in evaluation planning that can, if not dealt with, impede the planning process. Power can probably best be understood as the extent to which certain individuals or groups feel that they can exert influence over the outcomes and experiences of other individuals or groups. Broadly speaking, degrees of power are often perpetuated and sustained on the basis of certain status characteristics such as race/ethnicity, gender, age, socioeconomic status, and able-bodiedness. Having more power equates to having more control. Power can be visible, invisible, or hidden (VeneKlasen & Miller, 2006). Visible power is in the public sphere involving formal rules, structures, authorities, institutions, and procedures of decision making. It plays out through formal decision-making processes such as laws, government regulations, and other policymaking by government bodies. Hidden power is exercised by powerful people and institutions to maintain their influence and vested interests by setting and manipulating agendas, marginalizing the concerns and voices of less powerful groups, creating barriers to participation, and excluding key issues from the public arena. This often takes place behind closed doors by elite individuals or institutions that control who gets to the decision-making table and what gets on the agenda. An example includes interest groups lobbing politicians behind the scenes to get their agenda passed. Invisible power shapes the ways issues are seen and the ability to control what people think is possible; it hides the fact that power is at work. This can be realized through internalized oppression (i.e., feelings of inferiority and the internalization of stereotypes) or the myth of meritocracy (i.e., the belief that anyone can make it if they work hard enough, making individuals feel that when they do not succeed, it is all their own fault). The effects of invisible power are evident in people thinking about issues such as poverty or racism, for example, as natural or "just the way things are." The power to oppress is often at its strongest when it is invisible.

Power, however, is contextual. That is, having power in one context (e.g., tribal leader) does not necessarily transfer to having power in another context (e.g., broader society outside the reservation). The following activity helps readers think about sources of power in their own lives and strategies used to counteract those sources.

Reflect and Discuss
Hidden and Invisible Sources of Power in Our Own Lives

As VeneKlasen and Miller (2006) point out, power can be visible, hidden, and invisible. Visible power is that which is observable and is exerted via formal rules, structures, institutions, and procedures. Hidden power, often exercised behind closed doors, is the power to set the agenda and include or exclude certain individuals and groups. Invisible power involves the adoption of dominating ideologies such that people embrace belief systems that are created by those with power. Essentially, invisible power is the power to create beliefs and assumptions that become evident through the things such as the adoption of dominant language, values, and norms.

Issues for Reflection and Discussion

1. Think about people who you would describe as powerful, and then think about the contexts in which these people might be powerless and why.
2. Give two or three examples of hidden and invisible sources of power from your own context (e.g., professional/social organization, work, school, community).
3. What actions were taken (or could have been taken) in response to the hidden and invisible sources of power identified?

In evaluations, funders have more control than the grantee. As such, a funder can have a major influence on how the evaluation is carried out, oftentimes determining, in large part, how the evaluation is (a) conceptualized (e.g., determining the questions to ask, deciding on criteria to determine progress or success); (b) implemented (e.g., determining who the evaluator talks with, and does not talk with, during the data collection process); and (c) disseminated (i.e., deciding who, how, and what to disseminate). Additionally, a particular stakeholder group (e.g., project administrators) generally has more control than other stakeholder groups (e.g., project staff and participants). With inherent power differentials evident, for example, between funder and grantee, between project administrators and project staff, or between project staff and project participants, power imbalance is often inevitable. Sometimes imbalances can manifest themselves through the relationship between/among different stakeholder groups as well as the relationship between the evaluator and various stakeholder groups. When there is a power imbalance, resentment, tension, and struggle between evaluation and stakeholders or between/among different stakeholder groups is likely to occur. Further, power imbalance can result in the exclusion and devaluating of the concerns and representation of less powerful groups. As a result, the voices of persons with less power may be silenced even though they have something important to contribute.

One of the American Evaluation Association's (AEA, 2018b) *Evaluators' Ethical Guiding Principles* states that evaluators should mitigate the bias and potential power imbalances that can occur as a result of an evaluation's context. The *Evaluators' Ethical Guiding Principles* adds that evaluators should assess their own privilege and positioning within that context. The evaluator can and should work toward a rebalance of power. In the early stage of evaluation planning, it is important to have representation from as many stakeholder groups as possible (and manageable) in evaluation discussions. Stakeholder groups that should be represented include, for example, funders, project administrators, project staff, participants/clients, partner organization(s), and community members. Oftentimes, stakeholders most likely to be engaged during evaluation planning are the most powerful, most vocal, most visible, and easiest to work with. Ignoring other relevant stakeholders can then result in the evaluator failing to capture critical contextual aspects of the project under study, which potentially can lead to inaccurate judgments and conclusions (Frierson, Hood, Hughes, & Thomas, 2010). In evaluation of projects serving tribal communities, not including key elders in the planning, implementation, and dissemination of project evaluations is oftentimes viewed as a serious affront to those involved as evaluation participants and is thought to have the potential for invalidating the results (LaFrance, 2004). Therefore, it is critical during the planning phase that the evaluator gathers multiple perspectives from a broad range of stakeholders about important issues rather than hearing the perspective of only a limited number, but oftentimes the most powerful, of stakeholders. Also, during evaluation planning and throughout, evaluators need to pay attention to their own and others' assumptions about the group(s) involved in the evaluation so that they do not inadvertently display stereotypical attitudes and/or behaviors.

Sensitivity to and skillful use of language are core evaluation competencies (Patton, 2000). Terminology and the language utilized in evaluation planning (and throughout) can either enforce or reduce power imbalances. Language can empower, or it can (further) marginalize certain groups. For example, the first author (Veronica G. Thomas) previously worked for the Center for Research on the Education of Students Placed at Risk (CRESPAR). "Students placed at risk," in contrast to "at-risk children," was the language all staff used within the context of their work at the research center and within the larger urban school community. Wade Boykin (2000), the Howard University CRESPAR director, often used the language "children placed at promise" or "children placed at risk" to describe students from low-income families or who were marginalized at urban schools as children inherently at risk not because of something inside of them but, instead, due to a variety of personal, community, and societal issues. The adjective *at-risk* has been (and continues to be) used to describe a particular kind of youth (typically students from low-income families and who are African American and Latino) and to sort youth into social groups by ethnicity and class (Madison, 2000). Power to coin language to describe social phenomena is invariably distributed among the intellectual elite, policymakers, evaluators, and service providers (Madison, 2000). Evaluators should be mindful of how they use language to describe social problems and define their target populations, especially if those populations come from marginalized and vulnerable communities. Doing so will help toward rebalancing power dynamics.

Planning for Culturally Responsive and Social Justice–Oriented Evaluations

Increasingly, evaluations are taking place in contexts that are quite diverse and may be unfamiliar to the evaluator or members of the evaluation team. Evaluators must plan for working in culturally diverse settings and not just assume everything will work out because of their technical expertise. Many evaluators who are keenly attuned to cultural responsiveness, often working with marginalized populations or communities of color, think about planning evaluations from a social justice and racial equity lens, as discussed in earlier chapters in this book. Rodney K. Hopson, in his Voices From the Field interview, suggests that part of evaluation planning, from this perspective, includes a good understanding of concepts, such as social justice, inclusiveness, and racial equity, and consideration of how the evaluator intends to integrate perspectives embodying these concepts into the evaluation process. He also provides the readers with resources (e.g., Mertens & Wilson, 2019) that he has found particularly helpful in thinking through these issues in the planning process.

Voices From the Field

Rodney K. Hopson: Planning Evaluation With an Eye Toward Social Justice, Inclusiveness, and Racial Equity

So, what does it mean to plan a social justice–oriented evaluation? When planning an evaluation from a lens of inclusiveness, social justice, and race equity, first it is important that these terms be defined and understood as to where they fit within a particular evaluation process. Such definitions need to be talked about, talked through.

I often find that part of the challenge is in defining terms and being clear what's being understood and meant throughout the evaluation. This is critically important because these concepts are not generally situated in fundamental discussions of evaluation, and while evaluators may be rigid in definitions, stakeholders may

(Continued)

(Continued)

be less so. An evaluation planning document, for example, might frame an evaluation by signifying how historical issues of discrimination; human rights; lesbian, gay, bisexual, transgender, and queer (LGBTQ) and disability rights; and so on are emphasized but without much discussion about what these issues mean in the context of the evaluation work.

When thinking about framing social justice, there should also be thinking about the purpose(s) of evaluations. In the context of planning for evaluation where we apply culturally responsive lenses, this is important in preparing for and engaging with stakeholders (Hood, Hopson, & Kirkhart, 2015). Evaluators who apply culturally responsive evaluation would ask questions that reveal or attune to ways in which these purposes reveal social justice, power, and other dimensions important in the context of evaluation.

I use Mertens and Wilson's (2019) book and its landmark addition of a social justice branch on the tree of evaluation approaches to provide insight into planning evaluations with an eye toward social justice. Culturally responsive evaluation (CRE) is one evaluation approach (of several) that intersects the social justice evaluation branch, and nine steps have been articulated for planning, implementing, and disseminating such evaluations (Hood et al., 2015). Ultimately, part of planning for social justice in evaluation is developing a deeper knowledge of what this means and how it looks in practice. This takes place through preparing for evaluation by developing a deeper understanding of the history of the evaluand and the place where the program or intervention takes place. Part of building this deeper cultural, organizational, neighborhood, or program context aims to focus on spaces where we may engage stakeholders in ways that go beyond the project timeline, or beyond the roles prescribed in the evaluation process. That is, engaging stakeholders with a culturally responsive lens means paying attention and being mindful of these important relationships through the process, especially where issues of power and inequity are realized.

Rodney K. Hopson is a professor of educational psychology in the College of Education at the University of Illinois at Urbana-Champaign. Veronica G. Thomas interviewed him in the fall of 2019.

The complexities associated with multiple social identities and group membership are reasons why it is important for evaluators to reach out to people or organizations that already have credibility with the people participating in the evaluation (i.e., bridge builders or cultural translators) (Colorado Trust, 2009). While having a shared lived experience or ethnic and cultural concordance between qualified evaluators and the people involved in the evaluation is important and valuable (Hood, 2001; Thomas, 2004), it is not enough to account for all the possible layers of diversity within the group of people (Colorado Trust, 2009). For example, although Black evaluators, who are likely middle class, share the same race with African American project participants, differences in socioeconomic status and values could impede the evaluation process if not handled properly. Evaluators who do not have a shared lived experience (e.g., same race/ethnicity or gender) with the individuals involved in the evaluation should seek out bridge builders, cultural translators, or cultural guides who can help them navigate divide challenges. Such individuals can help the evaluator understand cultural nuances that might go unnoticed or be misinterpreted by the evaluator.

In the following activity, readers have an opportunity to reflect on and discuss the potential impact of cultural differences between the evaluator and those individuals participating in the evaluation.

> ## Reflect and Discuss
> ### Hypothetical STEM Project on Indigenous American Reservations
>
> The evaluator (a white, middle-aged male evaluator from an elite West Coast university) planned an evaluation of a middle school science, technology, engineering, and mathematics (STEM) project being implemented on three Indigenous American reservations. Although he had completed previous evaluations of STEM projects, this was the first STEM evaluation that he conducted with Indigenous populations, in general, and Indigenous populations living on American reservations, in particular. As had been done in his previous successful evaluations, the evaluator designed the pretest/posttest study to assess students' task engagement, motivation, and competitiveness—all characteristics the evaluator believed are qualities of "good STEM students." Initially, the evaluator interviewed students (and their parents) to get them to tell what was and was not working well for them (and their children) in the project. After the first three interviews were done, some students were upset, and other students (and parents) refused to be interviewed by the evaluator or to complete subsequent posttest surveys.
>
> The evaluation plan prioritized one-to-one interviews that focused on how well individual children were doing and how well they did compared to others in their classes. The interview questions were designed to elicit short responses to specific topics. The survey items also targeted individual impact and were primarily questions that required yes/no answers, ratings on scales of 1 (*low*) to 5 (*high*), or making choices from existing response categories. The plan had worked in other contexts, was simply not working well here.
>
> In this case, the evaluator did not share salient characteristics with the students in the project.
>
> - How might the students have perceived the evaluation differently than the evaluator did?
> - In what ways might this evaluator's power and privilege have influenced his effectiveness as an evaluator?
> - To what extent do you think it was necessary for the evaluator to share salient characteristics with the students and/or the community being served? Why or why not?
> - What potential issues might have arisen during evaluation planning because of this dissimilarity?
> - How might the evaluator have better prepared himself to work in this community and plan a more useful and culturally responsive evaluation?

Evaluation Planning Activities

In the field, the activities during evaluation planning will sometimes, but not always, take place in a linear fashion as described. While some steps (e.g., identifying project and evaluation goals and priorities) must take place prior to others (e.g., identifying indicators), in some cases, several steps will take place simultaneously. Also, some of the evaluation planning activities, such as stakeholder involvement, will continue even on into the implementation and reporting and use phases of the evaluation.

Table 9.1 summarizes the various activities involved in planning the evaluation. It should be pointed out that not every planning activity specified in the table will be necessary for every type of evaluation. For example, evaluation of a single professional development workshop would require considerably less planning than evaluation of a National Science Foundation (NSF) multilevel, multisite project aimed at recruiting, retaining, and promoting more women and persons of color in STEM fields.

Table 9.1 Planning the Evaluation: A Comprehensive Listing of Activities Involved

- Analysis of context
- Understanding the project's purpose
- Clarifying objectives
- Identifying, prioritizing, and engaging stakeholders
- Focusing the evaluation
- Identifying indicators
- Defining success
- Formulating and refining evaluation questions
- Selecting measures
- Choosing an evaluation design
- Developing procedures
- Developing a timeline and other planning and management tools (e.g., logic models, Gantt chart)
- Identifying resource needs
- Assembling an evaluation team
- Finalizing the written evaluation plan

Identifying and Involving Stakeholders in Evaluation Planning

Stakeholder identification and engagement are discussed in detail in Chapter 8. One of the first things that must be done very early in planning for an evaluation is identifying the stakeholders. This involves determining the key individuals and groups that have an interest in the project and outcomes of the evaluation and those with whom evaluators must cultivate productive relationships to better ensure a useful evaluation. Stakeholders include funders or sponsors, project staff and administrators, project participants, community leaders and members, collaborating agencies, and others with a direct, or even indirect, interest in program effectiveness.

Identifying Stakeholders and Their Potential Role(s)

The identified stakeholder groups should be representative of the populations the project serves. This ensures that individuals from all sectors have the chance for input in the planning phase and that their perspective is taken into account during the preparation phase. Input from a broad range of stakeholders helps the evaluator (and others) be keenly aware of the diverse levels of interests and perspectives related to the project. Working with an appropriately constituted advisory board can be very helpful during the evaluation planning process. Key issues and questions that can be discussed with advisory board members include the following:

- Are there tensions within the community or between the community and the project (or project staff) that the evaluator should be aware of?

- Are there certain individuals and/or groups with whom the evaluator must engage to gain entry into and/or support from the community and/or the project for the evaluation?

- How can the evaluation be best used to promote justice and equity for the community being served by the project?

Mertens (2000), for example, reported working with an advisory board in a national evaluation of court access for people who are deaf and hard of hearing. This board included representatives from the deaf and hard-of-hearing communities who were diverse in various aspects such as choice of communication mode and language (sign language, reading lips, use of voice); hearing status (hearing, hard of hearing, deaf); and backgrounds with the courts (attorneys, judges, judicial educators, police officers, interpreters). Mertens noted that this advisory group needed guidance regarding the diversity of experiences that people who are deaf and hard of hearing encounter in the courts and emphasized the importance of understanding these diverse experiences to develop interventions that could improve access to these communities and evaluation of such interventions.

As covered in Chapter 8, in addition to identifying stakeholders early during the planning phase, the evaluator should also determine the role various stakeholders will play in the evaluation process. Some stakeholders, for example, might be represented by an evaluation advisory group; others may assist in recruitment and data collection efforts. Still yet, some stakeholders may not be directly involved in the evaluation but nevertheless have a role in the evaluation. These stakeholders or groups should still be informed about evaluation activities through meetings, reports, and other means of communication (Centers for Disease Control and Prevention, 2008; G. McDonald et al., 2001). In the end, the evaluation, as was covered in Chapter 8, is more likely to be successful and useful if all relevant stakeholder groups have input into its planning and implementation.

Involving Stakeholders

Stakeholder involvement has long been an expectation of good evaluation practice (Frierson et al., 2010), and evidence indicates that attention to and involvement of stakeholders enhances the design and implementation of the evaluation (Patton, 2008). Stakeholders need to be involved in evaluation planning, as well as other phases of the process, to minimize misunderstandings and confusion. Chapter 8 provided more discussion on stakeholder engagement. The following case study describes the Talent Development Evaluation Framework (Thomas, 2004) that provides an example of involving stakeholders in a school reform intervention.

Case Study
Talent Development Evaluation Framework: Making Community Connections and Involving Stakeholders in Evaluation Planning

This case study, the Talent Development Evaluation Framework, describes how evaluations of urban school reform initiatives serving underresourced urban school populations were planned. It is described more fully by Thomas (2004) and others in a publication by Thomas and Stevens (2004).

The Case for Planning Urban School Evaluations: A Brief Description

CRESPAR evaluators entered the urban school context gently, respectfully, and with a willingness to listen and learn in order to obtain stakeholder buy-in and to plan and implement a quality evaluation that could be of use to the program and the stakeholders. The evaluators attempted to get to know the school—its students, staff, parents, and surrounding community—prior to the implementation of any evaluations. During evaluation planning (and implementation), stakeholders were engaged in meaningful ways through various activities such as small group meetings, focus groups, and individualized discussions with key stakeholders to deeply understand their perspectives. In meetings with key stakeholders, CRESPAR evaluators asked and answered questions, listened to stakeholders' concerns, discussed issues, and recorded responses. The urban school stakeholders (e.g., students, parents, school staff) were given multiple opportunities to ask questions, critique evaluative efforts, and provide input.

Subsequently, stakeholders were engaged by soliciting input from them into framing evaluation questions, developing instruments, collecting data, interpreting findings, and using and disseminating the findings. All of these activities created a climate of trust and respect among the school reform design team, evaluators, and school/community stakeholders. Once stakeholders realized that their input was genuinely wanted, valued, and incorporated into the evaluation activities, they became open to viewing evaluation as a collaborative process.

Analysis of the Context

The complexity of social programs makes it critical that anyone who is tasked with evaluating such projects understand the context of the project and evaluation. Greene (2005) identified five specific dimensions to context in evaluation, including (a) demographic characteristics of the setting and the people in it, (b) material and economic features, (c) institutional and organizational climate, (d) interpersonal dimensional or typical means of interaction and norms for relationships in the setting, and (e) political dynamics of the setting, including issues and interest. Cultural contexts are also important elements of the project's milieu that the evaluator should try to understand early in the evaluation planning process (e.g., AEA, 2011; Frierson et al., 2010; SenGupta, Hopson, & Thompson-Robinson, 2004). The evaluator should gather information, through various means (observation, document reviews, key stakeholder interviews, etc.), that will provide a familiarity and good understanding of the environment where the project is located. During this time, the evaluator must pay close attention to how race, power, inclusion, politics, and privilege may be affected by the context or may, themselves, be affecting the context. Additionally, any previous evaluations of the program or of similar programs are also important contextual information to review.

Context is a force in evaluation, and it shapes practice; influences how evaluators approach, design, and implement studies; and determines how findings are reported (Rog, Fitzpatrick, & Conner, 2012). Since context can undoubtedly have an impact on the evaluation implementation and effectiveness, it is important for evaluators to learn what they can do about this context prior to finalizing an evaluation plan. In fact, one of the 2018 AEA evaluator competencies is that evaluators respond to the uniqueness of the evaluation context (AEA, 2018a). While an analysis and understanding of the context should take place early, this analysis is an ongoing and interactive process that should be attended to throughout the evaluation. The program context is not static but, instead, can change during the course of evaluation planning and implementation. An extensive review of documents (e.g., funding proposals, internal and external reports, project logs, pamphlets, brochures, project websites, relevant strategic materials), in particular, can contribute substantially to the evaluator's understanding of the context in which the project operates, as well as its history, philosophy, and functioning. Table 9.2 provides a useful guide, including sample questions, for performing a context analysis during evaluation planning (Conner, Fitzpatrick, & Rog, 2012).

Table 9.2 Context Analysis Guide for Evaluation Planning

Area	Examples of Relevant Guiding Questions
General phenomenon or problem	• What problem is the program addressing? • How did it emerge? • How long has it existed? • What groups prompted concern about it? • What is already known about it? • What are the dominant methods used for understanding the phenomenon/problem? • What tools exist for measuring change?
Particular intervention	• Where is the program in its life cycle? • How is the program structured? • What are the different components, and how do they fit in the broader environment? • Who does the program serve? • What are their characteristics, beliefs, culture, needs, and desired outcomes?
Broad environment and the intervention	• What are the different layers of environment that affect and can be affected by the intervention? • What aspects of these different climates are affecting the design and operation of the program? • What are important historical, social, and cultural elements of the community in which the program is conducted? • Are there political or social views that affect perspectives on the program, its clients, or decision makers?
Parameter of the evaluation	• What are the primary and secondary evaluation questions and their implications for possible methodology and design choices? • What resources are available to support the evaluation (e.g., budget, time frame, local evaluation capacity, evaluation ethos)?

(*Continued*)

Table 9.2 (Continued)	
Broad decision-making arena	• Who are the main decision makers/users of the evaluation information? • What are their views, values, and history about the program, and about evaluation? • What is the larger political culture in which they work? • What are the expectations of their organization? • What are the expectations of citizens they serve regarding government programs, and about evaluation? • What are the political expectations for evaluation?

Source: Conner, R. F., Fitzpatrick, J. L., & Rog, D. J. (2012). A first step forward: Context assessment. In D. J. Rog, J. L. Fitzpatrick, & R. F. Conner (Eds.), Context: A framework for its influence on evaluation practice. New Directions for Evaluation, 135, 89–105.

Identifying and Clarifying Project Goals

Early during evaluation planning, the evaluator needs to know that project staff have an agreed-on understanding of project goals. Subsequently, the evaluator must have a clear understanding of the project goals. The project goals should be used to help frame the questions guiding the evaluation, which are covered in more detail in Chapter 10. The evaluation planning process is a good time for project staff, along with the evaluator, to clarify the project goals as necessary. The evaluator should not assume that project goals are clear or realistic, even for projects that have been implemented across several years. Furthermore, evaluators should not assume that their understanding of project goals are clear or align with those of project staff. The major written sources of project goals (i.e., the project proposal, project plan, and other project-related materials such as websites and brochures) might represent the intended project but not the actual project taking place in the field. Therefore, a documents review of project goals (and activities) is insufficient to provide the evaluator an up-to-date and accurate understanding of the project's intended outcomes. It is important to get the perspectives of project administrators, staff members, and even clients on the goals of the project. The evaluator should not be surprised or alarmed if project goals need to be sharpened in response efforts to the evaluating activities that will be taking place.

During evaluation planning, the evaluator can assist project staff to clarify their goals by helping them to focus on the end results or accomplishments rather than simply the processes or steps leading to accomplishments. Evaluators can also help project staff modify goals so that they are realistic and measureable, as evidenced in the activity that follows.

Reflect and Discuss
Working With Stakeholders to Clarify Project Goals

Read the short scenario of a hypothetical childhood obesity intervention. Then, organize into small groups and discuss the questions posed at the end of the project description.

The Situation

Kamila Z interviewed project staff for a childhood obesity intervention that she was hired to evaluate. When asked about the project's goals, the staff simply said that they hoped that this project would result in young people having

> "better weight" outcomes. The evaluator used some guiding questions to help the project staff articulate more focused and measurable goals.
>
> Reflect on and discuss what might be some answers to these questions provided by project staff:
>
> 1. At the end of the intervention, we hope that the participants *will have learned what*?
> 2. At the end of the intervention, we hope the participants *will have developed what attitudes and beliefs*?
> 3. At the end of the intervention, we hope the participants *will do what or behave in what specific ways*?
>
> Now, in what ways have your answers to these questions provided more focus to the project goals?

It is during the evaluation planning phase that program stakeholders and the evaluator either develop or revisit the project's logic model. A logic model, as was discussed in Chapter 7, is a visual representation of how the program is supposed to work and achieve its goals. Due to the diversity of stakeholders involved in the project, they will sometimes have different and even contradictory views and interests. This can lead to different expected or desired end goals for the evaluation. Having the project staff, in collaboration with the evaluator if necessary, develop (and/or revise) the project's logic model is one way to help reconcile varying goals. It is an excellent tool for building consensus among stakeholders regarding how and why the project is likely to succeed.

Identifying the Purpose(s) of the Evaluation

One of the first things an evaluator needs to do in evaluation planning is to obtain a clear understanding of the purpose of the evaluation. In other words, the evaluator must be clear what sponsors and key stakeholders want when they say they "want an evaluation." This is necessary because different purposes require different approaches, different timelines, different questions, different methods and designs, and different resources. Understanding of the evaluation's purpose(s) and priorities informs evaluation planning. For example, if stakeholders want to know the changes that occur as a result of the project, this indicates that some baseline data need to be collected before the program begins and after the program ends or at an agreed-on interval of time during the project. If the program is already underway when the evaluator is hired, then the evaluator needs to determine if there is existing information that can be used as baseline data.

Part of identifying the purpose of the evaluation is specifying its scope based on determination of what the evaluation will (and will not) cover. Here, the evaluator needs to determine what intervention activities will (and will not) be evaluated, during what time frame, and where, if there are multiple project sites. Finding out what relevant stakeholder groups want from the evaluation is not always easy, especially when different stakeholders may prioritize different desired outcomes from the evaluation. Gaining consensus requires ongoing engagement with stakeholders very early during evaluation planning to get an understanding of their perspectives and to give them an opportunity to reach agreement.

Varying Stakeholders' Perspectives on Evaluation Goals and Priorities

It is important that key stakeholders agree on the main purpose of an evaluation. On the one hand, there are likely certain issues that all the key stakeholders want the evaluation to focus on (e.g., whether the project is achieving its intended results). However, on the other hand, there may be conflicts or potential conflicts regarding evaluation purpose and/or priorities among different stakeholders. Funders, project administrators, project staff, participants, collaborators, advocacy groups, and community members who have been involved in the project sometimes have competing interests that result in different priorities for the evaluation. As such, the evaluator must analyze the stakeholder landscape during the planning process to understand the varying stakeholders' goals and priorities for the evaluation. Since different stakeholder groups may want different things from the evaluation, they also may value different kinds of evidence, which requires different resources and expertise. Realistically, no single evaluation generally is able to fully meet the goals and information needs of all key stakeholder groups. Therefore, during evaluation planning, the evaluator must prioritize stakeholders and their goals for the evaluation.

There are various strategies that the evaluator can utilize to help gain consensus on the evaluation purpose when required. It should be noted, however, that engaging in this process requires additional resources (e.g., time, money, people). The following case study presents a process for gaining stakeholder consensus.

Case Study
Gaining Consensus on Evaluation Purpose Through Engaging Stakeholders

In their workbook *Getting to an Evaluation Plan: A Six-Step Process From Evidence to Engagement*, Iskarpatyoti, Sutherland, and Reynolds (2017, p. 13) suggest taking one or more of the following approaches to engage stakeholders during evaluation planning:

- *Conduct a series of [in-person] meetings:* Stakeholders are brought together in a series of in-person meetings to share experiences and knowledge, and to come to consensus on aspects of the evaluation plan. This approach requires resources to convene stakeholders in a single location, conduct detailed logistical planning, and secure the services of a strong facilitator(s) who can move the conversation along and ensure the optimal use of time. Because distractions can be minimized, conversations and consensus-building may be more productive and efficient in-person compared to virtually.

- *Achieve virtual consensus:* Stakeholders come together through an electronic medium (such as email, Skype, and/or web forums) to share experiences and knowledge, and to come to a consensus. This approach reduces the amount of resources needed to bring people together; however, consensus may be more difficult to reach. Facilitators need to be dynamic enough to keep the conversation moving, stakeholders engaged, and the discussion on track.

- *Conduct individual consultations:* A consultant [the evaluator] meets with stakeholders individually or in small groups and synthesizes their input. This is a quick way to develop a plan; however, because stakeholders are not aware of each other's input, misunderstanding or competition priorities may impede consensus building.

Source: Iskarpatyoti, B.S., Sutherland, B., & Reynolds, H.W. (2017). Getting to an evaluation plan: A six-step process from evidence to engagement. A Workbook. Chapell, NC: Measure Evaluation.

Funder's Priorities

The evaluator certainly cannot lose sight of the funder's requirements for the evaluation. After all, it is the funder who is financially making the project and the evaluation possible.

When a funder releases a program evaluation request for proposals, there may be a written request indicating the evaluation's goal, objectives, key questions, expected timetable, deliverables, and the amount of available funds. The evaluator who is awarded the evaluation has a contractual obligation to provide the agreed-on information. Even when the project director, coordinator, and/or principal investigator selects the evaluator, funders still generally have priorities for the evaluation. If they do not, an important task for the evaluator is to work with funders to achieve consensus on what they want from the evaluation, how the evaluation findings will be used, and who are the intended primary users of the evaluation results. Having this information is critical to evaluation planning because it helps the evaluator know what the funder has in mind for the evaluation.

Funders, federal and nonfederal, generally want the evaluation to inform them of what their grantees are accomplishing. So, identifying the extent to which projects are achieving their intended outcome(s) is a critical evaluation goal for funders. However, increasingly, funders also acknowledge the importance of understanding project processes and learning from failure or unintended results. Policymakers generally want an evaluation to led to improve outcomes for its intended beneficiaries, but also to provide them with information regarding the cost-effectiveness of project activities.

Project Administrators' Priorities

During evaluation planning, a considerable amount of evaluator time (either in person or virtual) is spent interacting with program administrators, and sometimes with program staff. These interactions should not only be focused on gaining an understanding of what they desire from the evaluation, but should also be a time for the evaluators to build trust and rapport between themselves and project staff and to establish (or further establish) themselves as credible and competent.

In addition to information on project accomplishments, program administrators and other staff generally want the evaluation to provide information that can be used for improvement purposes. Further, project staff members want the evaluation to provide information that allows them to craft an inspiring story on the work that they have been doing.

Evaluator's Priorities

Evaluators want the evaluation to be technically sound and lead to meaningful results for intended users. Evaluators generally aim for conducting an evaluation that provides information on project process and outcomes, but also contributes to the knowledge based on the social problem being addressed. In some instances, the evaluator's primary intentions for accepting the evaluation contract might not be aligned with the intended goals of the evaluation. For example, when evaluators want to use the evaluation context to ask research questions and test hypotheses of particular interest to them but not relevant to the evaluation questions, this is inappropriate and unethical, and it must be avoided unless accepted by all relevant parties as a secondary activity or project.

Defining Success in Evaluation Planning

Obtaining multiple perspectives on success from various key stakeholders during the evaluation planning stage increases the chances of having more inclusive definitions of success. The meaning of success is not standard but, instead, is a function of the project, its target population, and its context. Since "success" can mean different things to different stakeholders, there must be an agreed-on definition of success, certainly before measures of success can be established.

Projects focusing on broadening participation in STEM, for example, include a number of challenges related to defining success. P. B. Campbell. Thomas, and Stoll (2009) argue that defining success in terms of increases in absolute numbers or percentages is often insufficient, at best, and misleading, at worst. A 300% increase in, for example, Indigenous Americans receiving PhDs in engineering sounds very impressive, but it could be merely representing an increase from one to three. Defining success as an increase in both the number and the percentage of increase is better but not adequate in part because it does not set success within a broader context. It should not be seen as success in broadening participation efforts if the percentage of African Americans taking STEM Advanced Placement (AP) courses increases but the percentage of students taking STEM AP courses who are African American decreases (note this would happen if the numbers of other students taking STEM AP courses increased at a higher rate than those of African American students). Defining success as "reducing the gaps while all gain" puts change in context but does not provide an end point—a point when success is achieved (P. B. Campbell. Thomas, & Stoll, 2009).

The Problem With "Parity" as Success Definition

Another common definition of success that includes "end point" is parity; so, if African Americans are 12.8% of the population, then parity is African Americans being 12.8% of those studying STEM or in the STEM workforce. P. B. Campbell. Thomas, and Stoll (2009) argue that defining success in terms of parity should be defined as a range rather than an absolute number. Rather than having 12.8% be defined as parity or "success" for African Americans studying STEM, a range might be used, such as 10%–15%. A process and rationale would need to be developed to determine and justify appropriate ranges.

While "parity" can be an intriguing definition of success, even that is not sufficient (P. B. Campbell. Thomas, & Stoll, 2009). Success in broadening participation initiatives, as in other social justice– and equity-related initiatives, should include increases in absolute numbers as well. Perhaps success can be best defined as "achieving parity, as more participate overall." Since parity is about being equal or equivalent, there should be equal concern when a group is over the range as well as under the range in any definition of success (P.B. Campbell, Thomas, & Stoll, 2009). Overparticipation of a subgroup in a field should be as great a concern as underparticipation. In the case of gender, some scholars argue that the "feminization" of a field has traditionally resulted in a loss of status and income and may contribute to men's avoidance of fields they perceive as female dominated.

Beyond Quantitative Definitions of Success

Success does not have to be defined only in terms of quantitative terms or measures of quantities or amounts (e.g., a 50% decrease in school suspensions). There may also be qualitative definitions of success that do not involve numeric aspects but instead depict the status of something in qualitative terms. In some instances, an outcome is better captured by a qualitative rather than a quantitative success definition, such as obtaining clients' perceptions of the extent to which they are better off since project completion. Both success approaches have their value, and evaluators, along with stakeholders, should strive to find which one is more suited for which circumstance. Increasingly, more evaluations are using a combination of quantitative and qualitative definitions of success. The evaluator can play a substantial role in helping both funders and other stakeholders see the equal value of both quantitative and qualitative definitions of success depending on the situation.

The following activity provides an opportunity for readers to discuss different ways of defining success.

Activity
Defining Success

Organize into small groups and discuss different ways of defining success in intervention addressing the following social problems: health disparities, homelessness, and the achievement gap.

Now, address the following questions and other issues the group raised.

- Why did your group select these definitions?
- Do you think that achieving gender and racial/ethnic parity is a good indicator of success for these social problems? Why or why not?

Identifying Indicators

Once project goals and outcomes have been clarified and the evaluation questions are delineated, the next planning task is to develop indicators (see Chapter 1). In an ideal situation, indicators are identified during program planning. These are measures that demonstrate whether certain conditions exist or whether certain results have, or have not, been achieved (Horsch, 1997). An indicator is a marker of success, progress, or change. In other words, it indicates how we know a change occurred. Indicators provide the information needed to answer the evaluation questions, and can take the form of a measurement, number, or perception that can be used to document change over time (Mertens & Wilson, 2019). Also, the language used to operationalize indicators matters. For example, Mertens and Wilson (2019) provide an example where the U.S. Department of Agriculture previously used as an indicator the "number of people who are hungry" but recently changed the indicator to the "number of people who have low food insecurity." Here, while food insecurity and hunger are related, they are not the same thing. Food security is socioeconomic in nature, referring to a lack of available financial resources for food at the household level; hunger is physical in nature and refers to a personal, physical sensation of discomfort (U.S. Department of Agriculture, 2019).

Oftentimes multiple indicators are needed to answer a single evaluation question more accurately. Given the complexity of social variables, total reliance on a single indicator to address a particularly complex evaluation question could yield biased, incomplete, and/or incorrect results. For example, reliance solely on standardized test scores as an indicator of student success can be problematic, especially with certain populations of students, which is covered in more detail in Chapter 12. In addition to standardized test scores, success indicators can include increased attendance, higher persistence rates, positive student–teacher interactions, increased parental involvement, increased student self-esteem, and improved student attitudes about schooling (Hughes, 2000).

During evaluation planning, there should be a determination of the methods for data gathering and reporting. This includes identification of the information sources (e.g., project records, clients, service providers), data collection methods (e.g., questionnaires, observations), data analysis plans, and dissemination and reporting strategies. These issues are discussed in detail in Chapters 12, 13, and 14.

There are established criteria and general guidelines for selecting useful indicators, including the following, expanded from Schuller, Yaffee, Higgs, Mogelgaard, and DeMattia (2006, pp. 6–7):

- *Measurable:* can be quantified and measured by some scale
- *Direct and precise:* closely tracks results it is intended to measure
- *Reliable:* can be measured repeatedly with precision by different people
- *Relevant and useful to decision making and diverse stakeholders:* provide information that can be acted on or used to motivate action
- *Easy to interpret:* has a clear, well-documented or -understood link to particular attributes of the project
- *Sensitive to change:* has the potential to provide an early warning signal
- *Feasible, practical, and cost-effective to obtain:* can be collected on a timely basis, is accessible at low cost, and is feasible to collect in terms of terms of equipment, time, and expertise required to collect and analyze
- *Capable of being disaggregated:* can be broken down by various dimensions such as gender, ethnicity, age, geographical locations, and so on
- *Easily communicated to a target audience:* is understood by different audiences, such as decision makers, project staff, participants, and the general public, and can be summarized or compiled into simple indices, charts, or pictures

To identify indicators for the evaluation, the evaluator should (a) involve stakeholders to help define what success looks like and get their input on meaningful indicators to capture the required data, (b) consult the literature and other relevant resources for insights, (c) use the evaluation questions and the project's logic model or conceptual framework as a guide to develop meaningful indicators, (d) develop a possible list of indicators, and (e) use criteria (as specified earlier) as a guide to assess the possible indicators identified in the listing. Issues of culture and context certainly should be a major consideration when planning what indicators to use in the evaluation. For example, while an indicator might be an adequate measure for a white or male population, it might seriously misrepresent what in going on in a Black or Latino population. Traditional indicators of gender (dichotomous male vs. female) overlook people who do not identify as male or female or identify as gender fluid. After going through this process during evaluation planning, the evaluator can then select the best indicators to meet the project's information needs.

Understanding Different Types of Indicators

The literature has identified multiple indicators that may be the focus of an evaluation. These include the following:

- *Input indicators* measure the resources, contributions, and investments (both human and financial) devoted to a particular program or intervention;

examples include funding, staffing, facilities, and equipment allocated to the project. Input indicators answer the question, *What are the investments that make the project work?*

- *Process indicators* measure program activities, services, and goods; examples include training and participation rates. Process indicators answer the questions, *What did the project do?* and *Was it done as planned?*

- *Output indicators* measure the size and/or scope of activities, services, events, and products that reached intended individuals/groups; they are the goods and services generated by the project, and examples include number of workshops delivered, number of clients served, and number of newspaper mailings. Output indicators answer the question, *How many products were generated by the project?*

- *Outcome indicators* measure results or changes for individuals, groups, communities, institutions, and systems as a result of the project (actual benefits, impacts, changes); examples include improved health outcomes, increased school attachment, and reduction of recidivism rates. Outcome indicators answer the question, *What difference did the project make?*

Social justice–oriented indicators look at issues of opportunity, equity, and fair access. Answering the question posed in the following activity, reflect on and discuss these issues within the context of the intervention identified.

> ### Reflect and Discuss
> #### Social Justice–Related Outcome Indicators
>
> You are planning an evaluation of a health intervention in a low-income rural community, serving a large proportion of the white, African American, and Hispanic population. What kinds of indicators might you consider related to issues of access, fairness, and opportunity?

Levels of Indicators

Depending on the nature of the project and the information needs, indicators aimed at measuring success and results can be considered at various levels. P. B. Campbell, Thomas, and Stoll (2009) discuss three levels of indicators that can be identified for use during evaluation planning: individual, institutional, and funder. Indicators at each of these levels can be inputs, outputs, processes, and/or outcomes.

Individual-level indicators focus on changes at the participant level that result from the project. In evaluations of education projects, for example, individual-level indicators generally focus on issues of participation, retention, persistence, success, experiences, and attitudes. Institutional-level indicators focus on institutional-level transformation and change as a result of the project. Examples of institutional-level indicators include changes in staffing and/or institutional policies and programs. In community-based projects, there may be community-level, rather than institutional-level, indicators. Such indicators focus on population groups instead of individuals. An example would be monitoring smoking through the community-level indicator of sales of cigarettes in the community, rather than by polling people to find out how many cigarettes each person smoked daily (Community Tool Box, n.d.a). Funder-level changes include modifications the funder or sponsor has made to serve as a catalyst for the desired changes at the individual and institutional levels.

The following case study provides readers with specific examples of indicators at various levels.

Case Study
Broadening Participation Indicators at Various Levels

P. B. Campbell, Thomas, and Stoll (2009) provided a listing of indicators that could be used in broadening participation interventions funded by the National Science Foundation (NSF).

Level of Indicators	Examples
Individual-level indicators	Student-level data evidence, such as • participation rates (e.g., presence of URM* students in STEM majors and/or courses); • persistence or retention (e.g., number of URM students who return to college and remain in the STEM field); • student experiences (e.g., URM students involved in research experiences at key points during undergraduate and graduate training, student participation in bridge or mentoring programming, student presentations at scientific meetings); and • attitudes (e.g., URM students' perceptions and attitudes toward STEM fields, STEM interest and confidence).
Institutional-level indicators	Institutional-level evidence data, such as • staffing and institutional personnel (e.g., demographics of STEM faculty and hiring practices of new faculty from URM and non-URM groups); • policies, programs, and institutional commitments (e.g., presence of written diversity mission statement, institutional budget/resources dedicated to diversity and closing gaps); • accountability and rewards (e.g., presence of strategy for holding leadership, such as university vice presidents and deans, accountable, and inclusion of broadening participation accomplishments in faculty reports and institutional reports at various levels); and • collaborations (e.g., presence of a two-way partnership between minority and majority institutions, and presence of partnership with K–12 schools, communities, and organizations serving significant proportions of students from underrepresented groups).
Funder-level indicators	Funder-level evidence data, such as • diversity of professionals involved with NSF (e.g., number and percentage of program officers, division directors, and others with different demographic characteristics); • foundation resources devoted to broadening participation (e.g., staff allocated to broadening participation efforts, intervention programs, training opportunities, materials, and travel money); and • foundation resources devoted to research on broadening participation (e.g., number of research projects on broadening participation, and number of research projects with a focus on broadening participation).

* URM denotes underrepresented minorities.

Source: National Science Foundation

Developing Timelines

Development of a timeline should be part of evaluation planning. A good timeline depicts information sequentially, thus allowing users to visualize the flow of the evaluation process from beginning to end. During implementation, timelines may need to be modified inasmuch as project activities may be more complex and messier than anticipated. However, having a timeline prior to project implementation is still useful because it helps evaluators to work out as much detail as they can about what will be done and when. Considering the evaluation timeline, in totality, will help the evaluator identify potential challenges and, hopefully, handle them before they occur and become insurmountable.

Identifying Resource Needs

It is crucial to be realistic, during evaluation planning, about what will be needed to complete the evaluation. The amount of money and time needed to plan and conduct the evaluation is an important issue to clarify during evaluation planning. In terms of the resources needed to conduct an evaluation, there are typically four categories that the evaluator should consider during planning: staffing, materials and supplies, equipment, and travel. Chapter 15 provides a detailed discussion on preparing an evaluation budget.

Frequently, evaluation budgets do not come close to obtaining the often-recommended 10%–15% of the total project funds. There are many situations where an evaluator may be asked to conduct the evaluation on a "shoestring"—in other words, where time and other resources are severely limited (Robson, 2000). Bamberger, Rugh, Church, and Fort (2004) discuss two scenarios of **shoestring evaluation**: One occurs when the evaluator is not called in until the project is well advanced and there is a tight timeline for completing the evaluation frequently combined with a limited budget and without access to baseline data. The other scenario occurs when the evaluator is called in early, but for budgetary, political, or methodological reasons it is not possible to collect baseline data. If an evaluator agrees to take on a shoestring evaluation, there are considerations that must be reflected in evaluation planning such as simplifying the evaluation design, reducing sample size, reducing the costs of data collection, and simplifying and speeding up data input and analysis (Bamberger et al., 2004; Robson, 2000). These modifications can have a negative impact on the quality of the evaluation.

It is worth mentioning, however, that Bamberger et al. (2004) put forth the "shoestring evaluation" approach to provide tools for ensuring the highest-quality evaluation possible under constraints of limited budget, time, and data availability. While this approach was originally designed to assist evaluators working in developing countries, Bamberger and colleagues argue that the options embedded in this approach are equally applicable for planning and implementing evaluations under similar constraints in industrial nations.

Assembling an Evaluation Team

In many instances, a project may require an evaluation team rather than a sole evaluator. Assembling the right evaluation team for a particular evaluation endeavor is an important task. For programs that involve ethnically diverse participants, stakeholders can call for the creation of multiethnic evaluation teams to increase the chances of really hearing the voices of underrepresented groups (Hood, 2001; Stevens, 2000). For example, a group of African American evaluators working in predominantly African American urban school settings maintained that because of the shared racial and ethnic background they had with project staff and participants, the evaluation team was keenly aware of and sensitive to many of the contextual and cultural issues relevant to the lives of the children and family members being served (Thomas, 2004). These particular evaluators brought a different set of experiences than non–African American evaluators, which, the evaluators argued, increased their ability to engage stakeholders and better understand the verbal and nonverbal behaviors of the individuals being served.

Identifying the Evaluation Team's Roles and Responsibilities

Early in the planning stage of an evaluation, it is important to decide who is responsible for doing what during the evaluation. This might include a combination of the assignments to the evaluator/evaluation team as well as project staff. Roles and responsibilities should be allocated with input from all affected parties such that everyone knows who has responsibility for what and there is agreement on task allocations. Regardless of the number of individuals involved, everyone will need to work collectively to ensure timely completion of the various tasks related to the evaluation. There are management tools (discussed later in this chapter) that assist the evaluator in visually delineating team members' roles and responsibilities.

Internal vs. External Evaluators

There are multiple ways in which an evaluation team may be assembled. One possibility is to have an **internal evaluator** who serves as the evaluation team leader and is supported by internal project staff (internal evaluation). This internal evaluator works within the project (or the project's larger organization) and is generally familiar with the project and its staff. While internal evaluators have access to organizational resources and more opportunities for informal feedback with project stakeholders, they often lack the outsider perspective and technical skills of external evaluators (W. W. Kellogg Foundation, 2017a). Another possibility is to contract with an **external evaluator** who may assemble the evaluation team, not including any internal staff persons. External evaluators often come from universities, consulting firms, and research institutes. They generally have broader and more specialized evaluation expertise than internal evaluators and bring a different perspective to the evaluation because they are not affiliated with the project (W. W. Kellogg Foundation, 2017a). A third possibility is to have a **hybrid (or mixed) model** that combines an internal evaluator with the external evaluator, coupled with any additional evaluation team members the evaluators assemble. Based on a review of the literature, as well as our own situated knowledge, we summarize the advantages and disadvantages of having internal or external evaluators in Table 9.3.

Table 9.3 Advantages and Disadvantages of Internal vs. External Evaluators

Internal Evaluator Advantages	Internal Evaluator Disadvantages
• More familiarity, knowledge, and understanding of the project, its culture, and the broader context • Can be less threatening to staff, less disruptive to the project, and increase participation • Often better able to make recommendations project staff can/will commit to • Can be better positioned to facilitate learning within the program and build capacity of the program to conduct future evaluations • Generally done quickly and at lower cost	• May have difficulty criticizing the evaluand and more susceptibility to internal pressure to make the project "look good" • May have no special evaluation training or experience • Can impede candor among project staff being evaluated (particularly if they know the internal evaluator) • May be too close to be "objective" and thus not highly regarded by potential funders and other external bodies • Susceptible to internal political challenges and constraints
External Evaluator Advantages	**External Evaluator Disadvantages**
• Generally viewed as more objective • Bring specialized skills and expertise • May be more forthright in recommendations and willingness to criticize (offer fresh perspective) • Sometimes more able to act as facilitators between various stakeholder groups and project administrators/staff since they are not part of the existing organization power structure • Have greater credibility to funders and other external bodies • Can bring a fresh perspective to the evaluation context	• May be more time consuming since they need time to understand the project and its culture and context • More disruptive to normal project activities • May have more difficulty accessing the required data • May be more costly because of the external evaluator's particular expertise

Adapted from Freeman, "Gantt Chart vs. Pert Chart - What Are the Differences?" (2020).

In the end, a good evaluator and/or evaluation team includes those who

- have experience in the type of evaluation needed;
- have the ability to grasp the project quickly after an understanding of its context and relevant communication;
- demonstrate a willingness to work collaboratively with a wide variety of diverse stakeholders to meet project needs;
- have an understanding of research designs and statistical methods;
- demonstrate a willingness and skill set to address cultural/contextual factors in the evaluation (e.g., whether cultural competence for evaluation is being undertaken);
- will incorporate evaluation into program activities;
- can develop innovative approaches to evaluation while considering the realities affecting a program (e.g., a small budget);
- have the ability to develop data collection forms and/or use appropriate measures;

- will treat data confidentially;
- will educate program personnel in the importance of evaluation;
- can develop innovative approaches to evaluation while considering the realities affecting a program (e.g., a small budget);
- will give staff the full findings (i.e., will not gloss over or fail to report certain findings);
- are able to communicate in simple, practical terms;
- understand both the potential benefits and risks of evaluation; and
- have the time to do the evaluation (adapted and expanded from the U.S. Department of Health and Human Services Centers for Disease Control and Prevention, 2011).

Evaluation Planning and Management Visualization Tools

In addition to logic models, there are other evaluation planning and management tools available for use. Three commonly used evaluation planning tools include the **Gantt chart**, **Program Evaluation Review Technique (PERT) chart**, and **time and task chart**. There are comprehensive chart design software programs that make it easy to create Gantt charts, PERT charts, timelines, and calendars and allow users to schedule projects, track time, plan resources, and monitor performance in a single project management tool. These programs are compatible with both Mac and PC operating systems and have the cloud feature that allows users to share files and collaborate on projects. (See the Supplemental Resources at the end of this chapter for examples.)

Gantt Charts

During the evaluation planning phase, some evaluators use a Gantt chart to create a graphic overview of all the evaluation activities, when they will begin, and how long they will continue. A Gantt chart, named after its inventor, Henry Gantt, is a popular project planning and management tool consisting of a table or horizontal bar chart that lists project tasks and when they are to be completed. Sometimes referred to as a milestone chart or activity chart, the Gantt chart is useful for communicating the evaluation plan to nontechnical audiences and a common visual included in proposals. Each evaluation-related activity is represented by a bar or x mark; the position and length of the bar reflects the start date, duration, and end date of the activity. Some Gantt charts depict other features, such as milestones, which are represented by a triangle, and relationships, which are shown with arrows.

The advantage of creating a Gantt chart is that it allows the evaluator, and others, to monitor every stage of evaluation implementation to determine if it is on track and, if not, to be in a position to implement corrective action. Gantt charts can be created and updated using Microsoft Excel, Microsoft Word, or other online software (e.g., SmartDraw, GanttProject.biz).

In the case study that follows, readers are provided with an illustration of a simple Gantt chart for evaluation planning of a professional development project.

Case Study
Simple Gantt Chart for Planning an Evaluation of a Professional Development (PD) Project

Task	Month 1	Month 2	Month 3
1. Finalize PD evaluation design	x		
2. Develop online pretest/posttest surveys	x		
3. Attend planning meetings	x		
4. Review PD workshop materials		x	
5. Work with project administrators to develop embedded assessment of workshop products			x
6. Develop workshop evaluation forms			x
7. Observe workshop			x

Program Evaluation Review Technique (PERT) Charts

A PERT chart is another graphic representation of evaluation planning. As a project management tool, it can be used to schedule, organize, and coordinate tasks within the evaluation. The PERT chart demonstrates the order in which task are to be done. PERT charts are sometimes preferred over Gantt charts because they can more clearly illustrate task dependencies. In PERT charts, a network diagram shows the sequence of evaluation tasks and milestones. It can also illustrate how those tasks and milestones are prioritized or their precedence. Because of this feature, PERT charts are often referred to as "network diagrams" or "precedence diagrams." Illustrating a particularly complex evaluation schedule in a PERT chart makes it easier for stakeholders to identify dependent or sequential tasks and nondependent or concurrent tasks. Figure 9.1 provides an illustration of a simple PERT chart for the various evaluation tasks and the order in which they need to be done.

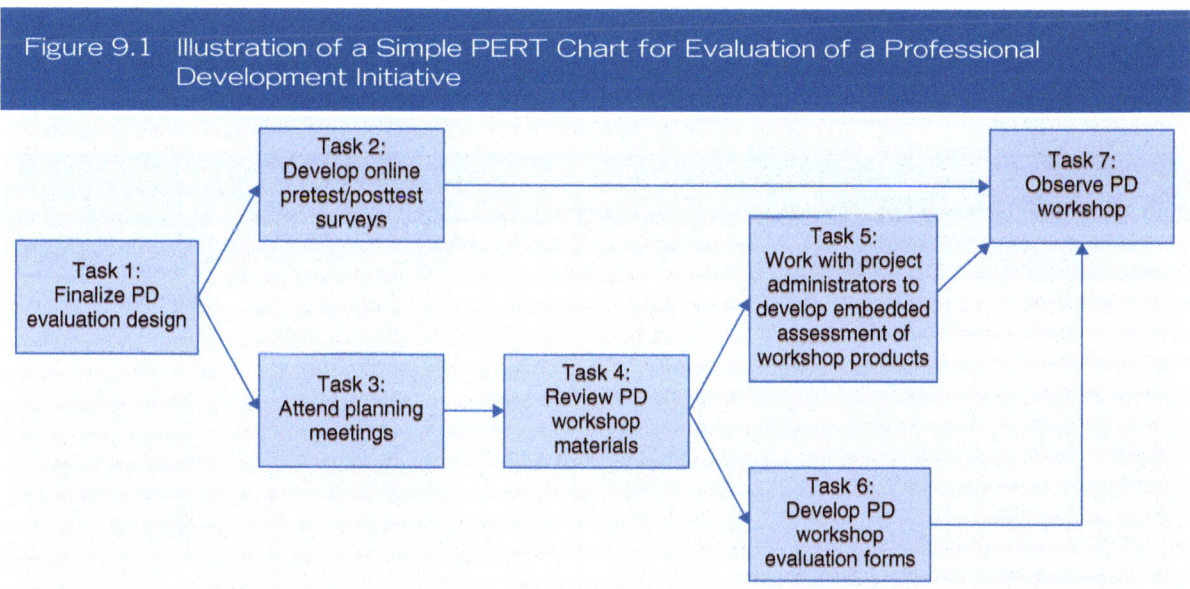

Figure 9.1 Illustration of a Simple PERT Chart for Evaluation of a Professional Development Initiative

Chapter 9 | Planning the Evaluation

Table 9.4 provides a comparison between Gantt and PERT charts. Gantt charts are more straightforward than PERT charts. In complex projects, a PERT chart can be much more difficult to interpret than a Gantt chart. As such, Gantt charts are more commonly used in evaluations than are PERT charts.

Table 9.4 Key Differences Between Gantt Charts and PERT Charts

Gantt Charts	PERT Charts
Represented with a bar graph	Represented with a flowchart (or network diagram)
More typically used for small projects	More typically used for large and complex projects
Provide accurate time duration and percentage complete	Need to predict the time
Do not display interconnecting tasks that depend on each other	Have numerous interconnecting networks of independent tasks

Source: Freeman, J. (2020, March 10). *Gantt chart vs. Pert chart—What are the differences?* Retrieved from https://www.edrawsoft.com/difference-gantt-chart-pert-chart.php

Time and Task Charts or Data Maps

A time and task chart, sometimes referred to as a data map, breaks down evaluation activities and provides a quick overview. The data map illustrates key evaluation questions, indicators associated with those questions, data collection methods, and expectations of when the goals will be accomplished, how, when, and by whom. Not all data maps contain all of these elements. Some may be relatively simple, focusing only on the planned methods, while others may include all the major tasks and activities related to the evaluation. Table 9.5 illustrates an abbreviated data map (or time and task chart) example developed by the first author, Veronica G. Thomas, for an evaluation of an environmental science/studies (ES/S) undergraduate degree program.

Table 9.5 Sample Data Map (Time and Task Chart)

Indicator	Data Source	Method	Responsible Party	Timing	Analysis Plan
Student interest in ES/S program	Enrolled majors and minors	Web-based survey	Evaluator	Beginning of each semester	Descriptive statistics
Changes in course enrollment	Institutional database	Review of records (i.e., institutional, department)	Principal investigator	End of each semester	Enrollment comparison over time
Faculty perceptions of project impact	Participating project faculty	In-person interviews	Evaluator	Annually	Inductive coding of interviews to identify themes

Note: ES/S denotes environmental science/studies.

Developing a Written Evaluation Plan

After doing preliminary work to understand the project's context, goals, stakeholders, information needs, and resources available for the evaluation, the evaluation plan is written. The ideal time to develop an evaluation plan is prior to project implementation. There are various evaluation frameworks and form templates available on the internet that can assist with developing a written evaluation plan. The U.S. Department of Education (www2.ed.gov/about/offices/list/oese/sst/evaluationmatters.pdf) and the Centers for Disease Control and Prevention (www.cdc.gov/eval/) are examples of agencies with accessible (online) evaluation frameworks, guides, and templates that can be used by evaluators to help guide their evaluation planning process.

The written evaluation plan may be done after substantial evaluation planning activities have taken place (e.g., engaging key stakeholders, prioritizing project and evaluation goals, performing context analysis), and it can be quite comprehensive; in other instances, due to time constraints and other limitations, the written evaluation plan might be needed shortly after the evaluator comes on board (maybe even within a week), and it only consists of the completion of a one-page template. In other words, the written plan does not necessarily have to be extensive and complex. The evaluation questions, information needs, and project context will determine the level of complexity and detail needed in the written plan.

A written evaluation plan is a vital part of most grant proposals, especially those requesting federal funds. The evaluator must have already defined the project's goals and objectives and the strategies or activities that will be used to achieve those goals prior to writing the evaluation plan. It is also crucial to involve key stakeholders in the development of the evaluation plan. This will ensure that important perspectives are being represented and that all the necessary parties are on board and willing to cooperate and collaborate during evaluation implementation.

The written evaluation plan provides a road map that clarifies the direction the evaluation will take based on goals, priorities, resources, and expertise required to accomplish the task. A comprehensive evaluation plan describes, in detail, each step of the evaluation process, indicating the purpose of the evaluation, key evaluation questions, what will be evaluated (e.g., processes, outcomes), how (e.g., indicators, data collection, analysis, and interpretation plan), and when (e.g., timelines). Ideally, evaluation plans are written during project planning. Here, the evaluator, in collaboration with program staff and other relevant stakeholders, develops the evaluation plan before the program begins. Having a written evaluation plan in place prior to project implementation will make collecting evaluation data much easier and likely produce more accurate data.

The evaluation plan guides the evaluation efforts throughout the life of the evaluation. Also, if shared, it fosters transparency and ensures that stakeholders have a mutual understanding of the evaluation's purpose (e.g., what it will and will not accomplish) and serves as a reference when questions arise related to priorities. Another benefit of having a written evaluation plan is that it guides the evaluator (and others) through each step of the evaluation process. It specifies, in writing, the what, who, how, and when. The evaluation plan clearly specifies the type of information stakeholders need, as well as helps the evaluator avoid focusing on and/or collecting irrelevant information. Further, the evaluation plan should outline the best-possible methodology, given realistic constraints, for gathering the necessary information and the end products (e.g., formal reports, journal articles, newspaper or magazine articles) generated from the evaluation. Good evaluation plans include a process detailing how and to whom the evaluation report, in whole or in part, will be disseminated.

The evaluation plan should be reviewed regularly over the life of the project to ensure the implementation activities are on track and, most importantly, that the evaluation questions are still relevant. Remaining flexible is important during evaluation planning, as well as throughout the evaluation life cycle. Situations may arise that necessitate updating, or even revising, the evaluation plan if project objectives change or there are modifications to project activities. Updating the evaluation plan should involve bringing in relevant stakeholders to gain consensus on the revisions to the original, agreed-on evaluation plan. The basic elements of an evaluation plan include the following components:

- Overview or background of the project (evaluand) (description of project, context, logic model, key stakeholders, target population and beneficiaries, key components, expected outcomes)
- Evaluation purpose (rationale, purpose, scope, who wants the evaluation and why, intended use)
- Evaluation questions
- Evaluation methods (design, ethical and cultural considerations, data collection procedures, data analysis plan)
- Reporting and dissemination plan
- Cost and resource needs
- Roles and responsibilities
- Timeline

Overcoming Pitfalls in Evaluation Planning

Good evaluation planning entails understanding the evaluand and its context, identifying and involving a broad range of stakeholders, having good definitions of success and appropriate indicators, poising relevant and useful evaluation questions, using an appropriate methodology that will answer these questions and provide credible evidence to stakeholders, and having the right evaluator (or evaluation team). An evaluation with a well-thought-out plan is more likely to get off to a good start and ultimately achieve its goals.

Pitfalls, or problems, can occur at any point in the life cycle of the evaluation. Pitfalls during the planning stage are particularly problematic because they can place the evaluation in peril early on. Hatry and Newcomer (2015) identified seven pitfalls that can occur during the planning phase and before data collection begins. These include

- failure to assess whether the program is evaluable;
- starting data collection too early in the life cycle of the program;
- failure to secure input from program managers and other stakeholders on appropriate evaluation criteria;
- failure to clarify program managers' expectations about what can be learned from the evaluation;

- failure to pretest data collection instruments appropriately;
- use of inadequate indicators of program effects; [and]
- inadequate training of data collectors. (pp. 703–708)

These pitfalls have methodological implications related to evaluation validity, reliability, and credibility. For example, failure to clarify program managers' expectations about what can be learned from the evaluator can limit the evaluation's credibility; similarly, inadequate training of the data collector not only impedes the evaluation's credibility, but also negatively impacts its potential internal validity, covered in Chapter 11; measurement validity, reliability, and generalizability, covered in Chapter 12; or transferability (Hatry & Newcomer, 2015).

Understanding and recognizing potential pitfalls in evaluation planning are vital to one's ability to either eliminate or minimize such pitfalls. It is certainly better for the evaluator to identify (and seek to ameliorate) a planning pitfall than to ignore it or have it pointed out by a funder or project administrator. A large part of this entails putting sufficient time and deliberation into the evaluation planning process.

SUMMARY

Evaluation planning is vital to good evaluation. Therefore, it is essential that evaluators formulate the overall evaluation strategy, from beginning to end, taking into account cultural and other contextual issues. This strategy is not static, but is subject to change and updates throughout the life of the project. In fact, evaluators must be patient and understanding and have a high tolerance for ambiguity and change (Thomas, 2004) because, in reality, despite thoughtful and careful planning, many evaluations will not be implemented exactly as planned. Evaluators should prepare for contingencies and the need to make adjustments to the changing dynamics (e.g., staff turnover, changing priorities, competing agendas) that often exist in projects—all of which might affect the evaluation as originally planned.

SUPPLEMENTAL RESOURCES

Community Tool Box

https://ctb.ku.edu/en/toolkits

This is a free, online resource for those working to build healthier communities and bring about social change. It offers thousands of pages of tips and tools for taking action in communities.

Gantt Project

www.ganttproject.biz/download

This free scheduling and management app for Windows, OSX, and Linux offers resources for creating tasks and milestones; organizing tasks in a work breakdown structure; drawing dependency constraints between tasks, like "start X when Y finishes"; and creating baselines to be able to compare the current project state with previous plans.

Project Chart Software for Both Gantt and PERT Charts

www.edrawsoft.com/projectchart/

Project Chart Maker provides templates for creating both Gantt charts and PERT charts. The software contains smart built-in symbols such as timeline, status table, Gantt chart, and calendar, which makes it relatively easy to use.

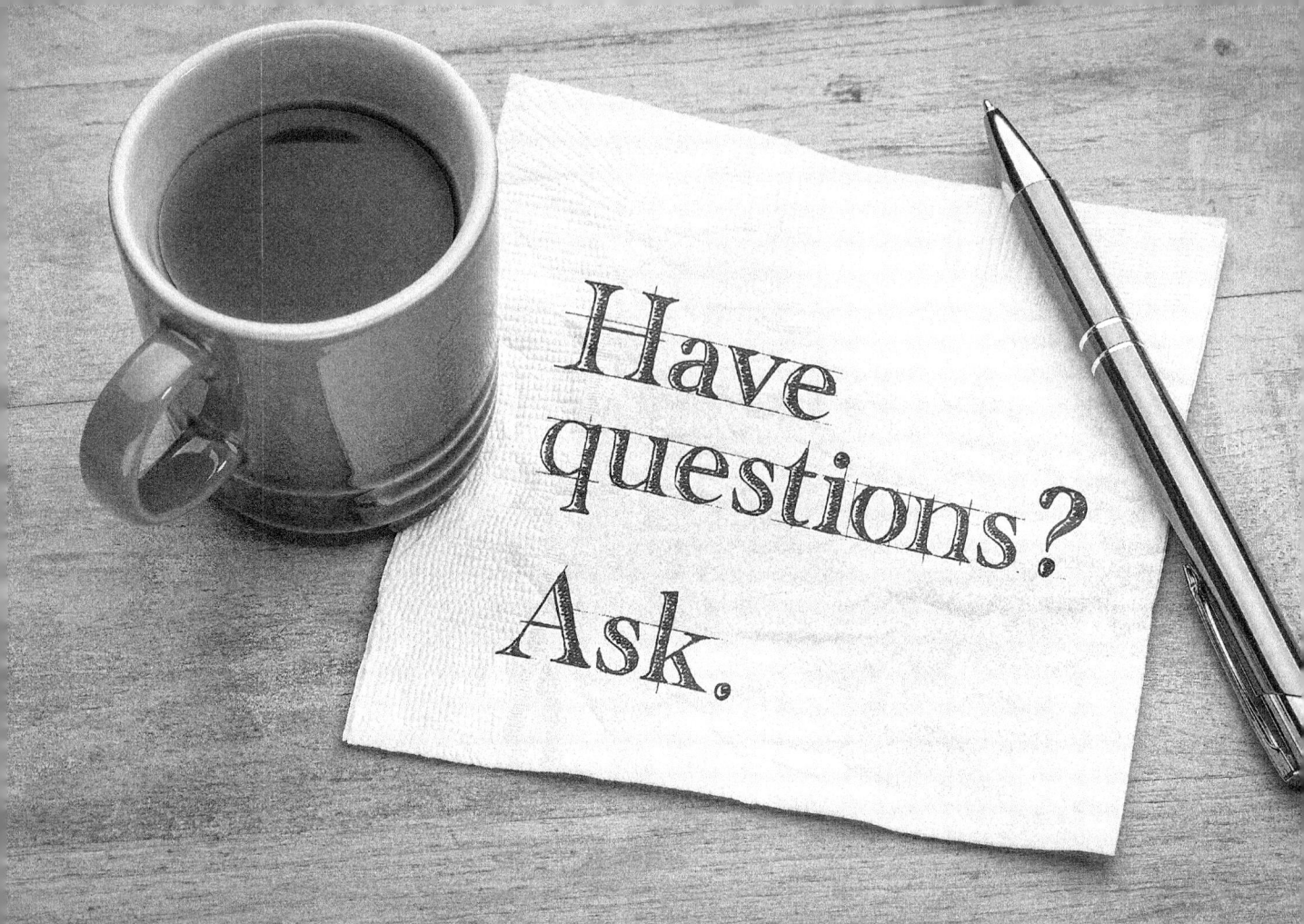

Shutterstock/marekuliasz

Evaluation questions that matter ask about important things that stakeholders care about, reflect local culture and diversity of stakeholder perspectives, and provide structure to the evaluation.

CHAPTER 10

Evaluation Questions That Matter

Evaluation questions that matter are those that provide key stakeholders and primary audiences with the information they want to know about the project by the end of the evaluation. These reflect multiple perspectives and include those that are relevant, appropriate for the context, and responsive to diverse stakeholders' concerns. In the end, a good evaluation provides clear and defensive answers to the important questions that matter.

After reading this chapter and participating in the activities, readers will be able to meet the following learning objectives:

- Understand the importance of generating evaluation questions that matter

- Engage diverse stakeholders in a process of identifying questions that matter

- Connect evaluation questions with the potential to yield useful and credible evidence Construct good and useful evaluation questions, including ones that address issues of cultural responsiveness and social justice, and evaluate those questions against specified criteria

- Know multiple sources of questions, different types of questions, and procedures for prioritizing and critiquing evaluation questions for diverse audiences

Introduction

Evaluation questions are central to evaluation planning, implementation, and dissemination of results since, at the most basic level, evaluations are designed to answer specific questions. The questions define the issues the evaluator will investigate, and they provide structure and refinement to the evaluation. Questions must be formulated and agreed on very early in the evaluation process since virtually all evaluation activities evolve from the evaluation questions. For example, identification of the evaluation questions will clarify the type of baseline data that a project will need to collect and will inform decisions on whether any comparison groups need to be established before an intervention begins. Additionally, evaluation reports are often structured around the evaluation questions with a section devoted to each question. There may be circumstances, as the project and evaluation unfolds, that require adjustments to the initial set of evaluation questions to reflect the reality of what is actually happening on the ground. The evaluator must be sensitive to emerging issues that require revision of the initial set of evaluation questions. However, if the evaluator formulates questions in a thoughtful and deliberate manner, with input from diverse and appropriate sources, there should be minimal modifications needed to the original set of evaluation questions.

Evaluators' philosophical assumptions, including those associated with methodology, can lead evaluators to ask certain questions and prioritize what questions and issues are most relevant to the evaluation (Mertens & Hesse-Biber, 2013). However, formulating good evaluation questions involves a continual interplay of

(a) finding out as much as one can about the project as well as its surrounding area's geography, history, politics, social and economic conditions, and cultural nuances; (b) developing an understanding of the intended processes and outcomes; and (c) engaging in ongoing dialogue and negotiation with diverse stakeholder groups to understand their perspectives and values to determine how best to meet their information needs.

Evaluation questions serve multiple purposes. They provide structure and focus to the evaluation, guide the evaluation planning process, and can reflect and determine evaluation goals. Using an analogy of a building's foundation, Robinson (2014) articulates three broad functions of evaluation questions, summarized in the following activity. In this activity, readers are asked to reflect on and discuss Robinson's analogy.

Reflect and Discuss
Three Critical Functions of Evaluation Questions

In a blog post, Sheila Robinson (2014) applies an analogy of a building's foundation to evaluation questions. A building's foundation, she stresses, is designed to bear the load of the building, to anchor it against potentially damaging natural forces such as earthquakes, and to shield it from other potential damage such as moisture. She argues that evaluation questions have three functions similar to a building's foundation:

1. They bear the load of the evaluation. The evaluation approach and social science theories that inform your approach, along with choices about evaluation design and selection of measures, rest squarely on the evaluation questions. These questions set the purpose for the entire evaluation.

2. They anchor the evaluation against potentially damaging "forces." What could potentially damage an evaluation? Looking for the wrong indicators (i.e., those most readily observable), selecting the wrong measures (i.e., the most readily available, cheapest, easiest to administer), collecting the wrong data, engaging the wrong stakeholders (i.e., those easiest to access), sampling the wrong respondents . . . You get the picture. Leveraging evaluation questions as the anchor lends critical purpose to all choices you make as you craft the evaluation.

3. They shield the evaluation from that which can seep in slowly and destroy it. Distrust, disdain, fear, misplaced expectations. These insidious dysfunctional attitudes towards evaluation can fester and erupt at any time in the evaluate life cycle. Clearly articulated questions give the evaluator the ability to defend against these and the potential to address them productively. (Robinson, 2014, para. 10)

Questions for Discussion

1. What do you think about Robinson's analogy? Is it helpful for better understanding the role of evaluation questions?

2. Under what circumstances might her analogy not work? For example, in what cultural and contextual environments might the evaluation questions fail to anchor the evaluation against "damaging forces"?

Why Evaluation Questions That Matter?

At the most basic level, good evaluation questions are ones that matter. Evaluation questions that matter ask about things that stakeholders and primary audiences value. In other words, these questions address key concerns of these groups. Questions that matter are relevant, appropriate for the context, and responsive to stakeholders' concerns. The stakeholders learn from clear answers to questions that matter, and therefore, they are more likely to use information gleaned from those answers. Good evaluation questions reflect multiple perspectives and take into account a number of factors. At a minimum, these factors include (a) the project's goals, objectives, and cultural context; (b) the project's logic model; (c) motivations for the evaluation; (d) the funder's requirements; (e) feedback from relevant stakeholders; and (f) the agreed-on focus and goals of the evaluation. Further, determining questions that matter must also take into consideration opportunities and constraints (e.g., time, cost, personnel, information access) the evaluator is likely to encounter in the process of addressing these questions. Ultimately, questions that matter are those that provide key stakeholders and primary audiences with the information they want to know about the project at designated intervals and by the end of the evaluation.

Questions can cover multiple aspects of the project although stakeholder interests and feasibility considerations may prevent the evaluator from focusing on all of these aspects in a single evaluation. For example, some questions that matter may focus on contextual characteristics of the project. Other questions that matter might focus on characteristics of project staff and participants. What the project is doing and stakeholders' views can also be the focus of questions that matter. Attention to project outcomes, including short-term, intermediate, and/or long-term, may be embedded in questions that matter. Questions related to equity and social justice concerns may be, and most likely should be, those that matter in virtually every evaluation. These and other types of questions will be discussed in greater detail later in the chapter.

Questions That Matter Meet Information Needs of Diverse Users

Questions that matter meet the information needs of key and diverse stakeholder groups and users. As introduced in Chapter 2, utility, or the extent to which evaluation processes and products are valuable in meeting stakeholder needs, is one of the five areas around which the *Program Evaluation Standards* (Yarbrough, Shulha, Hopson, & Caruthers, 2011) are organized. Good evaluations are expected to serve the identified and emergent needs of stakeholders. When stakeholders have authentic input into the formulation and prioritization of evaluation questions, they will be more likely to accept the conclusions of the evaluation and act on recommendations offered. Even in instances when the evaluation is driven primarily by the external demands (e.g., funders), it (including its questions) should be organized in a way that allows it to remain owned in the internal environment and creates useful knowledge for the community (Nelson-Barber, LaFrance, Trumbull, & Aburto, 2005).

Questions That Matter Set the Stage for the Collection of Credible Evidence

Evaluation questions are expected to produce answers that provide **credible evidence** that can be used for decision making around programs, policies, and practices. Credibility in evaluation is a multifaceted concept that involves consideration of diverse stakeholders' perspectives and purposes (Mertens, 2013). Credibility, in large part, is shaped by the context in which it resides. The ability of evaluation questions to yield credible evidence is, to some extent, subjective. The who, what, when, where, and how issues can shape the extent to which the evidence is viewed as credible. As is covered in Chapter 11, for many evaluators, credible evidence is primarily determined by the evaluation design (e.g., randomized controlled trial); however, Greene (2015) offered an alternative understanding to the nature of credible evidence in program evaluation, particularly democratic evaluation. She argues that credibility of evaluation evidence

> is not automatically granted via the use of particular methodologies, but rather is earned through inclusion, relational, and dialogic processes of interpretation and actions that happen on the ground, in context, and in interactions with stakeholders. (p. 206)

Since judging the legitimacy or acceptability of evidence can vary among various stakeholder groups with different assumptions and values, it is important that the evaluator has a good understanding of what the different stakeholder groups would accept as credible evidence for answers to the evaluation questions. The following case study provides an opportunity for readers to think about what credible evidence means to them within their own context.

Case Study
What Is Credible Evidence?

The Big Brothers Big Sisters of America (BBBS) Community-Based Mentoring (CBM) program has been evaluated and found to be effective by the National Institute of Justice (see Office of Justice Programs at www.crimesolutions.gov/advsearch.aspx). Review the brief description of the program and discuss the questions raised at the end of the case.

The Case

The goal of Big Brothers Big Sisters of America (BBBS) Community-Based Mentoring (CBM) is to support the development of healthy youths by addressing their need for positive adult contact, thereby reducing risk factors for negative behavior and enhancing protective factors for positive behavior. BBBS CBM offers one-to-one mentoring in a community setting for youth placed at risk. More specifically, the program is intended for youth between the ages of 6 and 18 who often come from single-parent households and low-income neighborhoods. In some cases, these youth are coping with the stress of parental incarceration. Youth targeted for this program are at high risk of exposure to violence and trauma at home and in the community.

> **Questions for Discussion**
>
> Now, imagine there is a BBBS CBM program in your community.
>
> 1. In thinking about an evaluation of this particular BBBS CBM program, what would be examples of credible evidence that could emerge from the evaluation questions?
>
> 2. On what basis (personal values and experiences, academic training, etc.) did you select these particular examples of credible evidence?

Power and Privilege Issues in Formulating Evaluation Questions

Issues of power and privilege can arise at any time during the evaluation process. It is important that evaluators be attentive to how these issues can impact the identification and prioritization of the program issues and ultimately the evaluation questions that emerge from this process. As covered in detail in Chapter 8, we acknowledge the reality that the issues and questions of those in power and those that sponsor the evaluation receive top priority in evaluation planning and implementation. However, the evaluator should also be concerned about the perspectives of the less powerful target individuals and communities likely impacted by the program. Defining these individuals' realities oftentimes requires an evaluator to have the ability and willingness to unmask the power inequities and outcomes of people in a program within the context of the (sometimes) racialized environments.

Mertens (1999, 2005) urges evaluators to prepare questions within a **transformative framework** where they exemplify power relationships that need to be addressed. The transformative paradigm, as was discussed in detail in Chapter 5, emerged, in large part, because of dissatisfaction with the dominant research paradigms and practices and partially because of a realization that much of sociological and psychological theory had been derived from the white, able-bodied, male perspective and was based on the study of male participants. Transformative questions address power and privilege, and they ask questions that place the locus of the problem in unresponsive systems with power inequities rather than in the individual without power. Mertens (2005) put forth examples of evaluation questions from a transformative paradigm that focused squarely on issues of power and privilege in an education setting, including serving students with disabilities. For example: *How has the institution or agency been unresponsive in meeting the needs of people with disabilities? Are resources equitably distributed? How can we teach and counsel students and clients so that they do not continue to be oppressed?* The answers to such questions are intended to reveal issues of inequity that need to be addressed.

Characteristics of Good Evaluation Questions: An Overview

Evaluation questions must reflect the agreed-on purpose of the evaluation. It is important to understand the characteristics of good evaluation questions. In general, a good evaluation question is one that focuses on an observable dimension of a project activity and/or outcome that can be credibly assessed. The evaluation literature has contributed to our understanding of the characteristics of good evaluation questions by delineating practical ways in which an evaluator can focus questions, formulate more effective questions, address the needs and concerns of stakeholders, and prioritize questions (e.g., Centers for Disease Control and Prevention [CDC], 2013; Davidson, 2012; Patton, 2012; Preskill & Jones, 2009; Rossi, Lipsey, & Freeman, 2004; USAID, 2013; Wingate & Schroeter, 2016).

Lori Wingate and Daniela Schroeter (2016) put forth the *Evaluation Questions Checklist for Program Evaluation* to assist evaluators in developing effective and appropriate evaluation questions and to assess the quality of existing questions. The characteristics of good evaluation questions that they identified were based on the relevant literature as well as their own experience with evaluation design, implementation, and use. Wingate and Schroeter (2016) point out that good evaluation questions should be

- *evaluative*, calling for an appraisal of a program or aspects of it based on the factual and descriptive information gathered about it;
- *pertinent*, including questions that are clearly related to the program's substance and evaluation users' information needs;
- *reasonable*, including questions that are linked to what a program can practically and realistically achieve or influence;
- *specific*, including questions that clearly identify what will be investigated in the evaluation;
- *answerable*, including questions that reflect the real-world constraints on the type and quantity of data that can feasibly be collected, analyzed, and interpreted; [and]
- *complete*—that is, the set of evaluation questions is complete when they, in totality, thoroughly address the purpose of the evaluation and evaluation users' information needs. (pp. 1–3)

This checklist offers a relatively easy guide that novice evaluators might find extremely useful. It can be found at https://wmich.edu/sites/default/files/attachments/u350/2018/eval-questions-wingate%26schroeter.pdf

In the next section, we offer a set of characteristics of good evaluation questions. Some of the characteristics identified certainly overlap with the characteristics offered by Wingate and Schroeter (2016), the CDC, and numerous others. These characteristics are put forth to help readers focus on important qualities of good evaluation questions.

Good Questions Align With the Funder's Requirements

If the funder has a Statement of Work (SOW), the evaluator will have very detailed guidance of the evaluation requirements. Some SOWs include a limited number of specified evaluation questions and their priorities. Good SOWs seek to guarantee that each evaluation question is answerable with the highest-quality and most credible evidence possible, given time and budget constraints. If there is not a SOW, the evaluator and funder, along with other stakeholders such as the program or project directors, must work together to determine the scope of the evaluation and the questions of interest.

Good Questions Are Useful and Ask About Important Issues

Davidson (2012) argued that one thing that makes an evaluation useless is a lot of tangential, barely related, wouldn't-it-be-nice-to-know stuff that seems to be more about the evaluator's interests than anything the primary users might need to know. Evaluation questions should be directly related to what primary users need to find out from the outcomes of the evaluation. They should not focus on minor, irrelevant, or superficial aspects of the project or stakeholders' interests. Sometimes the key stakeholders may agree on 10 evaluation questions that they wish to have answered. The evaluator, however, might indicate that there is insufficient time and resources to answer 10 questions and suggest that the set of evaluation questions be limited to 5. Therefore, it is wise to establish criteria that can be used to help stakeholders narrow down the questions' importance to the priority issues and to think about how useful the answers to those questions would be for taking action toward program improvement.

Good Questions Are Tailored and Appropriate to Local Needs

Evaluation questions must be tailored to the objectives of the project and the agreed-on goals of the evaluation in the localized context. Good evaluations provide clear link between the questions and the relevant issues/goals of the project. Furthermore, evaluation questions should address the local needs of the intended beneficiaries of the evaluation. Vague and general questions taken from another evaluation context should be replaced with contextualized questions that meet local nuances and interests at the particular place and point in time.

Good Questions Are Clear, Specific, and Well Defined

Evaluation questions must be specific enough to focus on the assessments, observations, and/or comparisons to be made. Questions should be sufficiently clear so that there is an understanding of the particular project components that will be investigated and the dimension of project performance that will be examined. Once the initial questions are written, the evaluator should scrutinize them with an eye toward making them even more specific. For example, stakeholders for a workforce development training project may want the evaluator to ask and answer the question, Was the project successful? However, this question, as stated, is too broad, is ill defined, and does not guide the evaluator toward what indicators of success need to be examined. In this instance, the evaluator must engage with stakeholders to understand what they mean by *successful*. In the case of the workforce development training project, a more useful question might be *Did project participants have greater employment rates than nonparticipants 12 months after participation?* Therefore, it is crucial that the evaluator avoid questions stated in overly broad terms that are unclear as to what aspects of the project need to be examined to answer the questions.

Good Questions Are Researchable (or Answerable)

Evaluation questions must be answerable with some degree of certainty. These include questions with answers that the evaluator can reasonably ascertain credible evidence for during the implementation phase of the evaluation. In considering whether questions are researchable or answerable, the evaluator takes into account a variety of issues including resources available to collect, analyze, and interpret data as well as issues of privacy, ethics, politics, and so on. If evaluation questions are too vague or broad, or require data that are unobservable or unavailable to the evaluator, they are not answerable.

For example, a question that intends to examine change in students' mathematics achievement within a school district participating in a teacher professional development program would be quite reasonable for an evaluation if the evaluator is provided access to the student math achievement scores. However, if such information is not available to the evaluator, this is an unanswerable question, and it should be avoided. In another example, where the community feels that the underlying assumption of some of the evaluation questions are problematic (e.g., marginalizing), the evaluator may not have the cooperation of certain segments of the community to obtain the data to answer the questions. For example, questions that are framed solely from a deficit perspective (e.g., problems in this community), rather than also seeking to uncover strengths, may ultimately be rejected by participants and members of the target community. In these contexts, such questions will not be answerable and therefore should be avoided.

Good Questions Are Realistic Considering Contexts and Project Realities

Questions must be answerable with the resources available to the evaluator. For example, if the time frame for collecting the required data to answer an evaluation question extends beyond the due date for the final evaluation report, then that is not a good question to include in the evaluation planning. Additionally, questions must be realistic given the realities of the implemented, not just the planned, project. Other realities that should be considered include how the project is structured, its maturity or stage of development, what activities are actually being undertaken, the roles and responsibilities of project staff, the demographics of program participants, and the cultural context of the project.

Good Questions Are Reasonable in Number and Scope

A single evaluation oftentimes cannot address every aspect of a project. As such, there should be a reasonable number of evaluation questions in a single evaluation project. While there is no minimum or maximum number of questions to have in an evaluation, the number should be reasonable considering the most important information to learn from the evaluation as well as available resources such as money, time frame, and access to the required data. As such, some evaluations may only have one, two, or three questions, whereas other evaluations may have five, six, or seven (or even more) questions. Nevertheless, it is also critical that evaluation questions are limited in scope. Since many projects have multiple objectives, a variety of tasks, and a diverse set of beneficiaries, it is crucial that the questions focus on the most critical issues where evidence is required to make a decision about current or future programming. The evaluator should work with relevant stakeholders to delimit and focus the evaluation questions. Questions that are reasonable in scope are more likely to be understood by others, and they are more likely to be answerable in depth.

Sources of Evaluation Questions

Evaluators must do a lot of frontloading, or working ahead, and find out as much as they can about a project before even starting to draft a set of evaluation questions. This can be accomplished through reviewing available written documents about the project, conducting key stakeholder interviews with diverse people who are knowledgeable about the project, and visiting the project and its surrounding community to better understand the project's culture and context. Project-related documents may be readily available on the internet or the project's website for review. Other documents, however, may not be publicly available and thus require some additional effort on the part of the evaluator to obtain.

Examples of documents to be reviewed include the project's funding proposal, brochures, stated goals and objectives of the project, the project's organizational chart, the project's logic model, progress or annual reports, past evaluations of this or similar programs, site visit reports, project minutes, and news articles, blogs, or any social media presence about the project. To learn more about the project, the document review might be followed up with key stakeholder interviews or focus groups with key individuals such as the project sponsor (or project officer), the project director, selected staff, advisory board members, influential community members, and selected project participants. Since good evaluation questions represent the views of people/groups that sponsor the evaluation as well as those affected, either directly or indirectly, by the project and/or the results of the evaluation, these interviews provide an opportunity for the evaluator to obtain this invaluable information. It also provides an opportunity to determine stakeholders' information needs, what they hope to learn from the evaluation, and how the results of the evaluation will be used and by whom.

In sum, sources of evaluation questions include information gleaned from a variety of sources. These include

- the original request for proposal to which the project responded to secure funds;
- the statement of work for the evaluation contract;
- key interviews, focus groups, and/or brainstorming sessions with key stakeholders such as project funders, project managers, administrators, project staff/volunteers, clients, and community leaders;
- adaptations of questions found in a review of the relevant literature;
- questions used in evaluations of similar programs;
- input from expert consultants and other professionals with knowledge of the project or the content area represented in the project;
- the project program theory or logic model; and
- the evaluator's own independent analysis of the program.

Prioritizing Evaluation Questions for Diverse Audiences

After input from relevant stakeholders, the evaluator must prepare for a multiple-step process of writing initial questions, refining these questions, and then prioritizing the questions. Once the evaluator and the relevant stakeholders have agreed on a list of co-constructed questions, those questions must be prioritized. In prioritizing questions, the evaluator should consider a variety of things, including (a) the extent to which the question reflects the project's goals, objectives, and cultural context; (b) the importance of the question to the funder, program staff, and other key stakeholders; (c) the extent to which answers to the question would yield actionable data for planning and decision making, particularly in the near term; (d) how much the information gleaned from the question can be leveraged to further the goals of the project; (e) the feasibility (e.g., time, money, staff) of gathering and analyzing the data yield from the question; and (f) the extent to which the answers to the question will contribute to filling a current knowledge gap.

In terms of prioritizing outcomes questions, the evaluator needs to think about which questions could yield outcomes most useful to understanding project success and guiding program improvements, most important for funders to know, and most important to program participants and diverse stakeholder groups. Equally important, the evaluator must put into place an equitable process to make sure that diverse voices are respected, heard, and acted on when prioritizing questions. This involves critical dialogue between the evaluator and diverse stakeholders with the goal of obtaining input from as many perspectives as possible to get a more complete picture before deciding on final evaluation questions.

Inclusion/Exclusion Criteria for Prioritizing Evaluation Questions: Two Approaches

Given limitations of time and resources (e.g., money, personnel), it is nearly impossible for a single undertaking to answer all the possible evaluation questions generated from various sources drawn on in an evaluation project. Therefore, some explicit criteria must be generated to help evaluators determine, in their own context, how to prioritize questions generated so that some questions included are selected through a thoughtful and deliberate process. Different organizations and evaluation scholars have proposed such approaches. In this section, we discuss two approaches that can be useful. The first approach was put forth by the U.S. Agency for International Development Office of Learning, Evaluation, and Research (2013). The second approach was put forth by staff at the CDC (2013).

U.S. Agency for International Development (USAID) Approach

The staff of the USAID Office of Learning, Evaluation, and Research (2013) developed a checklist to help USAID staff define, revise, and strengthen their evaluation questions. The USAID checklist recommends that evaluators ask themselves the following to determine which questions are most important to incorporate into the evaluation.

- Who would use the information?
- Who would be upset if the evaluation question was dropped?
- What is the level of interest [of the question] to key stakeholders?
- Would the information change or impact the course of events?
- Is it [information generated from the questions] of passing interest, or does it focus on a critical or major issue?

- Would the evaluation be compromised if this question were dropped?
- Is it feasible to answer the question?
- Can the evaluation users envision how they would actually use the evidence in response to each question? Can they specify decision-making scenarios for the response to each question? (pp. 1–2)

In addition to these questions, staff of the USAID include a personal factor for consideration. They suggest that evaluators ask themselves, *Do the key users really care about the evaluation questions, and are they really committed to having them answered?*

Centers for Disease Control and Prevention (CDC) Approach

The second approach to assessing and prioritizing evaluation questions is one developed by the CDC (2013) in a published checklist referred to as the *Checklist for Assessing Your Evaluation Questions*. The rationale for the creation of this checklist, according to its authors, is that many evaluators, especially those new to the field or those working with inexperienced evaluators, have difficulty applying broad principles of good evaluation questions in a manner that creates truly sound, meaningful questions. Therefore, to assist individuals to get to "good questions," the staff of the CDC aggregated and analyzed evaluation literature and solicited practical advice from evaluators working in the field.

The CDC checklist criteria encompass four areas to consider in evaluating potential questions, including the extent to which

- there was diverse *stakeholder engagement* in developing the question;
- there is an *appropriate fit* between the question and the project goals;
- the question is *relevant* to the project's purpose and needs; and
- it is *feasible* to obtain answers to the question in an ethical and reasonable manner considering one's resources.

These criteria are described in more detail in Table 10.1.

Table 10.1 CDC Criteria for Evaluating and Prioritizing Evaluation Questions

Evaluation Question Criteria	Description
Stakeholder engagement	Diverse stakeholders, including those who can act on evaluation findings and those who will be affected by such actions (e.g., clients, staff), were engaged in developing the question.
Appropriate fit	The question is congruent with the program's theory of change.
	The question can be explicitly linked to program goals and objectives.
	The program's values are reflected in the question.
	The question is appropriate for the program's stage of development.

(Continued)

Table 10.1	(Continued)
Relevance	The question clearly reflects the stated purpose of the evaluation.
	Answering the question will provide information that is useful to at least one stakeholder [or stakeholder group].
	Evaluation is the best way to answer this question, rather than some other (nonevaluative) process.
Feasibility	It is possible to obtain an answer to the question ethically and respectfully.
	Information to answer the question can be obtained with a level of accuracy acceptable to the stakeholders.
	Sufficient resources, including staff, money, expertise, and time, can be allocated to answer the question.
	The question will provide enough information to be worth the effort required to answer it.
	The question can be answered in a timely manner (i.e., before any decisions potentially influenced by the information are made).

Source: Abbreviated from CDC. (2013). *Checklist for assessing your evaluation questions* (p. 2). See supplementary resources at end of chapter for description and website location.

The CDC checklist not only identifies these four important criteria to consider, but also requests users to explain why a particular question might be suitable for inclusion even though it does not meet a particular aspect identified in the checklist. Additionally, the authors noted that, with the exception of the item addressing ethics, it is acceptable for a question(s) not to meet several of the criteria but still be retained if the evaluator has an acceptable rationale for doing so.

Steps to Identifying, Formulating, and Prioritizing Questions That Matter

Clearly, it is essential to have a clear vision of the evaluand, the purpose of the evaluation, and the information needs of users before drafting specific evaluation questions. In her Voices From the Field interview, Beverly Parsons stresses the importance of an evaluator not simply focusing on the project in formulating and prioritizing evaluation questions that matter, but also considering context, the situation, and relationships and boundaries surrounding the evaluand.

Voices From the Field

Beverly Parsons: Asking Questions That Matter

Before asking questions, one key thing evaluators must do is to understand the context they are working in and not just simply zero in on the evaluand. Evaluators should look at the situation, the nature of the context including the natural environment, the range of people involved and their varying perspectives, and what kinds of relationships and boundaries exist. As evaluators think of questions that matter, they must think about what is really meaningful to the people involved. It is important to think about what issues these people care about and if they can do something about those issues. An evaluation sometimes misses really important questions because, in part, it has gotten positioned as part of the formal organization and has become a tool to try to convince people to do something. It has gotten over-embedded in the hierarchical bureaucratic ways of operating. Instead, we need to get more grounded in the personal nature of change. Evaluation should be viewed not just as a mechanistic process but as a way of thinking and interacting. It is an ongoing, extended process through which we can learn from every evaluation activity that occurs. Evaluators should not get locked into their first evaluation plan; instead, the plan should allow opportunities to make change as we learn. There should be places for renegotiation of the plan and sharing of learning along the way.

Beverly Parsons is president and executive director of InSites, a Colorado-based nonprofit organization. InSites works through inquiry-based evaluation, planning, and research to support learning, growth, and change in formal and informal social systems. She also served as 2014 president of the American Evaluation Association (AEA). Veronica G. Thomas interviewed her in the fall of 2019.

The issues Parsons raises focus on some initial things the evaluator should do and be aware of before moving on to crafting evaluation questions. These issues will help the evaluator think about and frame questions that matter. Taking into consideration the advice offered by Parsons, and extensively found in the published literature, here we offer nine practical steps for developing and prioritizing evaluation questions that matter.

Step 1: Conduct a landscape scan and find out as much as you can about the project. Review available written documents and supporting materials about the project, including but not necessarily limited to project funding proposals, logic models, and interim/annual reports; also develop understanding of the project and its surrounding cultural and contextual context.

Step 2: Engage relevant stakeholders to get their input on the project, information needs, and expectations for the evaluation.

Step 3: Develop an initial set of evaluation questions based on the landscape scan, stakeholder input, and the evaluation's purpose.

Step 4: Share the initial set of evaluation questions with diverse stakeholders for their input and co-construct questions.

Step 5: Revise the set of evaluation questions, taking into consideration the input from diverse stakeholders.

Step 6: Reduce, fine-tune, and prioritize evaluation questions, taking into consideration project information needs, resources available to develop credible answers, and other feasibility (e.g., time constraints) concerns. Be sure the questions are relevant to the key diverse stakeholder groups.

Step 7: Submit the revised set of evaluation questions for review and approval by key stakeholders (e.g., funders, program administrators).

Step 8: Subject the revised set of evaluation questions to an established inclusion/exclusion and eliminate/add/revise questions as warranted.

Step 9: Finalize a feasible number of evaluation questions for focusing and structuring the evaluation.

In the following activity, readers are asked to generate a list of evaluation questions, then go back and prioritize their questions.

Activity
Generating and Prioritizing Evaluation Questions

Organize into several small groups. Choose from one of the topics listed to develop a hypothetical project, including a project name, mission statement, two or three goal statements, and objectives. The topics are education, health, employment, and criminal justice.

Let's say that your group has been selected to be the evaluator team for the project. Your group should brainstorm and come up with 7–10 possible evaluation questions for the hypothetical project created. Then, go back and prioritize the original set of questions to end up with a set of 5 key questions.

1. Identify the five prioritized questions.
2. Delineate the process or criteria your group used to prioritize the questions.
3. Provide a rationale for your criteria.

Types of Evaluation Questions

Evaluation questions must be tailored to the purpose of the evaluation and information needs to be met. Funders, for example, may have very specific expectations that must be fulfilled by the evaluator. Also, an evaluator might be expected not to evaluate the entire project at once, but instead to focus on the strongest or the longest-implemented components of the project. As such, it is important to ask the right types of questions for the intended purpose of the evaluation. A variety of different types of evaluation questions serve varied purposes and are appropriate at different stages of the project implementation. In the sections that follow, we discuss different types of evaluation questions, focusing on their meaning and purpose. For each of the major types of questions presented, the evaluator can include questions influenced by social justice and/or culturally responsive perspectives. We provide sample questions for each type including those from social justice and culturally responsive perspectives.

Program Theory Questions

Program theory evaluation assesses whether a program is designed in such a way that it can achieve its intended outcomes. Rossi, Lipsey, and Henry (2019) advocate that analyzing a program's theory, as discussed in Chapter 4, can assist in identifying potentially important evaluation questions. They further add that one aspect of evaluating a project is assessing how good the program theory is. Program theory questions, generally formative in nature, often focus on the logic and plausibility of a program theory and are most appropriately asked during project planning or the early stage of the evaluation.

Sample program theory questions, expanded from Rossi et al. (2019, p. 19), that might be asked include:

- What outcomes does the program intend to affect?
- How do the anticipated outcomes relate to the nature of the problem or conditions the program aims to change?

- What is the theory of action that supports the expectation that the program can have the intended effects on the targeted outcomes?
- How does the project theory-of-change compare and interact with the cultural values, lifestyles, and worldviews of its clients and the surrounding community?

Context Questions

Since projects and programs take place within a complex cultural, social, economic, and political environment, contextual factors may be an important aspect to focus on when determining questions that matter. Contextual factors can be either external (e.g., demographic shifts in the population surrounding the project, community norms, resources, and values) or internal (e.g., leadership style of the project director). Context questions, formative in nature, focus on how the project operates or will operate within a particular social, political, physical, and economic environment. Stakeholders are often interested in the extent to which certain contextual factors might be related to the outcome variables of interest. Two sample context questions include:

- What external factors (e.g., weather conditions, school leadership changes) influenced the delivery of the project's activities and services?
- What environmental (e.g., transportation access) or other contextual factors (e.g., community socioeconomic status, language barriers, unequal distribution of power, historic treatment of minorities or immigrant populations in the target community) are barriers to the participants' access to the project's services?

Process Questions

These types of formative question focus on what the project is doing and the extent to which the project is being implemented in a manner as intended. Process questions generally ask about effort, resources, activities, operations, and service delivery. These are the *who*, *what*, *when*, *where*, and *how* questions. Process questions consider things such as the number and types of clients served, number and types of services delivered, staffing characteristics, and stakeholders' views about the project (e.g., satisfaction, recommendations). Some process questions attend to structure-related issues—that is, how the project is organized—while others focus on activities-related issues. Examples of structure-related process questions include:

- To what extent does the project's administrative structure (personnel policy and hiring practices, organizational chart) support the project?
- Is the appropriate staff in place to offer the intended program?
- How well does the project access hard-to-reach populations? Who missed out?
- To what extent is there appropriate and equitable use of resources?
- What are the power dynamics operating within the project or between the project and the surrounding community?
- To what extent was the project implemented fairly, ethically, culturally appropriately, and in a way consistent with legal and professional standards?

Two examples of activity-related questions include:

- What types of activities take place? How often do they occur?
- Are the activities being offered as intended?
- How did different groups of participants experience the project activities?

Answers to process questions can yield immediate feedback to project administrators by monitoring the project's day-to-day operations and helping to identify problems faced in delivering services.

Relevance Questions

These types of formative questions focus on the extent to which the project's activities are consistent with the beneficiary's requirements, as well as the community's needs and priorities. Sample questions include:

- To what extent do stakeholders support (or value) the project?
- To what extent are the project's objectives still valid?
- Does the project meet the needs and priorities of participants?
- How valuable were the outcomes of the project to participants? To the community?
- How relevant is this project to the short- and/or long-term development needs of the target community?

Outcomes Questions

These types of questions, which are summative in nature, focus on the results or the effectiveness of the project in producing change. For projects providing direct services, the outcomes of interest generally focus on changes in the characteristics or circumstances of the target participants. Here, questions generally pay attention to changes in the participants' knowledge, attitudes, behaviors, and/or skills. Sometimes these questions focus on conditions (impact) that resulted from the intervention. In addition to project participants, other beneficiaries may include service providers and/or members of the community. Therefore, some outcomes questions might focus on these stakeholders as well. Projects might target changes beyond the individual level to include, also, changes at an organizational or community level such as increasing collaborations or partnerships across various community-based programs.

The outcomes questions may focus on short-term, intermediate, or longer-term outcomes. Questions concerned with short-term outcomes generally include questions related to immediate benefits or changes that the target groups are anticipated to experience or display as a result of their participation in (and/or completion of) the project. Here, the questions seek to identify the first meaningful changes that follow from the intervention and occur before more long-term results. Evaluation questions focusing on intermediate outcomes generally focus on changes in beneficiaries' behaviors and actions expected to result from or follow the short-term outcomes. Questions that focus on longer-term outcomes (or impact questions, discussed in the next section) focus on more distant benefits or changes as a result of the intervention. Sample outcomes questions include:

- Did the participants' motivation levels improve after participation in the project? (short and intermediate term)
- What unintended changes, positive or negative, did the project yield? (short, intermediate, or long term)
- Did participants' (desired) outcome levels change (or were they maintained) three years post–project completion? (longer term)
- How do outcomes differ across cultural (e.g., racial/ethnic, gender, language) groups? (short, intermediate, or longer term)
- To what extent are the burdens and benefits of the project distributed across different racial/ethnic and socioeconomic status groups? (short, intermediate, or longer term)

Impact Questions

These types of summative questions focus on broad and longer-term effects produced by the intervention. Whereas outcomes questions tend to focus on changes in the beneficiaries that occur as a result of the program, impacts questions typically focus on the broader changes that occur within the community, organization, society, or environment as a result of program outcomes. Impacts are generally not achievable during the life cycle of the project and are usually understood to occur later than, and as a result of, the short-term or intermediate outcomes. Impact questions seek to illuminate the project's wider story or the broader range of outcomes stemming from the project. Decision makers who request impact questions often want these answered to decide whether to terminate or scale up an intervention and to inform communities about the ways in which a project is benefitting them. The impacts under consideration in the evaluation questions can be intended or unintended, and they can be either direct or indirect. Unfortunately, many sponsors of evaluation do not have sufficient resources for their funded projects to undergo an impact evaluation. A few sample impact questions include:

- To what extent has the project influenced the target stakeholder community?
- What capacities have been built in this community as a result of the project?
- What outcomes in the community (intended and unintended) has the project contributed to?
- To what extent is the project impacting positively on key groups and issues that have been identified as important?
- How has the project produced changes to investment, policy, or practice that will enable change in infrastructure or scale?

The following case study includes a description of a project proposed by first author Veronica G. Thomas and her colleagues on the Secondary School Project at the Howard University Center for Research on the Education of Students Placed at Risk.

The description includes some potential process, outcomes, and impact questions. Readers are given an opportunity to add their own generated process, outcomes, and impact questions to this listing.

> # Case Study
> ## FACES Sample Process, Outcomes, and Impact Questions
>
> FACES (Families and Children Engaging Schools) was a project considered for implementation across secondary schools within a large urban district in the northeastern part of the United States. The project was particularly interested in improving school–parent–teacher relationships and increasing elementary students' interest and achievement in science.
>
> ### Sample Process Questions
>
> - How many elementary students and their parents or guardians participated in the FACES project?
> - What is the demographic profile of the participants in FACES?
> - What types of activities are taking place during project implementation?
> - In what ways, if any, do FACES activities align with the school science curriculum?
>
> ### Sample Outcomes Questions
>
> - Do students participating in the FACES project demonstrate improvements in their science grades and test scores over the course of the academic year?
> - Have parent–teacher communications improved since the FACES project has been in operation?
>
> ### Sample Impacts Questions
>
> - How has the FACES project improved school–community relationships?
> - Has the FACES project led to new school–community partnerships, coalitions, or other efforts to improve schools and communities?
> - What effects, if any, have the FACES program had on the 25 target schools, the school district, and the larger communities where the schools reside?
>
> After you review these questions, please critique the questions as well as add one or two additional process, outcomes, and impact questions to this listing.

Cost-Benefit and Cost-Effectiveness Questions

In some instances, summative questions ask about cost effectiveness and cost benefits. They seek to address the "bang for the buck" questions. Cost-benefit questions focus on the relationship between costs and monetary outcomes, whereas cost-effectiveness questions ask about the costs to gain a unit of a desired outcome (e.g., one year of life gained or death prevented) for one or more interventions. Sample cost-effectiveness and cost-benefit questions for a health intervention might ask:

- For every $100 spent on prenatal care for low-income mothers, how much is saved on neonatal intensive care? (cost benefit)
- To what extent does the obesity prevention and control program produce annual savings in reduced health care claims that are greater than the annual cost of operating the program? (cost benefit)

- What are the gains in health relative to the costs of different health interventions? (cost effectiveness)
- Do the economic benefits of providing this program outweigh the economic costs? (cost benefit)

Sustainability Questions

These types of evaluation questions, mostly summative in nature, focus on the continuation of benefits from the intervention after major development assistance or initial funding has been completed. The emphasis here is on identifying the long-term benefits of the project. It is generally difficult for an evaluator to reliably and directly assess sustainability because it cannot actually be determined until after the project is complete and the evaluation may be done. However, evaluators can obtain information on the likelihood of sustainability by asking questions such as:

- To what extent is there evidence that the project is likely to grow (scale up or out) beyond the project (grant) life?
- What are the prospects for the sustainability of the end results produced by this project?
- To what extent can the project survive or grow in the future without its current level of funding?
- What results appear to be less sustainable, and why?

In the following activity, readers are given an opportunity to generate different types of evaluation questions.

Activity
Generating Different Types of Evaluation Questions

In the activity on page 316, you were asked to organize into several small groups. Then, you were asked to choose from one of the topics listed to develop a hypothetical project, including a project name, mission statement, two or three goal statements, and objectives. The topics were education, health, employment, and criminal justice. You were asked to generate 7–10 possible evaluation questions for the hypothetical project created, then to go back and prioritize the original set of questions to end up with a set of 5 key questions.

If you responded to this activity, review, refine, and add to, as necessary, your questions for the hypothetical project and classify them into the types of evaluation questions specified as follows. If you didn't respond to the earlier activity, please complete and generate the various types of evaluation questions to include

- two context questions;
- two process questions;

(Continued)

(Continued)

- two outcomes questions;
- one cost-benefit question; and
- one impact question.

Be sure to include some questions that reflect culturally responsive and social justice perspectives.

Summary of Different Types of Evaluation Questions

Table 10.2 provides a summary of the various types of evaluation questions, along with their purpose.

Table 10.2 Summary of Different Types of Evaluation Questions

Type of Question	Purpose of Question
Program theory	To focus on formulation of the project's program theory of change and the extent to which the program theory presents a feasible and plausible plan for achieving its intended outcomes
Context	To focus on how the project operates or will operate in a particular social, political, physical, and economic environment
Relevance	To focus on the extent to which the project's activities are consistent with the beneficiaries' requirements and the community's needs for intervention
Process	To focus on how the project functions by examining the implementation of services and activities
Outcomes	To focus on effects of the intervention on the target population; examine the extent to which objectives were achieved and/or changes that occurred as a result of the intervention
Impact	To focus on the broader consequences (positive or negative, direct or indirect, intended or unintended)
Cost benefit and cost effectiveness	To focus on the cost of a program in relation to its economic and social benefits
Sustainability	To focus on extent to which benefits of the intervention are likely to continue after initial support (e.g., grant funds) has been completed

SUMMARY

Good evaluation questions include those that matter. They matter because good questions are appropriate to the project's circumstances and provide focus and structure to the evaluation. Good questions result from a collaborative and iterative process between the evaluator, key stakeholders, and primary users of the evaluation data. Good questions guide the design and conduct of the evaluation and ensure the information collected is important to sponsors, program implementers, beneficiaries, and other stakeholders. Good questions will always directly relate to what key stakeholders and the primary audience want to learn about the project from the evaluation. Additionally, good evaluation questions reflect a local culture and diversity of stakeholder perspectives. They are prioritized to address important aspects of the project and must be answered within the constraints of the resources available.

Numerous resources exist in the published literature and online for evaluating the quality of evaluation questions. These resources can be particularly useful in providing practical guidance to new evaluators, as well as experienced evaluators working in contexts where there is not consensus on the questions to ask or the priority assigned to each question. Ultimately, evaluators want clear, pertinent, and cultural and contextually relevant questions that yield credible evidence to answer those questions and increase the likelihood that this information will be acted on for making improvements and strengthening positive change.

SUPPLEMENTAL RESOURCES

Evaluation Questions Checklist for Program Evaluation

https://wmich.edu/sites/default/files/attachments/u350/2018/eval-questions-wingate%26schroeter.pdf

The purpose of this checklist, authored by Lori Wingate and Daniela Schroeter of Western Michigan University, is to aid in developing effective and appropriate evaluation questions and in assessing the quality of existing questions. It identifies characteristics of good evaluation questions, based on the relevant literature and the authors' own experience with evaluation design, implementation, and use.

Checklist for Assessing Your Evaluation Questions

www.cdc.gov/asthma/program_eval/AssessingEvaluationQuestionChecklist.pdf

This checklist, created by the CDC's (2013) National Asthma Control Program, offers a set of criteria for assessing and prioritizing evaluation questions. The criteria center on stakeholder engagement, appropriate fit, relevance, and feasibility.

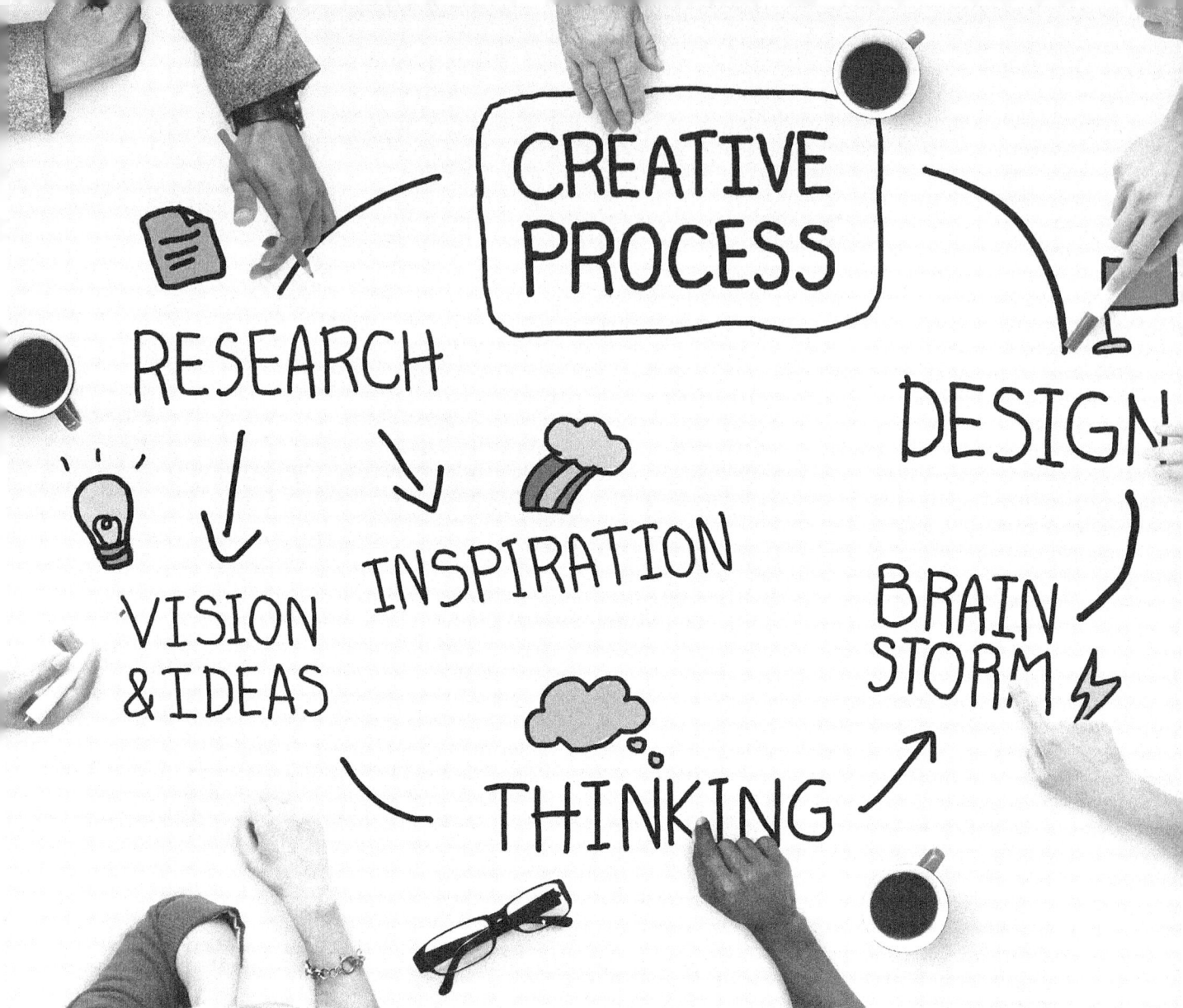

As complexity and context are introduced, there is less control, more uncontrolled variables, and thus less rigor. However, researchers and evaluators are looking for results that pay attention to context and can be applied in complex settings.

CHAPTER 11

Selecting Appropriate Evaluation Designs

We often say that there is no best design—there is only the best design to answer the questions being asked. While the statement is correct, it is incomplete. In evaluation, the best design is the one that not only can answer the questions but can do so within the budget, without compromising that which is being evaluated, while being ethical, being culturally responsive, and inconveniencing participants as little as possible.

After reading this chapter and participating in the activities, readers will be able to meet the following learning objectives:

- Discuss limitations to applying traditional definitions of methodological rigor to the choice of an evaluation design
- Develop criteria as to what is and isn't credible evidence for data
- Know the value and the challenges of the use of comparison and control groups and be able to determine appropriate comparison groups
- Discuss positive and negative impacts of the application of traditional definitions of rigor
- Describe what it means for an evaluation design to be culturally responsive
- Distinguish between experimental and quasi-experimental designs and describe their relative strengths and weaknesses
- Describe threats to validity that can be minimized by the choice of a design
- Select designs for different evaluations and justify their choices

Introduction

This chapter focuses on **evaluation design**—that is, the overall strategy used to integrate the different components of an evaluation in a coherent and logical way to ensure that the questions are effectively addressed. It constitutes the blueprint for the collection, measurement, and analysis of data. Braverman and Arnold (2008) described evaluation design as the "determination of how, when, and from whom data will be collected and the structure of the critical comparisons that will address the questions of interest" (p. 73). While some designs might be seen as stronger than others, in evaluation, as in research, the questions that the evaluation seeks to answer determine the type of design to be used. When selecting a design, the question the evaluator should be asking is not "What's the best design?" but "What's the best design for the question?" (De Vaus, 2001). While there are major differences between evaluation and research, the types of designs used are essentially the same depending on the questions asked and importance of generalizability and replicability.

The chapter begins with a discussion of methodological rigor, introduced in Chapter 5, and how a focus on rigor can potentially bias a study design and results. The value of control groups and comparison groups in evaluation designs is covered, as are some of the ethical issues tied to their use with different populations. Challenges and benefits of designs using longitudinal data are included, as are sources and limitations of such data. The chapter describes a variety of experimental designs, quasi-experimental designs, and case studies; their strengths and weaknesses; and their appropriateness for different evaluation questions. The chapter concludes with a discussion of threats to validity and a summary to help readers select the best design for the question.

Rigor

Rigor in evaluation designs and evaluation generally refers to scientific or methodological rigor, which the National Institutes of Health describes as compliance with "the strict application of the scientific method to ensure robust and unbiased experimental design, methodology, analysis, interpretation, and reporting of results" (Lauer, 2016, para. 1). This traditional definition of rigor has been thought to be the essence of scientific work. Evaluation, like other fields in the social and behavioral sciences, has substantially increased its emphasis on methodological rigor. For the last few decades, in particular, at virtually all levels, programs and their projects and interventions have been held more accountable for results than was formerly the case (National Institutes of Health, n.d.a). Substantial attention is being paid to methodological rigor, and evaluators are often pressured to employ methodologies that are seen to be the most "rigorous" and will stand up to scrutiny. Often the quality of an evaluation is measured by the rigor of the methods used in the evaluation (Institute of Education Sciences, 2003; Tucker, 2014). As will be discussed later in this chapter, traditional definitions of rigor are being challenged as limiting the quality, diversity, and usability of research and evaluation. For example, biologist Graciela Unguez (personal communication, April 10, 2019) points out that, traditionally, the more controlled a study is and the fewer uncontrolled variables there are, the more rigorous the work is considered to be. However, she says, that only happens in the simplest of studies. As complexity and context are introduced, there is less control, more uncontrolled variables, and thus less rigor. However, researchers and evaluators are looking for results that pay attention to context and can be applied in complex settings. Thus, there actually may be an inverse relationship between traditional definitions of rigor and usefulness.

In evaluation, while rigor should be considered, it is important to remember that the purpose is to assess program quality and/or effectiveness (P. B. Campbell & Hill, 2013). A good evaluation is one that is useful and relevant. Evaluators need to provide findings that can impact practice and policy. To do so, they need to use designs that can answer complex evaluation questions and do not harm participants whom projects are intended to benefit (E. Johnson, Kirkhart, Madison, Noley, & Solano-Flores, 2008). Debates about what counts as credible evidence in program evaluation and applied social science research have been ongoing for at least 20 years. Archibald (2018) points out that "seemingly esoteric methodological debates about credible evidence are in fact fundamentally important political questions about life" (para. 5). He goes on to quote William Trochim (para. 6) and Michael Scriven (para. 7):

> "The gold standard debate is one of the most important controversies in contemporary evaluation and applied social sciences. It's at the heart of

how we go about trying to understand the world around us. It is integrally related to what we think science is and how it relates to practice. There is a lot at stake." (W. Trochim, unpublished speech transcript, September 10, 2007)

"This issue is not a mere academic dispute, and should be treated as one involving the welfare of very many people, not just the egos of a few." (Scriven, 2008, p. 24)

Epistemological politics (the ways in which power and privilege position some ways of knowing as "better" and hierarchically "above" other ways of knowing) are inextricably linked with ontological politics (whose reality counts, and how some reals are made to be more or less real, in practice, through various tacit or explicit power plays). (Archibald, 2018, para. 8)

Bias

Over the past several decades, transformative- and culturally responsive–minded evaluation scholars and practitioners (e.g., LaFrance, 2004; Riley, 2017; Stanfield, 1993) have debated the potential negative impact of traditionally rigorous research designs and procedures on underrepresented and marginalized groups. In addition, as covered in previous chapters, philosophers and historians of science, most famously Thomas Kuhn (1962), have challenged the underlying premise that science is or can be objective and that more rigor makes results less biased or unbiased. Kuhn concluded that "practicing in different worlds, the two groups of scientists [or, in this case, evaluators] see different things when they look from the same point in the same direction" (p. 150).

This bias is present in how questions are asked and answered. For example, if one is evaluating a program to reduce achievement gaps between more and less marginalized groups, the focus of the evaluation could be to determine if the program "fixes" the underperforming students, or it could be to determine the extent to which the program, initiative, or opportunity increases the quality of the education these students receive, which should lead to better results. The evaluation design for the latter focus will be different from and much more complex than the design for the former focus (Ladson-Billings, 2006; Liston & Peoples, 2018).

Bias can be present in areas seen to be objective or even in what the definition of being objective is. Patterson (2018a) speaks of "the tyranny of quantification," pointing out that "when data and consequently empiricism is king, rationalism has been cast out into the wilderness" (para. 3). As Krause (2018) comments, "much of what we consider to be an objective science with 'best practices' is often simply one world view among many" (para. 1). For example, the **randomized controlled trial (RCT)**, in which individuals are randomly assigned to different groups to be studied, is often held up as the most rigorous and thus the best design, but there are many times when that is not the case. Goodman, Epstein, and Sullivan (2018) argue that the RCT is actually a poor design for evaluating social service programs, such as domestic violence programs, which "provide complex, individually tailored, flexible interventions and are embedded in large highly variable public systems and community contexts" (p. 59).

Practical Considerations

A variety of ethical and practical considerations must be considered when choosing a design for an evaluation study. Even if one wanted to randomly assign participants to different interventions or conditions, it might not be possible in the case of programs that provide an array of supports to meet different people's varying needs, rather than testing one or two distinct interventions (Goodman et al., 2018). This is the case, for example, with evaluations of graduate medical education programs.

> Residents and fellows usually experience rotations at different times: those experiencing the intervention later may learn from intervening experiences and no longer be comparable to those experiencing the intervention at an earlier time. Also, trainees have the option to refuse randomization, yet they cannot miss critical educational experiences. Residency and fellowship training are usually highly individualized, which makes the [RCT] model increasingly unsuitable as training advances. (Sullivan, 2011, p. 286)

A major practical consideration in design selection is "cost (amount of money that is available for the evaluation), time (uncompensated time from stakeholders and actual time in terms of how long it will take) and burden on participants (constraints on the services they receive and/or the amount of data they have to provide)" (Braverman & Arnold, 2008, p. 75). Other practical issues those who design evaluations commonly encounter include the following:

- *The appropriateness of the fit between the design of the program or "intervention" and the requirements of more rigorous evaluation methodologies.* The timing of the evaluation also has an impact on the design to be selected. Typically, more rigorous evaluation designs require certain compromises on the part of programs in order to facilitate key facets of the evaluation design. For instance, experimental design methodologies require the use of control groups from whom program services must be steadfastly withheld. Hence, one explicit trade-off involves the rigor of the evaluation design versus denying the potential benefit of the program to some "worthy" individuals or groups. When these more rigorous methodologies are considered, a decision must be made about the relative value of pursuing higher levels of evidence of program effectiveness. Consideration must also be given to the suitability of a program (given its design) to facilitate such an evaluation. For example, consideration must be given to many factors such as whether program participants can be randomly assigned and whether there are enough participants to have a control and intervention group. Additionally, if groups have already been selected in a broadening participation project, then random assignment is not possible, and if the intervention has already begun, pretest data will be limited to that which has already been collected.
- *The balance between the level of investment in the evaluation and the level of investment in and intensity of the intervention (they should be*

roughly commensurate). It probably does not make sense to invest in an elaborate or lengthy evaluation to study the effects of a relatively light intervention such as one that exposes students to a limited set of information that is expected to help them (e.g., a one-day career fair designed to expose students from underrepresented groups to careers in science, technology, engineering, and mathematics [STEM]). Conversely, it is likely quite worthwhile to consider whether very intensive interventions applied on a large scale may warrant serious evaluations to provide information about the efficacy of the approaches and strategy being funded.

- *The level of evidence expected given the nature of the intervention.* A social work curricular or instructional intervention that makes fundamental changes to what is being taught or how instruction occurs, for instance, may be one that particularly warrants rigorous study employing methodologies suited to produce high levels of evidence. There may be many competing explanations for results, and there may be opportunity costs associated with the foregone practices. In these instances, it is important to weigh the effectiveness of those traditional practices in relation to the new practices. Other types of interventions, like ones that promote change in institutional practices tied to program goals (e.g., staffing, policies, programs and institutional commitment, accountability and rewards), may not lend themselves well to rigorous measurements, and may produce changes that can be captured in less intensive studies.

- *The strength of rival hypotheses.* A **rival hypothesis** is a competing theory that might plausibly explain an outcome. As is noted earlier, a curricular or instructional intervention enters a crowded environment, and findings might be subjected to alternate explanations for results. However, in cases where criminal justice programs involve offering substantial scholarship assistance or unique supplemental support, there may not be a strong rival hypothesis that could plausibly explain the outcome (P. B. Campbell, Stoll, & Thomas, 2009, pp. 67–68).

Funders often explicitly spell out the components such as comparison groups and variables that must be included in the evaluation. For example, a federal program on increasing diversity in biomedical fields required the following from grantees, which had significant impact on the evaluation designs selected:

- Improve undergraduate retention rates of students in programs relevant to the project

- Increase participation in mentoring activities (students and faculty) in programs relevant to the project

- Increase in number of disadvantaged/underrepresented students retained in project biomedical research-related programs

- Increase in number of student research training opportunities for students and faculty in programs relevant to the project

- Increase in number of disadvantaged/underrepresented students enrolled in project biomedical research-related programs
- Increase interinstitutional collaborations to achieve project outcomes related to research, mentorship, and faculty development (e.g., linkages with community colleges or other partner institutions, collaborations and postdocs at research-intensive partner institutions) (P. B. Campbell & Kibler, 2017)

Theoretical and Cultural Considerations

Awareness of practical issues and constraints is related to selecting the most rigorous designs in evaluation. However, there are also theoretical and cultural considerations tied to rigor that should influence decisions about design. As mentioned earlier, traditionally, evaluators and researchers have conceived **methodological rigor** in a way described by Braverman and Arnold (2008) as "a characteristic of evaluation studies that refers to the strength of the design's underlying logic and the confidence with which conclusions can be drawn. An evaluation that incorporates attention to methodological rigor will be in a better position to afford evidence and conclusions that can stand up to critical analysis" (p. 72). On their website, Beyond Rigor: Improving Evaluations With Diverse Populations (www.BeyondRigor.org), coauthor Patricia B. Campbell and Eric Jolly (n.d.a) support this view with a caveat:

> It is not enough for evaluation to be methodologically rigorous. That is necessary but not sufficient to learn about what works for different groups of people. Including different groups of people in the samples studied is a start but without having evaluation methods targeted toward the needs, issues and goals of different subgroups, the results can be incomplete and even inaccurate. (para. 1)

Whitesell et al. (2018) agree, stressing the importance of integrating knowledge of cultural context in the design and evaluation of evidence-informed programming. "Without thoughtfully attending to context," they argue, "evaluations may fail to produce valid and reliable data and conclusions even when otherwise-rigorous study designs are faithfully pursued" (p. 25).

Riley (2017) challenges these views when she argues that "rigor is used to maintain disciplinary boundaries, with exclusionary implications for marginalized groups and marginalized ways of knowing" (p. 3). Rigor, in academic contexts, she explains, "connotes adherence to the protocols of a particular discipline, especially in methods and epistemology. Work is critiqued for lacking rigor if questions are not framed in particular ways, if certain tools are not employed, certain processes not followed, and certain modes of interpretation not applied," a point with which many would agree. Rigor, she says, "is socially constituted and reflective of mainstream presumptions and social hierarchies in a specific time and place," and "rigor restricts us to certain ways of knowing, specific to a particular discipline" (p. 3).

When thinking about rigor, Riley (2017) asks people to think about "What counts as evidence? Does theory count, or logical argument? What about evidence that is not empirical? What about evidence that is empirical but qualitative in nature?" When rigor standards are developed and applied, she concludes, "a key question is who decides what the standards are and how they are applied" (p. 14). In the following activity, readers are asked to reflect on and discuss what constitutes evidence and why.

> ## Reflect and Discuss
> ### What Counts as Evidence?
>
> Which, if any, of the following would you consider evidence? In small groups, discuss why you would or would not consider each of these as such:
>
> Theory
>
> A logical argument based on the research on class size
>
> Interview transcriptions
>
> SAT scores
>
> Meeting minutes
>
> Parole officers' perceptions of their parolees' chances of reoffending

What is and isn't rigorous is often decided by those who have power and influence. These can include those involved in policy decisions or funding decisions and those considered leaders in the appropriate academic disciplines, including evaluation. Riley (2017) points out "not only that rigor is discipline specific, but also that rigor is neither static nor objective. Rather it is socially constituted and reflective of mainstream presumptions and social hierarchies in a specific time and place" (p. 3). Mainstream presumptions that, for example, controlled quantitative studies are more rigorous and therefore more valuable than longitudinal interviews or ethnographies (discussed later in this chapter) limit the ability of evaluators to choose the best design for the question. As Yin (1984) explains, there is a common misconception that designs

> should be arrayed hierarchically, that case studies were appropriate for the exploratory phase of an investigation, that surveys and histories were appropriate for the descriptive phase, and that experiments were the only way of doing explanatory or causal inquiries. . . . This hierarchical view, however, is incorrect. Experiments with an exploratory motive have certainly always existed. In addition, the development of causal explanations has long been a serious concern of historians, reflected by the subfield known as historiography. Finally, case studies are far from being only an exploratory strategy. (p. 4)

In 2016, Preskill and Lynn proposed a redefinition of rigor for evaluation that balances the following criteria:

- Quality of the Thinking: The extent to which the evaluation's design and implementation engages in deep analysis that focuses on patterns, themes, and values . . . ; seeks alternative explanations and interpretations; is grounded in the research literature; and looks for outliers that offer different perspectives.

- Credibility and Legitimacy of the Claims: The extent to which the data are trustworthy, including the confidence in the findings; the transferability of findings to other contexts; the consistency and repeatability of the findings; and the extent to which the findings are shaped by respondents, rather than evaluator bias, motivation, or interests.

- Cultural Responsiveness and Context: The extent to which the evaluation questions, methods, and analysis respect and reflect the stakeholders' values and context, their definitions of success, their experiences and perceptions, and their insights about what is happening.

- Quality and Value of the Learning Process: The extent to which the learning process engages the people who most need the information, in a way that allows for reflection, dialogue, testing assumptions, and asking new questions, directly contributing to making decisions that help improve the process and outcomes. (para. 3)

While being interviewed for this book, Katrina L. Bledsoe (personal communication, December 13, 2019), explained that

> when we are trying to understand complex systems, if we consider rigor in the traditional sense, we are going to miss too much. It allows you to be marginalized, if you don't fit the structure. There has to be another way to think about how we can bring people together, that they can be themselves and contribute to the goal. When communities hear the term *rigor*, they think of a white male patriarchal model and shut down.

She went on to say that

> rigor says to me, and I have heard this from many communities, that there is a particular structure that you must abide by and if it doesn't fit, then the process is not considered valid. The word *rigor* is a trigger for many people that makes them feel that they are not good enough. I would rather use the term *robust*. *Robust* means that there is depth to the work, that we have looked at every aspect that we possibly can, and all is represented to the degree we possibly can do it.

In her Voices From the Field interview, Donna Riley speaks about what led her to challenge traditional definitions of rigor and what her perceptions are about what rigor can and should mean.

Voices From the Field

Donna Riley: The Myth of Rigor

Rigor is focused on concepts like objectivity and control. It is based on the myth that the harder the math, the truer the results must be. I began to think about what was behind the concept of rigor when I was helping to establish the first engineering program in a women's college. We were under a lot of scrutiny about how rigorous our program would be. Our leader felt that we needed to accept that premise and respond with lots of rigor. I would have preferred an approach that would challenge the assumption that by definition an engineering program in a women's college would be lacking in rigor.

This started me thinking about how rigor is used to police who's in and who's out and what's accepted and acceptable and what's not. Rigor has been used to exclude certain populations and certain ways of knowing. We need a bigger tent. We have boxed ourselves in, based on artificial hierarchies of what are the "best" designs. When we hold a standard that has only one type of scholarship, which supports objectivity and control, we are missing out on valuable conversations that could be held across different approaches. We need a definition of scholarship that includes any kind of systematic and critical inquiry.

Donna Riley was a founding faculty member of the Picker Engineering Program at Smith College, a National Science Foundation program director, and a professor and interim head in the Department of Engineering Education at Virginia Tech. She is currently the Kamyar Haghighi Head of the School of Engineering Education at Purdue University. She was interviewed by coauthor Patricia B. Campbell in the fall of 2019.

As covered in detail in earlier chapters, unlike many fields, evaluation, as a discipline, confronts some of these presumptions and hierarchies, particularly in its work in such areas as cultural competence (American Evaluation Association, 2011) and cultural conflict of interest (Thomas & Campbell, 2017). However, there is still much to unravel about the roles that culture and social hierarchies play in determining which designs to use. As is discussed in the next section, this has implications for the use of comparison groups.

Control and Comparison Groups

Without a comparative context, it is difficult to accurately evaluate program outcomes (Glover, 2002); or, to put it in the vernacular, the role of control and comparison groups is to answer the question "Compared to what?" **Control** and **comparison groups** are groups that must be as similar as possible to the group(s) participating in that which is being evaluated. Traditionally, there has been a distinction between a control group, which does not receive any intervention, and a comparison group, which receives a different intervention. In evaluation, that distinction tends to be moot, because people in both groups are generally participating in related activities, even if the activities are minimally related. For example, in an evaluation of an after-school program, students in a comparison group would not be involved in that after-school program; however, they would be doing something after school. More frequently in evaluation, a control group is defined as a group that has been randomly assigned not to participate in a program or an intervention, while those in comparison groups are not randomly assigned (BetterEvaluation, n.d.). The following case study helps to show the value of using control or comparison groups.

Case Study
The Impact of Comparison Groups on Data Interpretation

Table 11.1 shows the results from an evaluation done by coauthor Patricia B. Campbell, who was looking at the impact of a summer math review program for entering engineering students. The outcome measure was the college math course students enrolled in based on scores on a math placement test.

Table 11.1 Math Courses in Which Participants Placed

Course	Percentage of students in each course
Math Fundamentals	30%
Intro to Math Analysis	21%
Pre-calculus	23%
Calculus	26%

(Continued)

(Continued)

Looking at these results, it is difficult to determine what they mean. See Table 11.2 for data from a comparable group of entering engineering students who didn't participate in the program.

summer program may want to place more emphasis on fundamentals of mathematics for students coming in with low math skills) and for summative evaluation purposes (i.e., the program appears to be having an

Table 11.2 Math Courses in Which Participants and Comparison Students Placed

Course	Percentage of participants in each course	Percentage of comparison participants in each course
Math Fundamentals	30%	8%
Intro to Math Analysis	21%	49%
Pre-calculus	23%	26%
Calculus	26%	13%

The second table provides significantly more information both for formative evaluation purposes (i.e., the impact on the number of students placed in Calculus) (P. B. Campbell, Price, Chubin, Carson, & Kibler, 2006).

Ethical Issues

There can be political and/or ethical challenges to generating control or comparison groups including concerns about not offering services to groups in need because of the desire to evaluate the quality and impact of the services. The American Evaluation Association (AEA) said in 2003 that random assignment

> should sometimes be ruled out for reasons of ethics. For example, assigning experimental subjects [sic] to educationally inferior or medically unproven interventions, or denying control group subjects [sic] access to important instructional opportunities or critical medical intervention, is not ethically acceptable even when [RCT] results might be enlightening. Such studies would not be approved by Institutional Review Boards overseeing the protection of human subjects [sic] in accordance with federal statute. (quoted in Patton, 2008, p. 429)

Even when there are not ethical concerns, there can be a feeling that control or comparison groups are "unfair" because they deprive some people of access to services. This concern is based on the assumption that a program or intervention has value, which, if that is the case, somewhat negates the need for the evaluation. In these cases, the evaluator can play an important role in helping program administrators and others better see the importance of evaluation because it could be unethical to expand interventions that have not yet been demonstrated to be effective, may be ineffective, and/or may even have negative effects.

Ethical Use of Control and Comparison Groups

There are several ways to deal with ethical concerns. One thing that can be done is to provide different services to the comparison group. So, for example, in a study of the effect of nutritional training on diet, the comparison group might be given training in another area such as media training. This also helps to ensure that members of comparison groups don't become disgruntled because they feel the intervention group is getting more. If comparison group members become disgruntled, they may be more apt to provide less data or even stop participating in the evaluation.

Another strategy is to give the comparison group access to services one or two years after those initially receiving the program or service. One can also include in the treatment group of participants a higher percentage of those in need than are included in the control or comparison group. For example, the group receiving services might be composed of 70% of those in need while the control or comparison group would be composed of 30% of those in need. The outcomes of treatment group participants in need would then be compared to the outcomes of comparison group participants in need. Similarly, comparisons would be done between treatment group and comparison group participants not in need.

As indicated earlier in the chapter, randomly assigning people to a control group or to a group participating in an intervention is one way of making the groups as similar as possible. While that is often possible in some types of research, it is not often feasible in evaluations that are being done in real-life settings. Using the earlier example of an after-school program, in an evaluation, it would not be possible to randomly assign children to participate in an after-school program or not. However, it could be possible to randomly assign children to the after-school program or a control group if more children applied for the program than there was space and if children were selected for the program randomly from the applicants. Even then, it would be important to check that those in the control group are similar to the after-school program participants in terms of variables that are important to the evaluation—perhaps, in this case, children's age and gender. It is also crucial to know what the children in the control group are doing after school. The following case study provides another example of different ways control and comparison groups can be used.

Case Study
Using Control and Comparison Groups

Imagine that a charity working with a group of offenders finds that only 30% of its service users have reoffended. This may seem like a good result, but in truth you can't tell whether it is or not, for two related reasons:

1. You do not know what the reoffending rate would have been without the intervention. You could look at the national reoffending rate, but this would not be comparing like with like—reoffending rates vary for different groups. Alternatively, you could use reoffending rates for more comparable groups or predicted rates, but this still does not confirm that it is the intervention that is responsible for the difference.

2. Other factors may have influenced the result. The user group may differ from the average by chance, some of them may have received another intervention, there may have been changes in police recording procedures, the local job market may have improved, or there may be other factors that have affected their chance of reoffending (e.g., it is widely known that as people get older they are less likely to offend). (NPC & Clinks, n.d.)

Looking at the reoffending rate of a comparison group with which the charity isn't working can help resolve both points.

When it is not possible or even useful to randomly assign people to comparison and intervention groups, there are ways to find non–randomly assigned comparison groups including asking participants to suggest one or more people who are like them in terms of the variables that are important to the evaluation who are not participating in that which is being evaluated. For example, participants who are starting fitness training can be asked to suggest people who are at similar levels of fitness to them but who are not in training. In another example, preschools that include hands-on science could be compared to preschools serving similar populations with similar philosophies that don't do hands-on science. The following activity provides readers with an opportunity to provide their own arguments to explain to a client why a comparison or control group should be used.

Activity
Justifying Using Control or Comparison Groups

With a partner, make a list of arguments you could use to persuade a client to include comparison groups in an evaluation of a program to decrease cigarette use.

There may be times and programs in which comparison groups are neither possible nor feasible. This can be the case where programs are designed to be responsible to varied community needs, values, strengths, and limitations or where services are substantially shaped by such factors as local politics, cultural practices, and available community resources (Goodman et al., 2018).

A great deal of data is already being collected that can be used for comparison purposes, including

- historical data—for example, data on retention rates and weight loss in diet support programs before and after implementation of a new support strategy;
- data collected by college and university institutional research offices—for example, data on those who applied and enrolled in undergraduate and graduate programs or data on alumni; and
- other existing data such as that collected by individual states or the federal government.

The biggest limitation of using existing and/or historical databases is that variables for these studies have already been established and may not include what is needed for specific evaluations.

Longitudinal Data

According to Thomas R. Bailey, "being able to follow students longitudinally is the key to any sophisticated understanding of how colleges are doing and what's happening to students" (quoted in Glenn, 2008, p. A10). While Bailey was speaking about evaluations tied to educational programs and policies, being able to track participants and others is important for evaluations in a number of other areas including those tied to workforce development, health, and criminal justice. Without longitudinal data, the generation and testing of causal models in a variety of areas is difficult, if not impossible, to achieve. While it is possible to collect longitudinal data in individual evaluations, that is costly in terms of both resources and time. Collecting longitudinal data over control or comparison groups is even more difficult.

There are, however, a number of existing longitudinal data sets. The largest and best known is the U.S. Census (www.census.gov/data.html). The Census Bureau collects longitudinal data in a variety of areas, including population demographics, the economy, employment, education, business, health, housing, family and living arrangements, and income and poverty. The Census Bureau also collects and uses data from a number of other federal and state sources. While summary data are available to all, researchers and evaluators can submit proposals to the Census Bureau to request specific data sets. As the web page "How do I access and use data?" (www.census.gov/about/adrm/linkage/guidance.html) indicates, the proposal needs to include the project's methodology and objectives, anticipated output, and data sets required.

In the following activity, readers learn some ways to access and use U.S. Census Bureau data.

Activity
Using U.S. Census Bureau Data

Go to "How do I access and use data?" at www.census.gov/about/adrm/linkage/guidance.html. Then, using Census Bureau data, find some communities that are similar to Newark, New Jersey, in terms of race/ethnicity and socioeconomic status that could be used as comparison sites for an evaluation of a community development effort being done in the city of Newark.

There are more specialized databases that evaluators can access as well. For example, the National Center for Education Statistics (NCES) provides longitudinal data in a variety of areas, including the academic performance of the nation's students, adult literacy, the condition of public schools, libraries, and postsecondary education (see https://nces.ed.gov/). The National Science Foundation (NSF) has several sources of longitudinal data, many of which can be accessed through the National Center for Science and Engineering Statistics (NCSES) (www.nsf.gov/statistics/data.cfm). These include longitudinal data on business, federal, state, and higher education research and development and survey data from college graduates, graduate students, and doctoral recipients. They also have a "table tool," which allows researchers and evaluators to develop their own data tables (https://ncsesdata.nsf.gov/ids/). A data source that is of particular value to those evaluating projects and interventions tied to broadening participation in STEM is "Women, Minorities, and Persons with Disabilities in S&E" (www.nsf.gov/statistics/women/). Other data sets include the U.S. Department of Justice Open Data Inventory Program (www.justice.gov/open/open-data#s1) and the U.S. Department of Health and Human Services Health Data Sets (www.hhs.gov/about/agencies/omha/about/health-data-sets/index.html).

Whatever data sets are used, it is important to determine the sample over which the data were collected and the degree to which that sample is representative of the group that is receiving the services being evaluated. For example, if an evaluation is being done of a program to reduce homelessness and the comparison data are annual city homeless counts, it will be important to check out the methodology that was used for the counts to determine if the group counted is similar to the group receiving services.

For other data sets, it is important to check for response rates and **response bias**, which occurs when those who agree to respond to a survey or participate in another data collection effort are different from those who don't respond or don't agree. For example, because of concerns about personal or family member immigration status, surveys that ask for citizenship status may have a different set of nonrespondents than surveys that don't ask that question.

The following activity provides readers with an opportunity to determine appropriate comparison groups.

Activity
Selecting Comparison Data

Select what you feel would be appropriate comparison groups for each of the following evaluations and explain why you made that choice. If your comparison group is from an existing data set, please describe the data set you would use. If you feel there is no need for a comparison or control group, please explain why.

An evaluation of a program to reduce recidivism among parolees convicted of nonviolent crimes

An evaluation of program to increase preschoolers' academic success in elementary school

An evaluation of a rural economic development program in terms of increases in employment

Evaluation Designs

The following, adapted from P. B. Campbell and colleagues (2009) and D. T. Campbell and Stanley (1963), is a discussion of the major evaluation design options that may be appropriate for different types of programs. The strengths and weaknesses of each type of evaluation design, along with the feasibility of its successful implementation, are provided, including factors that may enable or inhibit the successful application of the evaluation approach. As was covered in Chapter 9, it is important to note that for any evaluation, a planning process that integrates program and evaluation designs is important, and serious consideration should be given to planning and initiating programs/projects and evaluations simultaneously.

Experimental Designs

Optimally, a summative evaluation captures outcomes and links them to an intervention in a manner that establishes a **causal relationship**. When this is done well, it is possible to draw conclusions about a program's impact. This is done by separating out or "isolating" the effects of a particular intervention. However, as indicated earlier, this is not always possible or even appropriate. **Experimental designs** can offer the most promise for establishing causal relationships, where the occurrence of something such as the intervention causes something else, such as cessation of smoking, to happen. However, experimental designs can leave out some important pieces tied to context. It is often assumed that experimental designs need to be quantitative. This is not the case. Qualitative data, including interviews and observations, can be collected under experimental designs as well.

As discussed earlier in the chapter, the experimental design that is seemingly most commonly discussed is the randomized controlled trial, or RCT. This approach can be summarized in the following manner:

$$R \quad O \quad X \quad O$$
$$R \quad O \quad \quad O$$

R denotes random assignment; *O* denotes the measures used; and *X* denotes participation in a program, a project, or activities/interventions within a program or project. Taken together, the symbols reflect that members of a group are randomly assigned to two groups; one of these groups participates in an intervention while the other does not, and pretest/posttest data are collected over both groups.

This evaluation design offers numerous methodological strengths that are valued by many evaluation stakeholders. Most notably, if implemented effectively, it rules out numerous rival hypotheses that could otherwise be seen as plausible causes of an outcome. It does so by demonstrating the difference between the performance on an outcome or other measure of a group participating in an intervention or activity and the performance of a comparable group not participating. The random assignment procedure is generally seen as the best way to construct a truly comparable group for comparison purposes. However, if the groups are relatively small, random assignment can lead to important differences in the composition of the groups. Theoretically, if the groups were perfectly comparable, the only difference observed would be due to the intervention.

While it's not statistically likely, it is possible to randomly divide a group that is half women and half men into two groups, one of which is predominantly female and the other of which is predominantly male. If there are variables that may confound the evaluation results—for example, previous experience in the area—then it might be necessary to do stratified or matched random assignment where the random selection is done within the important variables so comparison and intervention groups are similar in terms of such variables as levels of previous experience in the area.

To explore the application of this and other designs to evaluations, we use the following prototype of a program for middle school students developed by the Harlem Children's Zone (https://hcz.org). The goal of the out-of-school program is to get students to successfully transition to college. It seeks to support students in several areas of growth—foremost their academic growth—with tutoring, help with homework, and standardized test preparation. Students are expected to participate in gender-specific discussion groups aimed at fostering their social and emotional development, to do community service, and to participate in enrichment programs. There are workshops to help parents better understand the particular academic and social-emotional challenges faced by middle school youth, how to help their children confront these challenges, and what to expect when their children go to high school.

If this program is implemented in one or more communities and such communities are interested in participating in an experiment, it seems plausible to consider an experimental design. For instance, in one or more middle schools, students could be randomly assigned to intervention and control groups, or the schools themselves could be assigned to intervention or comparison groups. The intervention students would participate in the program along with being in middle school, while the control group would be in middle school without the program.

Feasibility of Implementation

Many conditions would have to be in place to facilitate successful implementation of this type of experimental design. In the example provided, the participating communities would have to place value in the lessons learned from studying this broadening participation strategy. The funding agency would need to devote considerable resources and make a sustained commitment to an expensive evaluation approach and to the program strategy. The intervention would have to be thoroughly implemented and applied only to the intervention group, and the intervention could not spill over to the control group. In practical terms, in our example, this would mean teachers and others in the community would have to be careful not to offer those services to comparison group students. In addition, a commitment on the part of all stakeholders would be needed to ensure the collection of quality longitudinal data. As will be discussed in Chapter 13, group sizes sufficiently robust to support the analyses would be necessary for the evaluation to be carried out, and comparison and intervention group response rates would need to remain high over the duration of a longitudinal project.

Another issue with random assignment, raised earlier, concerns providing services to some and not to others. The **delayed treatment design**, described as follows, addresses that issue. As with the earlier design, participants are randomly assigned to groups, and the same pre- and posttest data are collected from them. At that point, members of the control group become participants, and after their participation, additional data are collected.

$$R \quad O \quad X \quad O$$
$$R \quad O \quad \quad\quad O \quad X \quad O$$

While it is easy to envision many of these conditions being hard to meet, as the following case study indicates, it can be done.

Case Study
Opening Doors

In Opening Doors, MDRC worked with community colleges in several states to design and implement new types of financial aid, enhanced student services, and curricular and instructional innovations, with the goal of helping low-income students earn college credentials as the pathway to better jobs and further education. The evaluation used a random assignment design in which the experiences of students who received the Opening Doors interventions were compared with those of students who received existing services. The study tracked students for at least two years and measured the effects of Opening Doors on outcomes such as continued enrollment in college, academic performance, credential attainment, labor market success, and measures of individual well-being (MDRC, n.d.).

While these designs can control for a number of factors, one they don't control for is pretest effect. **Pretest effect** occurs when taking the initial measures has an impact on how participants respond to the intervention and/or how participants and control group members respond to the posttest measures. For example, if a pretest is a vocabulary test, those taking it might become interested in learning about words they didn't know from the pretest, which could impact their scores on the posttest.

There are several variations of the basic experimental design that control for the pretest effect. In the first variation, a posttest design using random assignment, participants don't take the pretest measures, which means there can be no pretest effect.

$$R \quad X \quad O$$
$$R \quad \quad O$$

However, it also means that it is not possible to determine if the groups were comparable originally; nor is it possible to determine the amount of change. Theoretically, if the participants were randomly selected from the same population, they are presumed initially equivalent.

A second variation, called the **Solomon four-group design**, controls for the pretest effect by adding two more groups, one intervention group and one control group, whose members don't take the pretest measures.

$$R \quad O \quad X \quad O$$
$$R \quad O \quad \quad O$$
$$R \quad \quad X \quad O$$
$$R \quad \quad \quad O$$

This allows the evaluators both to look at the pretest effect and to look at change. However, this adds a significant amount of complexity and cost to the design.

Quasi-experimental Designs

Quasi-experimental designs offer another set of methodological approaches for summative evaluations seeking to link outcomes to interventions. When these designs are executed effectively, they provide strong information about program effects. The difference between experimental and quasi-experimental designs is that experimental designs have control groups into which members are randomly assigned and quasi-experimental designs have comparison groups whose members are not randomly assigned.

The pretest/posttest version of quasi-experimental designs can be summarized as follows:

$$O \quad X \quad O$$
$$O \quad \quad O$$

O denotes the measures, and *X* denotes the participation in a program, a project, or activities/interventions within a program or project. The symbols reflect that pretest and posttest data are collected over both groups while only the participants are involved in the intervention.

Like experimental designs, quasi-experimental designs, if executed well, can provide evidence of program effects through comparisons of performance on outcome measures between a group exposed to an intervention and a comparison group that has not been exposed to the intervention. The logic underlying quasi-experimental and experimental design approaches is essentially the same. The strength of the quasi-experimental approach, in many ways, depends on the extent to which the comparison group is comparable to the participants. It is generally difficult to construct comparison groups that are well matched to the treatment group, and certain characteristics such as a self-selection bias may not be controlled for. Self-selection bias occurs because participants have chosen to participate while people in the comparison group have not chosen to participate. This can indicate a difference between the groups. Chapter 13 covers some ways some group differences can be controlled statistically.

An advantage of a quasi-experimental design, when contrasted with experimental designs, is that it is much less intrusive. People are not assigned to participate or to be in the comparison group, and it is possible to employ quasi-experimental methodologies without denying people support and services. Quasi-experimental designs are often used when programs are already underway prior to the start of the evaluation. They can offer a reasonable alternative when random assignment is not feasible or even possible.

This evaluation design might be applied to the Harlem Children's Zone program if the intervention were made available to students in one or more communities and not to others. For this to have a chance of providing useful information, the intervention and comparison groups would need to be comparable based on characteristics important to the evaluation such as socioeconomic status, school quality, and crime rates. Similarly, students in the intervention and comparison groups would need to be comparable in terms of variables important to the evaluation such as grades, test scores, general health, and educational aspirations. With comparable communities and students, differences between the two groups on outcome measures and indicators would be expected to be tied to the intervention.

Feasibility of Implementation

This methodology makes a serious attempt to isolate the effects of the program and thereby address rival hypotheses, other possible explanations for the outcome. In the example provided earlier, since the students were in different communities, the possibility of the intervention spilling over to the comparison group would be relatively small. However, there could be outside factors that affected one community but not another that could impact the results and would need to be documented and accounted for to the degree possible.

Quasi-experimental designs, like experimental designs, are well suited to situations where funding agencies and program operators and participants are committed to study the effectiveness of a strategy. The program and evaluation would have to be well resourced, and a high level of sustained commitment on the part of all evaluation stakeholders would be required.

A variation on this design is posttest-only intact group design in which no pretest data are collected from participants and comparison group members and their results are compared.

$$X \quad O$$
$$O$$

This design can be useful if there is some indication that the groups are comparable and if the posttest or outcome data are actions, like going to college or getting a job, where there is not an appropriate pretest measure.

A related, but not widely used, design is **regression-discontinuity (RD)**, in its simplest form

> a pretest-posttest program-comparison group strategy. The unique characteristic which sets RD designs apart from other pre-post group designs is the method by which participants are assigned to conditions. In RD designs, participants are assigned to program or comparison groups solely on the basis of a cutoff score on a pre-program measure. (Trochim, 2008, para. 2)

So if, for example, the impact of a gifted and talented program was being evaluated, and teachers were asked to rate students' eligibility for the program on a scale of 1 (*low*) to 10 (*high*), and it was decided that only those with a mean rating of 7 or higher would be in the program, those who scored between 6 and 6.9 would be the comparison group for participants who scored between 7 and 7.9. The assumption is that the groups are approximately equal. RD designs can be useful "when we wish to target a program or treatment to those who most need or deserve it" (Trochim, 2008, para. 2). This approach can be summarized in the following manner:

$$C+ \quad O \quad X \quad O$$
$$C- \quad O \quad \quad O$$

C denotes assignment by cutoff score, with *C+* being those who scored just above it and *C−* those just below; *O* denotes measures; and *X* denotes participation in a program, a project, or activities within a program or project. A "common implementation has been in compensatory education evaluation where school children who obtain scores which fall below some predetermined cutoff value on an achievement test are assigned to remedial training designed to improve their performance" (Trochim, 2008, para. 3).

Pretest/Posttest Designs

Under this approach, changes are tracked by comparing participants' performance on an outcome measure prior to their participation in an intervention and again after their participation. This design can be summarized as follows:

$$O \quad X \quad O$$

O symbolizes the measures, and *X* denotes participation in a program, a project, or activities/interventions within a program or project. Taken together, the symbols reflect that members of a group participate in an intervention and pretest and posttest data are collected from them.

This methodological approach does not address rival hypotheses. That is, it does not attempt to isolate the effects of the intervention, which is a limitation because it is always possible that something other than the intervention is causing any change detected on outcome measures. However, the approach does offer the promise of being able to capture whether change on an outcome measure has occurred. Applied to our prototypical program, one could look for change in such areas as student grades, student interest in going to college, or parent strategies for dealing with teenage behavior.

A key consideration when deciding on the appropriateness of this approach pertains to the need to deal with rival hypotheses. Pretest/posttest designs do not establish causality. In some situations, other summative information about outcomes, such as the number/percentage of students going to college or the number/percentage of parolees who don't violate their parole, may suffice and prove quite useful. Pretest/posttest designs do not interfere with the program operations (i.e., no one has to be denied participation). Because this design only involves participants, it takes fewer resources and is easier logistically, making it more feasible to conduct such evaluations across a larger set of projects or even an entire program initiative.

Feasibility of Implementation

A pretest/posttest design can be employed most easily when a project or an intervention is starting up. However, it can also be used for efforts that are already underway, assuming that data from participants before their involvement in the intervention are available or can be constructed. The pretest/posttest design will not be the first choice for evaluation stakeholders interested in establishing whether or not a strategy is effective. That said, for some programs, where there is not an array of plausible competing explanations, it may provide enough evidence of program effectiveness to be compelling to stakeholders and decision makers. It offers an option for studying whether desired outcomes are occurring and an approach that can be applied on a larger scale than is practical for more complex evaluation approaches.

A variation on this design is a **time-series design** where data are collected at several points prior to participation in the program and at several points after. Taking multiple measurements is essential for understanding how any given behavior unfolds over time, and doing so at equal intervals affords a clear investigation of how the dynamics of that behavior manifest at different times (Swanson, 2016).

$$O_1 \quad O_2 \quad O_3 \quad O_4 \quad X \quad O_5 \quad O_6 \quad O_7 \quad O_8$$

Retrospective Pretest Designs

The **retrospective pretest design (RPT)** can be a useful approach to collecting self-reported changes in knowledge, skills, intentions, behaviors, and attitudes of participants. In these designs, data are collected once at the end of the project. At that time, individuals are asked to assess their current level of knowledge/attitudes/skills/intentions *after* experiencing the intervention and to reflect on their previous level of knowledge/attitudes/skills/intentions *before* experiencing the broadening participation intervention.

$$X \quad O_{\text{retrospective pretest}} \quad O_{\text{posttest}}$$

This design is most useful when the results will be used in conjunction with other data. This relatively underutilized design is particularly useful when time or access constraints allow the evaluator only a single opportunity to gather data from participants. A traditional pretest is administered before the program and again at the end of the program (posttest) with the notion that intervention effects are demonstrated by differences in the two measures. However, in some evaluations, use of the traditional pretest/posttest approach (with two data collection points) is not feasible and prohibitively expensive. In such situations, the retrospective pretest design (RPT) is a good alternative and is a viable option to estimate pretest/posttest change (Moore & Tananis, 2009).

The design can be more robust if the retrospective pretest is given at a different time than the posttest—or at least in different parts of the questionnaire, which, if done electronically, could prevent editing of initial responses (Taylor, Russ-Eft, & Taylor, 2009). The design provides information about the intervention not available in posttest-only measures, and it is a fairly common practice in some areas of program evaluation such as evaluations of short-term intensive interventions (Moore & Tananis, 2009). Further, this design permits participants an opportunity to reflect on how much they have changed as a function of their work in the intervention. For example, in our prototype example, this design offers the opportunity to assess self-reported changes in students' attitudes toward going to college or in parents' perceptions of the efficacy of their interactions with their teenagers.

Feasibility of Implementation

This design clearly challenges traditional methodological logic, since both pretest data and posttest data are collected *after* the intervention has taken place. The design is simple, reduces the costs and time required for data collection, and is well suited to evaluations interested in assessing changes on a range of cognitive, attitudinal, and skill-based variables in instances when the intervention has already begun before the evaluation begins, thereby eliminating the possibility of collecting baseline data.

A major drawback of this design is that it does not address rival hypotheses. Similar to the traditional one-group pretest/posttest design, this design will not allow the evaluator to assess causality since it does not include a group that did not receive the intervention. Another limitation to the retrospective design is the recall period. For example, asking people to reflect back to the time prior to their participation can pose problems in terms of how accurately they can remember over time, with certain groups (e.g., elementary school–aged children) likely having more difficulty in accurately recalling pre-intervention knowledge, attitudes, behaviors, and skills than others. A final limitation is that in this design data are only collected over those who complete the intervention or remain in the program, possibly skewing the results.

As the following case study indicates, it is possible for the design to change over the project period.

Case Study
An Accidental Design

Coauthor Patricia B. Campbell was designing an evaluation for a multisite program for adults who had dropped out of high school and wanted to get a GED (general equivalency diploma). The program model consisted of three components: (a) instruction, (b) social supports and career exploration, and (c) the inclusion of six youth development principles. The measure was scored on a GED-preparedness test. The design was a pretest/posttest design with all sites implementing the complete model.

$$O\ X_{a,b,c}\ O$$

However, while all sites implemented (a), some implemented (a) and (b), others (a) and (c), and others the complete model. The design became more complicated:

$$O\ X_{a,b,c}\ O$$
$$O\ X_{a,b}\ O$$
$$O\ X_{a,c}\ O$$

(Continued)

(Continued)

And then later on in the project all the sites began implementing all three components, which meant there were components of the design as follows:

$$O \; X_{a,b,c} \; O \qquad\qquad O$$
$$O \; X_{a,b} \; O \; X_{a,b,c} \; O$$
$$O \; X_{a,c} \; O \; X_{a,b,c} \; O$$

While the analysis became a lot more complicated, the different levels of implementation meant that it was possible to look at the effectiveness of the model and its components. The results indicated that the full model was very effective while implementing only two of the three components was much less so.

Case Studies/Ethnography

A **case study** can be defined as an up-close, in-depth, and detailed examination of a subject of study, over time, and its related contextual conditions (Wikipedia, 2020b). Case studies should be done when "you deliberately wanted to cover contextual conditions—believing that they might be highly pertinent to your phenomenon of study" (Yin, 1984, p 13). Case studies can and often do include both qualitative and quantitative methods. Indeed, Stake (2005) feels that a case study is defined by "interest in the individual case, not by the methods of inquiry used" (p. 443). A case study can—and many say should—include such factors as triangulation of data in order to address issues of validity, reliability, and objectivity (Stake, 2005). However, some scholars disagree. For example, White, Drew, and Hay (2009) regarded "Stake's assessment of case study research as primarily situated in a post positivist tradition" (p. 20) that did not match well with feminist and **postmodern** views of case studies. They view a case study design as one that

- allows you to gather rich, detailed data in an authentic setting;
- is holistic and thus supports the idea that much of what we can know about human behavior is best understood as lived experience in the social context; [and]
- can be done without predetermined hypotheses and goals. (Willis, 2007, p. 240, quoted in White et al., 2009, p. 21)

In the Harlem Children's Zone example described earlier, a case study might be used to follow the members of a particular family as they participate in the various aspects of the project being evaluated, documenting changes in family dynamics, interactions, and behaviors. As seen in the following case study, case studies can have long-ranging impacts.

Case Study
An Exemplary Example

Street Corner Society (1943, 1955) by William F. Whyte has, for decades, been recommended reading in community sociology. The book is a classic example of a descriptive case study. Thus, it traces the sequence

> of interpersonal events over time, describes a subculture that had rarely been the topic of previous study, and discovers key phenomena—such as the career advancement of lower-income youths and their ability (or inability) to break neighborhood ties. The study has been highly regarded despite its being a single-case study covering one neighborhood ("Cornerville") and a time period now more than 50 years old. The value of the book is, paradoxically, its generalizability to issues on individual performance, group structure, and the social structure of neighborhoods. Later investigators have repeatedly found remnants of Cornerville in their work, even though they have studied different neighborhoods and different time periods. (Yin, 1984, p. 4)

Feasibility of Implementation

Case studies may provide detailed, complex, comprehensive data over time that are difficult to obtain under other designs; however, they have limited generalizability. Good case studies are very difficult to do. As Yin (1984) commented,

> The problem is that we have little way of screening or testing for an investigator's ability to do good case studies. People know when they cannot play music; they also know when they cannot do mathematics; and they can be tested for other skills, such as by the bar examination in law. Somehow, the skills for doing good case studies have not yet been defined, and as a result, most people feel that they can prepare a case study, and nearly all of us believe we can understand one. (p. 11)

There is some question as to whether ethnography is a form of a case study. White et al. (2009) feel that

> in the development of our project, the terms "case study" and "ethnography" were used interchangeably and the team discussed the strategic use of one term over the other at different times. In the funding and ethics applications there is little mention of ethnography and much mention of a case study approach. (p. 5)

Sociologists define **ethnography** as "a sociological method that explores how people live and make sense of their lives with one another in particular places. The focus might be on people and the meaning they produce through everyday interactions, or places, and the organizational logics that guide our activities" (Columbia University Department of Sociology, 2020, para. 3), which is reflective of the earlier definitions of case studies. However, while a variety of qualitative and quantitative data can be collected in case studies, ethnography most commonly collects data through participant observation where the ethnographer becomes immersed in the culture as an active participant and records extensive field notes. While in a traditional observation the observer stays in the background, being as unobtrusive as possible, a participant observer is actively involved. If the participants lift weights, take a test, dance, fix a car, or whatever, the participant observer does it too. These researchers experience the program and the context firsthand. When cultural anthropologists conduct ethnographies, it can take them years. Evaluators usually serve as participant observers for only a few weeks or even days. Ethnography provides very rich data but is time consuming, and since evaluators doing ethnography experience the program and context themselves, they need to be able to be very clear about their biases and perceptions and how they may be impacting their participation and observations.

Rival Hypotheses and Threats to Validity

In 1963, in their classic work "Experimental and Quasi-experimental Designs for Research," Donald T. Campbell and Julian C. Stanley summarized some of the basic **threats to validity** of the data collected and conclusions drawn. They grouped those threats as threats to two different types of validity, internal and external:

> **Internal validity** is the basic minimum without which any experiment is uninterpretable: Did in fact the experimental treatments make a difference in this specific experimental instance? **External validity** asks the question of generalizability: To what populations, settings, treatment variables, and measurement variables can this effect be generalized? (Campbell & Stanley, 1963, p. 5)

As will be seen as follows, some of their threats can be controlled or eliminated by the design selected for the evaluation. Threats to validity must be viewed within a cultural context—one that in today's world is very different from that of 1963. For example, Nelson-Barber, LaFrance, Trumbull, and Aburto (2005) argue that potential threats to validity are magnified in situations where evaluators are not members of the community they are working in. Too, while Kuhn (1984) was speaking about historians, his comments hold for evaluators as well:

> Historians must approach the generation that held them as the anthropologist approaches an alien culture. They must, that is, be prepared at the start to find that [those of that culture] speak a different language and map experience into different categories from those they themselves bring from home. And they must take as their object the discovery of those categories and the assimilation of the corresponding language. (p. 246)

The following is a summary of threats that are directly tied to design choice, adapted from D. T. Campbell and Stanley (1963).

- *Maturation:* This is a particular problem when evaluations are being done on interventions with children or young people. Over the period of a year or more, one would expect to see changes in participants regardless of whether or not they were in an intervention. This is particularly serious when the evaluation is being done with young children—children change very quickly. Control or comparison groups can help control for maturation.

- *Testing:* As indicated earlier, taking a pretest or other pre-assessments can influence participant response on a posttest. The Solomon four-group design, the posttest-only design, and the retrospective pretest or "then-post" design can control for the impact of testing on the results.

- *Selection:* Differences in the characteristics of participants and those in the control/comparison group can impact the validity of the evaluation.

Random assignment or stratified random assignment can help with this, if the numbers in the groups are large enough. Even if random assignment is used, it is important to check to make sure there is comparability between participants and control or comparison group members on variables that are important to the evaluation.

- *History:* Events, other than the intervention, influence results. Comparison groups can help reduce the impact of history; however, being aware of and documenting events outside of the intervention can be important.

The Best Design for the Question

Table 11.3 provides a summary of the designs described in this chapter, as well as other popular research designs, and their strengths and weaknesses. When making choices as to the design to use, it is important to keep in mind Whitesell's (2018) thought that rigor should be defined both by the integrity of the data and its value in answering meaningful questions.

Table 11.3 The Best Design for the Question

Design Type	Design	Representation1	Strengths and Weaknesses
Experimental	Pretest/posttest design with random assignment	R O X O R O O	R can increase comparability of the groups. Allows for analysis of changes in outcome measures across groups. Does not control for pretest effect.
Experimental	Solomon four-group design	R O X O R O O R X O R O	R can increase comparability of the groups. Allows for analysis of changes in outcome measures across groups. Controls for pretest effect.
Experimental	Posttest design with random assignment	R X O R O	R can increase comparability of the groups. Does not allow change to be measured.
Experimental	Delayed treatment design	R O X O R O O X O	R can increase comparability of the groups. Allows for analysis of changes in outcome measures across groups. Provides services to all involved. Does not control for pretest effect.
Quasi-experimental	Pretest/posttest intact group design	O X O O O	Allows for analysis of changes in outcome measures across groups. Does not control for pretest effect. Groups may not be comparable.
Quasi-experimental	Posttest-only group design	X O O	Allows for analysis of outcome measures across groups. Does not allow for analysis of changes. Groups may not be comparable.
Quasi-experimental	Regression-discontinuity	C+ O X O C− O O	Allows for analysis of changes in outcome measures across groups. Does not control for pretest effect. Appropriate when one wants to target a program or treatment to those who most need or deserve it.

(Continued)

Table 11.3 (Continued)

Pretest/posttest	Retrospective pretest or "then-post" design[2]	X $O_{\text{retrospective pretest}}$ O_{posttest}	Allows for analysis of perceived changes in outcome measures. Does not control for rival hypotheses.
Pretest/posttest	One-shot pretest–posttest design	O X O	Allows for analysis of changes in outcome measures. Does not control for rival hypotheses.
Pretest/posttest	Time-series design	O_1 O_2 O_3 O_4 X O_5 O_6 O_7 O_8	Examines change over time. Does not control for rival hypotheses.
Case study	Case study exploration of a case (or multiple cases) over time	N/A	Provides in-depth knowledge including a focus on context. Has limited generalizability.
Mixed methods	Use of more than one of the above designs	N/A	Weaknesses of any single design are minimized.

[1] X = intervention/treatment; O = measure/effects; R = random assignment. C = cutoff score assignment.

[2] There is disagreement among evaluators as to whether this design is a quasi-experimental study.

Source: Adapted from D. Campbell & Stanley, 1963; P. B. Campbell, 2008; Ingersoll, 1982.

The following activity can help readers apply what they have been learning about designs to real-life evaluations.

Activity
Choosing Designs

Earlier in the chapter, an example was given of two possible focuses for an evaluation of a program to reduce achievement gaps between more and less marginalized groups. The first focus of the evaluation was to determine the impact of the program on achievement gaps between groups of students while the second focus was to determine if the program increased the quality of the education these students received, which should lead to better results. Choose an evaluation design for the first and second focus and justify your choices.

While being interviewed for this book, Donna Riley (personal communication, November 4, 2019) gave readers some advice to consider when choosing an evaluation design:

> When choosing a design, we should ask what is being missed. If I chose this method, not that, what stories aren't I going to tell? If there is an opportunity to tell a more complete story, then I want to. However, a more complete story doesn't come without resources. Being able to say what is being lost by choosing to do one method rather than one or more others can help evaluators chose the design(s) they want to use and justify their choice to the client.

SUMMARY

Selecting the "right design for the question" was at the core of this chapter. Readers should now be able to select an appropriate design for different questions and provide a solid rationale for their choice, including the role that their definitions of rigor, comparison groups, and the availability of longitudinal data played in their decision.

SUPPLEMENTAL RESOURCES

"How to Solve U.S. Social Problems When Most Rigorous Program Evaluations Find Disappointing Effects"

https://www.straighttalkonevidence.org/2018/03/21/how-to-solve-u-s-social-problems-when-most-rigorous-program-evaluations-find-disappointing-effects-part-one-in-a-series/

This series, *Straight Talk on Evidence*, does just that—providing information on challenges of making evaluation rigorous and useful.

Research Methods Knowledge Base: Design

www.socialresearchmethods.net/kb/design.php

This short, but comprehensive, online overview of quantitative designs covers the following areas:

- Introduction to design
- Types of designs
- Experimental design
- Quasi-experimental design
- Relationships among pre–post designs
- Designing designs for research
- Advances in quasi-experimentation

Research Ready: Qualitative Approaches

https://cirt.gcu.edu/research/developmentresources/research_ready/qualitative/approaches

This module from the Center for Innovation in Research and Teaching at Grand Canyon University describes the most common types of qualitative research approaches—narrative, phenomenology, grounded theory, ethnography, and case study—and discusses how to select an appropriate approach.

StudentTracker for Outreach

www.studentclearinghouse.org/colleges/studenttracker-for-outreach/

This resource for tracking students from the National Student Clearinghouse covers areas such as participants' college enrollment, retention, degree attainment, and major.

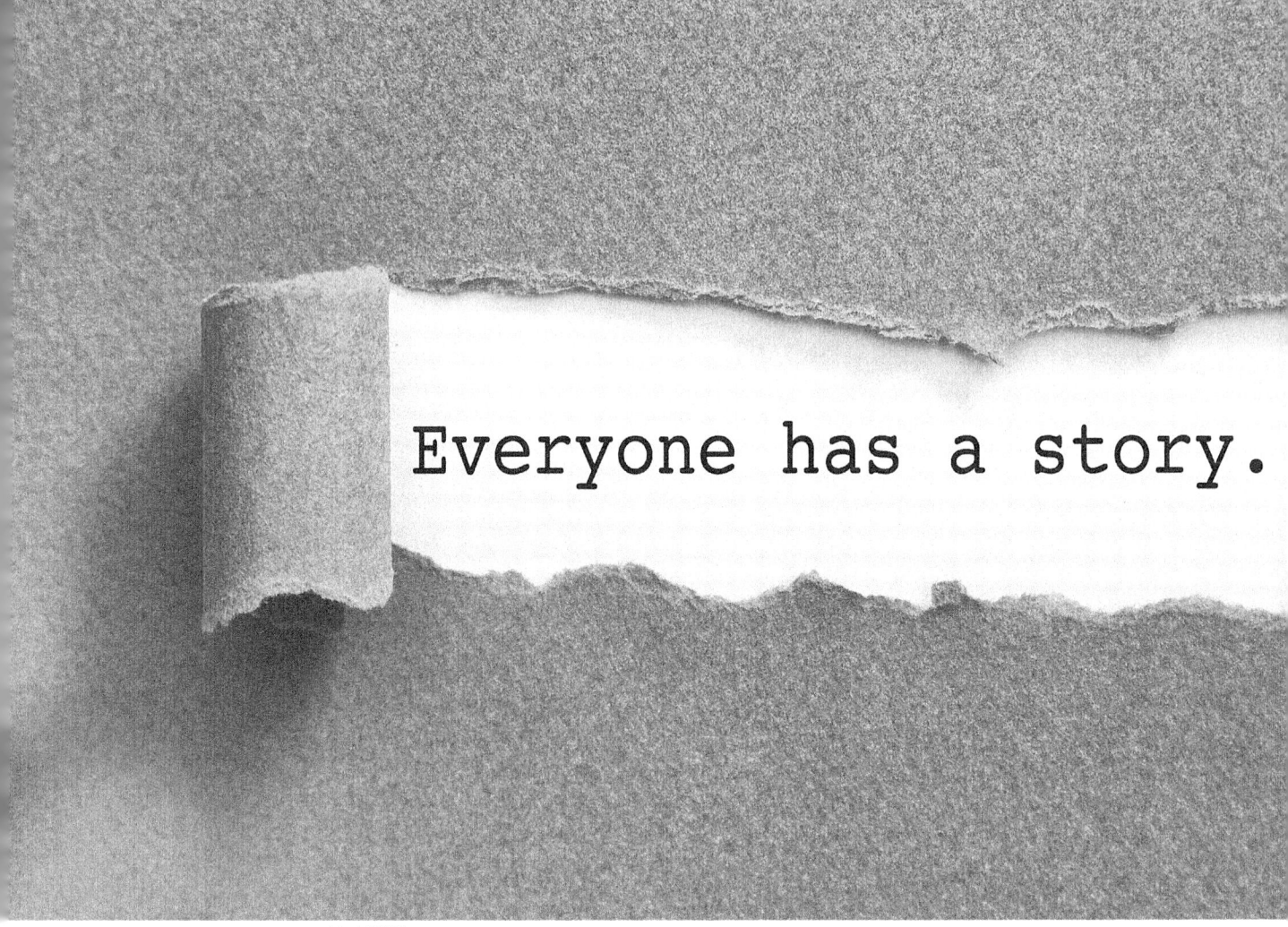
Istock/1001Love

Hearing the voices of those who haven't been heard and learning about their experiences from their perspective can have a big impact on the data to be collected and on the data itself

CHAPTER 12

Defining, Collecting, and Managing Data

The information technology world has an expression: Garbage In, Garbage Out (GIGO). It means that no matter how accurate a program's logic is, the results will be incorrect if the input is invalid. GIGO is true in evaluation as well. Our questions may be on target, our designs strong, and our analysis plan outstanding, but if the data we collect are inaccurate, culturally inappropriate, or incomplete, the results will be wrong. The goal of this chapter is to ensure that the data evaluators collect are as accurate and complete as possible.

After reading this chapter and participating in the activities, readers will be able to meet the following learning objectives:

- Know the strengths and weaknesses of different types of data and of different ways to collect data
- Discuss how cultural differences and inequalities can impact data and data collection
- Describe different types of reliability and validity and how to assess the reliability and validity of different measures for use with different populations
- Describe the basic principles of institutional review boards and their role in the protection of human participants
- Discuss major issues to be considered in managing data

Introduction

This chapter focuses on data—definitions of data, sources of data, data collection and management, and ways to ensure that the right data are collected. Collecting and managing accurate and appropriate data contributes to the soundness of evaluation findings and the usefulness of the evaluation to stakeholders. Along with examining strategies for the collection and management of quantitative and qualitative data, the chapter highlights the advantages and pitfalls of using existing measures versus adapting and/or developing measures for data collection. It also covers the measurement concepts of reliability and validity and, most importantly, the protection of human participants in data collection.

Qualitative and Quantitative Data

Merriam-Webster (2020a, para. 1) defines data as "factual information (such as measurements or statistics) that are used as a basis for reasoning, discussion, or calculation." As will be covered in greater detail in Chapter 13, there are two major types of data, qualitative and quantitative. Basically, qualitative data are words, and quantitative data are numbers. For example, participant ratings of the usefulness of a workshop on a scale of 1 (*not at all useful*) to 10 (*extremely useful*) are quantitative data, while participant descriptions of how useful the workshop was are qualitative data.

Sources of Qualitative Data

There are a variety of sources of qualitative data, including data that already exist and data that will be collected during the evaluation period. Existing data can include project reports, meeting minutes, websites, newspaper articles, video, or basically anything that is already there and available. Qualitative data that are collected as part of the project may include interviews, focus groups, observations, and video feedback as well as project or program documentation and participant written responses. Written responses can be collected as open-ended questions that are part of a survey or other measure or as part of journal entries or other stand-alone writing efforts. Regardless of how the data are collected, it is important to determine if there are potential barriers to the understanding of the data by observers, interviewers, focus group facilitators, coders, or reviewers. Whenever possible, the data collector should be fluent in the language(s) of the participants. If that isn't possible, translators will need to be used. When working with deaf populations, it is important to know the communication mode that is used, such as American Sign Language (ASL), another sign language, an assistive listening device, and/or lipreading and speech.

The following is an overview of qualitative data collection methods. Ways of analyzing the resulting data are covered in Chapter 13.

Interviews

Interviews are structured or semistructured conversations between two people, one of whom is the interviewer and the other the interviewee. The interviewer generally has a series of questions—an interview protocol—to ask, often with follow-up prompts to encourage the interviewee to speak more about a topic. Follow-up questions can be asked to clarify interviewee responses or to expand on unexpected responses. Interviews should be recorded, if permission is given, and/or extensive notes should be taken. For complex interviews or when responses may be misinterpreted, it can be useful to transcribe the interviews.

Whether the interview is in person or by phone or video, the interviewer needs to put some effort into establishing some rapport with the interviewee. This may involve engaging in short conversation at the beginning of the interview, perhaps by having the interviewer tell the interviewee a little about the purpose of the interview and what will be done with the results and thanking the interviewee for the time and effort. We have found that several things are important for the interviewee to know:

- There are no right or wrong answers to the questions; it is the interviewee's opinions and perspectives that are needed.

- If there is any question that an interviewee doesn't feel comfortable answering, the interviewee should feel free not to answer it, and the interviewer should move on to another question.

- All responses are confidential, and no individually identifiable responses will be released.

- The interviewee must be made aware of any individuals or groups who will have access to the interviewee's responses.

Prior to conducting interviews, it is important to pilot-test the questions with people who are similar to the participants. This can help the interviewer identify and refine questions that are confusing or that don't get at the information that is wanted. It can also give the interviewer some idea of the range of time the interviews may take. Letting interviewees know in advance about how much time the interview will take is helpful. It is difficult to say what the "right" length for an interview is. If one is collecting data on perceptions of a program, 15 or 20 minutes should be enough. However, if an interview is being used to, for example, look at differences in individuals' ideas, plans, or attitudes before and after participation in a program, it could take longer, maybe even 45 to 60 minutes. It is also important to remember that asking the same questions of different participants can take a very different amount of time. For example, we found in one of our studies that while the average interview length was 35 minutes, individual interview times ranged from 25 to 90 minutes.

Focus Groups

Focus groups started as marketing tools to provide businesses with information on people's responses to just about anything—products, movies, packaging, and even ideas. These groups are typically composed of 5–7 people brought together by a facilitator, for periods of 30 to 60 minutes, to, collectively and individually, provide a variety of ideas about and responses to a given topic. A focus group is a structured conversation. Its major strength is that people can build on the ideas of others in the group. In a good focus group, the whole is greater than the sum of its parts. This makes focus groups particularly valuable in finding out people's perceptions in a variety of areas, including why some people come to, stay, or leave programs or why different outreach programs seem to work better than others.

One of the biggest challenges for the focus group facilitator is to keep participants on task while making sure that individual perspectives are heard. The gender or racial makeup of the focus group may have an impact on participant responses. If the demographic breakdown of participants does not allow for balanced groups, or if there is concern that one group may dominate the focus group, one possibility is to consider collecting the data in all-male or all-female groups, in all-minority or all-majority groups, or in individual interviews (Stewart, Shamdasani, & Rook, 2002). Focus groups are not useful for collecting information for pre/post comparisons because the information one gets from an individual may have been influenced by the group members or by the dynamics of the group.

Focus groups are not appropriate for collecting personal or sensitive information. Sharing sensitive information is difficult, and at times even unwise, in a group setting. Confidentiality cannot be guaranteed in a focus group. Unlike individual interview questions, good focus group questions don't focus on the individual. For example, one might ask focus group participants, "Why do you think participants aren't coming to the program anymore?" rather than asking, "Why aren't you coming to the program anymore?" The following are some tips we have utilized to conduct a good focus group.

- Have all participants in the group introduce themselves. As they make these introductions, the facilitator should write down everyone's name. It greatly improves the conversation and the questioning if individuals are called by name.

- Ask the first question and then ask people what they think. It may take what seems like a long time for them to start talking, but they will. You can shorten the time by asking individuals, by name, what they think. It is useful to make this a request, such as "[Name], may I ask you what you think?" If that doesn't work, consider asking individual participants in turn what they think.

- Interrupting people can discourage others from speaking. Consider, instead, waiting until an overly talkative person takes a breath, say thank you, and ask another person for a response.

- To keep people on task, usually all that is needed is to say, "Thank you, that was very interesting, but I think we need to get back to talking about [the current topic]."

Observations

There are a variety of different types of observations that can be done. Some are naturalistic observations where a data collector unobtrusively observes participants interacting in a real-life setting. In this case, the observer tries to be as much a part of the background as possible. In other naturalistic situations, the observer may be a participant observer, where instead of being unobtrusive, they participate in whatever activities the participants are doing. Unobtrusive and participant observers can also be used in more structured observations where participants are responding to specific prompts or are participating in project-related activities.

Observers have several choices as to how they collect data. These include taking free-form field notes, selecting an existing coding scheme, or developing a new coding scheme (Siminoff & Step, 2011). With participants' permission, or with their and their parent/guardian's permission if the participants are minors, the observer can video or audio record the observations so that coding and/or field note–taking can be done later or rechecked.

Bias is a serious concern in observations. Observers have been found to rate the same behaviors differently based on the perceived characteristics of those being observed. For example, female musicians were more likely to be hired when a "blind" audition process was used, where the hiring committee was not aware of the auditioning musicians' gender (Goldin & Rouse, 2000). Observers, too, were found to rate the behaviors of those who were of their own sex differently from those who weren't (Pellegrini, 2011). Even accents made a difference. People viewed speakers with accents like theirs as being more knowledgeable than different-accent speakers, even when the different-accent speaker was more knowledgeable (Dahlback, Wang, Nass, & Alwin, 2007). While providing the observer with as little demographic information as possible about the participants may help, it is also important to make observers aware of their possible biases and to use other data sources to triangulate the ratings or findings.

Participant-Generated Visual Data

Participant paintings and drawings are an evaluation tool that has been used primarily with children. The artwork itself can be coded and/or used as a prompt to get the artist to speak about what is represented in the artwork. For example, in the evaluation of a museum exhibit for preschool children that focused on plants and animals living under the water, coauthor Patricia B. Campbell asked children to do a drawing of life under water before entering and after leaving the exhibit. The pretest/posttest drawings were compared in terms of what was included in the drawings and how accurate the presentations were. This helped the children's museum better understand what children were taking away from the exhibit. The children could also have been asked to describe their drawings, and why they drew what they did, which could give further insight.

Using drawings and paintings with participants other than young children can be challenging. Many people are self-conscious about their drawing and painting skills and uncomfortable creating art. Other ways participants can generate visual data include, for example, making collages out of existing pictures and drawings. Also, they can take photographs that express their attitudes and perceptions of the impact a project has had on them. Again, the visuals can be used alone, or participants can be asked to describe the visuals and what the visuals mean to them.

Wang and Burris (1997) describe a version of participant-generated visual data that they call photovoice. Photovoice is

> a process by which people can identify, represent, and enhance their community through a specific photographic technique. It entrusts cameras to the hands of people to enable them to act as recorders, and potential catalysts for change, in their own communities. It uses the immediacy of the visual image to furnish evidence and to promote an effective, participatory means of sharing expertise and knowledge. (p. 369)

Video can be used as well as still photography, but video is more expensive and can be more time consuming to analyze.

Keisha Farmer-Smith (2018) summarized a number of benefits to using the visual arts as an evaluation tool with young people:

- *Drawing artwork together builds rapport and engages program participants.* Young people may feel uncomfortable talking to unknown evaluators/adults. Art-based activities are a fun, nonthreatening way to break the ice.

- *Art is a great communication tool.* When young people explain their art, relevant and meaningful information about programming is shared. During this process, it is incredibly important for adult evaluators to actively listen as youth share the intent and meaning behind their artwork.

- *Art can be a strength-based tool.* When young people make art it affirms their vision, voice, and opinion. As the artist, the young person has power to explore topics that are important to them.

- *Using art as an evaluation tool helps evaluators collect rich, interesting and valuable information.* Sometimes, it is easier to express emotions and experiences while drawing. Art-based evaluation should always be accompanied by a listening or discussion session.

- *Using art as an evaluation tool is not difficult.* From stick figures to complicated images, art is fun for everyone! The artist's skill level doesn't matter because the story behind the art can still be shared. (paras. 10–14)

Sources of Quantitative Data

Surveys and Other Structured Questionnaires

Surveys are one of the most widely used forms of data collection. We define a survey as a series of closed- and/or open-ended questions about a topic or topics to which the participant responds in writing. Closed-ended questions are questions that are answered by ratings or other forced-choice responses, while open-ended questions are questions that are answered in words or sentences. For example, "In what ways, if any, did your attitudes toward eating sugar change after attending the workshop?" is an open-ended question, while "Please rate the change, if any, in your attitudes toward eating sugar after attending the workshop, on a scale of 1 (*made my attitudes toward eating sugar much more positive*) to 5 (*made my attitudes toward eating sugar much more negative*)" is a closed-ended question. Open-ended questions are qualitative data, but when used in surveys, they are usually coded and/or ranked into quantitative data. Coding is covered in greater detail in Chapter 13. Open-ended questions can provide more information, but they are more time consuming to complete and more complex to analyze.

It is useful for inexperienced survey designers to design surveys in conjunction with a more experienced person, or at least have a more experienced person review the draft survey. There are several common pitfalls to avoid in developing survey items. One is to only give neutral to positive options so that, for example, the choices range from 1 (*no impact*) to 5 (*strong positive impact*). That gives the respondent no option to report a negative impact. A second pitfall is to write questions that are ambiguous or combine several questions into one. For example, a survey question might ask, "On a scale of 1 (*very negative*) to 5 (*very positive*), how would you rate the impact of the program on your attitudes and behaviors tied to healthy eating?" If respondents felt the program had a positive impact on their attitudes but no impact on their behaviors, it would be impossible for them to answer the question accurately.

Asking a large number of open-ended questions in a survey can be a problem as well. Generally, the more open-ended questions asked, the shorter the answers become. Having too many open-ended questions—we often say more than five—can impact the response rate (discussed later in this chapter) negatively as well. For both open- and closed-ended questions, evaluators need to know how they will be using the responses. If evaluators aren't clear on how they will use the responses to a question, then the question shouldn't be asked.

Surveys should ask for demographic information *only* at the end of measures, although there may be exceptions for people with disabilities who need accommodations to complete the measures. Research has found that asking demographic information at the beginning of a measure can impact the response of participants, particularly people of color and white women, in a variety of areas, including

- how participants think they will be viewed by others;
- how participants view themselves; and
- academic performance, including AP Calculus scores (Danaher & Crandall, 2008; Sinclair, Hardin, & Lowery, 2006).

Some survey designers ask demographic questions at the beginning of a survey because they think these questions are easy to answer. However, there are other questions to ask as a survey begins—such as "How did you first hear about this program?"—that will have less impact on responses to other questions.

When asking demographic questions, it is important to have participants define their own race/ethnicity and disability status rather than having the identification done by data collectors or project/program staff. There are a variety of reasons for this. People are not very accurate in their identification of the race/ethnicity of others. Definitions of race/ethnicity can be inconsistent; for example, the child of one Black parent and one white parent is often categorized as Black, and a person with a "Hispanic- or Latino-sounding" last name is more apt to be categorized as Hispanic than a person with a similar background with an "Anglo-sounding" last name (Goldenberg & American Anthropological Association, 2011). Race is basically a social rather than a genetic concept. Scientifically, the genetic variation in populations such as Europeans and Asians is actually a subset of the variation in the African population, and skin colors—whether light or dark—are due not to race but to adaptation to life under the sun (Goldenberg & American Anthropological Association, 2011).

Also, while some disabilities are relatively easy to identify, others are not, and many disabilities (including those tied to learning, mental health, and disease) are "invisible" to researchers or evaluators. If a standard set of categories for race/ethnicity and/or disability is required to be used, surveys should also, in an open-ended question, ask participants to indicate their own race/ethnicity and disability status. Often standardized categories do not present a complete or accurate picture of one's race/ethnicity. This is particularly true for multiracial people who often end up having to choose one group to belong to or choose "Other." Similar issues arise when asking people about their sex or gender. Too, as covered in Chapter 1, there may be a distinction between individuals' sex at birth and their current/legal sex, and people may self-identify in a variety of categories such as female, male, nonbinary, nongendered, or bigendered.

Survey development, implementation, and analysis is not a simple task. Libraries of books have been written, and many graduate courses and professional development trainings have been developed and conducted, on how to develop valid surveys. Resources for readers who would like to know more about survey development include the following:

- The Pew Research Center (www.pewresearch.org/methodology/u-s-survey-research/questionnaire-design/) draws on research on surveys and questionnaire design to discuss the pitfalls and best practices of designing questionnaires.

- The New Jersey Agricultural Experiment Station at Rutgers University (https://njaes.rutgers.edu/evaluation/resources/survey-instrument.php) provides a number of resources tied to survey development, including how to craft questions with less bias, how to develop a cover letter, and what to consider when deciding the order of questions.

- Online survey company SurveyMonkey (www.surveymonkey.com/mp/survey-guidelines/) provides a variety of resources on survey development and how to get a higher response rate.

Records and Other Archival Data

Records or archival data refer to information that has already been collected by someone else other than the evaluator and already exists in someone else's files. For example, in evaluations of educational programs, evaluators often rely on student standardized achievement data, quarterly report cards, or suspension and attendance data. Records and other archival data can be particularly valuable in evaluations where one of the goals is to look at changes in policies and procedures over time. It is important to check any archival data for authenticity and for completeness. Missing records may indicate that the surviving data do not tell the complete story.

Evaluators can use records kept by the program delivering the service being evaluated or by other agencies or departments (e.g., school district, public health department, police department, U.S. Census Bureau) that have records relevant to the work of the program being evaluated. Hatry (2015) identified a number of examples of different types of records or archival data used by evaluators across a variety of program types, including

- client characteristics;
- which services are used, and how much of each;
- quantity of work done or amount of output;
- school attendance and number of school dropouts;
- student grades and test scores;
- number and categories of reported crimes;
- number and type of complaints;
- recidivism;
- response times; and
- number of reported cases of child abuse.

Archival data have certain practical advantages such as being easier to obtain and less time-consuming and costly than collecting data yourself. However, evaluators need to be aware of potential problems that can exist in such data. For the most part, the usefulness of records and archival data depends on whether they are accessible and accurate. Some specific potential problems of these types of data include missing or incomplete data, data inaccuracy, data available in overly aggregated form, and confidentiality and privacy considerations (Hatry, 2015).

It is often not clear under what circumstances the data were collected and what, if any, attention was paid to context including cultural context. It is generally recommended that evaluators not rely exclusively on the use of archival data when conducting an evaluation but, instead, always juxtapose archival or record data with other types of data such as surveys, observations, and interviews (Spaulding, 2014).

Strengths and Weaknesses of Qualitative and Quantitative Data

Qualitative data allow for the collection of rich, in-depth detail where participants can elaborate on their responses. They can contribute to a deep understanding of situations and help evaluators to understand and define context. Qualitative data are useful in evaluations where detailed contextual and other understandings are needed. These data can help evaluators see events and program components more holistically.

In qualitative data, much of the focus is on individuals and their words and/or actions. This focus, if done well, can allow individual voices, including the voices of those from marginalized groups, to be heard. Allowing participants to voice their own reality is an important aspect of qualitative methodology (Frierson, Hood, Hughes, & Thomas, 2010). Evaluations that utilize a culturally responsive evaluation lens often use qualitative data to learn more about the cultural contexts of the project and/or community under study. As was covered in detail in Chapter 4, those who are collecting data need to be attuned to the cultural context in which the project is situated to better understand participants and to increase the quality of the data collected.

While qualitative data can provide vivid, richly detailed accounts of participants' experiences, there are some challenges related to qualitative data. The collection of qualitative data can take considerable time and effort in relation to training of data collectors, the actual data collection process, coding data, and analysis of qualitative data. The collection of qualitative data may be particularly challenging when the evaluator is examining a project with a large number of participants and there is a need to hear from as many individuals as possible. Because of the focus on the individual and the complexity of the data that are collected, the number of individuals from whom qualitative data are collected tends to be relatively small. There can be a legitimate concern that the relatively small sample sizes when collecting qualitative data can yield a biased or skewed depiction of a program and its participants. The smaller sample size and the focus on the individual can limit the **generalizability** of the findings.

> Generalization, which is an act of reasoning that involves drawing broad inferences from particular observations, is widely-acknowledged as a quality standard in quantitative research, but is more controversial in qualitative research. The goal of most qualitative studies is not to generalize but rather to provide a rich, contextualized understanding of some aspect of human experience through the intensive study of particular cases. (Polit & Beck, 2011, p. 1451)

With quantitative data, the evaluator can collect information from a number of individuals in a relatively short period of time. Synthesis and analyses of such data can be done more quickly than with qualitative data. Furthermore, quantitative data provide the potential for greater generalization. Statistical analysis can be done, and **statistical significance**, the probability that the findings are real and not due to chance, can be determined. The size of differences and relationships can be determined, and the data can be used to make systematic, standardized comparisons. Too, as will be discussed in detail later in this chapter, the assessment tools used to generate quantitative data can be tested for explicit types of reliability and validity. Definitions of validity and reliability are somewhat different for quantitative and qualitative assessments and the resulting data. **Validity** in quantitative assessments and data refers to accuracy while in qualitative assessments and data it refers to "appropriateness." In quantitative assessments and data, reliability refers to replicability, but in qualitative areas, reliability is tied more to consistency. Leung (2015) points out that

> a margin of variability for results is tolerated in qualitative research provided the methodology and epistemological logistics consistently yield data that are ontologically similar but may differ in richness and ambience within similar dimensions. (p. 325)

As indicated earlier, one of the advantages of qualitative data is that it has potential for the voices and experiences of individuals to be heard; however, while it may be more difficult, it is possible for this to be done with quantitative data as well. As was covered in Chapter 5, hearing the voices of those who haven't been heard and learning about their experiences from their perspective can have a big impact on the data to be collected and on the data itself. Underlying the field of women's studies is the assumption that "girls and women matter, and our own assessment of our experiences constitutes the starting point for discussion, analysis, and the production of knowledge" (Schweitzer, 2017, p. 331), which is or should be the case for all marginalized groups. Considering this and, as was covered in Chapter 5, the negative impact of the application of the deficit model on individuals, programs and evaluations can have a major impact on what data are collected and how, for both qualitative and quantitative data.

In such instances, data need to be collected about the assumptions program staff and participants have about participants of different genders, races/ethnicities, and/or socioeconomic statuses. Both qualitative and quantitative data can be collected about the equities and inequities tied to gender and other demographic characteristics within a program and the context in which the program operates. An evaluation designed through the lens of these assertions could take a more systemic view of programs and program impacts and would have more of a focus on "fixing the system" than on "fixing the individual" (P. B. Campbell, 1995). Overall, the strengths of qualitative data can include providing contextual and cultural data that help explain complex issues. Such data can also complement quantitative data by explaining the "why" and "how" behind the "what." The limitations of qualitative data for evaluation may include lack of generalizability, the time-consuming and costly nature of data collection, and the difficulty and complexity of data analysis and interpretation (Patton, 2002).

In the following activity, readers select the qualitative and quantitative data they would like to collect and justify their choices.

Activity
What Data Would You Collect?

You've been asked to conduct an evaluation of the quality and impact of a multisite program, similar to the one described in Chapter 11 (page 345), for adults who have dropped out of high school and are working toward earning a GED (general equivalency diploma). The program model consists of three components: (a) instruction, (b) social supports and career exploration, and (c) the inclusion of six youth development principles.

In small groups, decide what other types of data you might collect to assess quality and impact and provide justification for your choices.

Ensuring Data Quality

Validity

Karen Kirkhart (2005) points out that validity addresses the fundamental correctness of evaluation, references the accuracy and limits of understandings, and guides what can and cannot be appropriately concluded from evaluative inquiry. For data to be appropriate and accurate, the assessment tools used to collect those data need to be both valid and reliable. While, as indicated earlier, validity refers in quantitative areas to accuracy and in qualitative areas to "appropriateness," in both areas a measure or an assessment tool is valid if it measures what it is supposed to. In any assessment, validity is the most important construct (Linn, 1997).

In her 2019 Voices From the Field interview, Karen E. Kirkhart speaks about ways we need to think about validity.

Voices From the Field

Karen E. Kirkhart: Thinking About Validity

In 1993, as American Evaluation Association (AEA) president, I picked evaluation and social justice as the theme for the annual meeting. The theme was to be the topic of my presentation, but it was such a huge topic that I stepped back and started to think about what was a prerequisite for social justice that is relevant to evaluation. The concept of validity came to mind, not just validity specific to measurement or causality or a type of inquiry, but validity as a broad concept tied to fundamental issues of trustworthiness. I see validity as the adequacy and appropriateness of understanding and action.

Social justice depends on the ability to have valid exchanges among people—exchanges that are trustworthy and honest and truthful. Without that, there will be no collaborations that will move social justice forward.

Social justice requires action. So often inaction is supported by critiquing the methodology and challenging its findings and then calling for more research and evaluation to justify inaction. Validity, in the past, has worked to make evaluators and policymakers more cautious about moving ahead. Yes, understandings are partial and imperfect, but that doesn't mean they are unworthy of action.

Karen E. Kirkhart is a professor in the School of Social Work at Syracuse University, where she teaches courses in program evaluation and clinical practice evaluation. She is also an affiliated faculty member of the Center for Culturally Responsive Evaluation and Assessment (CREA) at the University of Illinois at Urbana-Champaign. She was interviewed by coauthor Patricia B. Campbell in the fall of 2019.

Types of Validity

Content validity refers to the content of an assessment and asks if the measure covers the appropriate subject matter. In, for example, an evaluation of a program to reduce smoking, one would expect questions, whether they are interview questions or survey questions, to focus on such areas as smoking, smoking-related behaviors, and smoking triggers. In another example, in an evaluation of the impact of an earth science curriculum on earth science knowledge, to have content validity the test used would need to cover the topics covered in the curriculum. If the test covered areas not included in the curriculum being evaluated, it could be a good test, but it would not have content validity for use in that evaluation.

Before using an existing measure, whether it is a test, a survey, a set of interview questions, or an observation protocol, it is key to determine the degree to which the individual items reflect the areas needed for answering the evaluation questions. One way to do this is to construct a table of specifications. This is a matrix or a two-way chart in which the topics or areas to be covered are the column headers and the items or questions to be asked are the row headers. The evaluator then maps the items or questions to the topics to make sure that each item or question is related to at least one topic and that each topic is covered by at least one item or question.

Table 12.1 is a segment of a table of specifications for the earlier earth science example. As shown, questions 1–3 each fit into a topic and should be included in the measure, while question 4 doesn't fit into a topic and therefore shouldn't be included in the measure.

Table 12.1 A Partial Table of Specifications

Questions to Be Asked	Topic: The Structure and Scale of the Solar System	Topic: The Transfer of Energy Through Radiation and Convection
1. When air near the ground is warmed by sunlight, what happens to the warm air?		X
2. Why isn't Pluto a satellite of Neptune?	X	
3. Why do areas in the middle of a large continent generally have more extreme differences in temperature than areas near the coastline?		X
4. How many elements are there in the periodic table?		

A second form of validity of interest to evaluators is **predictive validity**. This is an indicator of whether the measure predicts what it purports to. Often a program's longer-term outcomes will not be able to be measured during the evaluation period. In that case, measures can be used that are good predictors of the longer-term outcome. For example, in the evaluation of the smoking cessation program described earlier, the evaluation may not last long enough to determine if participants quit smoking. In that case, measures of the intent to quit smoking could be used if they had predictive validity (Hummel et al., 2018). That is, researchers could give smokers a test designed to measure their intent to quit smoking and then some length of time later could go back to the people and determine whether they had attempted to quit smoking and, if they had, if they were successful. The researchers would then analyze the data to determine if participant responses to the intent-to-quit test predicted whether participants tried to quit or not and if they were successful or not. If the intent-to-quit measure has predictive validity, then the evaluator could use it and be reasonably sure of the conclusions as to whether the smoking cessation program was effective or not.

Two other common forms of validity, concurrent validity and construct validity, tend to be of less importance to evaluators. **Concurrent validity** is the degree to which the results of one measure reflect the results of other validated measures with similar content. This may be of interest to evaluators if they have to choose between different measures of the same concepts, such as self-efficacy or fitness. If the measures have concurrent validity, the evaluator may choose the measure that, for example, is less expensive or takes less time to complete. If the evaluator is concerned about pretest effect, and therefore decides to use different pre- and posttests, those tests will need to have good concurrent validity. **Construct validity** is the degree to which the results of a measure reflect existing theory. Evaluations tend not to include validations of theories, but if they do, then construct validity can be an important criterion in the selection of assessments.

A newer form of validity, multicultural validity (Kirkhart, 1995, 2005), is particularly important for evaluators to consider. **Multicultural validity** is based on the recognition "that cultural factors shape the sensitivity of evaluation instruments and the validity of the conclusions on program effectiveness" (Solano-Flores, 2011, p. 4). It focuses attention on how well the evaluation captures meaning across dimensions of cultural diversity. There are five components to multicultural validity:

- Methodological
- Interpersonal
- Theoretical
- Experiential
- Consequential (Hopson & Kirkhart 2011; Kirkhart, 2005)

While being interviewed for this book, Karen Kirkhart (personal communication, December 17, 2019) spoke about what led her to develop the concept of multicultural validity:

> Threats to internal and external validity are well documented and ingrained in researchers and evaluators, so I started thinking, *What about having a set of threats to validity from a cultural lens?* and set out to explore that.

The following, adapted from Hopson and Kirkhart (2011), provides some sample questions to ask to determine multicultural validity:

Methodological

Whose values are represented in the evaluation questions chosen?

What procedures will be used to gain multiple perspectives?

How do the sources of information included in the evaluation permit more than one perspective?

Interpersonal

What roles have been created for stakeholders to participate in the evaluation?

What steps are being taken to establish trust with participants in the program?

Do evaluators understand their positions vis-à-vis the local community (are they seen as insiders or outsiders?) and the program itself (what authority do they hold)?

Theoretical

Did the program theory take culture into account?

Experiential

Was a "cultural guide" needed or used? Why or why not?

How did your own personal characteristics and cultural location impact the evaluation?

How do participants and/or providers of the program contribute to the interpretation of the data? Are findings being "checked" with them?

Consequential

> In what ways has evaluation historically interfered with or supported the program?
>
> How does this evaluation itself support the goals of the program?
>
> How does the evaluation relate to social justice (or does it)?
>
> Did the evaluators build in any "giveback" to the community?

When looking at the validity of a measure, it is important to determine if the measure has been tested and validated with groups similar to the groups who will be given the measure. If the groups similar to those who are in the evaluation were not included in the development and testing of a measure, then the measure and its items may not be valid for that group. Measures developed and validated with, for example, white, middle-class groups may not be valid for other groups. Even geographic location can make a difference. For example, in measures of knowledge, personal familiarity with the context of individual items has been found to be tied to performance (Chipman, 1991). Thus, students in Montana are more likely to do better on a test item tied to skidding and sliding on the ice than are comparable students in Florida. Similarly, students in urban areas have very different intuitive views of what an elevator is than do students in rural farmlands (i.e., building elevator vs. grain elevator) (Patterson, Busch-Vishniac, Campbell, & Guillaume, 2011).

While this is important for all groups, it is particularly important when working with groups that include people with disabilities. Many measures are designed inadvertently for individuals who are able-bodied and may not be valid for those with disabilities. If one's sight, hearing, or movement is impaired, one's knowledge and understanding of—as well as familiarity with—items incorporating certain experiences may be minimal. For example, a person who is blind has different conceptions of color than a person who is sighted (Young, 2019).

Of course, if participants can't access a measure, it isn't valid for them. If a survey, test, or questionnaire is difficult for people with limited visibility, colorblindness, or learning disabilities to read and understand, they are less likely to respond to the questions, and even if they do respond, their responses may not be as complete or even as accurate as they would be if the measure had been more accessible.

To make evaluation, in general, and assessments, more specifically, more accessible, Jennifer Sullivan Sulewski and June Gothberg (2013) developed the Universal Design for Evaluation Checklist, which includes the following points tied to data collection:

- Provide for different communication preferences or needs.
- Use simple language, ask concrete questions, and show cultural competency.
- Meet low-vision and colorblindness requirements.
- Avoid acronyms, jargon, slang, and colloquial terms.

In her Voices From the Field interview, Jennifer Sullivan Sulewaski talks about the importance of universal design in evaluation and how the checklist came to be.

Voices From the Field

Jennifer Sullivan Sulewaski: Applying Universal Design to Evaluation

The Universal Design for Evaluation Checklist grew out of some discussions a group of us were having at the AEA about the importance of having more evaluators who understood how to work with people with disabilities as well as with other vulnerable populations. Often people don't think of disability as a form of diversity, but it is.

I want evaluators to know how common and pervasive it is to have a disability—to know that people with disabilities are everywhere. Whatever the topic of your evaluation, you will be running into people with disabilities, and you will have to have some awareness of how to accommodate them.

People with visual impairments may need the assessments in different formats, while people with hearing impairments may need interpreters, and there may need to be physical access for people with mobility issues. In addition, there are a lot of people with hidden disabilities. While there may be no one in a wheelchair in the group, there may be people with learning disabilities or a health condition who need accommodation to be part of your data collection.

We chose to focus on universal design because it isn't just for people with disabilities; it is about making things accessible for the broadest part of the population possible. Knowing where people are coming from, meeting them where they are, and making sure you are not putting barriers to the participation of any population, but particularly disenfranchised populations, is key.

Jennifer Sullivan Sulewaski is a senior research associate at the Institute for Community Inclusion at the University of Massachusetts Boston. She was interviewed by coauthor Patricia B. Campbell in the fall of 2019.

Language is another factor to be considered when addressing issues of validity. A number of programs and projects work with participants whose first language is not English. This can mean that written measures need to be in the first language of participants and interviews need to be done by those fluent in that language. Without accurate translations, the collation of accurate data from participants is virtually impossible. It is essential that translators be bilingual, bicultural, and familiar with the target population. In assessing the validity of the translated instruments, it is recommended that, at a minimum, the evaluator seek semantic and content equivalence. **Semantic equivalence** refers to the agreement between different language versions of the instruments. **Content equivalence** ensures that each item's content is relevant in each culture. Some common translation strategies include the following:

- Forward/backward translation (FBT) is where an individual translates an instrument into, for example, Spanish and a second person translates the Spanish version into English. The two English versions are compared. The extent to which the two English versions are equivalent is an indicator of the quality of the Spanish translation.

- Translation by committee (TBC) is often more suitable to complete in a short time frame and involves using a bilingual panel to translate the instrument into the desired language.

- Multiple forward translations (MFTs) occur when translators create two or more forward translations, and then reconcile them by a third (Frierson et al., 2010; Marin & Marin, 1991).

Another validity issue to consider is the obviousness of the measure. People's responses to some measures can be different when the purpose of the measure is obvious, particularly when social desirability bias can come into play (Campbell & Jolly, n.d.b). Social desirability bias is a form of response bias where individuals misrepresent their self-reported behaviors by overreporting behaviors considered socially desirable and underreporting undesirable behaviors. It is one of the most significant and common threats to validity of self-reported responses (King & Bruner 2000; D. Phillips & Clancy, 1972). When people, for example, grossly overrate the amount of time they spend brushing their teeth and underrepresent how much they smoke (Sanzone et al., 2013), social desirability bias is in play. In another example, job application ratings were higher when raters thought the candidate had a disability because it was felt that the raters realized the study was investigating attitudes toward workers with disabilities (B. Bell & Klein, 2001).

The use of indirect or less obvious questions can reduce the impact of social desirability bias. For example, white people's answers to multiple-choice survey questions about race were found to be different than their responses to in-depth open-ended questions on race and gender differences. These differences were greater on tests when it was very clear that gender-related concepts, like empathy, were being measured (Bonilla-Silva & Zuberi, 2008; Eisenberg & Lennon, 1983).

When there is concern that skewed responses due to obviousness may happen, it can be useful to have members of the target population review the measures for clarity and say what concepts they think are being measured. If what is being measured is obvious and there are gender, race, or disability stereotypes or socially desirable or undesirable variables seen to be associated with the measure, the evaluator should consider using a less obvious measure or use more than one measure and compare or triangulate the data. For example, both participants and staff could rate participant skills or interests, or participants could respond to both closed-ended questions and open-ended questions about the subject and comparisons could be made.

Reliability

Reliability of Quantitative Data

Reliability of quantitative data is the degree to which responses to items or questions on measures are consistent. Test/retest reliability is the degree of similarity and difference between individuals' responses the first and the second time they respond to a measure. Similar responses to questions or items when the circumstances are the same is a strength for a measure. However, in evaluation, where one is often looking for change, a measure with a high test/retest reliability may not be the best choice. Similar responses to items or questions when circumstances change could mean that the measure would not be useful in assessing program impact. Before using a measure in evaluation, it is important to know if the measure is sensitive to change. To do that can involve triangulation, or a variation on the concurrent validity described earlier, where changes in participants' responses to the items or questions are compared to other measures of change such as change in their behavior or other people's perceptions of changes in them. Two forms of reliability that pertain more to quantitative data are alternative-form reliability, which refers to the degree of similarity and difference between an individual's responses on different forms of the same test, and split-half reliability, where the scores on half the measure are compared to the scores on the other half to determine if the test is consistently measuring the intended concept.

Reliability of Qualitative Data

For qualitative data collection, several other forms of reliability are important to consider. One of the most common forms of qualitative data reliability is **interrater reliability**, which is the degree to which different raters score or code the same response or behavior the same way. Two other related reliabilities are **interinterviewer reliability**, the degree to which interviewees would give the same response to the same questions posed by two different interviewers, and **interobserver reliability**, the degree to which two observers "see" the same thing when they are doing the same observation.

If more than one observer or rater is going to be used in data collection, it is important to work with these individuals to increase their reliability as much as possible. In observations and ratings, this may involve having them observe the same setting or interpret the same response, determining the degree of agreement in their responses, discussing differences in their responses, and, as appropriate, establishing rules or guidelines about how different codes are applied or scores are given. Providing raters with samples of written responses and their ratings or videos of observations and how they were coded can help as well. These can also be helpful to increase **intrarater reliability**, which is the degree to which individual observers and/or raters are consistent in their ratings or codings over time.

A number of factors can impact interinterviewer and interobserver reliability, including data collector and participant demographic characteristics (D. Davis & Silver, 2003). For example, there is some inconsistency in the literature on the impact of similarities and differences in the race and gender of the data collector and the participant. Hood (1998, 2001) and Thomas (2004) argue that a shared lived experience could and probably should be accepted as important and valuable in the evaluation of programs serving members of racial minority groups. In particular, Hood (1998, 2001) notes that evaluators of color are more likely to have direct experiences with their own racial and cultural group that inform their evaluation of programs serving these groups, resulting in less time required in translating the cultural nuances and nonverbal communications in observations, interviews, and interpretations that go beyond quantitative indicators of what the programs appear to be. However, some scholars say that "there is surprisingly little evidence to indicate whether sociodemographic interviewer–respondent matching [e.g., gender, race] improves survey response rates or data validity" (Davis, Couper, Janz, Caldwell, & Resnicow, 2010, p. 14).

A major impact on interviewee responses is the relationship between the interviewer and the interviewee. As P. Ryan and Dundon (2008) explain,

> there is a simple rule of thumb: the better the quality of the relationship between interviewer and interviewee, the richer the quality of the data elicited. This is because experience shows that when interviewees are comfortable and trusting, they relate richer stories and elaborated explanations. (pp. 3–4)

Interinterviewer reliability is difficult to train for because interviewers are different people with different personalities, and some interviewers will relate better with some interviewees. However, helping the interviewers become skilled at building rapport with interviewees can help improve the quality of the interviews and hopefully increase interinterviewer reliability.

Pilot-Testing

Regardless of the data collection methods used, **pilot-testing** them with a sample of people like those in the target population tends to improve the quality of the data collected. In a typical pilot test, people complete the measure while being observed. Notes are taken on the comments people make to each other and the amount of time it takes different people to complete the measure. After they have completed the measure, in a focus group format, they critique the measure as a whole and the items in terms of clarity of the instructions and of that which is being requested, unnecessary technical language or jargon, and possible areas that could be perceived as offensive. Benefits to pilot-testing include

- finding logic gaps or flaws (e.g., unclear directions) in the measure or the collection procedure;
- identifying unintended redundancies, ambiguous words, or misinterpreted items;
- testing for **response set bias** (e.g., where possibly due to the order of items, people's response to one item biases their response to following items;
- checking for respondent burden or time constraints (e.g., the responder gets tired of answering questions and stops, gives one-word answers, or in rating questions rates everything the same); and
- finding culturally biased or inappropriate items or measures.

If problems are identified, refinements and adaptations of the measure should be made and retested so they provide reliable and valid information about the target population.

Response Rates

Another indicator of data quality is the **response rate**, the percentage of people who complete the data collection measure (e.g., survey, interview, focus group) relative to the number of people who were asked to participate. For example, if the evaluator contacted 100 project participants to complete a survey and 40 responded, the response rate would be 40%. While it is clear that higher response rates are better, it is difficult to say what is a "good" response rate. Fryrear (2015) estimates that internal surveys, those that are given to employees or project participants, generally receive a 30%–40% response rate compared to an average 10%–15% response rate for surveys sent to those with no investment in the institution or project sending them that survey. She says that

> response rates can soar past 85% . . . when the respondent population is motivated and the survey is well-executed. Response rates can also fall below 2% . . . when the respondent population is less-targeted, when contact information is unreliable, or where there is less incentive or little motivation to respond. (Fryrear, 2015, para. 9)

Reasons for low response rates include mistrust of research and evaluation, particularly among African Americans and Indigenous populations who have a history of being mistreated in research (Burns, Soward, Skelly, Leeman, & Carlson, 2008;

Han, Kang, Kim, Ryu, & Kim, 2007; Lindenberg, Solorzano, Vilaro, & Westbrook, 2001), and related perceptions that participation presented no personal benefit to respondents or their community and may cause potential harm, including possible social stigmatization and even legal ramifications (e.g., Hatchett, Holmes, Duran, & Davis, 2000; Lambert & Wiebel, 1990; Shedlin, Decena, Mangadu, & Martinez, 2014). Too, there tends to be lower response rates from hard-to-reach groups such as those who live in remote areas or without access to technology (Sydor, 2013).

Unless response rates are very high, say 90% or higher, it is important to check for response bias, as noted in Chapter 11, to determine if those who responded to the measure were similar to or different from those who did not. To determine the variables to check for response bias, the evaluator needs to know what information is available about all of those who were asked to complete the survey and what variables might have had an impact on the conclusions drawn from the survey (P. B. Campbell & Clewell, 2008). For example, if a survey was about racial attitudes and the response rate for white participants was much higher than that for Hispanic participants, response bias would have come into play. Particular attention needs to be paid to possible differences in response rates between dominant and marginalized groups. This can help evaluators to determine if some bias is present in the measure or in the data collection process.

We have used a number of strategies to increase response rates, including the following:

- *Know who your target respondents are and tailor your approach to meet them.* Some communities don't fill out surveys—if you want the information, you need to go to them and ask them. Some groups are not web savvy, so reaching them by paper or telephone is better. Have recruiting materials reviewed by members of the target population before they are sent out.

- *Use informants or cultural guides.* Target population members can help you figure out where to find target population members and how to get them to respond. For example, to follow up with a sample of high school dropouts, we hired some other dropouts to help. They knew where their friends "hung out" and how to get them to respond.

- *Explain the benefits and the risks.* Tell potential respondents why you are collecting the data and what will be done with it, including of what benefit it might be to their communities. Explain what will be done to protect them and the information they will share with you, and offer to send them a copy of the results.

- *Provide incentives.* Incentives can vary based on the group from whom you want to receive the data and the amount of time and effort it will take respondents to give you the data. Incentives can include being part of a raffle, a gift card, or access to a game. It is important that incentives offered are culturally appropriate and of interest to the target population. It is also important to check to see if funders and institutional review boards (discussed in the next section) allow incentives.

- *Follow up.* Gently remind nonrespondents that you really want their data. It is best to limit your reminders to two; however, consider sending out the two reminders at different times and on different days so that you can reach as many different respondents as possible.

Coauthor Patricia B. Campbell has found providing respondents something unique is an effective strategy:

> When I am collecting data in person, I always bring my homemade chocolate chip cookies, and when I am scheduling phone interviews, I remind people that three interviewees will be randomly selected to be sent a dozen of my cookies. The idea of homemade cookies makes people smile and makes them more apt to show up and/or respond.

In addition, lead author Veronica G. Thomas points out the value of providing something meaningful to participants by soliciting gift donations from vested stakeholders, if the evaluation budget does not provide funds for meaningful incentives:

> In previous surveys of university faculty, response rates were notoriously low, around 10%–15%. To encourage greater participation for a faculty development survey at a particular university, my team and I approached the university provost and requested that his office provide as an incentive six tickets (for three couples) to the university's annual Charter Day Dinner (valued at approximately $1,000 per couple) to raffle off to faculty members who completed the survey by the due date. Our response rate was considerably higher than response rates for this particular faculty body in previous surveys. It seems that having an opportunity to win tickets to this formal gala was a meaningful incentive to this population.

Protection of Human Participants

As was introduced in Chapter 2, ethically and morally, the evaluator has a responsibility to protect those from whom data are being collected and/or used. Acting ethically and morally can also build trust between the evaluator and participants, which can lead to the collection of better data. The fundamental principle of human subjects protection, called the Common Rule, is that people should not (in most cases) be involved in research (or evaluation) without their informed consent, and that participants should not incur increased risk of harm from their involvement, beyond the normal risks inherent in everyday life (U.S. Department of Health and Human Services, 2016). The Common Rule has been codified as the Federal Policy for the Protection of Human Subjects in separate regulations by 15 federal departments and agencies.

Evaluators need to "seek to maximize the benefits and reduce any unnecessary harms that might occur from an evaluation and carefully judge when the benefits from the evaluation or procedure should be forgone because of potential risks" (American Evaluation Association, 2018, pp. 164–165). As was covered in Chapter 2, rules for the protection of human subjects grew out of outrage at research studies in the United States, which put participants at great risk of harm without their informed consent. Informed consent is a voluntary agreement to participate in a study.

> Obtaining consent involves informing the subject about his or her rights, the purpose of the study, the procedures to be undergone, and the potential risks and benefits of participation. . . . The informed consent document must be written in language easily understood by the participant, it must minimize the

possibility of coercion or undue influence, and the subject [sic] must be given sufficient time to consider participation. (Office for the Protection of Human Subjects, 2014, pp. 3–4)

To provide informed consent, individuals have to be able to understand what they are being asked to do and what any potential risks might be. Some people, because of issues such as age or cognitive or emotional impairment, may not be able to give informed consent. However, someone who is able to understand the role an individual would play in the study and who has the legal authority (and, hopefully, the individual's best interests at heart), such as the parent of a young child, can sign on the participant's behalf. In other cases, power dynamics, such as those between an employee and a boss, a prison inmate and a warden, or even a student and a teacher, can raise concerns as to whether consent is truly voluntary. Special precautions must be taken to ensure that the consent is voluntary and that there will be no negative consequences for individuals who choose not to participate or who withdraw from a study.

In general, federally funded research that is or will be collecting or using data from people is required to be reviewed in terms of the potential risk to participants. The U.S. Department of Health and Human Services (n.d., para. 2) defines research as a "systematic investigation . . . designed to develop or contribute to generalizable knowledge," which also describes many evaluations. If a study involves intervention or interacting with individuals and/or the collection of identifiable private information about individuals, then it must be reviewed, regardless of whether the institution has an **institutional review board** to do the reviews. If a study is not classified as research, it does not have to be reviewed. Most colleges and universities and many school districts have their own institutional review boards. If neither the project nor the evaluator has an existing institutional review board, other institutions with institutional review boards will sometimes review research protocols from nonaffiliated community agencies. There are also private companies that review proposed studies for a fee.

Once a proposed evaluation is reviewed, it is classified into one of three levels: exempt, expedited, or full review. An **exempt study**, one that has no or very little risk to participants, still has to be reviewed, but the review is less rigorous and changes can be made to the study without having to get additional permissions. Most social science and educational evaluations, unless they are working with vulnerable populations such as prisoners, children, or pregnant women, are classified as "not research" or are classified at the exempt level. Otherwise, they are usually classified as **expedited studies**, which involve the collection of nonanonymous data that involves no more than minimal risk to those from whom the data are being collected. The third type of study, or **full review**, which requires the most stringent review, is one that does not fit into either the expedited or exempt category because it was deemed to pose more than a minimal risk to participants.

The following is an overview of the federally defined exempt categories, under which most evaluation studies will fall.

> Exempt studies involve human subjects research: research involving a living individual about whom data or biospecimens are obtained/used/studied/analyzed through interaction/intervention, or identifiable, private information is used/studied/analyzed/generated:
>
> > Exemption 1: conducted in an educational setting using normal educational practices.

> Exemption 2: uses educational tests, surveys, interviews, or observations of public behavior. Limited [institutional review board] review may be required.
>
> Exemption 3: uses benign behavioral interventions. Limited [institutional review board] review may be required.
>
> Exemption 4: involves the collection or study of data or specimens if publicly available or recorded such that subjects cannot be identified.
>
> Exemption 5: public service program or demonstration project.
>
> Exemption 6: taste and food quality.
>
> Exemption 7: storage of identifiable information or biospecimens for secondary research use. Broad consent and limited [institutional review board] review are required.
>
> Exemption 8: secondary research use of identifiable information or biospecimens. Broad consent and limited [institutional review board] review are required. (National Institutes of Health, 2019, paras. 1–2)

Determining if an evaluation study needs to be reviewed at all and if so, under what level, can be difficult, and judgments can be subjective. While the categories for qualifying for exempt and expedited studies are standardized, institutional review board policies and procedures differ by institution. The same study may be determined not to be "research" and therefore not have to be reviewed in one institution and determined to be at the exempt level at another institution and in need of review.

When there is any doubt, it is almost always better for the evaluator to contact the institution's institutional review board and follow its guidance. There can be consequences for doing a study without institutional review board approval, including the institution, and increasingly journals, not allowing the results of the study to be published. In extreme cases, federal funding to the institution can be threatened.

Federal agencies and most institutional review boards require those working with human participants to have training in their protection. The National Institutes of Health (n.d.b) does not endorse any specific programs to fulfill the requirement for education on the protection of human participants. The agency believes that institutions are in the best position to determine what programs are appropriate for fulfilling the education requirement. Institutions may require a particular program or may choose to develop a program to meet the requirement. One source of training, used by many colleges and universities, is the **Collaborative Institutional Training Initiative, or CITI** (www.citiprogram.org). To access CITI training, individuals must be affiliated with an institution that has a CITI subscription. In many cases, affiliated can mean working with an institution on a project. In the following activity, readers will read a proposed study, done by coauthor Patricia B. Campbell, and determine risks to participants and how they would categorize the study.

Activity
Exempt, Expedited, Full Review, or Not Research?

The following study was submitted for institutional review board approval. In small groups, decide what the potential for risk is to the human participants. How would you categorize the study? Why did you categorize it in that way?

> The National Institutes of Health has devoted much effort and great financial resources to increasing diversity among biomedical scientists. However, relatively little progress has been made, especially among science faculty. No studies have attempted to determine if this absence of increase in faculty diversity is due to inadequate preparation of trainees, ongoing discrimination, or active decisions of young minority scientists to not pursue academic careers. These possibilities will be studied using interview-based qualitative research methods to,
>
> - with a sample of students from National Institutes of Health–funded training programs across the United States, determine the processes and criteria for career decisions of students at several stages of training;
> - determine how activities of these training programs contribute to students' interests in academic careers;
> - compare the decision making of these students with that of nonminority students in the same or similar biomedical PhD programs; and
> - determine if themes shown to predict students who enter biomedical PhD programs also predict persistence to PhD completion and/or interest in academic careers.

Using Existing Measures or Developing New Ones

When choosing measures to use in an evaluation, evaluators can use an existing measure as is, adapt or modify an existing measure, or develop a new measure. If there are existing measures that are valid, meet the goals of the evaluation, and have been tested with groups who are similar to the target groups, it is better to use them. Developing good measures is not an easy task. It takes a lot of work and skill. And, as indicated earlier, new measures have to be tested for reliability and validity and possibly refined and retested. At an absolute minimum, the measures must be pilot-tested with individuals similar to those with whom the measure will be used.

Sources of Measures

There are a wide variety of developed measures covering many different areas that can be used. One of the most useful sources of measures is the Educational Testing Service (ETS) Test Link, (www.ets.org/test_link/about), a free searchable database of more than 25,000 tests and other measures. It provides information about the measure, validity and reliability references, and how to access the measure—including if it is downloadable and whether there is any cost associated with using it. An indication of the comprehensiveness of the database is that, for example, a search on self-efficacy measures found 63 different measures, and a search on measures of career interest found 16 different measures.

A second repository of measures specifically targets measures used in evaluation. The Online Evaluation Resource Library (http://oerl.sri.com/home.html), is a collection of qualitative and quantitative instruments developed for evaluations of National Science Foundation (NSF) projects. Measures cover such areas as technology, underrepresented populations, laboratory improvement, faculty development, teacher education, and curriculum development. R. L. Jones's (1996) two-volume *Handbook of Tests and Measurements for Black Populations* is a comprehensive resource manual for those who are interested in obtaining instruments, particularly psychological measures, for research with Black populations. Volumes I and II have over 80 survey and other research instruments, some of which include measures with infants, race perception, language perception, noncognitive measures, and a number of other measures that are pertinent to research with African American populations.

There are commercial sources of measures as well. The Mental Measurements Yearbook (https://buros.org/mental-measurements-yearbook) provides descriptive information about hundreds of measures, as well as reviews of the measures and their validity and reliability. The same publisher also has a collection of Tests in Print (https://buros.org/tests-print), which is a bibliography of commercially available tests in English.

Assessing Existing Measures

Before evaluators use any of these measures, it is important to check to see if the measure has content validity for the program or project in which it is going to be used. In addition, it is necessary if check if any tests of validity and reliability were done with populations that are similar to the groups with whom the evaluator will be using the measures. Some repositories like Online Evaluation Resource Library have as part of their mission to provide models for the development of new instruments and encourage evaluators to use or adapt instruments, sections, or individual questions to create instruments that are tailored to their projects. They, rightfully, caution users that sound instrument development requires further piloting of any instrument that has been adapted for use in a context that differs significantly from the context in which it was developed.

Measuring Complex Concepts

As important as it is to have a good, well-developed measure, it is even more important that the measure is measuring the right thing. According to Tom Kibler (personal communication, first quoted in Campbell, Hoey, & Perlman, 2001, p. 34), "Better a bad measure of the right thing, than a good measure of the wrong thing." His reasoning is that one can always improve a bad measure, but if the wrong thing is being measured, it doesn't matter how good the measure is—it's not going to be useful. If, for example, the goal of the project being evaluated is to increase participants' self-worth and there are no good measures of self-worth but there *are* good measures of self-efficacy, it will weaken the evaluation to use a measure of self-efficacy no matter how good it is. When measuring complex concepts, it can be better to use several different measures and report the results from all of them. The activity that follows provides a strategy, developed by coauthor Patricia B. Campbell, to help evaluators think about measures of complex concepts.

> ## Activity
> ### You Can't Measure Love, or Can You?
>
> To help people think more creatively about measures, I say to the group, "You all have someone who loves you, even if it's your dog. How do you know they love you?" As the discussion starts, I write down their answers and at times critique them. For example, if someone says, "They treat me well," I ask, "Treat you well how?" or "What do you mean by that?" Someone will say, "They say they love me." I might ask if that's always true. After about 10 minutes, a variety of responses have been given. I circle three or four and say, "Taken together, now we have a bad measure of the right thing, and we can always make it better."
>
> Take one of the following concepts and, in a small group, using the process just described, brainstorm possible measures and select those you feel are the best (and are measurable):
>
> Trust
>
> Health
>
> Empowerment
>
> Critical thinking
>
> Success

Individual definitions of concepts, including success, may differ including differences in funder and participant definitions. In Goodman, Epstein, and Sullivan's (2018) discussion of domestic violence survivors, they point out that survivors often have complex ways of defining "success" that do not necessarily reflect standardized outcome measures available to researchers. To adequately measure success, the perspectives of the participants and the funders will need to be considered.

Modes of Data Collection

There are five basic modes of data collection that can be used to collect quantitative and qualitative data. One of the most frequently used modes is online data collection. The ease of putting surveys online using tools like SurveyMonkey has made online data collection relatively inexpensive and easy to do. It is useful when data are being collected from many individuals or institutions and the surveys or measures being used are relatively short. Since participants enter their own data electronically, there is no need for the evaluator to do so. The evaluator will still have to check the data for obvious mistakes and inaccuracies. Online data collection is not at all useful for those who don't have web access or have a fear of technology. With an online or web-based data collection system, it is essential for it to be accessible so that data can be collected from people with disabilities.

Accessibility is also an issue with the second mode of data collection, **downloadable data collection templates**. These templates, most often generated in Microsoft Excel (discussed further in Chapter 13) or **Microsoft Access**, are very useful when existing data are being collected because those data can be electronically imported. Templates are also useful when it is important for respondents to be able to check previously submitted data for completeness and accuracy. The templates are less useful for collecting new data and are not useful for respondents with little technical knowledge.

Paper forms are a traditional way to collect data, and they are particularly useful when data are being collected from participants without access to or knowledge of technology. They are also used with other data collection formats to increase response rates. While paper forms are relatively inexpensive to produce, the data collected on paper need to be entered into an electronic template for analysis. The fourth mode, telephone data collection, is useful when more complex, open-ended questions are being asked and where there is a need for probing or follow-up questions. Telephone data collection is also a good way to follow up with nonrespondents.

Because it takes more time than the modes described earlier, collecting data in person is the most expensive mode of data collection and as such is used when there is no other reasonable way to get needed data. It is most often used for observations and focus groups and for in-person interviews when there is reason to believe that telephone interviews won't be as effective.

When collecting data in person, it is important to review the physical space to make sure that the space is both comfortable and inviting to the target groups, including people with disabilities, and does not reflect stereotypes. People's comfort/discomfort in an environment has been found to affect their responses to questions about interest in science, technology, engineering, and mathematics (STEM) fields and careers and their feelings of belonging (Davies, Spencer, & Steele, 2005). For example, women interviewed in a stereotypical male "nerd" space showed less interest in computer science careers than did women in other spaces (Purdie-Vaughns, Steele, Davis, Ditlmann, & Crosby, 2008). And when Black women and men were given a company newsletter that depicted the company as having a moderate amount of minorities, they were more apt to trust the company and feel that they belonged in that company at the same level that white respondents did (Cheryan, Plaut, Davies, & Steele, 2009; Cheryan, Meltzoff, & Kim, 2011). In the following activity, readers review possible data collection methods and make suggestions as to how to improve them.

Activity
Making It Better: Improving Data Collection Techniques

For each of the following data collection strategies, discuss changes that could be made to make the data collection process better and possibly improve response rates:

Using a web-based survey to collect data from residents in the Southwest on reasons why people chose to move into assisted living

Using a paper achievement test survey to collect pre- and posttest data from over 5,000 elementary school students

Data Management

Mapping Data Collection to Project Goals and Objectives

In a way similar to how a table of specification helps evaluators see if all of the concepts are covered and if there are extraneous items, mapping the data being collected to project goals and objectives helps evaluators see if there are data being collected that are not tied to the goals and if there are goals over which no data are being collected (Institute of Medicine Board on Global Health, 2014).

As the following activity, based on a project done by coauthor Patricia B. Campbell, shows, mapping the data to be collected can help the evaluator to see where new data need to be collected.

Activity
Mapping the Data

Match the existing data to the goals and determine what data are being collected but aren't needed and areas in which additional data need to be collected.

Data Currently Collected	Goal I: To build lifelong learners and lifelong users of the library	Goal II: To improve learner persistence rates with focus on increasing intensity of participation	Goal III: To develop program management tools	Goal IV: To develop strategies and support services that assist learners in overcoming barriers to more extensive participation
Comprehensive Adult Student Assessment System (CASAS, used by GED classes)				
Portfolio assessment (used by theme-based family literacy classes, small groups, and one-to-one tutoring groups)				
Participation in library literacy programs				
Attendance with children at story time				
Volunteering in the library				
Using public access computers to improve writing and/or computer literacy skills				
Participation in library community programs				
Input on the design of library programs and facilities from focus groups with learners				
Notes from monthly meetings with all program staff				
Monthly reports from volunteers				

Timing

A major component of **data management** is the timing of the data collection. The funder's deadline for needing the results of the data collection is one of the most important factors to consider when scheduling data collections. Ideally, knowing a funder's needs and timelines allows the evaluator to work backwards and schedule data collection so that there is time to collect and analyze the data, write up the results, and meet the funder's deadlines. This is not always easy or even possible. For example, in an evaluation of an undergraduate or graduate program, the timeline may indicate that institutional data from colleges and universities should be collected at the beginning of the academic year. However, most institutions don't have current data that early in the year, and even when they do have it, they tend to be too busy to give it to an outside agency.

Similarly, at the pre-college level, data collection scheduled during March and April tends to be doomed to failure. March and April are when state standardized tests are given, and it is a rare district that would allow any other student data collection during that period. And even though pre-college students take state standardized tests in the spring, test results are often not available until the fall or even the following winter, further impacting timelines (Campbell & Clewell, 2008).

While other organizations don't work on as strict a calendar as schools and other academic institutions, there are a variety of other factors that impact the timing of data collection including secular and religious holidays, vacations, and conflicts with other tasks, such as the closing of the organization's fiscal year.

Another area to be considered is the expected time for impact. If pre- and posttest data and follow-up data are being collected, then the time period that needs to elapse between the pretest and the posttest needs to be decided early in the process, and there needs to be a rationale to justify the choice. It is important to check if there are differences across target populations in terms of the average length of time it takes to achieve project/program goals. For example, if evaluations are being done on the efficacy of a program in getting graduate students to graduation, it could be important to note that white and Asian students took an average of 7.7 years to receive their PhDs while Black students took an average of 9.5 years (N. Bell, 2010). Similarly, professional advancement for minority workers is also slower. If evaluations in these areas and other areas don't take the time differences into account, they will show larger race/ethnicity differences than is actually the case (J. Jackson & O'Callaghan, 2011). Some possible things that can be done include

- extending the period of the evaluation;
- including benchmark measures/shorter-term measures that are good predictors of the longer term outcomes; and
- scheduling follow-ups with a sample of participants (Campbell & Jolly, n.d.b).

If data are going to be collected more than once, it is important that data collection procedures be consistent over time. This can be facilitated by recording in writing the data collection procedures, including the ways the data collection is being introduced. For interviews and focus groups, if it is at all possible, the same interviewers or focus group facilitators should be used.

Electronic Controls and Data Cleaning

If the data are being collected electronically, a variety of automated data-checking procedures can be incorporated into the data template, to improve the quality of the data, including the following:

Specify data type. Prohibit text when a response should be numerical. Error messages can then be shown on the screen explaining that the answer must be numerical.

Specify data range. Only allow data to be entered within the appropriate range (i.e., if it is a 1–5 scale, only 1, 2, 3, 4, or 5 is accepted). Error messages can then be shown on the screen describing the acceptable range.

Perform calculations. Automate all computations to reduce or eliminate respondent computation errors.

Prohibit contradiction. Do not allow impossible situations. For instance, a school should not have more students graduate than are enrolled. Error messages can then be shown on the screen explaining the problem.

Flag for follow-up. Highlight potentially anomalous situations such as very large increases or decreases in the numbers of students in a year. Email or telephone follow-up can then be done with respondents to check the accuracy of that particular subset of data (Campbell & Clewell, 2008).

No matter how clear questions are and how many electronic controls are added, the data will need to be cleaned. **Data cleaning** is the process of going through the submitted data, looking for inaccuracies, inconsistencies, misunderstandings, duplications, and general data anomalies. It may be the most painful and time-consuming part of the data quality and the general data management process. The most important thing that can be done to make the data cleaning process less painful is create, test, and retest all data forms and data collection templates to make them as clear as possible and easy to understand and complete. However, it is almost guaranteed that there will be some confusion and that data clearing will be needed. Most data cleaning must be done by hand, although some automation may be possible. For example, if names and some sort of individual identification numbers need to be matched across forms, the preliminary matching can be automated, but secondary matching for such anomalies as name shortenings (Susan/Sue, David/Dave), typos, inconsistent use of initials, and others need to be checked by hand.

Privacy

Protection of human participants includes the protection of their privacy, which in turn includes the privacy of the data they provide. The privacy ideal is when the data collected are anonymous; however, that is not possible when it is necessary to track individuals over time or to link individuals in groups. In those cases, an individual's data need to be confidential, and access to any individually identifiable information needs to be minimal. Using unique identification numbers for participants and storing the key that links the numbers and participant names in a place separate from the data files can help with this.

It is key to keep the data themselves secure. This means storing electronic data only in password-protected machines and/or files and not transferring any individually identifiable data over email attachments or unsecured websites. Data either should be transferred through a secure website or should be encrypted or both. Paper data should be secured in locked file cabinets and shredded when they are no longer being used. And, of course, data security and privacy criteria should be applied to any backup procedures that are applied. And these data should be backed up regularly. Evaluators may want to consider storing a copy of the backed-up data either on the cloud or in another location. Most of the data evaluators collect cannot be replicated. If they are lost, the data are gone.

Data Management Plans

It can be useful to put all of these pieces together as part of a data management plan including what will be done with the data after the project is over. At this point, the NSF requires all proposals to have a two-page Data Management Plan (DMP), which describes how the proposal will conform to NSF policy on the dissemination and sharing of research results. The requirements for the plan include

- the types of data, samples, physical collections, software, curriculum materials, and other materials to be produced in the course of the project;
- the standards to be used for data and metadata format and content (where existing standards are absent or deemed inadequate, this should be documented along with any proposed solutions or remedies);
- policies for access and sharing including provisions for appropriate protection of privacy, confidentiality, security, intellectual property, or other rights or requirements;
- policies and provisions for re-use, re-distribution, and the production of derivatives; and
- plans for archiving data, samples, and other research products, and for preservation of access to them. (National Science Foundation, 2014, section j, para. 4)

Regardless of whether an evaluation is funded by the NSF or not, these are things to think about in terms of data management and the archiving of data.

SUMMARY

This chapter focused on data, sources of data, and different ways to define, find, collect, and manage data. It covered ways of assessing measures used to collect data and ways that cultural and other assumptions can impact the quality and even the accuracy of the data being collected. The strengths and weaknesses of different data collection methods were discussed as well as the most appropriate data collection methods for different situations and the importance of high response rates. Forms of validity and reliability of particular concern to evaluators were covered as were sources of existing measures and ways of measuring more complex concepts. The chapter reintroduced the concept of protection of human participants and ways evaluators need to address the protection of people from whom they are collecting data.

As this chapter indicated, there are a number of issues that need to be attended to when collecting data with diverse populations, and, in reality, all populations are diverse. These include considering the collection of at least some qualitative data that can give a voice to those whose stories have not been told and whose experiences have not been valued. The negative experiences that some groups have had with researchers and evaluators needs to be considered, and strategies to acknowledge and deal with that history must be addressed. Measures used in evaluations must be culturally sensitive and must be valid for the populations with whom they will be used. Possible sources of bias need to be addressed and, to the degree possible, minimized. Data do not speak for themselves, nor are they self-evident; they are given voice by those who interpret them. The voices that are heard are not only those who are participating in the project, but also those of the evaluators and others who are interpreting and presenting the data. Deriving meaning from data in program evaluations that are culturally responsive requires people who have some sense of the context in which the data were gathered.

SUPPLEMENTAL RESOURCES

Overview: Data Collection and Analysis Methods in Impact Evaluation

https://www.unicef-irc.org/publications/pdf/brief_10_data_collection_analysis_eng.pdf

Peersman, G. (2014). *Methodological Briefs: Impact Evaluation* No. 10.

This 21-page overview provides a supplementary view of data collection methods and issues.

People or Systems? To Blame Is Human. The Fix Is to Engineer

www.ncbi.nlm.nih.gov/pmc/articles/PMC3115647/

Holden, R. J. (2009). *Professional Safety*, 54(12), 34–41.

This article provides a look at strengths and weaknesses of fixing the individual versus fixing the system from a very different perspective (safety).

Informed Consent in Human Subjects Research

https://oprs.usc.edu/files/2017/04/Informed-Consent-Booklet-4.4.13.pdf

Shahnazarian, D., Hagermann, J., Aburto, M., & Rose, S. (n.d.). University of Southern California Office for the Protection of Research Subjects.

This University of Southern California booklet on informed consent can help evaluators design acceptable informed consent forms.

Code of Federal Regulations Title 45 Public Welfare Department of Health and Human Services Part 46 Protection of Human Subjects

www.hhs.gov/ohrp/humansubjects/guidance/45cfr46.html

These are the National Institutes of Health regulations for the protection of human subjects.

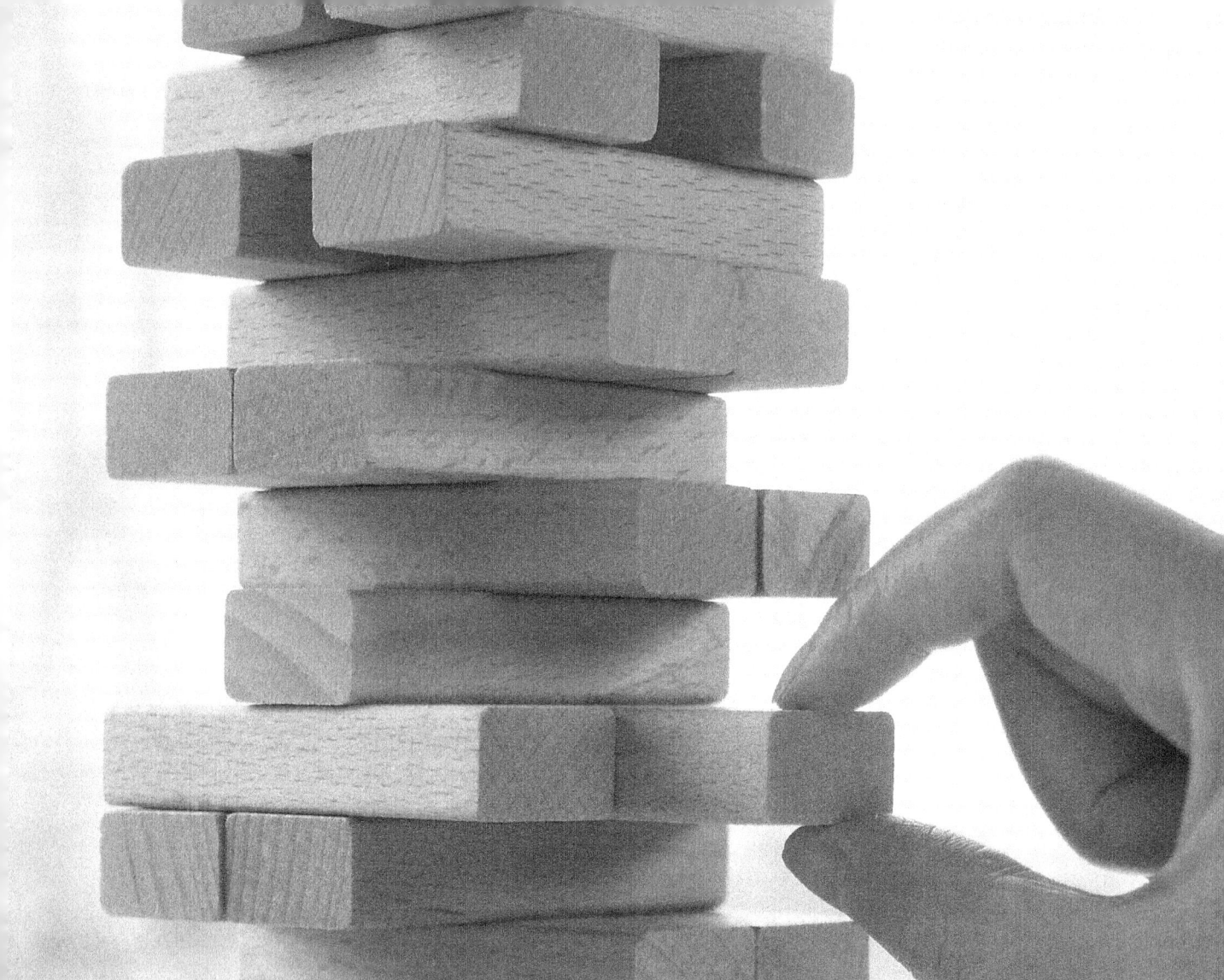
istock/xijian

Evaluators, like other researchers, must discern the best analysis given a number of statistical and methodological considerations. Equally important are considerations of ways to analyze data that uncover inequities that may be hidden from view and reveal findings that can facilitate discussions related to fairness and equity.

CHAPTER 13

The Best Analysis for the Data

As many research and evaluation faculty have found, students tend to be unhappy when quantitative and qualitative analysis topics are introduced. However, when the focus of the instruction is on the basics students need to know so they can make sense of the data they are or will be collecting, everyone becomes a lot happier. This chapter provides readers with those basics.

After reading this chapter and participating in the activities, readers will be able to meet the following learning objectives:

- Differentiate between inductive and deductive reasoning and explain when each should be used as an analytic framework

- Describe the interrelationships among statistical significance, effect size, and statistical power and implications for making Type I and Type II errors

- Describe the level of data being collected as dependent variables and, based on the level of data, suggest appropriate inferential statistics to analyze the data

- Describe the advantages and challenges of disaggregating data based on variables such as sex, race/ethnicity, and age

- Select and describe a qualitative analytic model and use it to code and analyze a sample of textual material

Introduction

This chapter is not meant to replace either a statistics or a qualitative methods textbook. Rather, it provides an overview of some of the assumptions, reasonings, and rationales behind the decisions that are made about the types of analysis used in evaluations. Beginning with an overview of the differences between deductive and inductive reasoning, we go on to an introduction to quantitative and qualitative analysis. The quantitative analysis overview includes those parametric and nonparametric statistics frequently used in evaluations and covers such concepts as statistical significance, effect size, Type I and Type II errors, statistical power, and difference-based and relationship-based analysis. The overview of qualitative analysis includes discussions of coding, codebooks, sample analysis models, and the generation of themes.

Deductive and Inductive Reasoning

An Overview of Deductive and Inductive Reasoning

The two basic types of analytic reasoning are deductive and inductive. **Deductive reasoning** begins with a possible theory or premise that is tied to the theory of change underlying the program to be evaluated. In deductive reasoning, one generally moves from theory to **hypothesis** to observation or another data collection method to confirmation. It is the basis of the scientific method. In deductive reasoning, there are two types of variables, independent and dependent. An **independent variable** is one that is changed or controlled to test the effects on the dependent variable. In evaluation, the intervention is often the independent variable. A **dependent variable** is that which is being measured, usually the outcomes of interest. In an evaluation question such as "What is the impact of participating in a community of practice on mental health professionals' interest in and ability to use behavior modification techniques with clients?" participation in a community of practice is the independent variable, and professionals' interest in and ability to use behavior modification are the dependent variables. In the example evaluation question, the theory of change, described in Chapter 4, or theoretical framework is social learning theory (Lave & Wenger, 1990), and a hypothesis could be "Participation in a community of practice will improve mental health professionals' ability to use behavior modification techniques with clients."

In **inductive reasoning**, which draws general principles from specific instances, the process is reversed. Here, one generally moves from the collected data to patterns based on the data to tentative hypotheses to hypothesis testing to theory. The process begins with observations and/or other collected data. Regardless of whether the data are numbers or words, they are examined to look for possible patterns, similarities, differences, and regularities. These results are then used to generate possible hypotheses, which can be tested and used to generate tentative conclusions and/or theories. As would be expected, inductive reasoning tends to be more exploratory and open ended—that is, evaluators go where the data lead them—while deductive reasoning is more confirmatory—that is, the data either support or don't support what evaluators hypothesize to be the case. The inductive process, however, can never be fully open ended. Decisions need to be made about the data that will be collected, including the questions to be asked, the measures to be used, and (for observations) the protocol to be used. The data collected will influence what is found. As such, when using inductive reasoning, it is particularly important to describe and justify the choices made (Herr, 2007). Trochim (2008) points out there is an interdependence between deductive and inductive reasoning. In inductive reasoning, possible hypotheses are generated that can be tested using a deductive reasoning process. Similarly, when results are found using deductive reasoning, it is useful to examine the results inductively to look for unexpected outcomes that can be used to formulate possible hypotheses to be tested. The case study that follows provides an example of this process.

Case Study
Generating Hypotheses

In an evaluation of an elementary school mathematics program, we found that in some of the schools students in focus groups were complaining about teachers, other than their own teacher, correcting their behavior, asking why they were out in the hall, and generally "getting into their business." From those data, we hypothesized that one of the factors impacting program success was the degree to which teachers felt responsible for the success of all of the students in their school. We then tested the hypothesis and found a relationship.

Source: P. B. Campbell, unpublished evaluation report.

As was covered in Chapter 12, there are two types of data: quantitative and qualitative. These data are analyzed very differently. Maxwell (2010) explains that quantitative data look at the world in terms of variables and correlations and qualitative data view the world in terms of events and processes. While quantitative analysis is often associated with deductive reasoning and qualitative analysis with inductive reasoning, it is possible to analyze qualitative or quantitative data with either reasoning model.

Using Deductive and Inductive Reasoning

When making choices as to whether to begin an evaluation using deductive or inductive reasoning, it is important to determine whether, in the areas to be evaluated, there are enough existing theories, results, and/or conclusions that can be used to generate hypotheses to be tested. This is not usually the responsibility of the evaluator; however, the evaluator may need to review program proposals and other materials and speak with program staff to determine if there is a theory of change and/or philosophy underlying the program and, if so, what it is. If there is, then a deductive reasoning process will be better. If there is not a program theory, then an inductive reasoning process may be better.

There may be times when, even though there are existing theories, inductive reasoning is the more appropriate reasoning to use. This can be the case when the perspective from which the existing theories have been built is skewed or biased. As was covered in detail in Chapter 1, a bias is a tendency that prevents unprejudiced, thoughtful, or deliberate consideration of a question (Pannucci & Wilkins, 2010). Over the past 50 years, considerable attention has been given to the impact of race and gender bias on social science theories (e.g., Gilligan, 1982; Guthrie, 1976, 2004; Shakeshaft et al., 1985). For example, in 1982, Gilligan criticized psychological theory, in general, and moral development theory, specifically, for the degree to which the theories were built based on studies where the participants were all boys and/or men and there was a greater valuing of men's lives and experiences over women's (Gilligan, 2011). Earlier, in 1976, Guthrie, in his book *Even the Rat Was White: A Historical Review of Psychology*, wrote about the infusion of racism in psychology leading to theories like "defective morality is a Negro characteristic," which, as Guthrie said, "undoubtedly laid the foundation for other research in the measurement of morality attributes in minority groups" (p. 43), the ramifications of which still haunt us today.

In 1984, Audre Lorde wrote that the "master's tools will never dismantle the master's house. They may allow us to temporarily beat him at his own game, but they will never enable us to bring about genuine change" (p. 111).

In evaluation as well as many other areas, much of what is known has been based on the theory and methods of the dominant culture and paradigms. As discussed in earlier chapters, the dominant culture often doesn't reflect the lived experience of many people. Trying to use existing theories and literature to define or evaluate those experiences can lead evaluators to incomplete or even inaccurate conclusions. Some, perhaps most, existing theories may be found to reflect the lives and experiences of those who are part of the dominant culture. Examining the experiences of those who are marginalized in the dominant culture, and seeing if those experiences reflect existing theories and results, is very different from starting with existing theory as a frame for understanding their lives and experiences. As is discussed in Chapters 2 and 5, when evaluators use their own perspective as a framework and assume others come from that perspective and fit that framework, misunderstandings can occur, and useful and important information can be lost or ignored. In the activity that follows, readers choose whether they would use inductive or deductive reasoning in an example.

Activity
Using Inductive or Deductive Reasoning

A big-city police department and several community-based organizations are designing a community outreach effort to improve police–community relations. You have been hired to work with them to design and conduct the evaluation. Much of the research conducted on outreach programs has been done by academics or by large research organizations.

When you are designing the evaluation of this community-based effort, you can choose to follow the deductive reasoning model and use existing research to generate and test hypotheses about program effectiveness and program components that make a difference. A second option is to use an inductive reasoning model where all the data are collected and you analyze them to determine potential patterns that can generate potential hypotheses about the more and less effective components.

Would you use an inductive or deductive reasoning model in this evaluation? Remembering that there is no one correct answer, please justify your choice.

Quantitative Analysis

Levels of Quantitative Data

In 1946, psychologist S. S. Stevens developed a classification scale still widely used today. In his classification, there are four different levels of quantitative data: **nominal**, **ordinal**, **interval**, and **ratio**. Understanding the level of the data is key in determining the appropriate statistical analysis to use. Table 13.1 provides a short summary of Stevens's four levels of data.

Table 13.1 Levels of Quantitative Data

Level	Definition	Examples
Nominal	Classification within a category. Labels can be numeric or alphabetic. If numbers are used as labels, they have no numeric value; they are just a unique name for the attribute.	Gender, ethnicity, country of origin
Ordinal	Rankings or order of a set of variables where the difference and/or distance among variables is not defined and cannot be determined if they are equal.	Risk factors (i.e., high, medium, low); student classification (freshman, sophomore, junior, senior); project manager effectiveness (most effective to least effective)
Interval	Along with variables being able to be ranked, the intervals between them are equal.	Grade point average, number of student credit hours
Ratio	Along with ranking and equal intervals, there is a true or absolute zero point.	Height, weight, unemployment rates; number of clients in the past 12 months

In the following activity, readers determine the level for a variety of different types of data.

> ## Activity
> ### Determining Levels of Data
>
> At what level of data would you categorize each of the following variables?
> - Level of education achieved
> - Number of years of education
> - Sexual orientation
> - Socioeconomic status
> - Annual income
> - Political orientation
> - Race
> - Strength of religious preference
> - Fahrenheit temperature
> - IQ (intelligence scale)

For ordinal-, interval-, and ratio-level data, there is a hierarchy of the levels of measurement, with ratio data being at the highest level. The category into which the data are placed is important because it determines the appropriate statistical test that can be used to analyze those data. Generally speaking, it is more advantageous to have higher levels of measurement, such as interval or ratio data, rather than the lower levels of nominal and ordinal data, because at the lower levels of measurement, data analyses tend to be less sophisticated and sensitive. A general rule is for the evaluator to aim for the highest levels of measurement feasible in a quantitative study.

Categorization of variables isn't always simple. Some categories are obvious; for example, money is ratio data because there is a true zero point of no money and the difference between $1 and $2 and between $150 and $151 is the same. Other classifications may be more difficult to determine. One should not automatically assume that nominal data cannot be numbers. Social Security numbers or numbers on a football jersey, for example, consist of numbers that are used as labels and not quantities.

Some things that are often classified at the nominal level may not be nominal data. For example, sexual orientation tends to be classified as nominal-level data. Some who do research on sexual orientation define it as a series of categories and thus nominal data; however, others have concluded that sexual orientation exists along a continuum that ranges from exclusive heterosexuality to exclusive homosexuality (Norris, Marcus, & Green, 2015), which would make it ordinal data. Similarly, level of education achieved (i.e., grade school, high school, some college, undergraduate degree) could be considered nominal data. However, since there are lower and higher levels of education achieved, it could be considered ordinal data.

Activity
Are Attitude Scales Ordinal or Interval Data?

Scales like the following are often used in evaluation.

Please indicate to what extent you are confident that you can complete the following tasks:

	1 = Not at All Confident	2	3 = Somewhat Confident	4	5 = Absolutely Confident
Identify what is known and not known in a problem					

Please indicate the degree to which you agree or disagree with the following statement:

	Strongly Agree	Agree	Neutral	Disagree	Strongly Disagree
Knowing bioinformatics will make me better at solving problems in biology					

The resulting data are at least at the ordinal level. To be interval data, an assumption would have to be made that, for example, the difference between "strongly agree" and "agree" is equal to the difference between "strongly disagree" and "disagree." Whether data are ordinal or interval has a big impact on the statistics that can be used and the conclusions that can be drawn from the analysis.

Would you classify these types of data as ordinal or interval? Why did you choose to classify the data as ordinal or interval?

Source: Adapted from unpublished surveys developed by P. B. Campbell.

In another example, centigrade temperature is at least interval data because the 10-degree difference between 40 and 50 degrees is equal to the 10-degree difference between 20 and 30 degrees. There is a 0 point, but it isn't a "real 0"; 0 degrees is the temperature at which water freezes. Since temperatures can go below 0, it is difficult to think of temperature as ratio data.

In the activity that follows, readers decide the level of data for attitude scales provided.

Descriptive Statistics

In quantitative analysis, data are analyzed using descriptive and inferential statistics. There are four major types of descriptive statistics that describe and summarize numerical data: measures of frequencies, central tendencies, variability, and position. An example of each type is provided as follows.

- *Measures of frequencies*
  - Count
  - Percentage
- *Measures of central tendencies*
  - **Mean** (the sum of the individual scores divided by the number of scores, commonly known as the average)
  - **Mode** (the most frequent score)
  - **Median** (the score in the middle where half of the scores are above it and half below)[1]
- *Measures of variability*
  - **Range** (the difference between the lowest and highest values)
  - **Standard deviation** (the variation among individual scores, computed by taking the square root of the averages of the squared differences from the mean)[2]
  - **Variance** (the square of the standard deviation)[3]
- *Measures of position*
  - **Quartile** (the data divided into four equal groups by value)
  - **Percentile** (the value below which a number of the data points fall—for example, half of the scores fall below the 50th percentile)

---

[1] In a normal distribution (a bell-shaped, symmetrical graph), the mean, mode, and median have the same value.
[2] In a normal distribution, about two-thirds of the scores are within one standard deviation from the mean.
[3] The standard deviation is in the same scale as the mean or the original data (e.g., feet or dollars) while the variance is the scale squared (e.g., square feet or number of dollars squared).

Descriptive statistics are at the heart of quantitative analysis. They provide information about the data and, because they summarize the data, make it easier to understand what is in the data and what the data say. The case study that follows is an example of the value of summarizing data.

Case Study
Summarizing Data

An evaluator asked health aides to rate the value of a two-day professional development workshop on a scale of 1 (*not at all useful*) to 5 (*very useful*). Their responses were as follows:

4 5 4 4 1 3 3 2 2 4 5 4 5 4 3 4 3 3 4 5

The mean is 3.6, the standard deviation is 1.05, the range is 1–5, the mode is 4, and the median is 4.

Descriptive statistics describe or summarize data; they do not indicate what can be inferred from the data. That is the role of the inferential statistics described next.

Inferential Statistics and Statistical Significance

Inferential statistics are designed to determine the odds (probability) that the descriptive statistical results from the group being analyzed (the sample) are real or random. To determine the "reality" of the results, their statistical significance needs to be computed. This is the likelihood that similar results would be found with a similar group in a similar situation. It is an estimation of the probability that the results were due to chance. Statistical significance does not indicate if a result is meaningful in a "real-world" sense, nor does it indicate how big any differences might be. It determines if a result is real, as in most likely able to be replicated. If the results are real, then they can be generalized to the broader group the sample represents (the population). While generalizability might not be the predominant concern in every evaluation study, Mark (2011) stresses that most evaluators hope or presume that evaluation findings have some implications beyond those directly involved with the evaluation and that, at the very least, evaluators hope that evaluation findings have meaningful implications for decisions about similar programs in the near future in the same or similar settings. Inferential statistics can help with that.

In inferential statistics, the standard for the acceptable level of chance, statistical significance, has been $p < .05$. The American Statistical Association informally defines a *p*-value as "the probability under a specified statistical model that a statistical summary of the data (e.g., the sample mean difference between two compared groups) would be equal to or more extreme than its observed value" (Wasserstein & Lazar, 2016, p. 131). In other words, the *p*-value is the probability that if the same data are collected from comparable samples, the results will be basically the same. The probability of $p < .05$ is not a magic number, nor is it an official standard; rather, it is a commonly accepted standard. In 1926, Fisher, the author of the statistical significance tables that continue to be widely reproduced in statistics textbooks, justified the $p < .05$ standard by explaining "it is convenient to draw the line at about the level at which we can say: Either there is something in the treatment, or a coincidence has occurred such as does not occur more than once in twenty trials" (p. 504). He acknowledged that some might feel that a 1-in-20 chance that the findings were not replicable was not rigorous enough and explained:

> If one in twenty does not seem high enough odds, we may, if we prefer it, draw the line at one in fifty (the 2 per cent point), or one in a hundred (the 1 per cent point). Personally, the writer prefers to set a low standard of significance at the 5 per cent point, and ignore entirely all results which fail to reach this level. (Fisher, 1926, p. 504)

Tests of statistical significance can be one- or two-tailed. In a one-tailed test, the evaluator is determining, for example, whether Program A is more effective than Program B. In a two-tailed test, the evaluator is determining if the effectiveness of

Program A is different from that of Program B—either more or less effective. In a two-tailed test, two tests of significance are done—one for either direction. Therefore, for the two-tailed test, to be significant at $p < .05$, each test in either direction has to be significant at $p < .025$ (UCLA Institute for Digital Research and Education, n.d.).

Statistical significance is related to sample size. Same-size differences in groups or relationships between variables are more apt to be statistically significant with larger sample sizes. This is because of the assumption that larger samples are more representative of the population to which the results will be generalized. In addition, levels of significance accumulate. Since statistical significance testing is based on a probability, the more statistical tests that are done, the more likely it is that some incorrect statistically significant results will be found (Hopkins, 2000). This is called **family-wise error rate** (Statistics How To, 2016). It is the probability of coming to at least one false conclusion in the series of statistical tests being run. If enough tests are run, it very likely that at least one of the statistically significant results will be false. Therefore, it is important to have a reason for doing each test that is done.

While it is important to be aware of family-wise error rate, it can also be used as a reason for not disaggregating the data in ways to look at possible differential program impacts on subgroups.

> For example, the Office of Adolescent Health evidence review excludes results of subgroup analysis of age and race/ethnicity categories. This exclusion arises out of concern for inflated error related to multiple comparisons but may have the effect of dismissing relevant and rigorous evidence that can be critical to understanding the impact of interventions across the developmental spectrum (e.g., enhanced impact of prevention efforts earlier in adolescence) or within specific ethnic/cultural populations, such as AIAN [American Indian and Alaska Native] communities. (Whitesell, Sarche, Keane, Mousseau, & Kaufman, 2018, p. 44)

Parametric and Nonparametric Statistics

Statistical significance is an important component of both of the two major types of inferential statistics: parametric and nonparametric statistics. **Parametric statistics** require that the data be interval or ratio data, while **nonparametric statistics** can be done over all levels of data. Unlike parametric statistics, nonparametric statistics do not assume that the data are **normally distributed**—that is, reflect the "bell curve." Nonparametric statistics can also be used with smaller sample sizes. In general, nonparametric statistics are less powerful than parametric statistics, which means they are less apt to find significant results. If data meet the requirements for parametric statistics, it is usually better to use them. Table 13.2 lists some common, comparable parametric and nonparametric statistics and when they can be used.

When comparisons are made between two groups and statistically significant results are found, it is clear where the differences are. However, when there are significant differences across more than two groups, additional statistical tests, called post hoc tests because they are done after the initial significance testing, must be done to determine where the differences occurred between individual groups. Post hoc tests are designed so they don't contribute to the family-wise error rate. Commonly used post hoc tests include the Newman-Keuls method, the Scheffé test, and Duncan's multiple-range test (Statistics How To, 2016).

Table 13.2 Using Common Parametric and Nonparametric Statistics

Task	Parametric Test*	Nonparametric Test
Test for differences between two related samples (i.e., pretest/posttest)	*t*-test for dependent samples	McNemar test
Test for differences among two or more related samples (i.e., pretest/posttest with comparison groups)	Analysis of variance with repeated measures	Friedman test**
Test for differences between two independent samples (i.e., posttest with treatment and comparison group)	*t*-test for independent samples	Chi-square test, Mann-Whitney test**
Test for differences among two or more independent samples (i.e., comparisons among people from five demographic regions)	Analysis of variance	Chi-square test, Kruskal-Wallis test**
Test for differences among two or more groups with two independent variables (i.e., comparisons among high- and low-income people from five demographic regions)	Two-way analysis of variance	
Test for correlations (i.e., the relationship between program participation and individual change)	Correlation coefficient	Spearman rank correlation

* Requires data at the interval level or above
** Requires data at the ordinal level or above
Source: Adapted from McKillup (2012) and Siegel (1956).

As the following case study shows, while evaluators may have their analysis planned out, when the design changes, the analysis most likely must change as well.

Case Study
An Accidental Design: The Analysis

As the design in Chapter 11's accidental design example (see page 345) changed, the analysis did as well. The initial design was $O\ X_{a,b,c}\ O$, where O represents the measures and X represents the intervention. What was being evaluated was the impact of a three-component model on scores on a GED (general equivalency diploma) preparedness test. This design could be analyzed using a related-samples *t*-test. That would tell if there were a significant pretest–posttest difference.

If the evaluator wanted to break out the results by site, then an analysis of variance (ANOVA) with repeated measures would be used. That would tell if there were

- a significant pretest/posttest difference;
- a significant difference among the different sites; or

- a significant interaction between site and pretest–posttest change—that is, if the program were more effective in some sites than in others.

Since some sites didn't implement all three components of the model, the design became this:

$$O\ X_{a,b,c}\ O$$
$$O\ X_{a,b}\ O$$
$$O\ X_{a,c}\ O$$

With this design, a two-way ANOVA with repeated measures, where one factor is the different sites and the other the exposure to different components of the model, would be used. That would tell if there were

- a significant pretest–posttest difference;
- a significant difference among the different sites;

- a significant difference based on the components used;
- a significant interaction between sites and pretest–posttest change;
- a significant interaction between pretest–posttest change and the components of the model implemented;
- a significant interaction between sites and the components of the model implemented; or
- a significant interaction among pretest–posttest change, sites, and the components of the model implemented.

If the measure were number of participants getting their GEDs after being exposed to different components of the model, as in the following design, the chi-square test would be used.

$$X_{a,b,c} \quad O$$
$$X_{a,b} \quad O$$
$$X_{a,c} \quad O$$

The chi-square test would tell if there were significant differences in the numbers of participants receiving GEDs in terms of the program components implemented.

Effect Size

In both parametric and nonparametric statistical analysis, statistical significance is one of the first factors to be considered when interpreting data results. However, it is key to remember statistical significance is *not* a measure of the size of the results but, rather, a measure of the likelihood that the results are replicable and not due to chance. Statisticians can agree on a level at which results are statistically significant (i.e., $p < .05$), but it is up to the individual evaluator, stakeholder, and client to determine if significant results are *meaningful*—that is, if the results are large enough to indicate if a program or an intervention is successful. As Gene V. Glass pointed out, "Statistical significance is the least interesting thing about the results. You should describe the results in terms of measures of magnitude—not just, does a treatment affect people, but how much does it affect them" (quoted in Sullivan & Feinn, 2012, p. 279).

One way of determining the size of the difference or relationship is through the computation of the effect size. **Effect size** is a simple way of quantifying the size of the difference between two groups where the differences have been found to be statistically significant (Coe, 2002). In social science and educational research and evaluation, one of the most common effect size computations is **Cohen's *d***, which is computed by subtracting the mean score of one group from the mean score of another group, then dividing by the standard deviation (Becker, 2000). Because Cohen's *d* is based on means and standard deviations, it can only be done with data that are interval or ratio. There are a number of online effect size calculators, including https://lbecker.uccs.edu/. Most statistical package programs also compute effect sizes. Some effect size computations can be done with nonparametric statistics, but they aren't well known, nor are they included in most statistical software packages.

Once the effect size is computed, it is still necessary to interpret what it means. One way to do that is to compare the effect size found to the effect sizes of differences that are familiar to people (Coe, 2002). For example, as Table 13.3 indicates, Cohen (1969, p. 23) calls an effect size of 0.2 "small" and explains that this reflects the difference between the heights of 13-year-old and 14-year-old American girls. In this example, one might see that there is little difference in height of 13- and 14-year-old girls, but it is so small that

Table 13.3 Cohen's (1969) Effect Size Interpretation

Effect Size (*d*) Found	Interpretation	Example
.20	Small	Difference in the heights of 13-year-old and 14-year-old girls
.50	Medium	Difference in the heights of 14-year-old and 18-year-old girls
.80	Large	Difference in the heights of 13-year-old and 18-year-old girls

you can only detect it through careful investigation. An effect size of 0.5, he describes, is "medium" and reflects the difference between the heights of 14-year-old and 18-year-old girls. Cohen describes an effect size of 0.8 as "grossly perceptible and therefore large" and equates it to the difference between the heights of 13-year-old and 18-year-old girls.

In this example, the difference in the height of 13- and 18-year-old girls is generally so large and consistent that you can observe the difference without much careful investigation. Cohen (1988) originally set values to interpret effect sizes because, at that time, there were no guidelines available. He warned that these values were somewhat arbitrary and stressed that the benchmark values were "recommended for use only when no better basis for estimating the index is available" (p. 25).

If an effect size is small, medium, or large, this can influence whether the evaluator, project staff, or other stakeholders consider the results as meaningful. However, Patterson (2018a) reminds us to be careful about the tyranny of quantification. Decisions cannot be made on a purely numeric basis, and judgment is needed to interpret the findings. Interpretations of the data should be based on substantive, theoretical, and conceptual considerations and not made on a purely statistical basis. "One such consideration is how the effect sizes compare to those of other interventions that seek to produce the same effect" (Glass, McGaw, & Smith, 1981, p. 104). Findings may be meaningful but not practical. Factors affecting whether the results have practical significance include cost of the intervention, interest of those in the target audience in participating in the intervention, and availability of those needed to implement the intervention. For example, the statistical analysis may show that the intervention group did significantly better than the comparison group on the outcome of interest and the effect size was medium. However, the project administrator may conclude that changing from the usual treatment to the new treatment (i.e., intervention) is not practical given its costs and the fact that the project will then have to serve fewer clients.

Effect sizes are useful for finding the magnitude of group differences. Means, standard deviations, and effect sizes, however, can mask individual results. As shown in the activity that follows, group data may represent numbers of participants not changing or even changing in a negative direction. In the activity, readers explore differences when the analysis focuses on group versus individual data.

Activity
Analyzing Group and Individual Differences

A project funded by a private foundation had a primary goal to increase math teachers' use of engineering and other math-related career materials in their classrooms. Teachers attended a one-week summer workshop where teams of teachers worked together to develop materials that could be used in their classes. As part of the evaluation, 108 teachers rated their use of engineering and other math-related career materials in their classrooms prior to their participation in the workshop and nine months later.

The data found that, on average, on a scale of 1 (*never*) to 4 (*almost always*), teachers increased their self-reported use of these measures from an average of 2.4 to 2.6. The level of statistical significance of the change was $p < .001$, and the effect size was .31.

Is this change enough for the evaluator to conclude the intervention worked?

In the same project, when individual teacher change was examined, it was found that

- 50% of the teachers increased their use of engineering and other math-related career materials;
- 23% of the teachers did not change their behavior; and
- 27% of the teachers decreased their use of engineering and other math-related career materials.

Individually or in small groups, please answer the following questions:

- Is this change enough for the evaluator to conclude the intervention worked?
- Did the type of analysis done impact your answer?
- Did knowing that for some teachers there was a negative effect on their behavior impact your answer?
- Does the positive change among 50% of the teachers outweigh the negative change in 27% of teachers?

Source: Adapted from P. B. Campbell and Carsen, unpublished evaluation report.

Decision Error and Statistical Power

Since hypothesis testing is not flawless, within quantitative analysis there are two possible decision errors, Type I and Type II. A **Type I error**, also known as a false positive, occurs when an effect was concluded as real but it was not. Type I errors are controlled for with the selection of a level of statistical significance. The greater the concern with making a Type I error, the more stringent the level of significance should be (i.e., choosing a level of $p < .001$ rather than a level of $p < .05$). A **Type II error**, also known as a false negative, occurs when an effect that is real wasn't found. As will be described later in the chapter, a Type II error can be controlled for by the level of **statistical power** applied. In evaluation, there can be real consequences when a Type I or Type II error is made (see Table 13.4). A Type I error can lead to decision makers not making needed changes or scaling up an intervention that isn't effective. A Type II error can result in decisions not to implement an effective intervention.

Statistical power is the probability that if there is a real effect, it will be found. Four variables are involved in computing statistical power: effect size (estimated), sample size, level of statistical power (which ranges from 0 to 1), and level of probability (most frequently .05) (P. Ellis, 2010). Knowing three of the four variables allows the computation of the fourth. The easiest way to compute statistical power is to enter the estimated effect size, the sample size, and the probability level into an online statistical

Table 13.4 Evaluator's Decision From Hypothesis Testing and Decision Errors

Statistical Decision by Evaluator	True State of the Null Hypothesis (Reality)	
	True	False
Reject Null Hypothesis	Type I Error	Correct Decision
Do Not Reject Null Hypothesis	Correct Decision	Type II Error

power calculator (e.g., www.danielsoper.com/statcalc/calculator.aspx?id=49). Sample size makes a big difference when statistical power is being computed. For example, with an estimated effect size of .5 and a level of probability of .05, for a sample of 30 the statistical power level is .4 while for samples of 100 and above the statistical power level increases to .8.

Hypothesis Testing

When thinking about the relationships among statistical significance, effect size, and power, it is important to understand that there are actually two competing hypotheses being considered. The hypothesis, based on earlier work or beliefs about the impacts of an evaluation, is called the **alternative hypothesis**. The other hypothesis is called the **null hypothesis**, or the hypothesis of no difference or no relationship. In inferential statistical analysis, the null hypothesis is tested. If the evidence is strong enough that there is statistical significance, then the null hypothesis is rejected, and the alternative hypothesis is accepted. If there are no significant differences, the null hypothesis is not accepted; instead, it "fails to be rejected." Failing to be rejected does not mean there are no differences or no relationships between groups. It means the probability that any differences found are due to error or chance is too high to be acceptable. If the alternative hypotheses are not accepted, it doesn't mean that the program staff are wrong or that the intervention was not effective; it means that there was insufficient statistical evidence to accept the hypothesis. If there are significant results, then it is often felt that there are results worth reporting, while if no statistical significance is found, the probability of being wrong is too high to report findings. Studies with statistically significant findings are even more likely to be submitted for publication and to be published (Hubbard & Armstrong, 1992).

It is tempting to report results as "approaching significance," but that is something to be very careful about. Evaluators have to ask themselves, "How big a chance do I want to take that I will be wrong?" The answer is dependent, in part, on the question being asked and the possible consequence of being wrong. In the evaluation of a program designed to facilitate weight loss, an evaluator might be willing to accept a level of significance of 1 chance in 10 of being wrong ($p < .1$). If there are greater consequences to making an error, say, in a program for recovering drug addicts, the evaluator may choose a more stringent level of significance such as 1 chance in 100 ($p < .01$) or even 1 chance in 1,000 ($p < .001$).

Difference-Based and Relationship-Based Analysis

In evaluation, the analytic process is often based on a search for differences. As was covered in Chapter 11, evaluation designs are often set up to look for pretest–posttest differences and/or differences between those who were in a particular program (i.e., the intervention) and those who were not. Evaluators often look at differences across different subgroups, as in whether there are differences in the responses of women and men or between high- and low-achieving students. Additionally, *t*-tests are used to look at differences between two groups, while ANOVA is used to look at differences among two or more groups over two or more variables.

Evaluators also look at relationships between variables. For example, one might be interested in the relationship or correlation between family income and response to diversity training or between grade point average and attendance at optional tutoring sessions. Correlations determine the strength of a relationship and whether it is positive (when the value of one variable increases, the other increases as well) or negative (when the value of one variable increases, the other decreases). Correlations range from −1.0 (*a perfect negative relationship*) through 0 (*no relationship*) to +1.0 (*a perfect positive relationship*). The correlation indicates if a relationship is present, it doesn't imply causality; that is, it does not indicate that a change in one variable causes a change in the other. For example, there is a strong correlation between the amount of ice cream sold and the amount of sunscreen sold; however, there are no data to indicate that an increase in the amount of ice cream sold caused the increase in sunscreen sales, or vice versa. Another factor—the weather—is most likely behind the correlation. When it is hot and sunny, people are more apt to buy ice cream and sunscreen; when it is cold and snowing, they are less likely to do so.

That example is silly; however, confusing correlation with causality can cause real harm. For example, in the 1800s, a strong negative correlation was found between women's level of education and the number of children that they had. It was concluded that this relationship was causal and that higher education caused women's uteruses to atrophy, leading them to have fewer children. This research was used as an argument against women's education for years (Clark, 1873/1972). The more probable causes, such as more highly educated women being less apt to be married and more apt to be aware of methods of avoiding pregnancy, which may have contributed to the correlation, were not considered. Much more recently, the correlation between race/ethnicity and incarceration rates has been used to conclude that being from a certain ethnic group causes one to be a criminal (Ye Hee Lee, 2015). Again, the more probable causes that were not considered include cross-race/ethnicity income disparities that impact ability to get a good lawyer, the different level of sentencing for the same or similar crimes, and racial/ethnic differences between who is arrested and who gets a warning for the same actions.

Another way of analyzing relationships is through social network analysis, which is

> the mapping and measuring of relationships and flows between people, groups, organizations, computers, URLs, and other connected information/knowledge entities. The nodes in the network are the people and groups while the links show relationships or flows between the nodes. [Social network analysis] provides both a visual and a mathematical analysis of human relationships. (Krebs, n.d., para. 1)

The case study that follows provides an example of a simple social network analysis.

> ## Case Study
> ### A Simple Social Network Analysis
>
> As part of an evaluation of a program to increase faculty collaboration, we looked at the degree to which nine faculty were working with faculty from other departments on the development of grant proposals. The letters are the faculty initials. The lines indicate which faculty are collaborating on grant proposals with other faculty. As the following illustration indicates, seven of the nine faculty have three or more collaborations. SH is the outlier having only one collaboration, and that is with AB who has the most collaborations, with only SH and LQ not collaborating with AB. Without AB, the collaboration pattern would look quite different.
>
>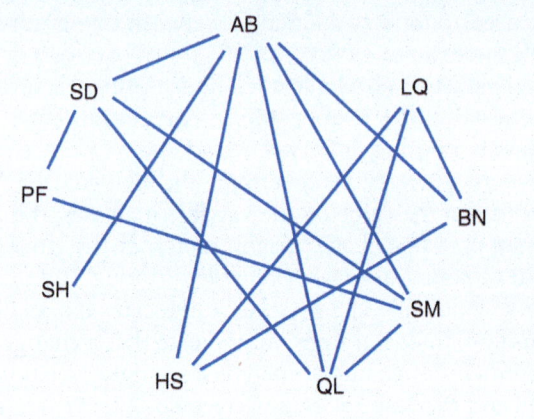
>
> *Source:* Adapted from P. B. Campbell, unpublished evaluation report.

Regardless of whether one is looking at differences or relationships, for quantitative data it can be useful to "play" with the data first. This playing can include graphing, using scatterplots, putting the data in tables, switching table columns and rows, or using ratios, modes, and medians as well as means and standard deviations. Playing with data can help evaluators determine the statistical analysis to use. It can also help them determine if they need to be concerned with **statistical regression**. This can occur when participants score at the highest or lowest level of a measure, be it one of achievement, behavior, or personality. In such cases, when measures are given a second time, there is a tendency toward pseudo-changes in outcomes, which is the lowering of extremely high scores and the raising of extremely low scores (regressing toward the average score). Playing with the data can help evaluators see if, in a pretest/posttest design, the differences are primarily caused by declines in the highest scores or increases in the lowest scores, which may mean that the change is due to statistical regression (D. Campbell & Stanley, 1963).

Disaggregating Data

A good evaluation looks at what works for whom in what context, which means a number of decisions need to be made about the ways the data can, or should, be disaggregated. Very often, data are disaggregated by such demographic variables as race, ethnicity, gender, or disability status. While this can provide very useful information, a number of issues need to be addressed, including intersectionality. Lexico.com (2020b) defines intersectionality, introduced in Chapter 1, as the "interconnected nature of social categorizations such as race, class, and gender as they apply to a given individual or group, regarded as creating overlapping and interdependent systems of discrimination or disadvantage" (para. 1). The term was first coined by Kimberlé Crenshaw

(1991), who "used the concept of intersectionality to denote the various ways in which race and gender interact to shape the multiple dimensions of Black women's employment experiences" (p. 1244). In the activity that follows, readers explore some of the different characteristics that define them.

> ### Activity
> Who Am I?
>
> Take 30 seconds to write down all the characteristics that define you. Then, in small groups, share your characteristics.

Everyone is defined by more than one characteristic. Gender, race, age, geographic location, socioeconomic status, educational level, hobbies—these are just some of the characteristics that define us as individuals. Breaking out the data by only one characteristic, such as gender, means that we don't look at interactions between gender and other demographic characteristics and therefore the results can be incomplete or inaccurate. Data are often disaggregated by gender and by race/ethnicity separately and reported out for "women and people of color" or for "women and minorities." However, as Niemann (2015, para. 2) points out,

> the phrases "women and minorities" and "women and people of color" can be seen and heard daily in newspaper articles, statistical reports, political rhetoric, and organizational statements in support of diversity. Yet the use of these phrases is highly problematic because these phrases irreverently and visibly ignore the reality that women of color are women *and* people of color—and they are also minorities. The phrases, thus, make women of color invisible while defining [W]hite women as the de facto norm. They minimize the intersectional realities that both link and separate [W]hite women, men of color, and women of color.

Demographic characteristics interact with other variables such as socioeconomic status, individual and family educational backgrounds, immigrant status, and place of residence. For example, in 2016, the Pew Research Center found the median net worth for white households was $171,000, while it was $20,600 for Hispanic households and $17,100 for Black households (Kochhar & Cilluffo, 2017), and the 2006 American Community Survey found median earnings for individuals who were able-bodied totaled over $28,000 compared to a $17,000 median income for individuals with disabilities (American Psychological Association, 2013).

There can be heterogeneity within subgroups as well. For example, people who are visually impaired, hearing impaired, or learning disabled are all classified as having disabilities; however, the differences among them are great, and often it might be appropriate to disaggregate by different categories of disability. Unless such differences are addressed, in any analysis, there is a great danger of generating inaccurate conclusions.

There are important reasons to disaggregate the data as much as possible, but there are statistical and privacy limitations to the amount of disaggregation that can be done. Cell size is an important factor in determining the degree to which disaggregation can be done. When disaggregating data by gender and by race/ethnicity, the number in one cell is the number of white women. The number of Black men is in another cell, and so on. If some cell sizes are very small at a specific level of disaggregation, then statistical analysis at that level may not be appropriate. For example, a nonparametric statistical test such as a chi-square test requires a minimum expected value of 5 for each cell to be valid (J. McDonald, 2014). For parametric statistical tests such as *t*-tests, a cell size of 30 is considered the minimum. In addition, in parametric statistics, as indicated earlier, the smaller the sample or cell size, the more difficult it is to obtain statistical significance (Wikibooks, 2020). This can be an opportunity to use the power analysis described earlier.

There are several techniques that evaluators can use to help determine the levels of aggregation and disaggregation that can be done. These include the following:

> Use crosstabs to break down the demographic characteristics of participants to help determine where levels of disaggregation can be done. If almost all of the participants are from one demographic subcategory, for example, the middle class, then it is not necessary nor [is it] perhaps appropriate to disaggregate data for analysis by socioeconomic status. However, the results could not then be generalized to other socioeconomic groups. . . .
>
> Do preliminary analysis of subgroup differences in areas of importance to the study. This can help inform disaggregation and aggregation decisions.
>
> There may be some cases where disaggregation is not needed. As Jolly explained, "when you mix ammonia and Clorox in a room, everyone gets sick. At that level it is not necessary to disaggregate." (Campbell & Jolly, n.d.g, paras. 1, 5–6)

Another technique is to review the literature tied to program goals to determine if there is potential for differential project/program impact for different subgroups and therefore a need for disaggregation. For example, since women students tend to exhibit lower skills in some spatial areas, such as 3D rotation, that are important to success in engineering (Metz, Donohue, & Moore, 2012), projects/programs tying improved spatial skills to increased retention in engineering should disaggregate their data by sex to determine if there are statistically significant interactions between sex and impact of program participation in a spatial skills training program. Too, since drug use is tied to prison recidivism, in an evaluation of a program to reduce recidivism the data may need to be disaggregated on participant previous drug use.

When findings do not reflect other work, it may be useful to explore if there are other variables by which the results should be disaggregated. For example, while being interviewed for this book, Jane Butler Kahle (personal communication, August 24, 2018) described an example where achievement data from white students in one school district did not reflect the data from comparable school districts in the rest of the state. The evaluator and the school administrators met together to discuss what might be behind the differences. In the district, it was found that a number of the students were from one geographic subregion. They then disaggregated the data by subregion and found white students from one subregion were scoring significantly lower than others, which had a major impact on recommendations for changes in the project.

For statistical reasons and often for confidentiality, some aggregation of data needs to be done even though information will be lost in each aggregation. For example, when aggregation is done across disability groups, the ability to determine if a project/program has different impacts on people with learning disabilities and people with mobility impairment is lost. Another example shows the aggregation of Indigenous

Peoples with other groups because of their small numbers means that less is known about Indigenous Peoples. While evaluators must assume responsibilities for capturing and correctly interpreting within-group variability for the groups under study (Nelson-Barber, LaFrance, Trumbull, & Aburto, 2005), types of disaggregation must be both meaningful and viable. If, for example, there is an interest in trend data, aggregation across years is not appropriate. If there is reason to think there might be different trends for different subgroups, it is important to disaggregate by those subgroups. As indicated in the earlier example, since there are gender differences in some spatial skills, if you are interested in the impact of a project/program to improve spatial skills, then it is important to disaggregate by gender. Based on the questions to be answered, it might be more appropriate to aggregate across subdisciplines, institutions, years, or some racial/ethnic or disability categories. Regardless of the choices that are made, it is important to provide a rationale for the decisions regarding which demographic categories are aggregated and which are disaggregated. In the activity that follows, readers determine the levels of disaggregation they would choose in different evaluations.

Activity
Disaggregating Data

For each of the following evaluation questions, please indicate how you would disaggregate the data and why.

- What is the relative impact of (a) financial support alone and (b) financial support and community-based counseling on first-time offenders' rates of recidivism?
- What is the impact of mandated company training on company harassment policies on employee turnover?
- What is the impact of academic and social supports on first-year engineering student retention?

This has been a basic overview of quantitative analysis that focuses on understanding some underlying concepts and assumptions and introducing some common inferential statistics. A wide variety of other statistics can be used that are beyond the scope of this chapter. They include, to name a few, regression, which describes the relationship between a dependent variable and one or more independent variables; cluster analysis, which combines sets of data in groups or clusters where they are more similar to each other, on some characteristic, than they are to others; and multivariate analysis, where the analysis involves more than one dependent variable.

A number of statistical package programs are available that can be used in quantitative analysis. The following are four of the most common quantitative statistical packages (University of South Australia, n.d.):

- **Microsoft Excel** (part of Microsoft Office) is easy to use and can be exported into other Microsoft products and other statistical packages. Its graphs are very good. However, while Microsoft Excel can compute many basic statistics, the need to perform more sophisticated statistical analyses requires the purchase of add-ons.
- **SPSS** (Statistical Package for the Social Sciences) is a commercial analytic package that is easy to learn and use. It focuses on statistical methods

mainly used in the social and behavioral sciences and market research. It excels at descriptive statistics, basic regression analysis, and ANOVA, and has some newer techniques such as classification and regression trees (CARTs). SPSS allows the user to generate reports and offers tables and charts for reporting.

- **SAS (Statistical Analysis System),** another commercial package, is more powerful but harder to learn and use than SPSS. Users must have some knowledge of code and be able to write lines of code to perform some SAS tasks. SAS is a statistical programming language, and it does not, like SPSS, allow users the copy and paste functionality for tables and charts.

- **R** is a free statistical programming language and environment. It is open source and free to use, and probably best used by people who have a reasonable knowledge of statistical analysis and programming.

Qualitative Analysis

Qualitative data have been described by Miles and Huberman (2009) as a source of well-grounded, rich descriptions and explanations of processes in identifiable local contexts. Flick, Von Kardorff, and Steinke (2004) describe qualitative methods as being concerned with how human behavior can be explained within the framework of the context where that behavior takes place. As covered in Chapter 12, qualitative data and analyses are used in evaluation to explore and explain the why and the how and to understand the context. Qualitative research methods can play a useful and powerful role in program evaluation. While this line of inquiry is currently receiving wider acceptability in the evaluation community, qualitative evaluations are still frequently misunderstood, which can give support to the stereotype that qualitative inquiry is not as rigorous or credible as quantitative methods and thus is of limited value. Qualitative methods in program evaluation focus on "how" and "why" questions rather than the "how many" and "how much" questions of quantitative inquiry. Further, qualitative inquiry is often used to capture participants' lived experiences and the meaning they attribute to those experiences. This approach has been used frequently when seeking to understand the experiences of people of color in programs from a culturally responsive perspective. In her Voices From the Field interview, Katrina L. Bledsoe discusses some things evaluators should consider when they are making decisions about the analytic procedures to use.

Voices From the Field

Katrina L. Bledsoe: Making Analytic Choices

Communities know best what information they want to gather and, by extension, what sources to gain that information are most credible to them. If the information gathered is credible, then they will be more apt to believe. If they don't want to believe the information, they won't, regardless of how well the evaluation is conducted and what data are yielded. Knowing what is considered credible evidence helps evaluators make decisions about the kinds of methods that they might use. In my experience, while community members often resonate with and trust qualitative data more, they want quantitative data to be collected and analyzed as well. The evaluator is hired to work with the team to help them understand or figure out what is considered valid and credible within that context and community, and to test the accuracy of the interpretations. Working within communities and with the stakeholders, the evaluator takes the lead on the analysis and bears the responsibility for that, but always in collaboration with the team.

Most of the evaluation projects I've conducted within the past 15 years have been mixed methods. New evaluators need to know both. They need to know the strengths and weaknesses of both types of methods, and they need to know how to integrate the data sets. You can be exceptionally good at one or the other, but you need to *know* both. Evaluators need a basic knowledge of how the different types of analysis work. However, it's not just about using and describing the results from two separate method types; it's really about how you integrate the data to understand the whole picture. Both analyses are useful on their own, but it is the integration of both that provides the robust story.

Katrina L. Bledsoe is a senior evaluation specialist and research scientist at the Education Development Center and principal consultant of Katrina Bledsoe Consulting. She was interviewed by coauthor Patricia B. Campbell in the fall of 2019.

Sources of Qualitative Data

Chapter 12 covered in detail the primary sources of qualitative data including observations, interviews, focus groups, and written materials such as meeting minutes, reports, policies, blog posts, materials that were developed, photographs, and videos. Data from observations are extensive notes taken by the observer that may be supplemented by recordings, either video or audio. The expectation is that interviews and focus groups will be reported and transcribed and/or extensive notes will be taken. Often in interviews and focus groups evaluators take their own notes in addition to the recordings. Sample notes like the following can provide context to the transcriptions.

- Interviewee seems very antsy about what impact participating in the project will have on his tenure chances.
- It took weeks to get her to schedule a time to speak with me about the project.
- With this interviewee and several others there were a lot of hesitations when I asked about their relationship with their supervisor.
- The nonverbal language of the focus group members seems to indicate indifference toward what the others are saying.

Coding and Codebooks

Just as descriptive statistics are used to reduce and summarize quantitative data, coding is used to sort or make sense of qualitative data. "A code in qualitative inquiry is most often a word or short phrase that symbolically assigns a summative, salient, essence-capturing, and/or evocative attribute for a portion of language-based or visual data" (Saldana, 2008, p. 3). At times, evaluators, especially when there are surveys with just a few open-ended responses, report the open-ended data with no coding or analysis. While this is better than nothing, it is not a particularly useful form of qualitative data analysis. If all the reader does is read the responses, there is a tendency to remember the most articulate replies or the most positive ones or even the strangest ones rather than getting a comprehensive picture. To arrive at a complete picture, responses, be they oral or written, need to be coded or collapsed into a smaller number of categories from which patterns and conclusions can be drawn. In the following activity, readers are introduced to ways to do this.

Activity
Applying Codes and Coding

The coder in a study of career decision making coded the following as LOCATION.

I want to be able to choose where I live. Where I live is really important to me. And that's guided where I've gone, everywhere from Seattle to Maine to San Francisco to back here. And I'm just—I know there are people who are so into the science that they can move to like . . . you know, University of South Dakota, because they've got a great lab there, [but] that's something I can't do.

The following response was assigned several different codes: RACE, GENDER, ROLE MODELS, and STEREOTYPES.

So, I don't know if it's because there seems to be a lack of women scientists—like, of Black women scientists—maybe that makes people more impressed with what I'm doing or more interested with what I'm doing. I'm sad that it's the case that we have, you know, this disparity. But I take it as a positive thing, and my goal is to be a role model for other minority students who are interested in doing something like this but have never seen someone like them do this particular career.

In small groups, discuss what you thought about the codes. Did you agree with them? Are there other words or phrases that you might have used? As Saldana (2008) commented, "It's all right if your choices differed from mine. Coding is not a precise science; it's primarily an interpretive act" (p. 4).

Coding can be done following either inductive or deductive reasoning processes. Coding done using inductive reasoning is called **open coding**. This is where the codes or categories grow out of the data, usually by reading the open-ended responses, field notes, transcribed interviews, or focus group or observation notes. While reading the material, the evaluator makes notes as to the categories or codes that appear to be coming up in the reading. When coding is done using deductive reasoning, an existing set of codes is used, or a set of codes is developed based on the theory behind the project and/or the hypotheses.

Regardless of whether the code list has been generated inductively or deductively, once there is a list, the evaluator reads the data and, for each section of the data, indicates the code or codes it represents. A section may be a line, a paragraph, a page, or in the case of an observation a time period such as a minute or five minutes. The coding can be done on paper, using a word processing program, or using a qualitative analysis program. Codes can be almost anything tied to the evaluation—family support, concerns about unemployment, things that make me angry, and so on.

As indicated earlier, a section of the data may fit into two or more categories. Also, as the data are being read, there may be instances where they don't fit into the existing coding schema. If that is the case, it is appropriate to add additional codes or refine existing ones. There is always a balance between having a few codes or categories that are so general they don't deliver any information and having so many that not a lot of progress has been made in summarizing the responses. Some feel that it is better to start with more, rather than fewer, categories and collapse across categories later; others feel that it is more efficient to start with more general codes and subcode within the more general codes as needed.

When more than one person is coding, as was covered in Chapter 12, steps need to be taken to ensure that different coders are consistent in their coding (interrater reliability). Each coder should be able to consistently rate sections of the data in ways similar to the other coders. A common way of computing interrater reliability is percent agreement, in which the number of agreement scores or codes are divided by the total number of scores or codes. To ensure interrater reliability, coders should read and code the same data and compare their results. If there are disagreements, they should keep practicing together and discussing their codes. This may lead to some refinement of some of the codes; for longer-term evaluations, this can lead to the development of a codebook. "A codebook is a set of codes, definitions, and examples used as a guide to help analyze interview data" (DeCuir-Gunby, Marshall, Mcculloch, 2011, p. 138). Most codebooks include the name of the code, a short definition of the code, as appropriate what it includes and excludes, and an example. Table 13.5 provides a sample codebook entry.

Table 13.5 A Sample From a Codebook for Interview Data in a Study of Graduate Student Career Decision Making

Class/Socioeconomic Status

Direct comments specifically about class or finances from their past, present, or future that have implications about class/socioeconomic status and/or implications for access to resources. Comments about what it was like to grow up in their family regarding neighborhood, number of siblings, type of schools attended, siblings/parents/family members' level of education or profession.

Based on ideas of privilege and access tied to cultural capital. "Family" may often be double-coded here.

Includes:
- Explicit relation to financial hardship
- Discussions of current salary or desired salary down the road
- Insurance gaps, access to health care—related to benefits/income
- Discussions of child care or household division of labor *explicitly* related to finances
- Mentions of low-income student programs

Excludes:
- General comments about funding related to graduate programs, training grants, and fellowships
- Comments about stipends in grad programs

Examples
- "I grew up in a middle-class neighborhood."
- "I was told I can't go to grad school because I have no money."
- "I hope to make enough in the future that my wife will be able to stay home with the kids, so that we will have that flexibility."

Nonexamples
- "My grant proposal was rejected, and I'm frustrated."

Source: excerpt from an unpublished codebook developed by scientific careers research and development group, Northwestern University, Rick McGee, group leader) if that would work

As Saldana (2008) says, coding is "primarily an interpretive act" (p. 4). As such, coders and therefore their coding can be subject to bias. For example, knowing the gender, the race/ethnicity, and even the first name of the person whose work, interview, or observation is being analyzed has been found to impact coders' or raters' interpretations in such areas as

- open-ended responses;
- job applications;
- research work;
- faculty evaluations;
- résumés; and
- coursework (Anderson-Clark, Green, & Henley, 2008; Correll & Benard, 2006; Pellegrini, 2011).

Good codebooks can help to reduce the impact of bias and can make the analysis procedures as anonymous as possible by separating, if the responses are written, names and other identifying information from the data being analyzed (Moss-Racusin, Dovidio, Brescoll, Graham, & Handelsman, 2012; Campbell & Jolly, n.d.c).

In the activity that follows, readers develop and apply some codes to interview responses.

Activity
Developing and Using Codes

Participants in a fellowship to help them develop as leaders in community management[1] were asked, at the end of the program, how their ideas about community management changed. The following are some of their responses. Based on these responses, develop a list of codes and code the responses.

- I am mindful that the organization itself is a community. Previously I had been thinking primarily with respect to the external community, and the team members were well aligned and on track without "community management" per se. I have enjoyed applying this lens to our organizational function.
- I think they have expanded more than changed. They have also become more structured, and I feel that I have been given an intellectual framework or lens through which I am now able to observe and influence the evolution of a community of science practitioners.
- I started with zero ideas or expectations, and they have all been 100% overwhelmingly replaced by "yes" in my mind. Yes, this career path really exists. Yes, I want to pursue it further and create my own niche in microbiome science.
- My idea of a community manager was exclusive to online community platforms. I realized in this fellowship that a community is not so black-and-white to define. A community does not have to operate on a platform. It could look like a mailing list or well-established digital community. It was humbling to learn that there are so many maturity levels of a community. My organization is very mature but has almost digressed back to mitosis.
- I really didn't know what community management was before the fellowship. Now I understand it both as a role that has been defined in the private sector and is being ported to science communities and as a set of skills and responsibilities that is valuable and impactful. I feel more able to describe what I do and to advocate for that work.
- I think of it is my major job description, now, whereas before I only saw a few things I do as specifically community management. I also see how a community manager is vital to success of a large science collaboration and how my work fits into the bigger picture of scientific discovery.

- I previously did not understand the level of planning and organization required for being an effective community manager.
- I have a better understanding of "community manager" as a role, and the different forms it may entail. I also feel empowered to talk about many of the skills that a community manager needs that I employ in my job that I wouldn't have considered "community manager" skills previously.

[1] Community managers are those responsible for an organization, institution, or company's social media presence. Their role usually focuses engaging members and/or target audiences.

Source: Courtesy of Campbell-Kibler Associates, Inc.

Sample Qualitative Analysis Models

B. Williams (n.d., p. 2) provides a humorous yet useful process for doing some initial exploration of the mass of data that have been generated. As he points out, it is easy to get lost in the raw data, and there needs to be some form of filtering and prioritizing the data. His process is to identify and discuss four aspects of the data:

1. *Generalizations and exceptions:* Usually . . . , but . . .
2. *Contradiction:* On the one hand . . . , but on the other hand . . .
3. *Surprise:* I'd expected . . . , but . . . [or] I didn't expect . . . , but . . .
4. *Puzzle:* Why . . . ?

B. Williams suggests evaluators invite some others to help analyze the data. The others are then provided with a fairly rich summary of the results that does not include conclusions. Together, the evaluator and others go through the data and identify generalizations and exceptions, contradictions, surprises, and puzzles.

The activity that follows provides readers with an opportunity to do that.

Activity
Following Williams's Four Steps

The following are transcripts from four different students as to how they first got interested in science. With at least one other person, go through the four steps from Williams (n.d.) and take note of what you find.

Student 1: I guess I got that influence from my sister because she's also in the science field, and my mom is a nurse—a baby nurse. So, it's sort of in the family, I suppose. And I have some uncles that are actually in the medical field. So, I've kind of been pushed towards this from the time I was young, and I just happen to be good at it and I like it as well. So then—that's what brought me into science, I guess.

Student 2: I guess interest in science dates back to my high school days. I was introduced to science courses. That was an intensive school. It's one of the prestigious schools in the Caribbean where I grew

(Continued)

(Continued)

up. And we had a natural science program where you were introduced to physics, chemistry, and biology. So I was introduced at, like, 12 years old to doing science and in a lab, too. We had a science lecture class (mechanical noise) and a science lab.

Student 3: To be honest, my first interest in science was in college. I used to be an economics major, but I decided that was not for me. Then I started taking math classes. And, through that, I started hearing about physics here and there, so from there, I went into physics. Prior to that, I usually took science classes in high school, but I never saw myself having a career in science until I went to college. At the end of my first year, that's when I went into physics.

Student 4: I think I felt like I'm different than everyone else—in the respect that I realized I wanted to go into science when I was about 8 or 9 years old, reading the newspaper at the breakfast table with my dad. We were reading—I was reading an article about the discovery of the human genome, and I found it so interesting that I figured that if I finished school in time, I would still be able to be part of it, and that's how I got into science.

Source: Quotes from unpublished data collected by P. B. Campbell.

Seidel (1998) viewed qualitative data analysis as "essentially a simple process. It consists of three parts: Noticing, Collecting, and Thinking about interesting things. It is, of course, an iterative process and one in which there is not necessarily a logical order of steps" (pp. 1–2). Noticing involves collecting the data and making a record of what has been noticed. The record is then read, often many times and as different things are noticed—that is, indicated—and a category or code is noted and named (Seidel, 1998).

> Analysis is a breaking up, separating, or disassembling of research materials into pieces, parts, elements, or units. With facts broken down into manageable pieces, the researcher sorts and sifts them, searching for types, classes, sequences, processes, patterns, or wholes. The aim of this process is to assemble or reconstruct the data in a meaningful or comprehensible fashion. (Jorgensen, 1989, p. 107)

Thinking about things means that

> you examine the things that you have collected. Your goals are: 1) to make some type of sense out of each collection, 2) [to] look for patterns and relationships both within a collection and also across collections, and 3) to make general discoveries about the phenomena you are researching. (Seidel, 1998, p. 5)

The case study that follows applies a model for qualitative analysis that is more comprehensive than what is normally used in evaluation, but that can provide comprehensive, accurate qualitative findings.

> ## Case Study
> ### A Comprehensive Qualitative Coding Process
>
> Interviews were transcribed and checked for accuracy with the audio recording. Throughout the analysis we utilized a content analysis approach and constant comparative coding procedures. Two of us began our coding by identifying themes from the data guided by, but not limited to, sensitizing concepts from the literature review and theoretical framework. As we each independently coded, we conferred to reach consensus on each transcript and then utilized QSR International's NVivo qualitative data analysis software. Through this process, we produced memos for each transcript; [we produced] theoretical memos about emerging patterns, themes, and additional literature; and we continually refined definitions of each node by reviewing NVivo node reports. As we refined the node definitions, we returned to transcripts for additional coding. We completed full coding of 26 transcripts in this iterative manner for this sample that represented a mix of gender, race, ethnicity, and PREP sites [a post baccalaureate program for underrepresented students]. This yielded a coding scheme and preliminary findings with four patterns that we presented, discussed, and further developed with our colleagues. Then we returned to the transcripts and found further distinguishing themes within our largest pattern to reveal a fifth pattern. With the final coding scheme, we jointly coded the remaining 26 transcripts for selected themes to substantiate the initial findings and test the five patterns in our analytical.
>
> *Source:* Dr. Lynn Gazley (2014, p. 7).

There are qualitative analysis software packages to facilitate evaluators doing qualitative analysis. The more commonly used commercial packages are **MAXQDA** (www.capterra.com/p/174104/MAXQDA/), **NVivo** (www.qsrinternational.com/nvivo/home), and **ATLAS.ti** (https://atlasti.com/). There are free open-source packages as well, including **Coding Analysis Toolkit CAT**, a text analysis service hosted by Texifter, that allows users to load, code, and annotate text data in teams (https://cat.texifter.com/), and **Weft QDA**, a package for the analysis of qualitative (unstructured text) data (www.pressure.to/qda/). Unlike quantitative software programs, which perform the analysis, qualitative software programs are tools to systematically organize, code, visualize, and annotate data.

While the common wisdom is that quantitative analysis analyzes numbers and qualitative analysis doesn't, in some cases qualitative analysis does include numbers. However, the use of numbers in qualitative analysis has been, as Maxwell (2010) pointed out, controversial, with some qualitative scholars "supporting the use of numbers as simple counts of things to make statements such as 'some,' 'usually,' and 'most' more precise" (p. 475) while other qualitative scholars disagree. For the latter group, the concern is that while "numbers give precision to statements about the frequency, amount, or typicality of particular phenomena . . . they do this at the cost of stripping away everything but the quantitative information" (p. 477). While Maxwell acknowledged that using numbers in qualitative analysis can be valuable, he also pointed out that they are "necessarily complementary to qualitative information rather than substituting for it" (p. 477).

SUMMARY

This chapter examined some of the assumptions, reasonings, and rationales behind the decisions that are made about the types of analysis conducted in evaluations. Differences between deductive and inductive reasoning were covered as were some basics about quantitative and qualitative analysis. Common parametric and nonparametric statistics were covered along with related concepts including statistical significance, effect size, Type I and Type II errors, statistical power, and difference- and relationship-based analysis. Also covered were different models of qualitative analysis and qualitative data coding and the development of codebooks. As the chapter indicated, a number of issues need to be considered when developing a data analysis plan. These include

- considering using inductive rather than deductive reasoning when the related literature does not include or reflect the experiences and perspectives of underrepresented populations;

- using demographic variables as independent variables without considering the variety of contexts and other variables, such as socioeconomic status, that may allow inaccurate conclusions to be drawn; and

- dealing with the well-researched impact of bias on coding.

SUPPLEMENTAL RESOURCES

Computational Handbook of Statistics (3rd ed.)

Bruning, J. L. (1968). Glenview, IL: Scott, Foresman.

Those with little access to quantitative analysis software may find this book a helpful tool.

Choosing the Correct Statistical Test in SAS, STATA, SPSS, and R

https://stats.idre.ucla.edu/other/mult-pkg/whatstat/

This resource provides guidelines for choosing a statistical analysis. These are general guidelines and should not be construed as hard-and-fast rules. Usually, data can be analyzed in multiple ways, each of which can yield legitimate answers.

Developing and Using a Codebook for the Analysis of Interview Data: An Example From a Professional Development Research Project

DeCuir-Gunby, J. T., Marshall, P. L., & McCulloch, A. W. (2011, May). *Field Methods*, 23(2), 136–155. https://www.researchgate.net/publication/254091978

This resource gives specific steps on how to create a codebook for coding interview data. The authors examine the development of theory- and data-driven codes through the discussion of a professional development research project and with practical suggestions from their experiences in creating a codebook.

How to Lie With Statistics

Huff, D. (1954). New York, NY: Norton.

This book is a humorous look at how descriptive statistics can be used so they are accurate but presented in such a way that the reader will most likely draw inaccurate conclusions. The book was written in the 1950s and still includes some valuable information. However, it should be noted that much of the context is considered sexist by today's standards.

Open Coding

Khandkar, S. H. (n.d.). University of Calgary Department of Computer Science.

http://pages.cpsc.ucalgary.ca/~saul/wiki/uploads/CPSC681/open-coding.pdf

This paper covers labeling concepts and defining and developing coding categories based on their properties and dimensions. It provides readers with examples and opportunities to practice developing codes from text.

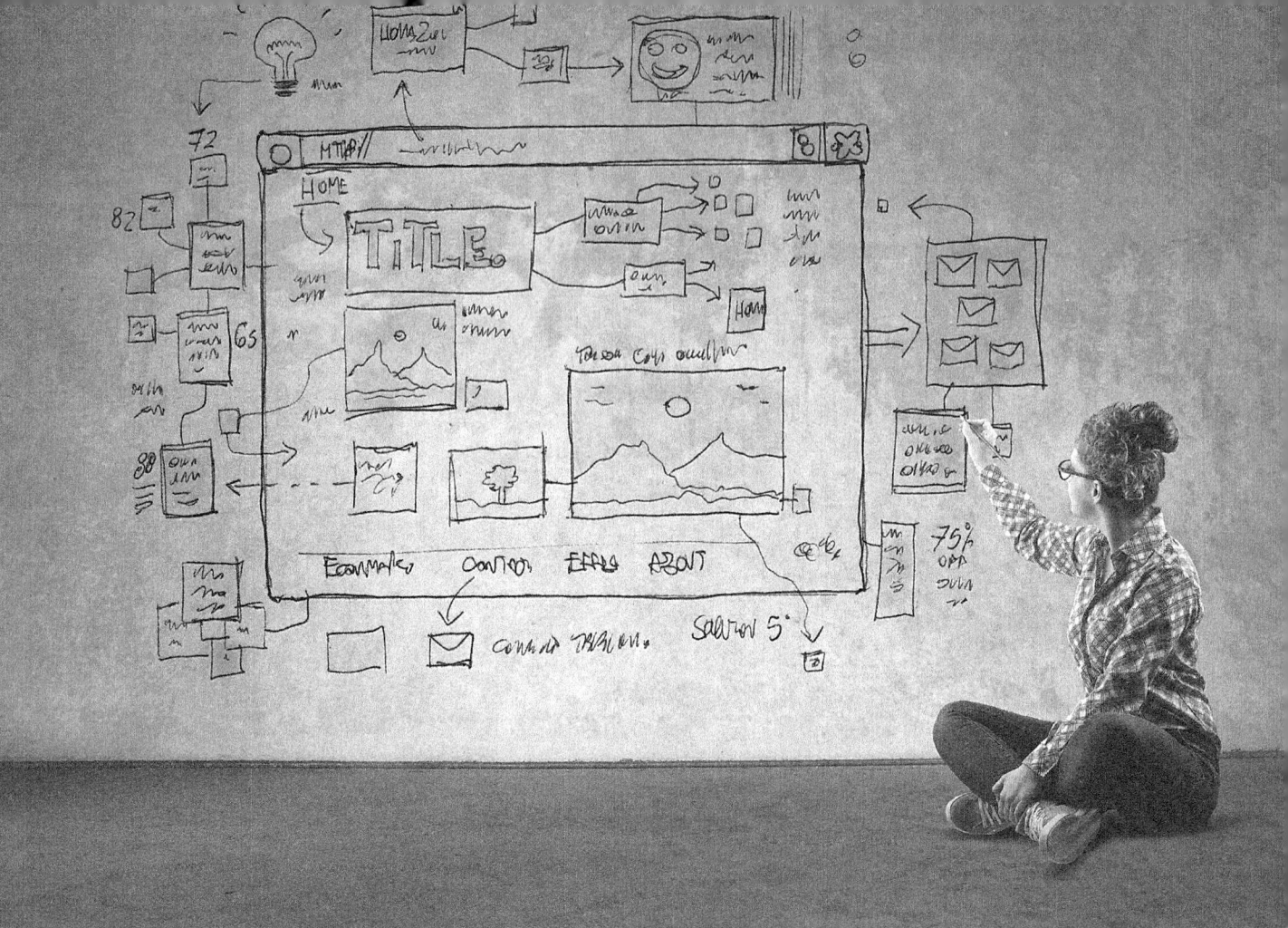
istock/ bowie15

Evaluation results, regardless of their quality and importance, are of little value unless they meet the needs of stakeholders and are reported in ways that are understood and can be used.

CHAPTER 14

Reporting, Disseminating, and Utilizing Evaluation Results

The report for one of the first evaluations I (coauthor Patricia B. Campbell) conducted concluded that there were real problems with the program and recommended it not be continued. Not only did the program get refunded, but the director asked me to do the evaluation again. To me, that meant that the report didn't well represent the findings, the appropriate people didn't get the report, and/or people didn't read the report. Since then, I always present evaluation results in multiple ways, including speaking directly with stakeholders about the results.

After reading this chapter and participating in the activities, readers will be able to meet the following learning objectives:

- Explain ways words and images can be understood and misunderstood by different audiences
- Outline the contents of an evaluation report for different audiences, including funders, project staff, and participants
- Determine appropriate visualization formats for different data sets
- Describe different modes for communicating results in culturally responsive ways and be able to identify possible target audiences for each mode, including audiences with disabilities
- Develop a realistic dissemination plan for an evaluation that targets different stakeholders
- List various ways evaluation results can be used

Introduction

If an evaluation report is not read—or read but not easily understood—the time and resources spent on the evaluation are wasted. The purpose of this chapter is to reduce the chances that this will happen by providing readers with skills and resources needed to report evaluation results in compelling and innovative ways. It focuses on ways to present information visually and textually to different stakeholders in valid and culturally appropriate ways and explores how evaluation can be **actionable** so results can be used to make important decisions (Davidson, 2012). The chapter also covers different modes for communicating and disseminating results, including ways to make findings accessible to people with disabilities.

It is expected that after completing the chapter and the activities, readers will be able to write up evaluation findings in ways that are accessible to and understood by different stakeholders. It is also expected that readers will have an understanding of basic principles of how to present data visually and how to use those principles to develop graphs and tables that report findings in meaningful and usable ways.

Reporting Results

Evaluation results, regardless of their quality and importance, are of little value unless they meet the needs of stakeholders and are reported in ways that are understood and can be used. Even if this is done, if the evaluation results are not reported in a timely fashion so the findings can be used in decision making and/or program improvement, they lose much of their value. Traditionally, evaluation results have been reported at the end of the evaluation. However, there are a variety of reporting mechanisms that can, and often should, be used to report results throughout the evaluation period. These include oral and written feedback reports and quarterly and annual reports. Timely feedback is key. Final evaluation reports should provide stakeholders with as few surprises as possible. Briefing stakeholders throughout the process and presenting a draft of the report before it goes public are effective ways to keep stakeholders abreast of evaluation processes and findings, which minimize the likelihood of surprises once the report is received. Having individuals from different stakeholder groups and communities review findings before they are widely disseminated also helps to decrease potential backlash (Frierson, Hood, Hughes, & Thomas, 2010). Community review and feedback also have the potential to increase the credibility and utility of the evaluation results and their benefit to involved communities (Hood, Hopson, & Kirkhart, 2015).

Table 14.1 provides an overview of the different types of reports and the primary audiences for them.

Table 14.1 Types of Reports by Primary Audience

Type of Report	Primary Audience/Intended Users
Full evaluation reports	Project staff, funders
Three- to five-page stand-alone summaries	Project staff, funders, staff from similar projects, interested members of the general public
One-page bullet point summaries	Participants, board members, senior managers
Summaries of conclusions and recommendations	Project staff, funders, policymakers
Feedback reports	Project staff, participants
In-person presentations	Project staff, funders, participants, staff from similar projects, interested members of the general public
Web-based presentations	Anyone interested in the results

Like many other evaluators, we believe that recommendations should be part of final evaluation reporting. As those with the best understanding of the data, evaluators are well placed to provide recommendations that will be useful to the program. However, some evaluators feel that the evaluator's role is to provide the findings and it is the program staff's responsibility to read the reports and develop their own recommendations. This may be something the evaluator and program staff should discuss early in the evaluation process.

The Full Evaluation Report

The full evaluation report is at the core of evaluation reporting. This report includes, either in the text or appendices, information on the program, the evaluation methods and measures used, and the results, conclusions, and recommendations. Many other modes of reporting, including summaries and presentations, are based on the content in the full evaluation report. While different summaries and/or presentations may be developed and used to report results, generally there is only one full evaluation report.

The following outline of a typical full evaluation report, adapted from Miron (2004), can also be used as a checklist to help determine the pieces that should be included in a full evaluation report.

I. *Title page:* a clear and succinct title, author names and affiliations, client and/or funder, and date

II. *Table of contents* (optional):

III. *Two- or three-page executive summary:* an overview of the project and the evaluation along with key findings and major recommendations

IV. *Introduction:* the project goals and objectives, the context in which the project is operating, and the evaluation questions

V. *Methods:* the evaluation model, design, instrumentation, and data collection methods, including sources of information and data analysis methods

VI. *Results:* the answers to the evaluation questions and/or an explanation as to why answers could not be found; other findings and tables and graphs as appropriate

VII. *Conclusions:* a summary of the results and the conclusions that are drawn from the results

VIII. *Recommendations:* suggestions drawn from the results and conclusions

IX. *Appendices (optional):* a more detailed description of the evaluation, including the design, data collection, and analysis; copies of the measures and interview protocols used; more detailed description of the results, which may in some cases include more detailed statistics; copies of interim reports and/or feedback reports

Other Reporting Mechanisms

Stand-Alone Summaries

Stand-alone summaries are three- to five-page summaries that include

- two or three paragraphs describing the project and its goals and objectives;
- two or three paragraphs stating the evaluation questions and design;
- major conclusions, with a short summary of the results that led to each conclusion;
- major recommendations; and
- a link to the full report.

A One-Page Bullet Point Summary

A one-page bullet point summary is the written equivalent of an **elevator speech** where one has 30 seconds, the average time of an elevator ride, to explain a concept or, in this case, evaluation results and recommendations (University of

California Davis, n.d.). The summary starts with a short paragraph about the project and its context and then bullets the top three takeaway points for the reader. Different summaries may need to be written for different stakeholder groups, but all should include how to get additional information about the project and the evaluation.

A Summary of Conclusions and Recommendations

The summary of conclusions and recommendations usually targets senior administrators or managers, board members, and others who are familiar with the project being evaluated and want to "get to the point" as to what was found and what it means. The following case study provides an example of a summary of conclusions and recommendations for an evaluation of the impact of different professional development strategies on teacher classroom behaviors, using a format where, for each conclusion, supporting data and an interpretation with recommendations are provided.

Case Study
A Summary of Conclusions and Recommendations

Conclusion

Teachers involved in these projects were significantly more apt to use math and science career information and student-centered teaching strategies if the interventions in which they participated included curriculum materials and resources, with or without professional development.

Supporting Data

Projects with curriculum components, regardless of whether or not they included professional development, were significantly more successful at increasing teachers' use of science and math career information in their classes. The inclusion of curriculum also significantly increased teacher use of student-centered instructional strategies, such as having students explain their problem-solving strategies, but did not have an impact on the third factor, teachers' comfort with the level of the content they were teaching. The inclusion of professional development was related to an increase in negative results.

	Changes in Teacher Classroom Use of Math and Science Career Information			Changes in Teacher Classroom Use of Student-Centered Instructional Strategies		
	Positive Change	No Change	Negative Change	Positive Change	No Change	Negative Change
Curriculum Alone (5 Projects)	52%	33%	15%	70%	10%	19%
Professional Development Alone (10 Projects)	39%	25%	35%	50%	9%	41%
Professional Development and Curriculum (14 Projects)	47%	30%	23%	61%	6%	33%

> **Interpretations and Recommendations**
>
> It is recommended that future projects include curriculum materials and resources and that the professional development strategies used be reviewed to explore what may have contributed to the increased negative results.
>
> Source: Adapted from P. B. Campbell, Price, Chubin, Carson, and Kibler (2006).

Feedback Reports

The types of reports described earlier are usually provided annually or at the end of an evaluation. Feedback reports can be provided whenever there is feedback that can be used to improve the ongoing project. They should be short, easy to read, and timely. For example, themes that came up during the visit can be provided to involved stakeholders a week or two after the visit. This allows those interviewed to see that they have been heard and allows projects to address issues that may have come up in a timely manner. The following is a section of a feedback report, after a site visit, focusing on cross-project efforts to infuse more computer programming into student coursework.

> There is potential for overlap across different aspects of the project. For example, a four-week Python [a programming language] module has already been developed and is being implemented. Since Python is going to be the basis for the revised CS 100 [an introductory computer science course], it could be useful to see the degree to which the materials in the Python module can be used in CS 100 and, based on how CS 100 is designed, what a revised Python module might include. (P. B. Campbell & Kibler, unpublished evaluation report)

Based on the feedback, the involved faculty came together and implemented a plan to reduce the overlap.

Another type of feedback reports on participant response to activities. The following are actual qualitative and quantitative summaries of participant responses (P. B. Campbell, unpublished evaluation report).

Sample qualitative summary

Fellows in the final several years of their graduate program found the professional development activities tied to job searches and postdoctorates very useful. These activities were less useful for those who were in the first years of their graduate programs. Fellows have suggested there be "developmentally appropriate" professional development, tied to where participants are in their programs.

Sample quantitative summary

While only 4 (8%) respondents joined the program to disseminate their research and resources, 9 (17%) were using the group to disseminate their research and resources. Other sources the respondents used to disseminate resources were as follows:

> Institution" websites (31; 60%)
>
> Disciplinary conference presentations (23; 44%)
>
> Conference presentations (20; 38%)
>
> Disciplinary journals (18; 35%)
>
> Personal website (14; 27%)
>
> Other online community libraries (10; 19%)
>
> Newsletters/mailing lists (7; 14%)
>
> Journals (5; 10%)

Oral Presentations

Results can, and often should, be shared with in-person and/or virtual presentations. One of the biggest advantages of presentations is that they are interactive so people can ask questions, findings can be clarified, recommendations can be discussed, and next steps can be brainstormed. For most presentations, it's useful to have visuals, such as PowerPoint slides, that highlight the major findings, conclusions, and recommendations. Having copies of a one-page bulleted summary that includes links to the full report can increase the impact of the presentation. Presentations can range from individual conversations to small group conversations to town halls and formal presentations at meetings of professional societies.

Whether live or virtual, the content and the structure of a presentation will vary based on the target audience and the goals for the presentation. Piloting the presentation with representatives of the target audience in advance provides feedback and helps to hone the presentation so it better meets audience needs. It is also important to "make sure that the messenger fits the message and the audience" (Gervin et al., 2014, p. 20). The evaluator may not always be the best person to communicate the findings. Instead, a community member who played an active role in the evaluation may be a better choice for some audiences.

Presentations, if they are engaging and done well, are excellent ways to get people interested in the evaluation findings. One way to make presentations engaging is to present the findings in a more conversational format. When people tell a story in conversation, they start with the main idea, and their story has a beginning, a middle, and an end. A good presentation should be a story. Storytelling matches people's natural talking expertise with their audience's natural listening process. The key question for presenters to ask and answer is, "How would I say this to someone who didn't already know what I was talking about?" (Aruffo, n.d.).

As is the case with other dissemination formats, presentations need to be accessible to people with disabilities. This may mean always using a microphone and/or having a sign language interpreter in live presentations or captioning or subtitling for virtual presentations when people with hearing impairments may be in attendance. Presenters can and should describe any visuals presented in presentations when people with visual impairments may be present.

Sharing of Raw Data

Traditionally, raw data, data that haven't been processed in any way, were not shared with others. However, that has been changing. The National Science Foundation (NSF, n.d.), for example, has a data-sharing policy that says "investigators are expected to share [their data] with other researchers, at no more than incremental cost and within a reasonable time (para. 1) The National Institutes of Health (NIH, 2003) has a similar policy, which says "data should be made as widely and freely available as possible while safeguarding the privacy of participants and protecting confidential and proprietary data" (para. 4). Evaluators need to anonymize raw quantitative and qualitative data, before they are shared. Individually identifiable data should not be released.

Evaluators need to check with project staff and funders about what data will be shared, with whom, and under what circumstances. If participants are not comfortable with their anonymous data being shared, they can choose not to participate in the evaluation. As covered in Chapter 12, this is something that should be considered in the protection of human participants. Information on what data will be shared, with whom, and in what format should be a part of participant informed consent.

Developing High-Quality, Accessible Reports and Presentations

Regardless of the audience, the American Evaluation Association's (AEA) *Guiding Principles for Evaluators* state that in reporting the results of evaluations evaluators must "communicate the approaches, methods and limitations of the evaluation accurately and in sufficient detail to allow others to understand, interpret and critique their work" (AEA, 2018b, p. 164).

While being interviewed for this book, Roger Nozaki (personal communication, October 10, 2018), vice president of the Barr Foundation, stressed that all reports, regardless of the target audience, should be clear and relatively jargon free. They should communicate the findings succinctly and clearly without requiring every reader to go through the methodology and nuances. Readers, Nozaki pointed out, should not have to figure out all of the implications of the results themselves. In *Actionable Evaluation Basics*, Davidson (2012) makes very similar points, explaining that good reports are succinct and straight to the point, but not simplistic. Good reports, she argues, are useful at strategic and practical levels, with results that don't get lost in the details and are oriented toward action and decision making. Poor evaluation reports, she says, are those that are excessively long and wordy, written in academic language, and either don't make the key points apparent or bury them at the end.

Grob (2015) points out that, to be impactful, the evaluation needs to convey a message for readers or viewers to take away from the reporting. A good message must pass what he calls the Mom Test, where in one or two sentences the message or takeaway from the evaluation can be explained in such a way that your mom would understand it. While his assumptions about what moms do and don't understand do not reflect the wide diversity of mothers, his point about having a message that most people can understand is important.

Readability

As indicated earlier, different presentations, summaries, and feedback reports will need to be developed based on the audiences for whom they are intended. For example, summaries for middle school students and/or target populations who are lower literacy should be shorter with less complex language than summaries written for funders. Checking the *readability*, the quality of writing being legible or decipherable and easy to read, is a useful way of matching the level of what is written to the target audience. A number of free readability tools are available to do that, including the Readability Test Tool (www.webpagefx.com/tools/read-able/), which tests the readability of websites, documents, and sections of documents. Readability tools provide information on the average grade level of education needed for the document text to be easily understood. For context, *New York Times* articles have, on average, a 10th-grade reading level while romance novels have about a 5th-grade reading level (Full Media, n.d.).

The appropriate level of readability should be based on the groups the materials are targeted toward. An upper high school level, 11th or 12th grade, is a good reading level for technical reports while reports for the general public are better written at a middle school level, 6th or 7th grade (Full Media, n.d.). All reports and summaries should be as jargon free as possible and any technical language used should be explained. Nontechnical reports and materials should be written such that they can be understood by members of the target audiences the first time they are read. There are resources to assist those wishing to write in plain language, including the government website plainlanguage.gov. *Writing in Plan Language: A Training Manual* (DuBay, 2008) is another useful resource. It can be downloaded for free from www.impact-information.com/Resources/working.pdf. The following activity provides an opportunity for readers to check the readability of their writing.

Activity
Testing Readability

Either take a paragraph you wrote earlier about evaluation or write a paragraph about why you think it is important for programs to do evaluations, and use a readability program such as www.webpagefx.com/tools/read-able/ to determine readability. If the readability level of your paragraph is 10th grade or higher, rewrite it to get it to the 7th-grade level or below. If the readability level is 8th grade or below, rewrite it to make it a 10th-grade level or higher.

Reports can be written in either an active or passive voice. "**Active voice** means that a sentence has a subject that acts upon its verb" (Traffis, n.d., para. 1), as in "Over half of the participants thought the program was successful." **Passive voice** means that a subject is a recipient of a verb's action" (Traffis, n.d., para. 1), as in "The program was thought to be successful by over half the participants." Using the active voice tends to make sentences clearer and less wordy, while the more formal passive voice has been more apt to be used in scientific writing. The choice of whether to use active or passive voice can be determined by who the target audience is and how formal a report is desired (Purdue Online Writing Lab, n.d.

Making the materials accessible is not just about the language used; it is also about formats and fonts that make it easier for those with low vision to read the materials. The following are useful guidelines for writers (VisionAware, n.d.).

- Use large print type with fonts with easily recognizable characters, either standard roman or sans serif fonts. A good choice is Arial.
- Avoid using italics or all capital letters. Both of these forms of print make it more difficult to differentiate among letters.

- Minimize the use of color. Different-colored lettering for headings and emphasis is difficult to read for many people with low vision.

- Print text with the best possible contrast. For many older people, light lettering—either white or light yellow—on a dark background, usually black, is easier to read than black lettering on a white or light yellow background.

- Use 1.5-line spacing between lines of text rather than single spacing.

- Use wide spacing between letters. For example, a mono-spaced font such as Courier, which allocates an equal amount of space for each letter, is very readable.

- Use a minimum of one-inch margins.

If digital versions of the reports and other materials are sent, save them if possible in formats that allow readers to change the font and font size. It may also be useful to add links to accessibility options within Windows and Apple operating systems such as those that can be found at www.afb.org/info/living-with-vision-loss/using-technology/using-a-computer/part-ii-for-the-experienced-computer-user-with-a-new-visual-impairment/windows-accessibility-options/12345.

In addition, reports—or, at a minimum, summaries—need to be provided in the dominant languages of the target audiences. As was covered in Chapter 12, generally the most accurate way to translate documents is to use forward/backward translation, where the report or other document is translated from English by one person and then translated back to English by another person and the English versions are compared to see where any mistranslations occurred. A second way is translation by committee where a panel of people who speak both English and the language into which the document is being translated translate the instrument into the desired language.

Two translation strategies were not included in Chapter 12 because when they are used there is an increased risk of mistranslation, which can seriously impact the quality of the collected data. One is simple direct translation, where the translation is done by a person fluent in both languages. The second is online translation, where the document is entered into a program and the program translates it. Neither of these methods may provide the most accurate, nuanced translations (Frierson et al., 2010). The activity that follows provides readers with an opportunity to try out and test the accuracy of an online translation program.

Activity
Trying Translation Software

Take a sentence or two you used for the readability test and, using one of the free translation programs, such as www.babelfish.com, translate it from English to another language. Then translate the sentence(s) from that language back to English and compare the original English and the translated English versions. How close are they to each other?

As indicated earlier, it is always a good idea to have one or more members of the target audience read draft summaries and provide feedback before the summaries are finalized and shared. LaFrance and Nichols (2009) urge that those writing and/or reviewing reports or findings make sure that confidentiality is ensured and that there is an emphasis on strengths as well as weaknesses and that solutions as well as problems and findings are set in a cultural context. While LaFrance and Nichols were speaking explicitly about Indigenous American populations, their recommendations hold for other underrepresented and disenfranchised communities as well. Robles, Venkateswaran, and Feldman (2018, para. 5) go even further, saying that

> the evaluation plan should clearly state that stakeholders will respond to drafts and the timeline should prioritize soliciting and integrating their comments as a way to lift up multiple voices. Making their inclusion a non-negotiable prevents potential gatekeepers from removing uncomfortable or negative findings. Feedback from different groups, even (especially!) when extensive, helps ensure participants' truths are told accurately and strengthens buy-in to the findings.

Words Matter

Sensitivity to and skillful use of language are core evaluation competencies and that the language used among evaluations and between evaluators and stakeholders, necessarily and inherently, shapes perceptions, defines reality, and alters mutual understanding (Patton, 2000). Whatever the type of report being written or the type of target audience, it is important to know that the words that are used make a difference. For example, two cars can "collide," or they can "smash into each other." Both phrases accurately describe what happened; however, they suggest very different images to the reader. Similarly, there is a great difference between calling the health care law the Affordable Care Act and calling it Obamacare. The words the evaluator chooses to describe a phenomenon can be powerful and denote different imagery of the issue under consideration.

In general, one thinks about words in relation to their meaning and the information they transmit. However, words can also convey things like how much we know about our topic, the perspective from which we approach it, where we stand on different issues, and how much we think our audience knows. The words we use influence our audience's feelings about us and, more importantly, about how relevant our message is to them and their interests. Since there's no single set of words that will work with all audiences, we need to choose the words we use consciously and carefully (Campbell-Kibler & Campbell, 2007). The following is an example of the power of words.

> There is a park in Washington DC that is called Meridian Hill Park, Malcolm X Park or sometimes both. The name of the park is sensitive enough that at least one local business owner switches "between calling it Meridian Hill or Malcolm X depending on who I'm talking to or what I'm talking about. (Kurzius, 2018, p. 3)

The words authors use can reveal their underlying beliefs about and/or knowledge (or lack of knowledge) of the communities to which they are reporting. For example, any one of the terms *undocumented immigrant, illegal alien,* and *foreigner in a country without authorized permission* could be used to describe an individual who is in a country without the proper documentation. While the terms could be considered synonyms, the choice of term to use could be seen as an indication of the author's attitudes toward people who fit that definition. If the term *illegal alien* is used, some readers, rightly or wrongly, assume that the author has some biases and stereotypes about people who are undocumented, which can impact the degree to which they trust or believe the findings. Words can marginalize or empower, as is the case when using the term *at-risk students* vs. *students placed at risk* or the term *mentally ill person* vs. *person with a mental illness* (Campbell-Kibler & Campbell, 2007).

How words are used can cause the message to be lost. For example, many would find the term *Mom Test* (Grob, 2015), described earlier in this chapter, patronizing and sexist. Even choosing how to best describe people from Spanish-speaking countries or their dependents—as Hispanic, Latino, Latino/a, or Latinx (a gender-neutral or nonbinary alternative)—can have an impact on the reader. Some may prefer *Latino/a* because it explicitly includes women and men, while others may find the relatively recent term *Latinx* off-putting because it's new. Some people find all of these terms too generic, feeling if a target group is predominantly Puerto Rican or Cuban American or Mexican American, using a more generic term like *Hispanic* or *Latino* can lead to inaccurate overgeneralizations.

Word choices are not just important in terms of how people are described. For example, consider the following word pairs:

paradigm shift vs. *change*

pedagogy vs. *teaching*

hegemony vs. *powerful influence*

If a target audience is likely to respect specialized vocabulary, the first choice of each word pair might be more appropriate. Otherwise, simpler words or phrases are better. As Jessica Chen (2018) points out,

> I cannot stress enough how important it is to recognize that lack of exposure to terminology doesn't mean lack of ability to understand. An audience, unfamiliar with a topic, can neither identify important info, nor follow a storyline because gaps in their knowledge were not addressed. So, invest time in getting to know your audience and building trust, the most important aspect of successful communication. . . . [C]redentials mean nothing if your audience doesn't know what you're saying. (para. 5)

Based on the target audience, evaluators should consciously make decisions as to the degree to which they are going to use "scientific" or "research" language. Responses to being told that a change in participants' behavior had an effect size of .4 would be quite different based on whether the evaluator was speaking with evaluators/researchers or speaking with community members.

Words can also change their meanings over time. For example, *bad* used to, and often still is used to, describe something that is unwelcome, unpleasant, or just not good, but today it can also mean good or great. *Gay* used to mean happy or joyous, but it is now a positive term for homosexuality (*HuffPost*, 2014). Words also can take on political connotations. *Scientifically based research* used to be a neutral term describing specific types of research designs but has now become a politically loaded term (Campbell-Kibler & Campbell, 2007).

There is no list of the right words to use. Evaluators need to do their homework and find out as much as they can about the kinds of words commonly used and the kinds avoided by their target audiences and learn what emotions, divisions, and concepts these words can evoke (Campbell-Kibler & Campbell, 2007). This information should influence the words that are used in reporting results and conclusions.

As evaluators, it is useful to understand that some words have a strong impact on us. In the following activity, readers think about some terms to which they have a strong reaction and explore replacement terms that are less incendiary.

> ### Reflect and Discuss
> #### Hot-Button Words
>
> Everyone has hot-button words to which they have strong, often visceral, positive or negative reactions. *Feminism* can be an example of a hot-button word, as can be *big government* or *climate change*. Most people have strong reactions to a hot-button word—some positive, some negative. Different groups will have different hot-button words.
>
> Individually or in small groups, discuss some of your hot-button words and brainstorm other words that could be used that are equivalent to your hot-button words but aren't as loaded.

Images Matter

While the words used in evaluation reports matter, so do the images. Images, including drawings and photographs, can be useful ways to break up the text and increase understanding of the context of the programs or projects being evaluated. It is, of course, important that any included images are related to the content being covered.

As discussed in Chapter 12, what is or isn't included in an image can have a major impact on the reader. When pictures in an organization's newsletter included a moderate number of minorities, minority group members felt more positive about the organization than when only white people were pictured (Purdie-Vaughns, Steele, Davis, Diltmann, & Crosby, 2008). When women viewed a video with equal numbers of women and men in it, they were more positive about the video's content than when the video had 3 times as many men and women in it (Cheryan, Plaut, Davies, & Steele, 2009).

While pictures and illustrations in the evaluation report should reflect the demographic characteristics of project participants, they should also reflect the context and values of the project that was evaluated. For example, images of people shopping at a grocery store would not fit well in an evaluation report about projects to increase urban farming, although images of people shopping at a farmer's market could. Images with mountains in the backdrop might be beautiful but wouldn't be helpful if the project being evaluated was about improving knowledge of coastal ecology. Irony and satire do not go well in evaluation reports, so, for example, using an image of people fighting alongside a finding that a program decreased collaboration is not wise.

It can be useful to use existing images from the project being evaluated or to create new images of participants and/or staff in action or of artifacts like products or logos. Before any images involving people can be used, there needs to be a signed release from anyone who can be recognized in the image. For participants under 18, their parent or guardian also needs to sign a release. Whatever the image, credit must be given in the report to the photographer and/or illustrator. If images specific to the projects aren't going to be used, there are a number of different places to access more generic images online. It is important to check to see if the images are copyrighted and, if they are, what permissions will need to be acquired before an image can be used. Some, such as Getty Images (www.gettyimages.com), a leading source of online images, will require a payment, or royalty, before an image can be used. Others may not. Regardless of whether a royalty is paid or an image is copyrighted or not, credit should be given to the illustrator, artist, designer, and/or photographer.

When using illustrations, it should be remembered that different illustrators have different styles, and illustrations in some styles may cause different responses in different target audiences. For example, the two illustrations that follow are conveying the same idea, but their style and tone are quite different.

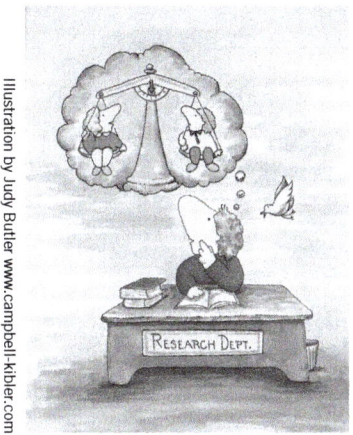
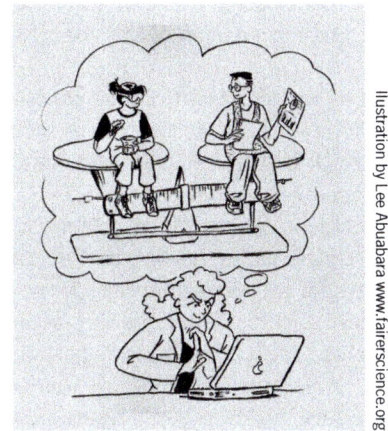

In the following activity, readers are asked to think about circumstances where they would use one or the other of these illustrations.

Reflect and Discuss
Who Likes What and Why

Individually or in small groups, think about the target audiences you feel would prefer the Butler illustration or the Abuabara illustration, and discuss why you think so.

Visually Representing Data

Data visualization refers to efforts to help people visualize and understand data by using visuals. It is "a process that (a) is based on qualitative or quantitative data and, (b) results in an image that is representative of the raw data, which is (c) is readable by viewers and supports exploration, examination, and communication of the data)" (Azzam, Evergreen, Germuth, & Kistler, 2013, p. 9).

"With visual representation of data, patterns, trends and correlations that might go undetected in text-based data can be exposed and recognized" (Rouse, 2012, para. 1).

The most common forms of data visualization are tables and figures. "Tables present lists of numbers or text in columns" and/or rows while figures may be "graphs, charts, drawings, photos, or maps" (The Writing Center, n.d., paras. 3–4). One reason data visualization is important is that it is easier for people to understand data using images, charts, or graphs than when it is presented as raw data or data described in text (Azzam et al., 2013).

Regardless of the type of visual presentation of data being used, as is the case in so much of evaluation, the first rule is to know your audience. As Rougier, Droettboom, and Bourne (2014) point out,

> problems arise when how a visual is perceived differs significantly from the intent of the conveyer. Consequently, it is important to identify, as early as possible in the design process, the audience and the message the visual is to convey. The graphical design of the visual should be informed by this intent. (para. 2)

Just as written reports of results often differ based on the target group, visual representations of data may need to as well. It is always important that a figure is correct and conveys all the relevant information to a broader audience; however, what that means can differ by audience.

Visual representations of data must convey a message. The message may be something as simple as the finding that over time most former smokers start smoking again or something more complex to show which programs are more effective for which groups such as the relative rates of former smokers smoking again based on the type of smoking cessation program they participated in and their age. As Rougier et al. (2014) explain, "it is important to clearly identify the role of the figure, i.e., what is the underlying message and how can a figure best express this message? . . . Only after identifying the message will it be worth the time to develop your figure" (p. 2). As always, it is useful to have members of the target audience(s) review the visuals and give feedback on what message(s) the images convey to them.

Tables

Tables can present both qualitative data and quantitative data in rows and/or columns. A good table allows the reader to easily understand the meaning of the presented data, displaying relationships between quantitative values and the categories to which these values are related (Few, 2012). As covered in Chapter 13, if quantitative data are included in a table and inferential statistics have been done, it is useful to include levels of significance and, for interval or ratio data, effect sizes in the tables. Tables should include a descriptive title and row and/or column labels that describe the data. While there is no consensus as to the number of decimal points in which quantitative data should be reported, we suggest that such data not be reported in more than one decimal place. For example, if the raw data are whole numbers, then means would be reported with one decimal place. However, often standard deviations (SDs) are reported with two decimal points (Habibzadeh & Habibzadeh, 2015). If tables are reporting frequency counts, it is useful to have both counts and percentages.

Using shading or bolding in a table can help highlight the key points. Table 14.2 is an example of a simple table, showing where project participants go to find diversity materials and other resources, which shows both the places that are most frequently used and differences between the two groups.

Table 14.2 Where Participants Go to Find Diversity Resources

(N = 50)*

	Colleagues**	Google or other search engines	Groups focused on diversity	Professional societies	Funder websites**	Online communities
People with diversity backgrounds (n = 25)	25 (100%)	19 (76%)	11 (44%)	10 (40%)	**12 (48%)**	2 (8%)
Others (n = 25)	13 (52%)	18 (72%)	8 (32%)	5 (20%)	**2 (8%)**	2 (8%)
Totals	38 (76%)	37 (72%)	19 (38%)	15 (30%)	**14 (28%)**	4 (8%)

*Participants could choose more than one option.

** $p < .05$

Source: P. B. Campbell, unpublished evaluation report.

One of the easiest and fastest ways to develop a table is to start to enter the numbers in a Microsoft Excel spreadsheet. With Excel, it is relatively easy to experiment with different ways of organizing the data and even different fonts and colors. While tables can be generated in Word, it is easier to begin a table in Excel, and once the basic table is developed, it can be imported into Word. In Word, table tools can be used to format the table in many different ways, and different shadings and border styles can be added. The following activity provides readers with an opportunity to make a table in Word and one in Excel.

Activity
Using Word and Excel to Make Tables

Replicate Table 14.2 using Word and then using Excel.

Even when the same data set is used, how data are presented in a table can have implications as to what conclusions are drawn. Using the same raw pretest/posttest data from 570 instructors who participated in a professional development training to increase their use of student-centered instruction, results can be reported in two different ways. Table 14.3a has mean pretest/posttest differences in teachers' self-report of their use of student-centered instruction, and Table 14.3b has the number

Table 14.3 Teacher Ratings* of Their Use of Student-Centered Learning

(a)

	Mean	Standard Deviation
Pretest	2.3	0.5
Posttest	2.2	0.5

* 1 (*daily*) to 5 (*rarely or not at all*)

(*Continued*)

Table 14.3 (Continued)

(b)

	Positive Change	No Change	Negative Change
Number	301	54	192
Percentage	55%	10%	35%

Source: P. B. Campbell (2006).

and percentage of instructors increasing, decreasing, or not changing the degree to which they used student-centered instruction in their classes. Table 14.3a shows a slight increase while Table 14.3b, using the same data, shows that a majority of the instructors changed in the desired direction but more than a third became worse.

In the following activity, readers reflect on and discuss the differences between the two tables.

Reflect and Discuss
Interpreting Different Tables

Individually or in small groups, discuss the messages that Tables 14.3a and 14.3b convey. Does the way the results are presented in either or both tables influence any conclusions you might draw about whether the program should be modified or continued? If yes, how?

Figures

Graphs and charts are the most commonly used figures in evaluation reporting; however, figures may also be diagrams, photographs, drawings, or even maps. If evaluation results are reported online in nonstatic ways, figures can be videos and/or interactive. Basically, "figures are visual presentations of results that provide visual impact that can effectively communicate your primary finding" (The Writing Center, n.d., para. 4).

Although there are many types of figures, like tables, they share some typical features. Figures need clear captions including explanatory titles, labels on each axis to let the readers know what the scale is, and a **legend** that describes the different data sets in the figure. Also needed is any necessary contextual information. That information may be in the title, a note, or the text surrounding the figure. The text should not repeat what is in the figure, but can explain it or point out some highlights to the reader (The Writing Center, n.d.).

In general, tables are better than figures for giving structured numeric information, while figures are better than tables for demonstrating trends, making comparisons, or showing relationships. Figures also present the overall shape of the data in ways that cannot be depicted in tables. For tables and figures, it is important to have enough contextual information that they can stand alone—that is, be understandable to the reader. While the surrounding text provides more elaboration, the reader should not have to go to the text to understand what a table or figure's message is.

There are a number of different types of figures. While the terms *graphs* and *charts* are often used interchangeably, graphs are a subset of charts. A chart is a graphic representation of data while a graph is a chart showing the relationship between two or more variables. Typical charts used in evaluation are line, column, bar, and area graphs and pie charts. Whatever chart or graph is used, it is key to keep it simple.

If the reader doesn't immediately understand a chart or graph, its message will be lost (The Writing Center, n.d.).

The following are standard tips to use in data visualization (International Development Research Center, 2012; Rougier et al., 2014; Usabilla, n.d.).

1. Keep it simple.
   a. Show the data and eliminate such things as background colors and borders.
   b. Avoid using special effects such as 3D graphs.
2. Have a message you want the visual to communicate.
   a. Use the title and the labels to support the message you want the chart to convey.
   b. Check with others to see if the visual presents the message you want.
3. Pick the chart type that best fits your data.
4. If you use color, remember that different colors may impact different people in different ways and there may be some readers who are color-blind and may not be able to make the needed distinctions to interpret the chart. The most common color blindness is red/green, where people mix up all colors that have red or green as part of the whole color.

Overall a clear message is more important than if the figure is beautiful. There exists a myriad of online graphics in which aesthetic is the first criterion and content comes in second place. Even if a lot of those graphics might be considered beautiful, most of them do not fit the scientific [or evaluation] framework. Remember, in science [and evaluation], message and readability of the figure is the most important aspect while beauty is only an option. (Rougier et al., 2014, p. 8)

Using the data from Table 14.2, line, area, column, and bar graphs and pie charts were developed, as was a combo chart in which two figures, in this case a column graph and a line graph, are combined.

Line graphs, as shown in Figure 14.1, are used to connect individual (quantitative) data points and to display the trend of a series of data points.

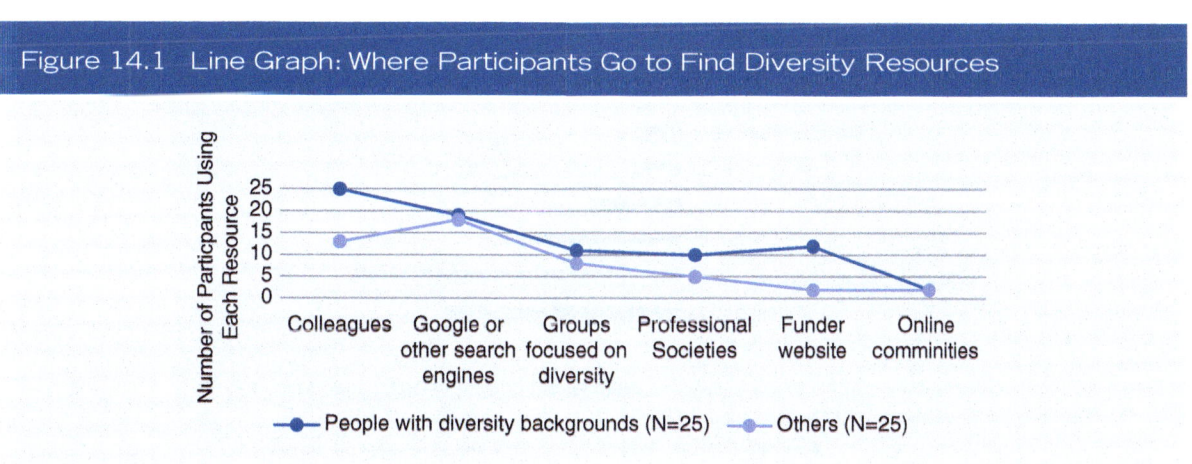

Figure 14.1   Line Graph: Where Participants Go to Find Diversity Resources

Area graphs are very similar to line graphs; however, as shown in Figure 14.2, the colors or different fillings may help readers better visualize changes over time, or in this case group differences.

Column and bar graphs, as shown in Figures 14.3 and 14.4, are good for doing direct comparisons of data sets. It often makes it easier to follow the chart if the numbers are sorted in some order such as highest to lowest or vice versa.

Figure 14.2 Area Graph: Where Participants Go to Find Diversity Resources

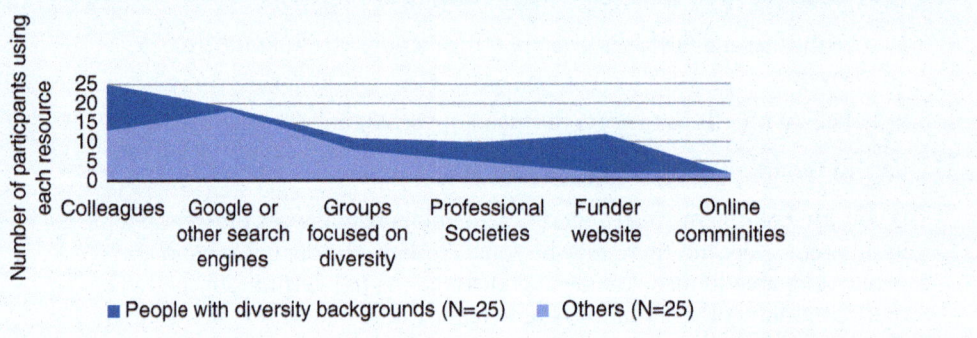

Figure 14.3 Column Graph: Where Participants Go to Find Diversity Resources

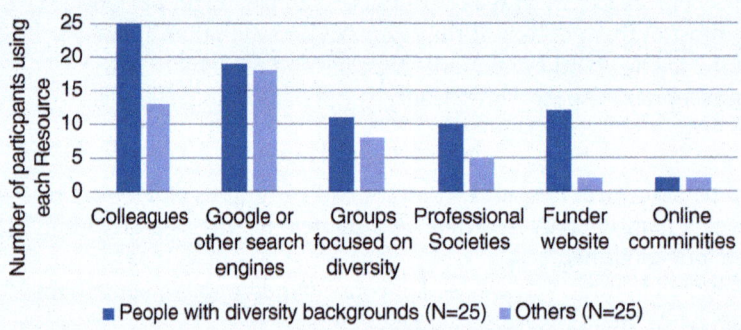

Figure 14.4 Bar Graph: Where Participants Go to Find Diversity Resources

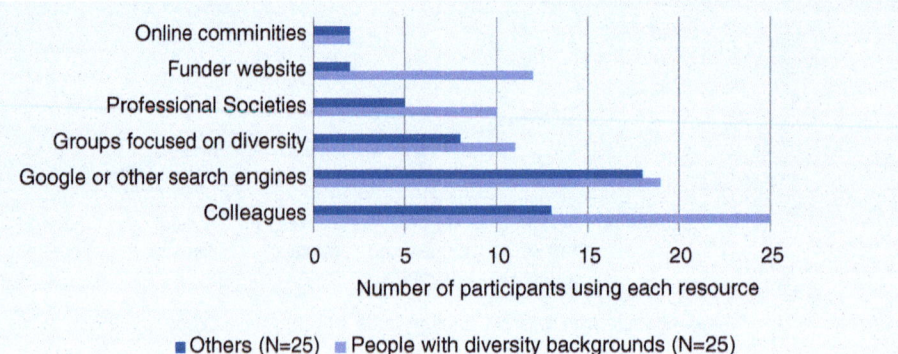

As indicated earlier, a combo chart is created when two charts, in this case a column graph and a line graph, are combined. Figure 14.5 uses the combo chart to highlight differences between two groups. It can also be used to place data from two different but related variables on the same chart.

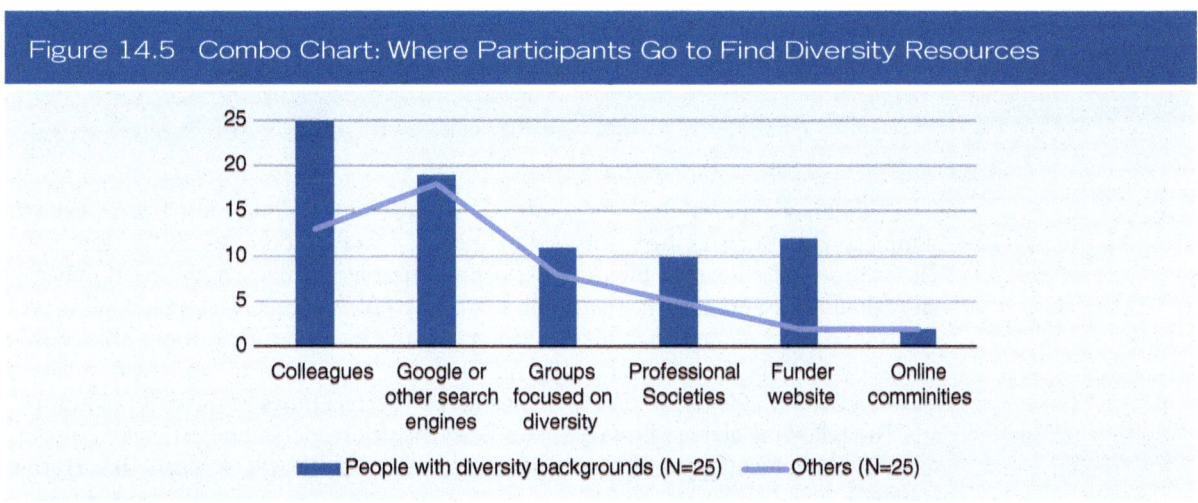

Figure 14.5   Combo Chart: Where Participants Go to Find Diversity Resources

The two data sets used in the earlier examples cannot be displayed together in a pie chart, because pie charts can't display comparisons among groups. However, the aggregated data can be reported as a pie chart, as seen in Figure 14.6, or as two pie charts—one for each group.

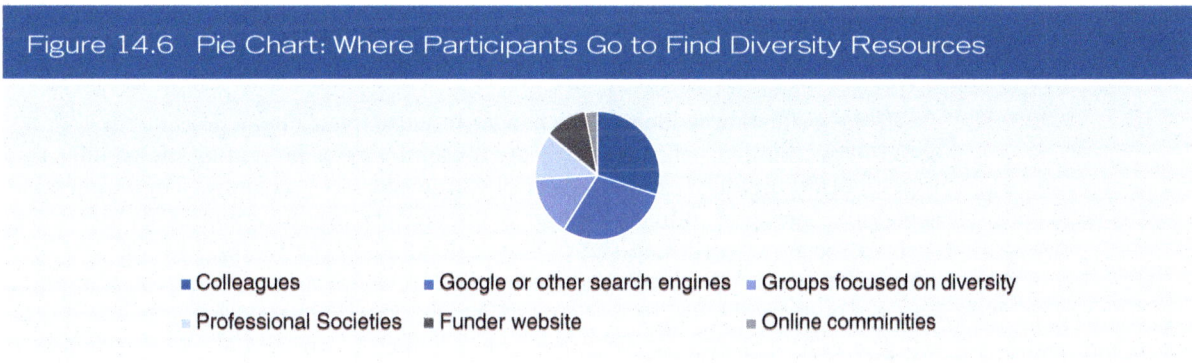

Figure 14.6   Pie Chart: Where Participants Go to Find Diversity Resources

The following activity gives readers a chance to reflect on and discuss some of the differences between the different charts in the figures.

Reflect and Discuss
What are Your Chart Preferences?

In small groups, discuss some of the differences among the chart types and the format(s) you feel best represents the data and why.

Chapter 14 | Reporting, Disseminating, and Utilizing Evaluation Results   433

Figure 14.7 Number of Participant Presentations vs. Publications

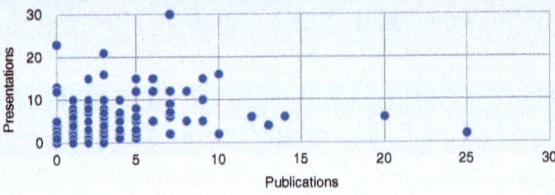

A different type of chart or graph is a **scatter plot**. While most figures present summary data such as frequencies and means, scatter plots present the raw data. The scatter plot shown in Figure 14.7, using unpublished data, maps the number of individuals' presentations to the number of their publications. The scatter plot gives much more information than just knowing that the mean number of presentations is 2.8 (SD = 3.4), the mean number of publications is 4.6 (SD = 4.6), and the correlation between two variables is .28. However, scatter plots can at times be difficult to interpret.

The following activity provides an opportunity for readers to reflect on and discuss some of the advantages and disadvantages of using scatter plots versus **descriptive statistics**.

> ### Reflect and Discuss
> #### Comparing Scatter Plots and Descriptive Statistics
>
> What are some conclusions that you might draw from the scatter plot in Figure 14.7 that you wouldn't have been able to draw if you just knew the means, SDs, and correlations? Discuss your conclusions with others.

If the evaluation is looking at changes in participant interactions of networking, social networking visualization tools are a useful way of presenting the results. This is particularly useful when the subject of your evaluation is a family, a department, or some other group of individuals. Rather than describing the group by its identifying traits, a social network map shows how individuals relate to and network with one another. It visually demonstrates natural leaders, connectors, and outliers through a series of nodes and lines that vary in size and density (DiLuzio, 2018).

The following illustration, taken from Chapter 13 (page 400), is an example of a social networking visual of the collaborations of nine faculty members from five departments in terms of their working together.

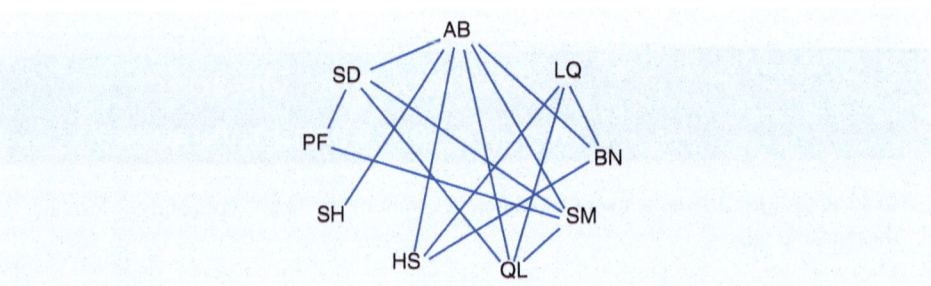

With the exception of the networking illustration, which was developed manually, the earlier charts were done in Excel. While a wide variety of data visualization tools are available, Excel is a commonly available tool that develops charts and graphs easily. Different formats, colors, and label options are available, and Excel charts and graphs can be easily imported into Word documents.

While the charts shown earlier are best for straightforward data stories, there are more esoteric charts, including

- slope graphs, a special type of a line graph where two (or more) sets of values are compared by connecting each group's values on one scale to their values on the second scale;

- alluvial diagrams, which show how various entities (or nodes) flow together or apart across stages representing multiple groups or time periods; and

- steam graphs, which show how the size or proportion of groups varies over time.

These types of graphs, which require more specialized software to create, are used for communicating more complex data stories (Sinar, 2016) and are beyond the scope of this chapter.

As discussed earlier, different presentations of data can influence readers' interpretations of the results differently, even when, as was the case here, the examples were unskewed presentations of the data. Often, however, as Darrel Huff describes in his classic 1954 book, *How to Lie With Statistics*, data are presented in figures that skew the interpretation of the results, which, as he points out, can be done intentionally, and unethically, to give readers the impression the difference is larger than it actually is. His examples show how changing the coordinates of the axis can change how the results are viewed. For example, in Figure 14.8, respondents rated their skills on a scale of 1 (*very weak*) to 5 (*very strong*), so that is the range on the vertical axis.

Changing the vertical axis scale to 2–4, as is shown in Figure 14.9, presents all of the data accurately, but the perception is of a much bigger pretest–posttest change than it is when Figure 14.8 is viewed.

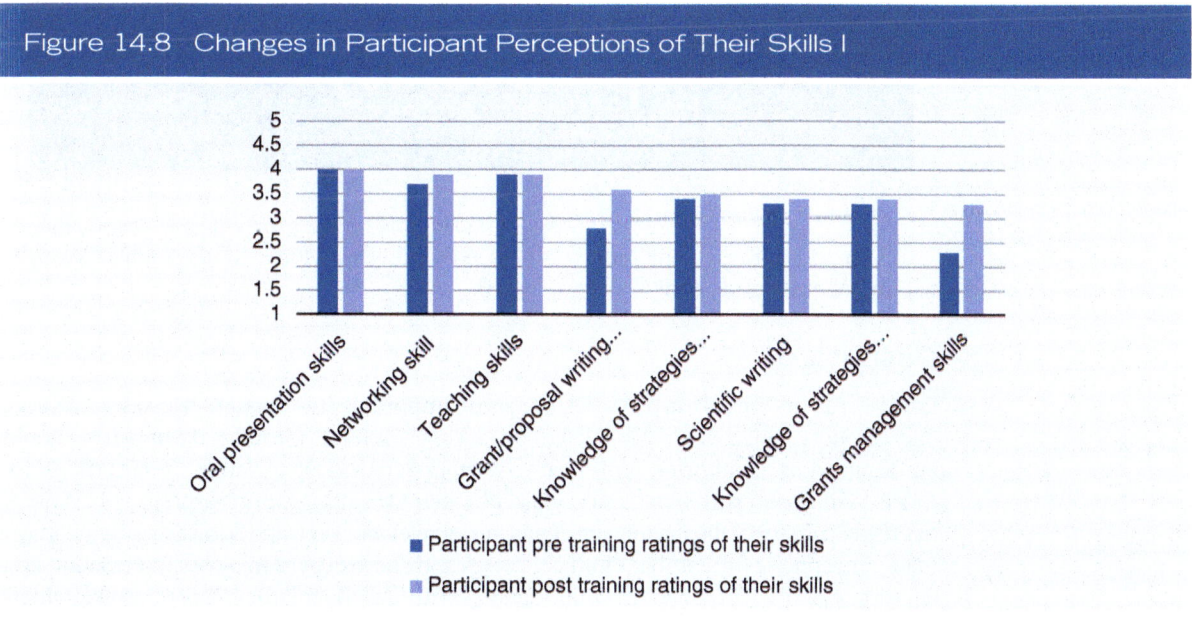

Figure 14.8 Changes in Participant Perceptions of Their Skills I

Chapter 14 | Reporting, Disseminating, and Utilizing Evaluation Results

Figure 14.9 Changes in Participant Perceptions of Their Skills II

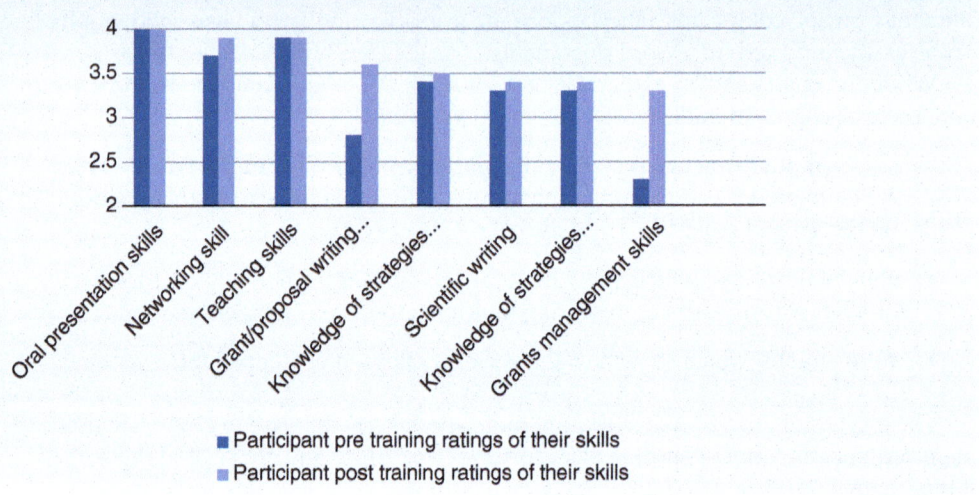

- Participant pre training ratings of their skills
- Participant post training ratings of their skills

As Edward Tufte (2001) points out in his principles of graphical excellence, it is important to show the data and avoid (unintended and intended) distorting what the data have to say.

Figures can also be used to present qualitative data. One popular figure is a **word cloud**, which is an image that shows the words used in interviews or other qualitative data in different sizes according to how often they are used. The following is an example of a word cloud from Chapter 5 (page 137).

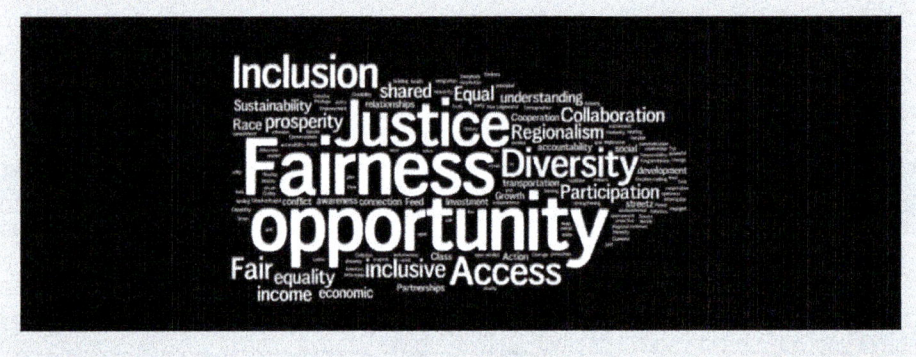

A variety of free online tools can be used to develop word clouds, such as Wordle.net and WordClouds.com (DiLazio, 2018).

Dashboards

Dashboards are visual displays "of the most important information needed to achieve one or more objectives consolidated on a single screen. Effective dashboards should be designed as monitoring tools that can be understood at a glance" (V. Smith, 2013, p. 21). The dashboard is particularly useful when evaluating complex projects because it has the capability of displaying large amounts of relevant, rich, and sometimes dense information in concise format that ultimately eases and speeds users' intake of information and decision making based on such information. With dashboard data displays, stakeholders are typically able to more quickly understand visualization of data compared to text presented in tables and lengthy reports. Dashboards also can indicate the degree to which the program and/or individual elements of the program are on track to meet their goals.

Dashboards typically include multiple visualizations, such as tables and figures, accompanied by minimal text to describe the indicators being displayed on the dashboard. By displaying such visualizations on a single screen, the user can directly compare and draw conclusions from the data "at a glance," which is not possible if the data are split across several screens or require scrolling to view. The example provided in Figure 14.10 is a dashboard based on hypothetical data from the educational component of the Georgetown–Howard Universities Center for Clinical and Translational Science (GHUCCTS), developed by lead author Veronica G. Thomas and dashboard consultant Veronica Smith.

As displayed in this sample dashboard, there are visual data on a number of metrics on a single screen, including, for example, number of applications received for selected educational and professional development offerings, scholarship production (e.g., number of publications, presentations, and posters of participants), disciplinary background and ethnicity of scholars and fellows, and outreach as operationalized, in this case, as the number of website visits across a particular time frame.

Dissemination

Why Disseminate

One of the guiding principles put forth by the AEA is for evaluators to "promote transparency and active sharing of data and findings with the goal of equitable access to information in forms that respect people and honor promises of confidentiality" (AEA, 2018, section E4). While dissemination is often seen as the responsibility of the project and the funder, as the AEA's guiding principle points out, it is also the responsibility of the evaluator. Ideally, program staff and the evaluator should collaborate on disseminating the results of the evaluation. However, project staff and even funders may not be likely to share results that can be seen as critical of the project. The ability of the evaluator to disseminate the results can be tied to the contract that the evaluator signed. As will be discussed more completely in Chapter 15, under some contracts the evaluator may have no rights to disseminate the results of the evaluation, without the permission of the project director or principal investigator(s) (PIs).

Dissemination Plans

As the Substance Abuse and Mental Health Services Administration (SAMHSA, 2019) points out:

> Evaluation results need to get into the hands of the people who can use them. Keep in mind that organizations don't use evaluation results; people do. The Department of Health, for example, isn't going to use the results of an evaluation, but "Cathy Smith" in the Department of Health may. So, unless you get the results of the program evaluation into her hands and explain how she can use the results, they will sit on a shelf somewhere in the Department of Health. (p. 43)

A major goal of the dissemination plan is to make sure that those who can use the results get them. Developing a dissemination plan is an important step in the dissemination—one in which the evaluator should be involved both to ensure that accurate information goes to appropriate target audiences and to provide opportunities for the evaluator's work to be known and shared.

Figure 14.10 Dashboard Design Example From the GHUCCTS Educational Component, 2013

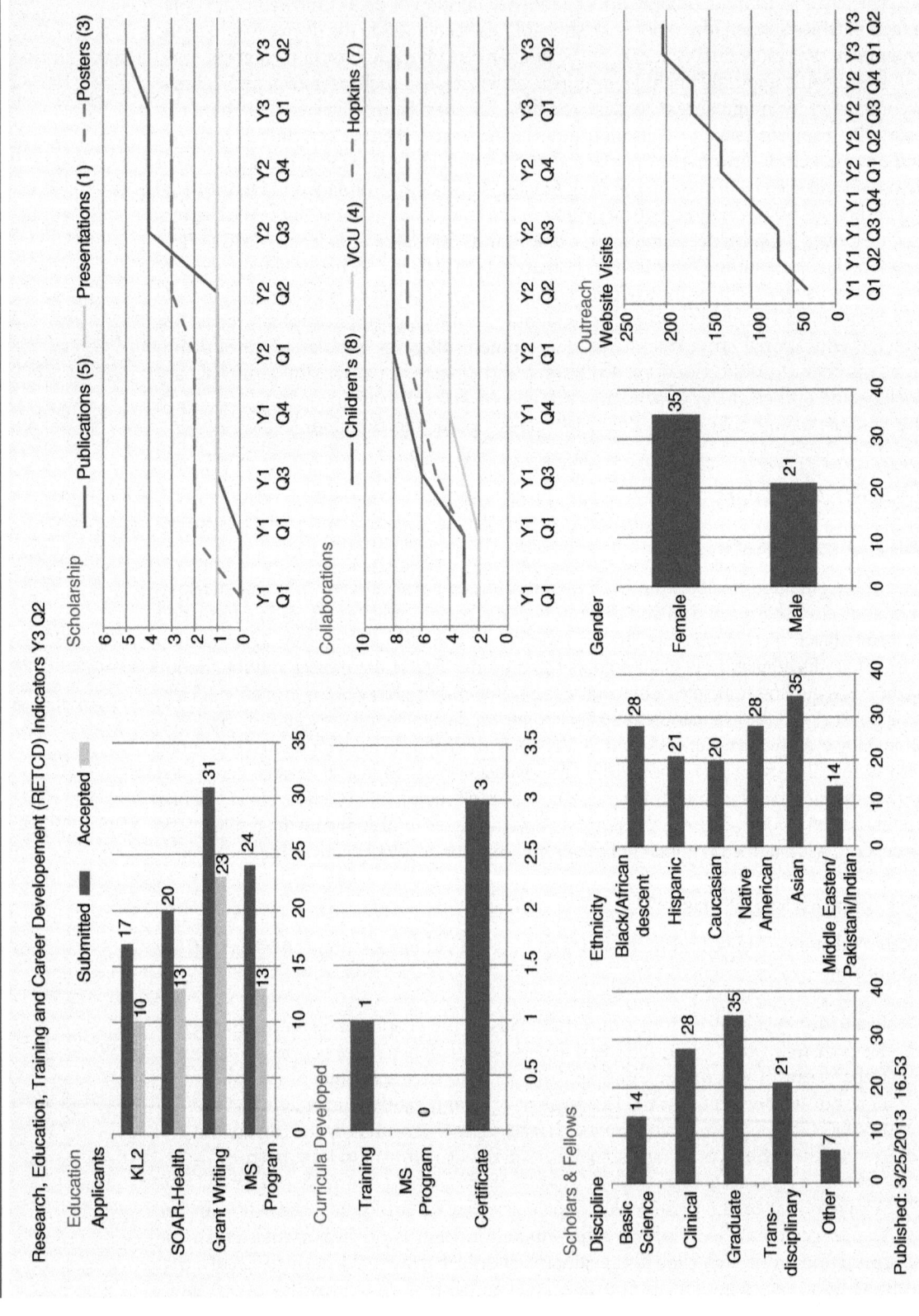

Source: Thomas and Smith (2013).

When developing a dissemination plan, Nancy Duarte points out it is all about the audience:

> The number one thing . . . is to be audience-centric. To take the time to think through who the audience is and develop all your material from a place of empathy toward them. . . . By flipping that paradigm to an audience-centric approach, your material will resonate and the audience can feel a deeper connection to you and your material. (Quoted in Torgovnick May, 2012, para. 4)

The activity that follows is a first step to thinking about different ways people access information that they need.

Reflect and Discuss
Sharing Information

In small groups, reflect on and discuss some of the most common ways you share information with others. Also discuss how these ways differ depending on the different groups with whom you are sharing information, such as the following:

- Friends and family members
- Coworkers
- Graduate students
- Professors
- Teenagers

Learning about how different modes of communication differ in different groups is key to a successful dissemination. If evaluators are not aware of modes target groups use to communicate and access information, they need to determine what the most common modes are for those groups. Traditionally, evaluation reports and summaries were printed on paper and distributed. However, they can be presented in a variety of formats. Paper copies, particularly paper copies of summaries, work well when in-person dissemination is being done. This could be in person as part of a presentation, debriefing, or a site visit. Sending print versions, via email, can supplement and dramatically expand the range of those who receive the results. If there are concerns about recipients receiving the reports changing report content and sending them on to others, it is important to send the reports as protected pdf documents or other protected documents rather than as documents that can be edited and changed such as Word documents.

Using Websites and Social Media

Reports may also be made available on the project or the evaluator's website if approved by the appropriate parties involved. There are a number of advantages to posting reports on a website. While reports can be put in as downloadable pdfs, highlights of the reports can also be posted in HTML documents with live links to difference components of the reports and/or to project descriptions, visuals and other materials.

Along with written reports, results from evaluations can be provided as audio reports or podcasts or as video reports. Audio reports and podcasts should be more than just reading the report. It might be useful to start with an overview of the report in a narrative style and then have more than one person engage in a conversation about the evaluation findings and their implications for the project. Video casts can work as well, but filming and editing can be time consuming and expensive. A cheaper, easier alternative to a video is to pair PowerPoint slides with audio.

It is often useful to copyright the reports and other products of the evaluation to protect the work from being used by others without permission (Copyright.gov, n.d.). As will be covered in greater detail in Chapter 15, a copyright is the exclusive legal right, given to an originator or an assignee, to print, publish, perform, film, or record literary, artistic, or musical material, and to authorize others to do the same. Whatever the format that is used, the materials need to be accessible to people with disabilities. The following is an overview of information and guidance from the Web Accessibility Initiative (WAI, 2019), which provides strategies, standards, and resources to make the web accessible to people with disabilities.

> Web accessibility means that websites, tools, and technologies are designed and developed so that people with disabilities can use them. More specifically, people can:
>
> - perceive, understand, navigate, and interact with the Web
> - contribute to the Web
>
> Web accessibility encompasses all disabilities that affect access to the Web, including:
>
> - auditory
> - cognitive
> - neurological
> - physical
> - speech
> - visual

The following are basic principles of web content accessibility from the WAI (2019):

- Principle 1, perceivability: Information and user interface components must be presentable to users in ways they can perceive.
- Principle 2, operability: User interface components and navigation must be operable.
- Principle 3, understandability: Information and the operation of the user interface must be understandable.
- Principle 4, robustness: Content must be robust enough that it can be interpreted by a wide variety of user agents, including assistive technologies.

Social media can play an important role in dissemination. The percentage of adults in the United States who use at least one social media tool grew from near 0% in 2005 to 69% in 2016, and it continues to grow. Too, unlike other modes of dissemination, there is little difference in social media use by race/ethnicity, sex, income, education, or community type (Allen, Stanton, Di Pietro, & Moseley, 2013). Even for academics, social media can be an effective dissemination technique. For example, Peoples, Midway, Sackett, Lynch, and Cooney (2016) found a strong positive relationship between Twitter activity (i.e., the number of unique tweets about an article) and the number of citations. Twitter activity was a more important predictor of citation rates than five-year journal impact factor, although it must be remembered that this is a correlation and does not mean causality (Brownson, Eyler, Harris, Moore, & Tabak, 2018).

However, social media may not be a viable dissemination method for some groups, especially marginalized ones. If a community has limited internet access, then dissemination should include sharing paper copies of the summary findings and recommendations by mail or making them available at community meeting places.

Distrust of social media as well as research and evaluation can be an issue. In some target groups, elders or trusted others in their community are among the most-used sources of information. It is important for evaluators to involve elders and trusted others in their dissemination of results, as well as, as indicated in earlier chapters, in the evaluation design and results.

Using Mainstream Media

Mainstream media can play an important role in reaching broader populations, especially populations composed of people who are not on social media and who may not be on the internet. Mainstream media includes local, regional, and national newspapers and radio and television stations. As might be expected, it is easier to get interviews and articles in local media, but what is reported in local media may be picked up by regional and national media. Press releases sent by the program to media outlets are a good first step. Having the evaluator be interviewed, along with others such as program staff and participants, can help increase the probability that the story/interview accurately reflects the findings. The following are some tips that print, web, and broadcast journalists gave to researchers. However, their advice holds for evaluators as well.

Keep It Simple

> *Your research will be simplified in the story; either you simplify it or the journalist will.* Who do you want to simplify the story? One of you will and for your sake and the sake of your research, it had better be you.

> *Simplification differs based on the publication.* The sound bite that you would give to a journalist from a local tabloid should be quite different than one you would give to a journalist from *Science* magazine. Whatever the sound bite, decide on it in advance, practice saying it and don't let unexpected or uninformed questions take you off message.

> *Many journalists won't have a lot of background knowledge in your field.* Start out at an extremely basic level, with no assumptions about what the journalist already knows

> *Very few of your caveats about your work will be published.* Decide in advance the caution you want people to hear and work it into your main message.

Journalists need highlights. Don't get so lost in your data that the journalists can't hear the high points of your results. Decide in advance what you consider the most important points to get across, write them down, and be sure to say them in the interview. (P. B. Campbell, 2006, paras. 2–6)

Keep It Interesting

Journalists are storytellers. They need a story to tell. They care about your work, but they also care about the human reaction; about how you felt. Be able to explain why your work is important and why the average reader/listener should care.

Journalists need quotes from people, not from publications. Most journalists aren't going to be allowed to quote your written work. They need a quote from you, so sending them your publications is not enough. You need to be available to speak with them.

Journalists are interested in broader impacts. Be sure to have some.

Different media have different requirements. In print, people read and can read again. In radio, they listen once. In TV, they listen and view once. On the web they can listen and view more than once. Your statements need to reflect those different ways of delivering and receiving information. (P. B. Campbell, 2006, paras. 7–10)

Creative Dissemination Modes

Some groups are using the arts to disseminate results and engage audiences. For example, science writer John Bohannon (2011) demonstrated how using dancers along with verbal presentations helped people's understanding of research results. His work led to the American Association for the Advancement of Science (AAAS) annual contest "Dance Your PhD" where researchers submit videos of their PhD research. Finalists work with professional chorographers, and the resulting dances provide useful contexts for the results and generate interest (Travis, 2020). For example, a dance about the evaluation of creative ideas received over 20,000 views on You Tube (Pétervári, 2017).

Actor and science communicator Alan Alda has some excellent advice about science communication that holds for the communication of evaluation results as well:

> Effective science communication happens when we listen and connect. It happens when we use empathy. Communication is headed for success when we pay more attention to what the other person is understanding rather than focusing solely on what we want to say. (Alda, 2019, p. 1)

Working With Others

Reflecting one of the central themes of the book, engaging others, the Agency for Healthcare Research and Quality (2014) points out:

You do not have to work alone to reach your end users! Consider working with professionals who are trusted opinion leaders and are influential in their fields. Think about formal and informal networks that you can tap into to spread the word about your research findings or products. Consider also how you might develop working partnerships with organizations to which your end users belong, or that can influence them through their credibility, expertise, or licensing powers. These individuals and organizations can serve as dissemination intermediaries, amplifying your reach into your target audiences. (Section III, para. 1)

For example, to reach parents with information about the success of a statewide education initiative in partnership with the state parks, Jane Butler Kahle (personal communication, August 24, 2018), while being interviewed for this book, described how her evaluation team developed a one-page summary of the findings of the evaluation, copies of which were put in the same boxes as state park maps, both of which were available to people entering a state park. Tens of thousands of summaries were disseminated that way.

Sometimes, such as when target audiences include the more general public, it can be useful to draw on the expertise of marketing and public relations professionals. Many universities have marketing departments where professors may be willing to have their students provide assistance to community-based organizations or other nonprofit organizations. Most universities and larger nonprofits have a press office, which focuses on publicizing the organization and may be able to provide some advice. The following activity provides an opportunity for readers to unleash their creativity.

> **Reflect and Discuss**
> **Effective Dissemination Strategies**
>
> In small groups, brainstorm the most creative and feasible ways to disseminate the results of an evaluation to each of the following stakeholders/target audiences:
>
> Participants
>
> Funders
>
> Policymakers
>
> Groups not usually reached by traditional dissemination strategies such as people living on Indian reservations, people with disabilities, people with low literacy, and people of lower socioeconomic status

Using Evaluation Results

Regardless of the specific objectives of individual evaluations, the overall purpose of evaluation is for it to be useful and used—that it provides meaningful information from which decisions about programs and related policies can be made. In his Voices From the Field interview, Roger Nozaki, vice president of the Barr Foundation, explains why evaluation is important to him.

Voices From the Field

Roger Nozaki: Why I Care About Evaluation

Evaluation is important because:

- Resources are limited. Whether funders or practitioners, we are doing mission-driven work with limited resources. So we need to maximize the impact of those resources and direct them to the strategies and approaches that demonstrate impact.

- Data-driven culture is important. The GE Foundation [where Nozaki was the executive director] was very data driven, like the company it represented. The board expected the staff to clearly articulate the goals of any strategy or program and why they thought programs would reach those goals, collect the data to see what was changing, and make appropriate decisions and adjustments.

- The "common sense" answer isn't always right. There are times when it just seems obvious that something will work, so why waste time and money on an evaluation, when you know the strategy will work? For example, it seemed like common sense that having volunteers who worked in the sciences could go into classrooms and get students excited about science careers. But [co-author Patricia B. Campbell] then showed me the data that not only did this strategy not always work, it could even have a negative impact on student interest.

Roger Nozaki is the vice president of the Barr Foundation. Formerly, he was a senior policy advisor in the U.S. Department of Education, an academic dean at Brown University, and executive director of the GE Foundation. He was interviewed by coauthor Patricia B. Campbell in the fall of 2018.

Evaluation results can be used in a variety of ways, including

- to improve ongoing programs;
- to inform individual decision making about continued participation in programs;
- to improve program outcomes;
- to inform the development of new programs;
- to inform organizational decisions about future directions;
- to influence the probability of getting additional funding;
- to generate awareness of programs;
- to inform funder decision making;
- to influence the public's perceptions of programs;
- to inform policymaker decision making; and
- to move the knowledge base about the content area and/or discipline forward.

The following activity can help readers add to the list.

Reflect and Discuss
Using Evaluation

What other ways do you think evaluation results can be used? Are some of these ways a higher priority for you? If so, what are they? And why do you feel they are higher priorities for you?

While there are many valuable ways evaluation can be used, there has been some question as to the degree to which evaluation results are used. For example, a 2006 survey of over 1,100 evaluators found that 68% felt that nonuse of evaluation findings was a major problem (Fleischer & Christie, 2009).

Based on research on utilization, Patton (2008, p. 66) determined 11 factors that could impact evaluation usage: methodological quality, methodological appropriateness, timeliness, lateness of report, positive or negative findings, surprise of findings, central or peripheral program objectives evaluated, presence or absence of related studies, political factors, decision maker/evaluator interactions, and resources available for the study. When evaluators and those for whom the evaluations were done were asked to "pick out the single factor you feel had the greatest effect on how this study was used," two factors emerged: political considerations and the personal factor. Patton defines the *personal factor* as

> the presence of an identifiable individual or group of people who personally care about the evaluation and the findings it generates. Where such a person or group was present, evaluations were used; where the personal factor was absent, there was a correspondingly marked absence of evaluation impact. The personal factor represents the leadership, interest, enthusiasm, determination, commitment, assertiveness, and caring of specific, individual people. These are people who actively seek information to learn, make judgments, get better at what they do, and reduce decision uncertainties. (pp. 66–67)

Fleischer and Christie (2009) cluster possible barriers to evaluation use into three factors: human factors (relating to user or evaluator characteristics; e.g., knowledge, experience, perceptions), contextual factors (relating to the context surrounding the evaluation; e.g., political background, organizational background), and evaluation factors (relating to how the evaluation is conducted; e.g., ethics, design, methods). Fleischer and Christie also argue that "is likely that human and contextual factors are contributing to nonuse more so than evaluation factors" (pp. 171–172).

While this can suggest that major factors tied to evaluation usage are outside of the evaluator's control, there are things the evaluator can do that can influence whether the evaluation results are used. If the evaluation is not well done, the findings aren't clear, and the recommendations don't focus on ways the findings can be used, or the findings aren't provided before decisions have to be made, then the evaluation is less apt to be used. To increase the use of evaluation findings, some have suggested adding a section in the report called "Use of the Evaluation" or "Use of This Report" where the evaluator and the readers can "start thinking of the 'So what?' once the evaluation exercise is finished" (Vaca, 2018, para. 4). Another suggestion from Sara Vaca (2018) is to modify

> the Recommendations section, but not in a prescriptive manner. Usually I would analyze all the evaluation ideas for improvement, and I would prioritize them according to their relevance, feasibility and impact. This time, I pointed out the priority areas I would focus on, and a list of ideas to improve each area, without clearly outlining what to do. Then I invited the organization to discuss and take that decision internally, and maybe forming internal teams to address each of the recommendations. (para. 5)

As the following case study indicate, under the right circumstance, evaluations can make a difference.

Case Study
Evaluation Can Make a Difference

Evaluations of the HighScope Preschool program found participation improved children's chances of living a better life through adulthood. After participating in the program, children

- were less likely to be placed in special education programs (through age 14) or retained in grade (through grade 4);
- showed a significant decrease in self-reported delinquent behavior at age 14 and officially reported crime and delinquency at age 19;
- had significantly higher grade point averages and were more likely to graduate from high school, enroll in further training or education, and be employed at age 19; [and]
- had significantly better educational outcomes, averaged significantly fewer lifetime criminal arrests, and had higher mean monthly earnings at age 27. (Blueprints for Healthy Youth Development, 2019)

These results impacted the design of early childhood curriculum.

Evaluation of the Louis Stokes Alliances for Minority Participation (LSAMP) found LSAMP increased the quality and quantity of students who successfully completed LSAMP-supported science, technology, engineering, and mathematics (STEM) baccalaureate programs and "produced underrepresented minority students who enroll in and attain graduate degrees in STEM at a higher percentage rate than that of a national sample of underrepresented minority students, and a national sample of [W]hite and Asian STEM baccalaureate degree recipients." The results led to the continuation and expansion of the program and "a critical advance in the knowledge base of intervention program models" (Clewell et al., 2005, p. 2).

SUMMARY

The focus of this chapter has been to provide the reader with the skills and knowledge to be able to report and disseminate the results, conclusions, and recommendations of evaluations in ways that are culturally and contextually appropriate, accessible, and usable. This included ways to present information visually and textually to different groups and in ways that the results can be used in decision making. Covered were issues tied to accessibility, including making results available in formats for those with visual and hearing impairments as well as to those with different levels of literacy skills and speakers of languages other than English. Attention was paid to the meaning and impact of different words and images on people with different backgrounds. Readers are now aware of formats to report evaluation results to different audiences and of the ways to develop and implement a dissemination plan to share the results, using old and new media, in ways that the results are most likely to be used.

SUPPLEMENTAL RESOURCES

Tableau Public
https://public.tableau.com/en-us/s/gallery/visual-vocabulary

This data visualization website allows users to design charts based on nine types of relationships they want to show such as correlation, deviation, and change over time. It also provides sample data sets and free training videos and webinars.

Potent Presentations Initiative: p2i Tools and Guidelines

www.eval.org/page/p2i-tools

This website provides free tools and resources to strengthen and enhance evaluators' message, design, and delivery and improve their presentations. These include guidelines for developing handouts and slides and keeping on message.

AEA Data Visualization and Reporting: Websites and Tools

http://comm.eval.org/datavisualizationandreporting/tigresources/websitescombined

This website presents a wide variety of tools and resources, including webinars, to help develop useful and visually appealing charts and graphs.

Gapminder

www.gapminder.org/tools-offline/

Gapminder is an independent Swedish foundation that promotes a fact-based worldview everyone can understand. It presents trend data in a variety of creative, easy-to-understand visuals and provides free downloadable tools for people to create their own videos of trend data.

Edward Tufte

www.edwardtufte.com/tufte/

The works of Tufte, an eminent scholar on data visualization, including *Visual Display of Quantitative Information*, *Envisioning Information*, and *Visual Explanations: Images and Quantities, Evidence and Narrative*, are excellent resources on displaying data.

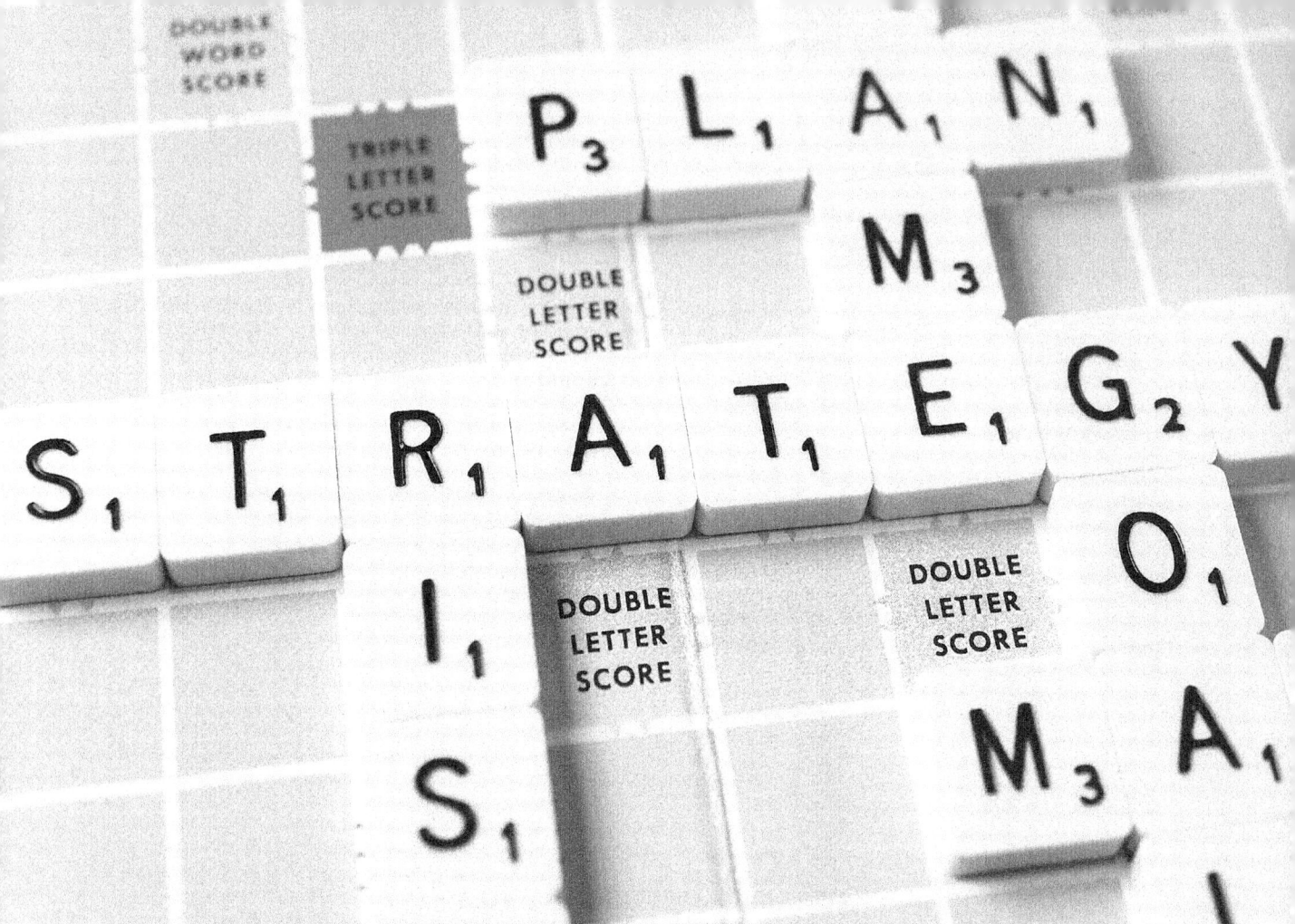

Translating your passion into a successful business takes hard work, resilience, and the ability to multitask, but the results can be truly fulfilling

CHAPTER 15

Evaluation as a Business

Evaluation is a field, a discipline, and a possible career. For some, evaluation can also be a full- or part-time business. Running your own small business is both challenging and rewarding. If doing evaluation as a business is for you, there are a number of things you can do to increase the probability that your business will be successful. Translating your passion into a successful business takes hard work, resilience, and the ability to multitask, but the results can be truly fulfilling.

After reading this chapter and participating in the activities, readers will be able to meet the following learning objectives:

- Discuss some of advantages and disadvantages of doing evaluation as a business
- Describe some ethical areas that may be more difficult for someone doing evaluation as a business
- List major components of an evaluation proposal and key areas to be covered in an evaluation budget
- Describe the components that should be included in an evaluation contract
- Describe advantages and disadvantages of different business entities and select a business entity that you feel would be most appropriate for you and provide a rationale
- Develop an overview of a possible evaluation business plan including possible ways of marketing your business and/or yourself as an evaluator

Introduction

This chapter covers many of the areas that practicing evaluators and those who may be considering doing evaluations full-time, part-time, or even occasionally should know. It covers such areas as how to market yourself as an evaluator, as well as how to prepare an evaluation proposal and a budget. It provides an overview of some of the advantages having a contract can provide. Additionally, the chapter examines advantages and disadvantages of different possible business entities for evaluators to consider if they want to set up a business. Ethical issues that are particularly relevant to those doing evaluations as a business are addressed, as are things that evaluators need to consider to make their business financially viable. While most of the areas covered in this chapter are important for all practicing evaluators, other areas such as deciding on a business entity, writing a business plan, and making the business financially viable are more relevant for those who are planning to go into doing evaluations on their own or with a partner or partners, part- or full-time.

Perspectives on Doing Evaluation as a Business

There are a number of reasons to consider doing evaluations either part- or full-time. For example, faculty members who do evaluations part-time (such as lead author Veronica G. Thomas) gain "real life" evaluation experiences, applying evaluation theory and concepts to practice, which can positively impact their teaching, research, and service at their university. Faculty and others who are employed may consider doing evaluations part-time for the experience or the extra money and/or to expand their networks. Germuth (2019) lists the following benefits to working as an independent evaluator: One can choose "how to work (intermittently, part-time, full-time), with whom to work (non-profits, public schools, private corporations) and where to work (in an office, at home, in a co-working space)" (pp. 44–45).

If you are employed, before doing any evaluations outside of your job requirements, it is important to check with your employer to make sure that conducting evaluations outside of your job is allowed. In some institutions no outside work is allowed, while in others employees can work on outside projects for up to a maximum number of days or a maximum amount of money. Breaking employer rules and policies can lead to termination and a lack of references for future employment. And, of course, even if outside work is allowed, it should be done independently, not during working hours and not using the employer's resources (supplies, office space, etc.).

In their Voices From the Field interviews, Mary Moriarty and Jane Butler Kahle discuss some of the reasons they started doing evaluation as a business.

Voices From the Field

Mary Moriarty and Jane Butler Kahle: Why I Do Evaluations

At this point in my life I wanted the flexibility to travel a little bit and still work. With my own business, I have the flexibility to work from wherever I want to work. I have projects in Georgia, Texas, Massachusetts, and Washington, DC. I'm not tied to being in one place. Working at the National Science Foundation (NSF) gave me an incredible opportunity to be involved in multiple projects. After leaving I didn't want to be narrowed to one institution working on one project. I wanted to be able to be involved in a variety of projects that were of interest to me. Having your own business gives you the ability to do that. It also gives you the ability to choose the work you do. I can say yes when I really want to do a project that is something I believe in. When you work for an organization, you do what is in front of you. I get to choose what I do. There are times when you need to work and work and work. There will be times when you can't say I'm taking the weekend off. But running your own evaluation business is worth it. It's given me the opportunity to have some really interesting projects and work with some great principal investigators (PIs) and I'm learning a lot of things.

Mary Moriarty was an evaluator at Smith College and an NSF program officer and now has her own company, Moriarty Research and Evaluation Associates, LLC. She was interviewed by coauthor Patricia B. Campbell in the fall of 2017.

I got into evaluation out of intellectual curiosity. It was so interesting to me. I wanted to continue evaluating projects so I could see what works and advise people on what to try. I would say having a career as an evaluator was more satisfying than being a professor, and it was more satisfying than being a teacher or bringing a student of biology through a master's thesis. It's something where you feel you can understand a problem and maybe do something about it.

Jane Butler Kahle was a professor of science education and the founding director of Ohio's Evaluation and Assessment Center for Mathematics and Science Education at Miami University of Ohio. Since her retirement, she has worked as an independent evaluator. She was interviewed by coauthor Patricia B. Campbell in summer of 2018.

Ethics

Every evaluator should be concerned about ethics and ethical behavior. As was covered in Chapter 2, the American Evaluation Association (AEA, 2018b) has ethical standards tied to integrity and honesty to ensure that "evaluators behave with honesty and transparency in order to ensure the integrity of the evaluation" (p. 3). The AEA's Evaluators' Ethical Guiding Principles with a special relevance for those who are doing evaluation as a business include the following:

- Communicate truthfully and openly with clients and relevant stakeholders concerning all aspects of the evaluation, including its limitations.
- Disclose any conflicts of interest (or appearance of a conflict) prior to accepting an evaluation assignment and manage or mitigate any conflicts during the evaluation.
- Clearly communicate, justify, and address concerns related to procedures or activities that are likely to produce misleading evaluative information or conclusions.
- Consult colleagues for suggestions on proper ways to proceed if concerns cannot be resolved, and decline the evaluation when necessary.
- Disclose all sources of financial support for an evaluation, and the source of the request for the evaluation. (AEA, 2018b, p. 3)

Ethics can be of particular concern to those who are doing evaluations independently. Evaluators who are working in universities, in government, or in nonprofits usually have a series of institutional guidelines that, as employees, they have to follow. The areas covered by these guidelines usually include such ethical areas as conflicts of interest, protection of human participants, and nondiscrimination. Independent evaluators, however, need to develop their own guidelines or procedures in these areas.

Conflicts of Interest

As covered in detail in Chapter 2, a conflict of interest (COI) is

> a situation in which a person has a duty to more than one person or organization, but cannot do justice to the actual or potentially adverse interests of both parties. This includes when an individual's personal interests or concerns are

inconsistent with the best for a customer, or when a public official's personal interests are contrary to his/her loyalty to public business. (Law.com, n.d., para. 1)

Evaluators must always be concerned with actual and potential COIs and must deal with them openly and honestly so that they do not compromise the evaluation processes and results. COIs include situations in which financial or other personal considerations may compromise, or have the appearance of compromising, an evaluator's judgment in conducting the evaluation and/or reporting the findings. A COI exists regardless of whether the evaluator's judgment and behavior can be demonstrated to have adversely influenced the evaluation; instead, it exists simply as a condition of the evaluator having competing interests (Thomas & Campbell, 2017).

Usually, COI forms request a listing of any relationships that might impact the evaluators' work. These may include

- personal relationships—where the evaluator is evaluating a project or program where the evaluator, family members, or close friends are staff or participants;

- financial relationships—where the evaluator or a close family member has a financial interest in the success or lack of success of that which is being evaluated; and

- professional relationships—where the evaluator or a close family member is working on other non-evaluation-oriented projects with key staff of the program being evaluated (Yarbrough, Shulha, Hopson, & Caruthers, 2011).

In addition, as discussed in Chapter 2, we proposed an additional COI, a cultural conflict of interest, which occurs when an individual's culture mores (social or cultural rules) are seen as the norm or even the only way. An evaluator's inability to recognize other ways can mean that outcomes are defined, conclusions are drawn, and/or policies are made that, usually unintentionally, benefit the evaluator either directly or indirectly through the validation of the evaluator's culture (Thomas & Campbell, 2017).

Often clients and funders require that evaluators and other contractors have COI guidelines or that evaluators agree to abide by the client's COI guidelines. Since different clients may have different guidelines, it is often useful for evaluators working for themselves or with a small group of others to have their own guidelines or policies. Sample guidelines, covering traditional COIs, can be downloaded from the Web and adapted to meet the needs and concerns of those doing evaluation as a business. The National Council of Nonprofits provides information on COIs and sample guidelines at www.councilofnonprofits.org/tools-resources/conflicts-of-interest.

Protection of Human Participants

As was covered in detail in Chapters 2 and 12, the protection of human participants is one of the highest ethical concerns and is required in research projects and programs that receive federal funding. To ensure the protection of human participants, most colleges and universities and many school districts have their own institutional review boards (IRBs) to review proposed research plans. There are also private companies that review studies for risk to participants for a fee. If a study is not classified as research, it does not have to be reviewed by the IRB. Technically, evaluation studies are not research studies; however, there can be a great deal of overlap between evaluation and research. If the evaluation is being done for a client whose organization has an IRB, it is most appropriate to contact that IRB and describe the evaluation and ask whether the proposed evaluation needs to be reviewed.

While Chapter 12 went into detail about the U.S. Department of Health and Human Services (DHHS) criteria for protection of human participants, Oregon State University (n.d., p. 1) provides some suggestions as to when an evaluation may not need to be submitted for IRB approval. An evaluation may not need IRB approval if

- the intent of project is to evaluate a specific program only to provide information for and about that program;
- the project is not initiated by the evaluator and occurs regardless of whether individual(s) conducting it may benefit professionally from conducting the project;
- the project is not designed to develop or contribute to generalizable knowledge and does not involve randomization of individuals, but may involve comparison of variations in programs;
- the evaluation is mandated by the program, usually its funder, as part of its operations;
- there is no benefit to participants expected, as the evaluation concentrates on program improvements or whether the program should continue; and
- there is no intent to publish or present, other than to program stakeholders and participants or to suggest potentially effective models, strategies, or assessment tools rather than to develop or contribute to generalizable knowledge.

If these criteria do not describe the evaluation being planned, then it should be submitted for IRB review. Even if it does meet those criteria, it can be useful to contact the IRB to be sure.

Nondiscrimination

Unfortunately, discrimination claims have an integral part of the landscape of businesses in this country. Under many state laws, and some federal laws, certain employers are required to establish and maintain nondiscrimination policies to protect their employees. Even if not specifically required by law, it is a generally good idea for any business owner to have these policies in place. A nondiscrimination policy is just that—a policy indicating that the individual and/or organization doesn't discriminate against various populations. The following is a sample nondiscrimination statement from The Denver Foundation.

> [ORGANIZATION] does not and shall not discriminate on the basis of race, color, religion (creed), gender, gender expression, age, national origin (ancestry), disability, marital status, sexual orientation, or military status, in any of its activities or operations. These activities include, but are not limited to, hiring and firing of staff, selection of volunteers and vendors, and provision

of services. We are committed to providing an inclusive and welcoming environment for all members of our staff, clients, volunteers, subcontractors, vendors, and clients.

[ORGANIZATION] is an equal opportunity employer. We will not discriminate and will take affirmative action measures to ensure against discrimination in employment, recruitment, advertisements for employment, compensation, termination, upgrading, promotions, and other conditions of employment against any employee or job applicant on the bases of race, color, gender, national origin, age, religion, creed, disability, veteran's status, sexual orientation, gender identity or gender expression. (The Denver Foundation, n.d., paras. 1–2)

Cultural Respect

Being ethical is an important step, but it is not the only step. As an evaluator doing evaluations as a business, it is important to consider how evaluators and evaluation can unwittingly play into the power of the status quo and what can be done to minimize or eliminate that (Hall, 2018b). This requires that evaluators maintain a high degree of self-awareness and self-examination to better understand how their own backgrounds and other life experiences serve as assets or limitations in the conduct of an evaluation and that evaluators work to avoid reinforcing cultural stereotypes and prejudice in their work. This includes being honest about whether the evaluation will benefit participants in the long run and, if not, whether there are changes that can be made in the evaluation that will make it of greater value or benefit to the participants and their communities (Zahra, 2018).

When doing evaluation as a business, evaluators can be confronted with the ethical questions of whether they agree to do an evaluation when the possible client/program's philosophy is in conflict with their own philosophy and/or beliefs. During a 2017 AEA think tank meeting facilitated by coauthors Veronica G. Thomas and Patricia B. Campbell, Michael Morris, a participant in the think tank, pointed out that differences in opinions that are not important to the evaluation may not be an issue; however, when they are tied to the evaluation, there can be a conflict. His example was a situation where the evaluator has a strong belief against the physical disciplining of children, and the client/program/project participants believe in physical disciplining of children and see it as necessary. The greater the extent to which that difference is tied to the evaluation focus, which is the degree to which the physical disciplining of children is central to the evaluation, the greater the conflict. If the evaluator is judging the participants in a negative way, this is influencing the evaluation, and the evaluator should not be doing an evaluation of that program.

However, in that same 2017 think tank, participant Henry T. Frierson pointed out that using the notion of the benefit to the evaluator, particularly from the evaluator's cultural lens, cultural conflict of interest can cut both ways. If the evaluator is in cultural agreement with the program's milieu, the evaluation study may be fully slanted in a favorable, but possibly unwarranted, direction. By the same token, but at the opposite end, Frierson contends, if the evaluator has cultural issues with the milieu in which the program is based, the evaluation study may be fully slanted in a more negative direction and likely unwarranted as well. It may also be the case that evaluators are not aware of their bias or are aware but feel it will not be a problem because they believe they are "objective" and therefore feel there will be no issues in terms of how they interact with the program.

While these conundrums can impact all evaluators, they are of particular concern to those evaluators who are doing evaluation as a business because when turning down work, they are turning down income that may be needed to keep the business going. The activity that follows can help readers think more about COIs for an independent evaluator.

> ## Activity
> ### Thinking About Conflicts of Interest
>
> Answer the following questions in writing and then, in small groups, discuss your responses.
>
> - Can or should one do the evaluation if one is opposed to the culture or some of the values embodied in that culture?
> - Is it enough to simply inform the client of one's position?
> - Is it necessary or even feasible to indicate one's biases in the report and how those biases may impact the evaluation?
> - Should the evaluator present the clients' views as well as the evaluator's views in the report?
> - Is it the responsibility of the client or the evaluator to explore, in advance, if there is a cultural or values conflict?
> - Can, or should, a client break a contract based on such a conflict?

Business Knowledge and Skills

Marketing

"If you build it, will they come?" is a question that should be asked of anyone who is planning to start their own business, even if the business is a one-person evaluation company. Marketing, of course, increases the probability that clients will come. The type of marketing evaluators do is dependent on how their target client pool is defined. Evaluators don't need to be expert in the content areas of the programs, practices, businesses, or institutions that they will be evaluating, but they do need to have a working knowledge of those areas. If one has little knowledge of or experience with public health issues or programs, those running or funding such programs should not be considered potential clients. However, if one has some science or math knowledge as well as some knowledge about efforts to broaden participation in science, then the target client pool could include programs to diversify the scientific workforce, even if the evaluator does not have a deep knowledge of the specific science, technology, engineering, and mathematics (STEM) area being covered.

Content knowledge is important, as is knowledge of the communities and cultures in which the program or project is being implemented and with whom the evaluation will be done. Community and cultural knowledge is often not generalizable (AEA, 2011). An evaluator who is well prepared to work with a particular community is not necessarily prepared to work with a different community.

Developing a knowledge and experience table like Table 15.1 and marking the cells, where the evaluator has enough knowledge of content and context to do an evaluation, can help evaluators define a target client pool.

Table 15.1 Sample Knowledge and Experience Table

Sample Organizations*	Sample Topic Areas*					
	Administration/ Management	Athletics	Diversity/Broadening Participation	Finance	STEM	Training/Teaching
Armed Services						
Colleges and Universities			X		X	X
Federal Government			X			
Health Services Organizations						
Industry						
Criminal and Juvenile Justice Programs						
Pre-college Education						X
Sports Organizations						
State Government			X			

* It is important to note that these are sample organizations and topic areas. This table can be used as a model, but individuals need to develop their own organization and topic area lists.

In Table 15.1, one target client pool would be government programs to increase diversity and broaden participation while a second target client pool would be colleges and universities with STEM teaching and training programs. In the activity that follows, readers develop their own experience and skills table.

Activity
Evaluation Tools: Developing Your Own Skills and Experience Matrix

Based on the template in Table 15.1, develop and fill out a personal skills and experience matrix and determine possible target client pools.

While Table 15.1 focuses on topics and institutional areas, there is another important area of experience that needs to be addressed. This includes evaluator knowledge of and experience working with the types of people who are participating in the project as leaders, staff, and/or participants. Just as evaluators who have had no experience with military-based programs or projects should not include these programs in their target client pool, evaluators with no experience working in and with different nondominant communities should not include programs or projects working with specific nondominant communities in their target client pool. However, evaluators can expand their target client pools by developing and implementing plans to increase their knowledge of and experience with different communities. As covered in earlier chapters, the plan can include working with members of the communities as cultural guides, liaisons, and/or critical friends and increasing one's own understanding of the community's history and cultural values.

Marketing plans should be based on the target client pool; however, there are some things any evaluator who is starting a business or working as an independent evaluator should do. The first is to "get your name out" as an evaluator. Electronic business cards attached to email messages, often called **vCards**, and paper business cards, both of which identify an individual or a business as doing evaluations, are easy and inexpensive ways to reach potential clients. If email is being used as part of a marketing plan, either through business cards or the emails themselves, it is important that the email account used be the evaluator's personal business or personal account. Using an employer's email account for personal business without the employer's permission is unethical and can lead to termination.

Joining the AEA is an excellent marketing strategy for evaluators. The AEA is an important source of information and networking. It also has a "Find an Evaluator" website (www.eval.org/findanevaluator) where, as the name implies, potential clients can find evaluators. AEA members can complete a form that asks for contact information, including a website and a short description of their areas of expertise. This information is then added to the searchable website. While the AEA is an international organization, it has many regional, state, and local affiliates whose contact information is listed on the website (www.eval.org/affiliate). Among them are regional affiliates such as the Eastern Evaluation Research Society and the Evaluation Network for the Missouri River Basin; state affiliates such as the Arizona Evaluation Network and the Michigan Association for Evaluation; and affiliates at the local level such as the Greater Boston Evaluation Network and the Washington (DC) Evaluators (AEA, n.d.). Participating in affiliate activities provides opportunities for local and regional networking, at little or no cost.

Presenting and being active in the AEA can help relatively new evaluators become known by other evaluators. This is a valuable way for new evaluators to get contacts or even clients. When evaluators turn down potential clients, they are often asked for recommendations for other evaluators. If they do make recommendations, it is usually someone whose work they know. The case study that follows describes one evaluator's experience networking though the AEA.

Case Study
Marketing Tips From the AEA365 Blog

Through the AEA "Find an Evaluator" link, I found two people living in my area and sent them an email asking if they wanted to meet for coffee.

The first lived right around the corner. After several coffees and good conversations about evaluation, she asked for help with one of her projects.

(Continued)

> (Continued)
>
> I said yes . . . and when she moved away to greener pastures she passed on what, to this day, is my favorite client.
>
> I reached out to the second person after admiring her website. We have met for coffee and lunch over the years. During our first meeting, she provided me with inspiration, friendship and some excellent resources related to evaluation consulting.
>
> Recently, she asked "Can you help with conducting an interview?"
>
> I said yes . . . and was exposed first hand to an evaluation of a complex initiative where networks of people and organizations are changing systems in local communities and I saw a very innovative use of graphic presentation. (Clavijo, 2018, paras. 1–6)

The kind of networking described in the case study can help reduce isolation as well. While being interviewed for this book, Mary Moriarty (personal communication, September 7, 2017) explained that,

> in the beginning, I was working on my own. I would have very little contact with other people, and it was difficult. I've learned to have a mix of projects, some of which are local, so I go to meetings and see people. Having one or two people who work with me in the business helps with that as well.

Being active in the professional societies of those in the target client pool is another way to market an evaluation business. Results from a completed knowledge and experience table such as Table 15.1 can help identify appropriate professional societies. For example, those interested in evaluating STEM outreach and/or diversity programs should consider joining the Women in Engineering ProActive Network (WEPAN) (www.WEPAN.org). Being a part of WEPAN is an excellent way to meet people who run programs at the college and pre-college level to increase women students' interest in engineering and increase the diversity of those doing engineering. Based on their target client pool, other professional organizations that evaluators could consider joining include the Academy of Criminal Justice Sciences (ACJS) (www.acjs.org), which promotes criminal justice education, research, and policy analysis for both educators and practitioners, and the National Association of Social Workers (NASW) (www.socialworkers.org), which works to enhance the professional growth and development of its members, to create and maintain professional standards, and to advance sound social policies. Many of the members of these and other organizations run programs, and most of those programs will need evaluators.

Publishing, even self-publishing, nontechnical pieces that might be of interest to potential clients and sharing those pieces with them is another way for evaluators to get their name out and to provide potential clients with information that will be useful to them. These client-oriented pieces could include lessons learned from previous work done in their field, ways potential clients can use evaluation results, or even what their rights and responsibilities are as evaluation clients. The following is a sample piece to share with potential clients.

Your Rights and Responsibilities as an Evaluation Client

I. You have the right to a written contract describing the tasks and products of the evaluation, a timetable, and a budget.

II. You have the right to see the data supporting negative and positive conclusions about your project.

III. You have the right to receive interim reports on aspects of the evaluation needed for planning, proposal writing, and other activities.

IV. You have the right to describe the general direction of the evaluation and the major areas it will cover.

V. You do *not* have the right to demand a positive evaluation.

VI. You have the right to include your own explanations in an evaluation report, as long as they are labeled as such.

VII. You have the right to withhold payment until the products of the evaluation, described in the contract, are delivered to you.

VIII. You do *not* have the right to withhold payment because you do not like the results of the evaluation.

IX. You have the right to an ethical and professional evaluation that uses valid methods, employs solid analyses, and does not violate confidentiality.

Source: P. B. Campbell, 2003, p. 1. Your Rights and Responsibilities as an Evaluation Client 2003

The efforts described earlier are relatively inexpensive. There are other, more traditional and more costly, marketing strategies that can be done as well. For example, many professional organizations provide conference attendees with a bag full of swag, free promotional items. For a fee, a brochure about an individual evaluator or an evaluation business can be included in the bag. Pens, small notebooks, or pretty much anything with a business name, email address, and website on them can all be included in the bag. Of course, along with the fee paid to the organization, the **swag** needs to be paid for. If a major target client pool is, for example engineering education programs, doing this at the annual meeting of the American Society for Engineering Education (ASEE) (www.ASEE.org) could be of value.

Without a website, it is not clear how useful brochures and swag are. In our experience, potential clients are more apt to go to a website to find out more about evaluators and their work than they are to email them. Having an online presence is important, but it can be time consuming and may require assistance. A poorly designed, hard-to-use website with typos and/or inaccurate information can be worse than having no website at all. If an evaluator wants to have a website, there are some free online guides to get started. Entering phrases such as "how to make your own website" into search engines will provide a variety of resources. Before any website goes live, it is important to have colleagues go through the website, to ensure everything on the site is working and easy to navigate and the information is accurate and useful.

Advertising, including putting an advertisement in journals or newsletters of the professional organizations of primary target client pools, is another marketing strategy. As with a website, any advertisement needs to be clear, correct, and well written and provide useful information. The activity that follows is designed to help readers think about ways to market themselves as evaluators.

> **Activity**
> Developing a Marketing Plan

In small groups, develop an initial marketing plan for an independent evaluator starting out in one of the following areas:

- Criminal justice
- Public health
- Child development
- Programs to increase diversity in the sciences

Preparing a Proposal

For those doing evaluation as a business, the evaluation process usually starts with a request to submit an evaluation proposal. If the evaluation proposal is part of a larger proposal being submitted for funding, the client or the client's funder most likely will have requirements as to what needs to be included in the evaluation proposal. In some cases, the description of what needs to be covered in the evaluation section will be fairly specific, as is the case for the National Institutes of Health (NIH) grants announcement for the Research Initiative for Scientific Enhancement (RISE):

> It is expected that the RISE Program will undergo regular evaluation, in order to promote innovation and progress, as well as to bring attention to any deficiencies that arise, and that reviewers will be asked to answer the following question: "Is the plan for evaluation sound and likely to provide information on the effectiveness of the program?" (U.S. DHHS, 2016, p. 1)

This grants announcement also requires that information be provided about previous evaluations:

> Describe the progress made in improving outcomes for students (with attention to the unique needs of UR [underrepresented] students), such as, but not limited to, persistence in the major, increase in overall GPA, and increased progression to a Ph.D. program or, where relevant, postdoctoral appointment. Describe what has been learned through the program evaluation and any changes made in the program as a result of the evaluation. (U.S. DHHS, 2016, p. 17)

Private foundations also often specify what needs to be included in an evaluation, as can be seen in this example from the W. K. Kellogg Foundation (2017b):

> The Kellogg Foundation uses evaluation as an essential tool to capture the impact of grantees' work and to generate learning. Our approach to evaluation is aligned

with and guided by our grantees' needs and priorities. A significant portion of our evaluation resources are applied to build grantee organizations' internal abilities to conduct and use evaluation so that over time, we can co-create and share actionable knowledge about improving children's well-being with the broader field.

Describe your organization's existing capacity/ability (staffing, financial resources, etc.) to evaluate this work; or your plan to build the capacity.

(Optional) If you have a draft evaluation plan for this funding request, please upload it. (p. 4)

The activity that follows is designed to help readers determine the evaluation requirements of those who tend to fund projects and programs from the evaluator's target client pool.

Activity
Finding Funder Evaluation Requirements

Do a Web search and find funder evaluation requirements for one government funder and one private funder who funds proposals in one of your target client pool areas identified in an earlier activity (p. 456).

Funders, particularly the federal government, often have other requirements for the proposed evaluator including a letter of support/commitment from the evaluator, the evaluator's résumé in a format specific to that agency, and often a statement listing the evaluator's other funded or submitted projects. If evaluators will be working with projects funded by agencies, such as the NIH and the NSF, it is useful to have up-to-date copies of résumés and projects in the agency's required formats. While most funder descriptions of evaluation requirements don't specify the inclusion of a logic model, which was covered in Chapter 7, including one can add to the quality of the evaluation plan as well as the competitiveness of the overall proposal.

The process of writing an evaluation proposal for a project that has already been funded is quite similar to writing an evaluation plan for a proposed project. While it is still necessary to know and follow the funder's guidelines for evaluation, there is no need to worry about page limits or impressing external reviewers. Before writing an evaluation proposal for a project that has already been funded, it is useful to meet with the project director to discuss the level of detail that should be included in the proposal.

There will be times when an evaluator will be asked to take over the evaluation of an existing project. There are a variety of reasons that might happen. The client may not have been satisfied with the work that another evaluator was doing, or the evaluator, for health or other reasons, may not have been able to continue. However, another reason the evaluator may have left was because the client didn't like the findings. While being interviewed for this book, Jane Butler Kahle (personal communication, August 24, 2018) recalled that "we had a couple of projects that weren't doing very well. We wrote honest reports, and we got fired. If you report a project is failing, you are at their [clients'] mercy and they can fire you." Evaluators may also make the choice to leave a project because they feel the situation has become such that there is no way they can do a good or even adequate job.

If one is considering taking over an evaluation already in progress, an early step should be getting copies of the original evaluation proposal, any existing evaluation reports, and any funder evaluation requirements. Finding out why the client is no longer using the original evaluator can help other evaluators decide if they want to take the evaluation on. If the original evaluator was fired because the client was not satisfied with the work, finding out what the dissatisfactions were is key. Even if the original evaluator was not fired, it is useful to ask the client if there were any concerns with the evaluation as it was being done and if any parts of the evaluation were particularly useful to the client. A next step is to find out the status of any data that have been collected— that is, whether you will have access to the data and, if so, in what format(s). If you will not be given access to the data already collected, the evaluation will have to be, at least in part, retrospective. Additional questions to be answered include the following:

- Is there enough time remaining in the project for needed data to be collected and to write a useful evaluation report?
- If there is access to existing data, is there enough documentation to allow the data to be analyzed?
- If the client had dissatisfactions with the existing evaluation, can they be corrected or eliminated?
- Is the evaluation budget adequate?

If possible, it is often useful to speak with the former evaluator or a trusted informant. When all of this information is collected, you can make an informed decision as to whether you should take over an existing evaluation. At that point, writing the proposal is relatively easy. Basically, the proposal will describe the parts of the evaluation that will continue and the changes that will be made and why.

Making a Budget

A key part of an evaluation proposal is the budget. Finding out from the client the approximate dollar figure for the evaluation, and planning an evaluation that can be done for that amount, saves both time and money. Otherwise, one runs the risk of having to rewrite the original design to cut it back.

If a client does not have an estimated amount budgeted for the evaluation or is not comfortable giving out a figure, then the potential evaluator should ask for the approximate overall cost of the project. Total evaluation costs usually range from 5% to 10% of the overall project budget but can be less or more based on the extensiveness of the evaluation. Speaking with potential clients about what they expect to get from an evaluation can help evaluators decide if they should be designing an evaluation closer to the 5% or 10% budget figure. Whatever the budget figure is, the budget needs to cover evaluator time and costs.

The most important step to making a good budget is to determine how much it would cost to do the proposed work. It is rare to have an evaluation project where the budget is not determined in advance. Especially when there is a contract, the expectation is that obligations will be fulfilled regardless of whether the budget covers all the tasks or not. If the proposed budget costs are significantly higher than the estimated figure given, then the evaluation proposal will, most likely, not be competitive. If the budget costs are significantly underestimated, then if the proposal is accepted, the evaluator will lose money.

Once the evaluation plan is developed, the next step is to break the plan into specific tasks, determine who is going to do each task, and estimate the amount of time it will take to do these tasks. One way to do this is to use a time and task chart, which was introduced in Chapter 9. The time and task chart in Table 15.2 is for a relatively small formative and summative evaluation of a series of workshops for youth workers.

In the activity that follows, readers develop their own time and task chart.

Table 15.2 Sample Time and Task Chart

Year 1 Tasks	Evaluator Hours	Staff Hours	Consultant Hours
Sum of total hours	86	72	20
Meet with staff/participate in monthly calls	18	4	
Develop formative evaluation measures	2	1	
Develop surveys/interview protocols	4	3	
Develop coding schema for open-ended responses to the formative measures	2	2	
Set up evaluation database	2		16
Work with project staff to set up the data collection process	4	12	
Collect data	4	24	
Analyze data	16	16	4
Write annual report	24	8	
Provide feedback	10	2	

Activity
Developing a Time and Task Chart

Assume that you have been asked to do a formative evaluation of an after-school program to encourage children's interest in reading. Construct a time and task chart for the evaluation.

To determine personnel costs, as shown in Table 15.3, multiply the number of hours by the person's daily rate, as done here based on the time and task chart provided in Table 15.2.

Table 15.3 Sample Calculation of Personnel Costs

Year 1	Evaluator Hours	Staff Hours	Consultant Hours
Sum of total hours	86	72	20
Hourly rate	$65	$30	$100
Cost	$5,590	$2,160	$2,000

There is a value in having multiple people involved in an evaluation. It allows the evaluator to have access to needed skills, and it can also make the evaluation more cost-effective. As Jane Butler Kahle (personal communication, 2018) pointed out while being interviewed for this book,

> it was always cheaper to have me, the person in charge, outsource parts of the project to experts, such as statisticians or designers, and charge the project at their rates. It was cheaper and gave the client more value for the dollar.

When one is computing an hourly rate, it is important to be clear what it covers. The independent evaluator is also an employer. As employers, evaluators pay the employer's contribution to Social Security for themselves and any staff (6.4% of salaries up to $132,900 for 2019) and the employer's contribution to Medicare (1.45% of salaries with no limit) (Social Security Administration, 2019). The employer is also responsible for paying a state unemployment tax (the rate varies by state and by the number of unemployment claims that have been filed by former employees) and **workers' compensation** (the amount varies by employee risk of being harmed at work and previous employee compensation claims).

The employer can also contribute to other benefits such as health insurance and pension plans. If individuals are doing evaluations as a full-time career, they need to seriously consider providing health insurance and a pension plan. Decisions need to be made as to how comprehensive, and expensive, the plans will be and what share of the cost will be covered by the employer and what share will be covered by the employee. If evaluator–employers are providing health insurance and/or a pension plan for themselves, they are legally obligated to provide the same benefits to their employees. Small Business Health Options (SHOP) is a federal program to help small businesses (from 1 to 50 employees) provide their employees with health insurance. SHOP resources are available online at www.healthcare.gov/small-businesses/employers/.

There is a simple pension plan that small businesses can set up. The Simplified Employee Pension Plan (SEP) allows employers to contribute to traditional, tax-deferred individual retirement accounts, which employers set up for themselves and their employees. As of 2020, a business of any size, even a one-person business, can establish an SEP (Internal Revenue Service [IRS], 2019).

Mandated and optional employer contributions are considered fringe benefits and should be added to personnel costs. As can be seen in Table 15.4, this can be done with adding fringe benefits as a separate budget line (a) or including the costs of fringe benefits in the hourly rate (b). Fringe benefits are only added to employee salaries, not to fees paid to consultants.

After the personnel costs have been estimated, it is necessary to determine additional costs. These may include the following:

- Travel—Will there be travel? If so how many trips? To where? For how long? What are current airfare and hotel rates?

- Participant costs—Will participants be given gift cards or other incentives to participate in the evaluation? If so, how much will the incentives cost, and how many will be needed?

Table 15.4 Sample Presentation of Fringe Benefits as Part of Personnel Costs

(a)

Year 1	Evaluator Hours	Staff Hours	Consultants Hours
Sum of total hours	86	72	20
Hourly rate	$65.00	$30.00	$100.00
Total salaries	$5,590.00	$2,160.00	$2,000.00
25% fringe benefits	$1,397.50	$540.00	
Personnel costs	$6,987.50	$2,700.00	$2,000.00

(b)

Year 1	Evaluator Hours	Staff Hours	Consultants Hours
Sum of total hours	86	72	20
Hourly rate with fringe benefits included	$81.25	$38.00	$100.00
Personnel cost	$6,987.50	$109.50	$2,000.00

- Equipment—What equipment needs to be purchased to do the evaluation? How much will any needed equipment cost?

- Supplies and communication costs—Are any unusual supplies needed to do the project? Are additional phone lines needed? How much will these cost?

These costs, including personnel costs, are called direct costs because they are directly related to the project. There are other costs, referred to as indirect costs, that are not directly tied to an individual project but are part of the costs of doing business. These include such expenses as rent, utilities (e.g., heat, electricity, telephone, internet services including Wi-Fi), and professional fees (e.g., bookkeeping and tax preparation). Indirect costs need to be included in the budget. This can be done by adding the costs to daily/hourly rates, by breaking out the costs in the budget (i.e., rent, utilities, professional fees), or by charging the costs as a percentage of direct costs.

A spreadsheet in the following format can help estimate the budget. However, it is necessary to check with clients and/or funders to determine if they have a format in which they want the budget to be presented. The budget shown in Table 15.5 is for a relatively small program evaluation with a $25,000 budget.

Once the proposed evaluation design proposal and budget are completed, if a potential client wants to cut the budget, then a decision needs to be made to determine the parts of the evaluation that will need to be cut to reflect the reduced budget. It is rarely wise to agree to do the same amount of work for less money. If one does, it indicates to the client either that the original budget was too high or that the evaluator is willing to lose money doing the evaluation. Evaluators may choose to do an evaluation pro bono, or for a reduced cost, as a way of giving back to the community or to build capacity or for other reasons, but that is very different from losing money on an evaluation because the budget wasn't high enough to cover the activities outlined in the evaluation plan.

Table 15.5 Sample Budget for a Small Program Evaluation

	Hours	Dollars*	Percentage	Months	
Evaluator	250	$65	0.14	1.65	$16,250
Other	40	30	0.02	0.26	$1,200
Total Salaries					$17,450
Fringe Benefits 20% of Salaries**					$3,490
Salaries and Fringe Benefits					$20,940
Supplies/Communication					$250
Travel					$1,700
Consultants					$250
Equipment					$0
Participant Costs					$0
Other Direct					$100
Total Direct					$23,240
Indirect*** (10% of salaries)					$1,745
Total					$24,985

* Hourly rates will vary.

** Percentage for fringe benefits will vary based on the benefits offered.

*** Percentage for indirect costs will be based on what is included in indirect costs.

Contracts

For the protection of the evaluator and the client, it is useful to have a signed contract. The contract is a legally binding document that should make clear the evaluators' and the clients' expectations as to what will be done, in what time frame, and for what cost. It can also cover procedures for what the clients and/or evaluators have to do if they wish to break the contract as well as procedures for modifying the contract. Contracts can also include a variety of issues such as confidentiality, COIs, and intellectual property.

Contract Components

In varying amounts of detail, contracts should include the following components:

- A statement of work and deliverables, including the explicit tasks that will be done by the evaluator (these should come from the task and time chart described earlier). The deliverables may include annual reports, periodic oral and written feedback, and copies of measures that are developed. Dates when the deliverables are due should also be included.

- Budget and payment, including the amount the evaluator will be paid, which in most cases is broken out by categories listed earlier in our discussion of making the budget. It also should include how the fees will be paid, which may be a cost reimbursement where invoices for costs incurred are submitted and paid or where proportions of the total budget are paid to the evaluator upon receipt of different deliverables. For a small business, it is not usually good idea to receive the total amount after the evaluation is done and the final report submitted. In this instance, evaluators must pay all the costs associated with doing the evaluation themselves and wait to be reimbursed, which can be a financial burden for an individual or a small business. Also included should be any requirements for what should be included in the invoice and to whom the invoices should be sent and, if necessary, a listing of allowable costs.

- Terms for termination, including the length of the contract and conditions of termination by the client and/or the evaluator.

- Resolution of disputes, including the procedures that will be followed in case of conflicts.

- Financial record-keeping requirements, including the types of records the evaluator needs to provide to the client upon request and the length of time the evaluator needs to keep the records.

Intellectual Property

The contract should spell out who owns the intellectual property, that which is developed by the evaluator doing the evaluation. The intellectual property may be owned by the evaluator or the client, or it may be in the public domain, which means it is available to all at no cost. Usually, in the contract, there is an assignment of copyright, which, as indicated in Chapter 14, gives the holder the exclusive right to print, publish, and use the developed material. If the contract gives the copyright only to the client, the evaluator will have no right to use any materials developed without getting the client's permission. It is usually best for evaluators to have copyright of the work that they have authored and then give the client the right to use that work. An alternative is that the client has the copyright but the client gives the evaluator the right to use that work. While copyright has been the traditional way to protect intellectual property, in recent years there has been a move toward a more flexible concept of copyright that allows individuals to choose how they share their work. Creative Commons copyright licenses and tools allow options other than the traditional "all rights reserved" setting that copyright law creates (Creative Commons, n.d.). Under Creative Commons (https://creativecommons.org), you can choose, for example, if adaptations can be made to the original work as long as attribution is given, or if adapters can market their adaptations of the original work commercially.

The contract can, and should, indicate who owns the data from which the reports and other products were generated and who can use those data for other purposes. For communities that are outside the dominant power structure, there are often very legitimate concerns about how data about them and their communities will be used, and they may require that they own their data and control who has access to the data and where the data are stored (Whitesell, 2018). This needs to be decided before evaluation data are collected because it might mean that the evaluator cannot guarantee the confidentiality of the data.

Making a Business Financially Viable

Once a business is started, there are upfront costs. Even when there are clients and projects, it may be several months before invoices are paid. Without other sources of financial support, it may be necessary for evaluators starting out to keep their salaried job or get another job and work on starting an evaluation business part-time until there is an adequate client base and income. While being interviewed for this book in 2017, Mary Moriarty said,

> If you are setting up your own business, you need to plan a development year. You don't just walk out of a job into having contracts. It can be frustrating particularly in the first months when you are writing a lot and you are not seeing anything coming in either financially or in other areas.

In a small business, there are times when there is a great deal of work and other times when there is less. When there is a great deal of work and income is coming in, it is important to put money aside for leaner times. Keeping track of the end dates of current evaluation projects, so that not all, or even most, projects finish at one time, can also help with finances. Having staggered end dates means when one or more projects end, there will still be money coming in until new projects start.

Evaluators need to understand that "time is money." For example, doing **pro bono** evaluation—that is, doing an evaluation at no cost to the client—can be valuable; however, before doing pro bono evaluation, it is important to determine the approximate amount of time to be donated and the impact it may have on the business's bottom line. Unpaid professional time can also be an issue when an evaluation is being designed "on spec." **On spec** means that a document, in this case an evaluation plan, is submitted without a contract, in the hope that it will be accepted. Along with approximate number of unpaid hours it will take to develop and write an evaluation plan and budget, a judgment needs to be made as to the probability that the evaluation proposal will be accepted. Often an evaluator will be asked to design an evaluation for a proposal that is being submitted with the understanding that, if the proposal is funded, the evaluator will do the evaluation. If the overall proposal does not appear to be competitive, the evaluator's time spent designing an evaluation will, most likely, not lead to a contract.

Other times, evaluators will be asked, by a project or program that already has funding, to propose an evaluation plan. In those cases, it's useful to see if this is an open competition to which a number of evaluators are expected to respond. If it is an open competition, evaluators should try to determine if their proposal will be competitive. Unless they have reasons to believe their proposal will be competitive, it may not be worth the unpaid time it takes to develop and submit an evaluation proposal. If it is an open competition to do the evaluation for an effort that hasn't yet been funded, the probability of getting one's evaluation plan selected, and of the overall proposal getting funded, tends to be too low to make the work of planning an evaluation worth it.

Whenever an evaluation plan is submitted and either the overall project is not funded or the design is not selected, the evaluator needs to make it clear that the design and any other submitted materials cannot be used without the author's permission. As Mary Moriarty explained in her 2017 interview, those who are doing evaluation as a business need to learn "when to say no."

I needed to learn when to say no. Particularly in the beginning when someone asked me to write an evaluation proposal I would jump on it. I'm more thoughtful about that now. I think about whether or not it's a good match. I think about whether or not I have the time. I think about whether or not it's a good proposal. If it's great people but not a great proposal, that's a lot of time for me to put in that may or may not pay off. Sometimes I'll try to help strengthen a proposal, but that's extra time that I don't get paid for. Spending that extra unpaid time could be tough when starting out. Principal investigators are from organizations or universities. It is part of their normal work routine to write proposals. They don't always have an understanding that you aren't getting paid for extra work. They don't understand that I am doing work that I'm not getting paid for.

Those who are new to doing evaluations on their own may think that one submits a bill and then gets paid. Very often it doesn't work out that way. There will be times when payments will not be received in a timely manner, or perhaps at all. It may seem obvious, but if one doesn't get paid, one's business will probably fail. Some clients are "slow payers," allowing months to go by before an invoice is paid. Sometimes that is because they are having cash flow problems and don't have the funds to pay all of their bills. Other times the problem is with the client's bureaucracy and/or the complexity of the client's financial system. There may be forms that haven't yet been submitted, invoices in the wrong format, or approvals from senior administrators that have not been received. Regardless of the reason, if invoices are not being paid in a timely manner or at all, it is important to speak with the client, regularly if necessary, and determine what must be done to get the invoice paid.

Individuals must either pay their bills promptly or pay additional fees. If those bills and fees aren't paid, companies stop providing services. This is something for evaluators to consider as well. However, before an evaluator decides to stop providing services because of nonpayment, it is wise to contact the client in advance and explain the consequences if payment is not received by a certain date. Consequences might include temporarily stopping the analysis of data or the writing of reports, or not submitting reports until payment is received. It is also possible to collect data that otherwise would be lost but not share the data with the client until payment is received. If none of these strategies work, it may be necessary to terminate the evaluation. This is not an easy decision to make, and there are no hard-and-fast answers. The question is, What do evaluators owe the people/institution who hired them but didn't pay them for their work? Some may say that as in the case of other professionals, such as lawyers and accountants, if the work isn't paid for, then the evaluator stops working on that evaluation. Others might say that just as medical doctors keep treating a patient regardless of whether they are getting paid, the evaluator should complete the evaluation. Complicating the decision is the seriousness of impact of not getting paid on the evaluator's finances and financial security.

Selecting a Business Entity

An early decision that evaluators have to make is under what business entity they will be working. The purpose of this section is to provide the reader with an overview of different types of business entities. It is important to note that we are neither attorneys nor accountants. Readers should not decide on a business entity without checking with an attorney about possible legal ramifications and with an accountant about possible tax ramifications.

Employee

If an evaluator is a full-time evaluator for a university, corporation, or government, then the decision has already been made. In this case, the evaluator is an employee. That means the evaluator provides services to an employer who controls what will be done and how it will be done. The employer has the right to control the details of how the services are performed (IRS, n.d.).

Sole Proprietor

The simplest way to start doing evaluations, other than an as employee, is in a sole proprietorship. A sole proprietorship is an unincorporated business owned and run by one individual with no distinction between the business and the owner. You are entitled to all profits and are responsible for all your business's debts, losses, and liabilities (Small Business Administration [SBA], n.d.a).

No formal action is required to form a sole proprietorship. If a person is the only owner, this status automatically comes from that person's business activities. One can be a **sole proprietor** for one's own business, while working at another job, if that doesn't violate the employer's rules. Individuals can operate as sole proprietors under their own name or can give the business another name (known as "doing business as" or **DBA**). While there is no formal action that needs to be taken with the federal government to start a sole proprietorship, state and/or local governments may require licenses to be obtained. If the evaluator has a DBA, the name may need to be registered with local or state governments. It will be necessary to check and see what are the state and local regulations.

As sole proprietors, individuals and their businesses are one and the same, so the business itself is not taxed separately. The income one gets as a sole proprietorship is the individual's income. Because the sole proprietor and the business are the same entity, that individual is responsible for withholding money for federal, state, and possibly local taxes and for withholding both the employer's and the employee's share of Social Security and taxes. Sole proprietors are also responsible for getting whatever licenses and permits might be required by their local or state governments for unincorporated businesses owned and run by one individual.

The advantages of a sole proprietorship are that it's easy to form and, other than any state or local licenses needed, it's free and, as the sole owner, the proprietor has complete control of the business. Since the money that sole proprietors make in their business is added to their other earned income, it is not necessary to file additional sets of federal and state tax returns.

The biggest disadvantage of being a sole proprietor is the sole proprietor has personal liability. Because there is no legal separation between the individual and the business, the proprietor can be held personally liable for the debts and obligations of the business. It also means that if the proprietor is sued by a client, the client can go after the proprietor's personal assets, including personal bank accounts, houses, and cars. If a sole proprietor has employees, the proprietor is personally responsible for any liabilities incurred because of employee actions (SBA, n.d.a).

Partner in a Partnership

A **partnership** is basically a sole proprietorship with more than own owner. Each partner contributes to the business in such areas as money, property, labor, and skill. In return, each partner shares in the profits and losses of the business. Legally, there is no requirement to have a written partnership agreement, but thinking about all the things that could go wrong, it would be very risky not to have something, in writing, that covers areas such as profit sharing, dissolution of the partnership, conflict resolution, and so on. The document should be written, or at least reviewed, by an attorney (SBA, n.d.a).

Limited Liability Company

For those who are concerned about the personal liability of being in a sole proprietorship or a partnership, there are other more complicated options to consider including a limited liability company. A **limited liability company (LLC)** is a hybrid type of legal structure that provides the limited liability features of a corporation and the tax efficiencies and operational flexibility of a sole proprietorship or partnership. All LLC profits and losses are "passed through" the business to individual LLC owners (called members) who then report profits and losses on their personal federal tax returns, just like the owners of a partnership would. Rules for setting up an LLC vary by state, and this is not something an individual should do without legal assistance (SBA, n.d.a).

Corporation/S Corporation

At the next level is a corporation. A **corporation** is an independent legal entity owned by shareholders. This means that the corporation itself, not the shareholders who own it, is liable for the actions and debts the business incurs. There is a particular type of corporation, called an **S corporation** or S corp, that is worth considering for those starting a business. Unlike a traditional corporation, in an S corp profits and losses are passed through to the shareholders' personal tax returns. Consequently, the business is not taxed itself; only the shareholders are taxed. To incorporate, there needs to be more than one person or existing business entity involved to start a corporation, and each person or entity controls an assigned amount of shares of the corporation. Corporations are registered through individual states and need to be set up by an attorney. Corporations also need to have an accountant or certified public accountant to assist with taxes (SBA, n.d.a).

Nonprofit Organization

Evaluators may work for a nonprofit organization, but setting up their own nonprofit to do evaluations is not a particularly viable option. Nonprofit organizations are granted tax-exempt status by the IRS and need to be set up to do some kinds of charitable, educational, scientific, or religious work. It is difficult and time consuming to become a nonprofit, and there are major reporting requirements. Realistically, if one is setting up a small evaluation business, it is rare that it would qualify for nonprofit status.

In the activity that follows, readers determine what they think what might be the best business entity for them if they choose to do evaluation as a business.

Activity
Exploring Different Business Entities

Assume that you are planning to start an evaluation business. After going through the various options for setting up a business entity, select the option that you feel would be best for you and the one that you feel would be the worst. Provide a rationale for your choices.

Regardless of the business entity chosen, evaluators should do several things as they set up their business:

- Get an Employer Identification Number (EIN), also known as a Federal Tax Identification Number. It can be acquired from the IRS online or by phone, and it's free. Sole proprietors with no employees and no pension plan can work under their Social Security number. However, because of the potential for people to use Social Security numbers for identity theft, it is best to get an EIN and use it for business.

- Set up a separate checking account for business income and expenses. As with the EIN, it is not required for a sole proprietor, but it makes tracking finances easier and reduces the accidental misuse of funds.

- Have a mechanism to deposit funds to cover federal tax liabilities, including tax withholding and Social Security and Medicare taxes (for both the employee and employer shares) either quarterly or monthly. This is the case regardless of whether the evaluator has another job. For individual sole proprietors, this withholding can be quarterly payments of estimated taxes. Otherwise, they will need to do monthly or biweekly deposits.

Bookkeeping and Record Keeping

Regardless of the business entity, there is a great deal of paperwork and record keeping. The first step is to set up the books for the business. There are a variety of online and desktop programs to help you do that, the best known of which is QuickBooks. QuickBooks and similar programs keep track of revenues and expenses, pay employees, and generate reports and required federal forms. An accountant can set up the books and each year be sent an electronic copy of those books to prepare the business's taxes. Individuals can keep the books themselves or hire a part-time bookkeeper or a bookkeeping service. One of the best early purchases someone starting a business can make is an inexpensive scanner so that paper receipts, signed contracts, and other paperwork can be kept electronically.

Developing a Business Plan

As the SBA (n.d.b) explains,

> There's no right or wrong way to write a business plan. What's important is that your plan meets your needs.

Most business plans fall into one of two common categories: traditional or lean startup.

Traditional business plans are more common, use a standard structure, and encourage you to go into detail in each section. They tend to require more work upfront and can be dozens of pages long.

Lean startup business plans are less common but still use a standard structure. They focus on summarizing only the most important points of the key elements of your plan. They can take as little as one hour to make and are typically only one page. (pp. 1–2)

The following is an overview of the pieces that are included in a specific type of business plan, the Business Model Canvas (SBA, n.d.b, adapted from Osterwalder & Pigneur, 2010). However, these pieces can be used in other plans as well.

- Key partnerships: Note the other businesses or services you'll work with to run your business.
- Key activities: List the ways your business will gain a competitive advantage.
- Key resources: List any resource you'll leverage to create value for your clients. Don't forget to leverage business resources that might be available to women, veterans, Indigenous Peoples, and HUBZone businesses.
- Value proposition: Make a clear and compelling statement about the unique value your company brings to the market.
- Client pool: Be specific when you name your target market. Your business won't be for everybody, so it's important to have a clear sense of who your business will serve.
- Cost structure: Will your company focus on reducing cost or maximizing value? Define your strategy, then list the most significant costs you'll face pursuing it.
- Revenue streams: Explain how your company will actually make money.

Using some of these components of a business plan, in the activity that follows, readers will begin to develop a business plan.

Activity
Developing a Business Plan

In small groups, outline a business plan that includes at least three of the components of the Business Model Canvas.

SUMMARY

The chapter focused on introducing readers to the practical realities of doing evaluations. Some of the content, including preparing a proposal and preparing a budget, is for every evaluator who will be doing evaluations. Other content, such as marketing, contracts, and ethics, was targeted more toward those who will not be doing evaluations as employees of a larger organization. Still other content areas, such as selecting a business entity, developing a business plan, and making the business financially viable, were targeted toward those who are or will be doing evaluations individually or as members of a small group regardless of whether they are doing evaluations full-time, part-time, or even occasionally. It is expected that readers now know some of the ins and outs of ways to do evaluations, outside of being a part of a larger institution, and have a greater chance of being successful if this is what they want to do. Because they have a better understanding of how to build a viable budget, how to make choices about the evaluations they bid on and/or do, and how to stay financially solvent, they can develop a business plan if they choose to do so.

SUPPLEMENTAL RESOURCES

AEA Graduate Student and New Evaluators Topical Interest Group (TIG)

http://comm.eval.org/gsne/home

This TIG, also available on Facebook, seeks to develop activities for, and represent the interests of, AEA members who are completing graduate degrees and/or are new to the field of evaluation. The intent is to foster communication and networking among graduate students, new evaluators, interested faculty, recent graduates, potential employers, and other AEA members.

AEA Independent Consulting TIG

http://comm.eval.org/independentconsulting/home

The members of this TIG are sole proprietors or have formed LLCs, partnerships, or corporations. They network and work together to inform one another of contract leads and seek one another out to join forces in completing contracts.

Small Business Administration (SBA)

www.sba.gov

The SBA was developed in 1953 to help Americans start, build, and grow businesses. It provides a series of step-by-step guides to plan, launch, manage, and grow your business. While the information provided is not specific to a business devoted to evaluation, its information, including its step-by-step guide to developing a business plan, can be very useful.

System for Award Management (SAM)

www.sam.gov

One needs to be registered with SAM to do business with the federal government. This website provides everything you need to register for free, including how to get a Dun & Bradstreet number for those who are required to register with the federal government for contracts or grants.

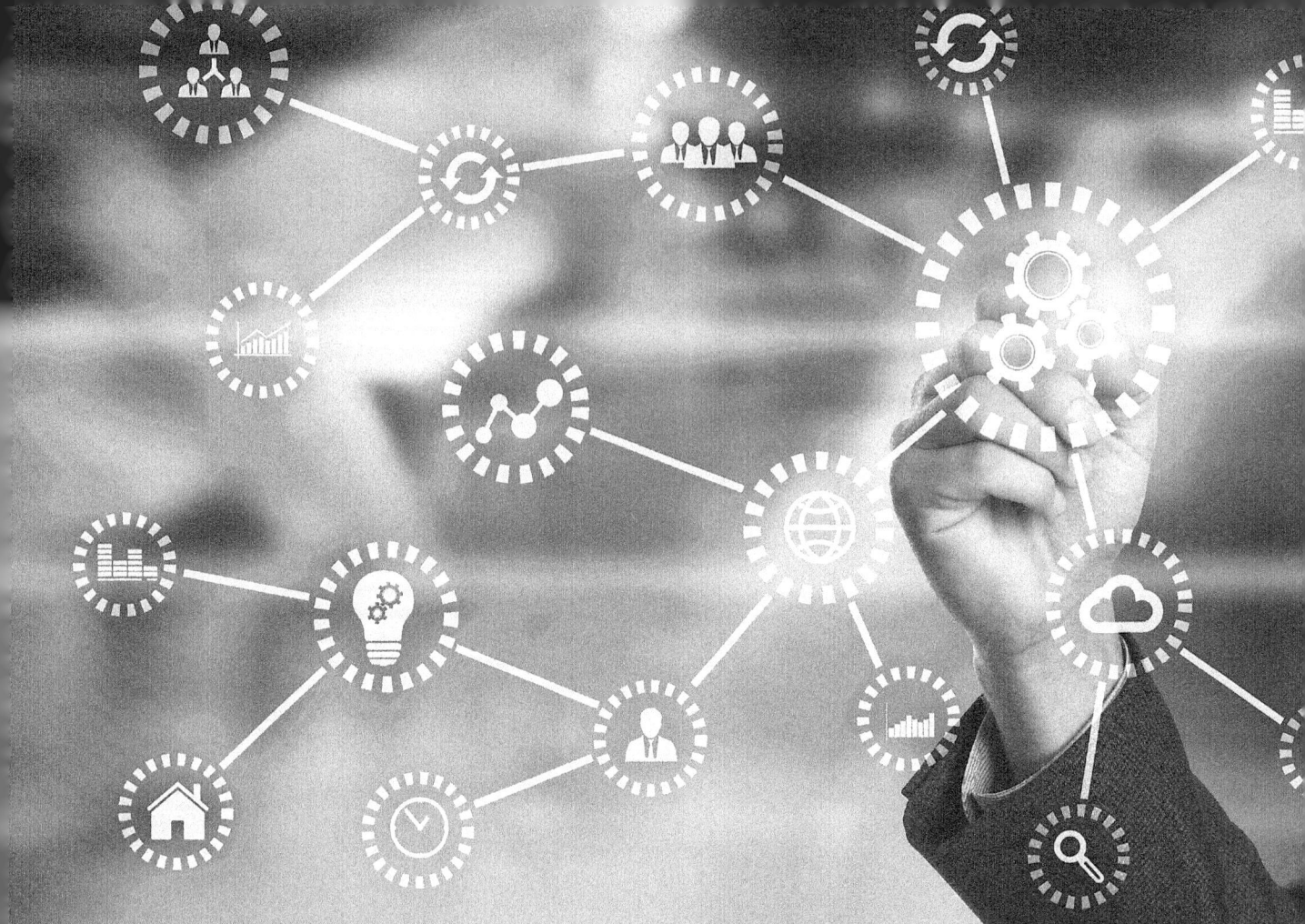
Shutterstock/Wright Studio

Understanding and becoming aware of one's own cultural values, beliefs, attitudes and judgments becomes central when we have to interact with people from different cultural backgrounds. Our values and beliefs shape our perceptions; they define the ways we see the world.

CHAPTER 16

Interconnections and Practical Implications

> As evaluators, we are given the awesome responsibility of speaking for those who cannot speak for themselves to, in essence, define their reality. At times, this might involve unmasking the power inequalities that are typically veiled under the language of institutional neutrality . . . We must forge an evaluation practice that serves broad democratic ideals of diverse participation, justice, and equity by meaningfully engaging, understanding, and uncovering (a) the quality of the program experience for diverse participants, (b) the appropriateness and contextual fit of the program design and theory of change, and finally (c) the outcomes of people in programs within the context of their racialized environments.
>
> —Thomas, Madison, Rockcliffe, DeLaine, and Lowe (2018, pp. 516–517)

After reading this and earlier chapters and participating in the activities, readers will be able to meet the following learning objectives:

- Describe ways to reduce bias and increase cultural competence
- Describe what is involved in being a culturally responsive evaluator
- Explain how doing a culturally responsive evaluation impacts decisions made about evaluation planning, implementation, and dissemination
- Discuss possible relationships between bias and ethics
- Reflect on possible differences in your own responses to evaluation and social justice issues raised in the earliest chapters and in this chapter

Introduction

In many ways, the opening comments from first author Veronica G. Thomas and colleagues reflect our goal for this book. The goal is not just to provide readers with the knowledge, skills, and experiences necessary to be evaluators, but to provide them in such a way that readers question traditional methods and assumptions and make conscious decisions whether to accept, reject, or refine those methods and assumptions. The book seeks not only to answer Melvin Hall's (2018b) concern, raised in Chapter 5, "that the training evaluators receive may not provide the skillset necessary to efficaciously handle the thorny issues of race and class when they emerge through an evaluation process" (para. 3), but also to expand the concern to include such areas as gender, disability, and sexual orientation.

In this, the final chapter, we take another look at bias and cultural competence, introduced in Chapter 1, and how bias and a lack of cultural competence can impact evaluation decision making. Also included are ways that readers can reduce their own biases and increase their cultural competence and how that can lead to evaluators becoming more culturally responsive. Reflecting on what was covered in earlier chapters, in this chapter we explore some of the impacts of cultural responsiveness on decision making in such areas as the models and frameworks used, how stakeholders are engaged, and design, data collection, and data analysis choices. Also included are ways cultural responsiveness can impact responses to ethical dilemmas and the evaluator's responsibilities in disseminating the results and facilitating their usefulness.

We expect that after completing this chapter and the activities, readers will have a greater understanding of ways to reduce their own biases and the biases of others as well as ways to increase their cultural competence. Drawing on the work here and in earlier chapters, it is expected that readers will have the ability to begin to become culturally responsive evaluators and an understanding of how this affects the evaluation decisions they make.

Objectivity and Bias

As was indicated in Chapter 1, while we, as evaluators, would like to see ourselves as objective and unbiased, that is not the case. We all see the world through our own lens, which is colored by our lives, experiences, hopes, and fears. As eminent statistician Maurice Tatsuoka pointed out, "It's about time we outgrew the notion that science is value free" (quoted in Huberty & Olejnik, 2006, p. 31). Years earlier, poet and writer Anaïs Nin noted, "We don't see things as they are, we see them as we are" (quoted in Kukolic, 2017, para. 1). A lack of awareness of our subjectivity can easily lead to bias. Bias is a particular tendency or inclination that prevents reasonable, knowledgeable, thoughtful consideration of a question (Harmon, 1973). With bias, we accept things as true without question or evidence.

While bias can be intentional, it often is not. Bias can grow out of one's assumptions, and as Goldratt and Cox (1986) point out, our assumptions are often wrong:

> When I was a physicist, people would come to me from time to time with problems in mathematics they could not solve. They wanted me to check their numbers for them. But after a while I learned not to waste time checking the numbers—because the numbers were almost always right. However if I checked the assumptions, they were almost always wrong. (p. 157)

Impacts of Bias on Evaluation

As has been pointed out throughout this book, there are a variety of ways that bias and the assumptions made based on bias can impact how we do program evaluations. Being a member of the dominant culture—that is, one of those who are in the majority and/or wield more power than other groups—can mean one assumes or accepts unquestioningly the values and/or systems of thought in a society that are most standard and widely held at a given time. With this unquestioning acceptance comes an inability to value or even recognize that there are other, different systems of thought and values (Thomas & Campbell, 2017) and a mindset of "'I think it, therefore it's true' where people assume that their own beliefs and introspections are, by definition, valid and therefore worthy of being acted on" (Uhlmann & Cohen, 2007, p. 207). These assumptions and the related mindset can lead to unintentional unethical behavior. As pointed out in Chapter 2, unethical behavior can stem from actions that individuals don't recognize as unethical. For example, assuming that those who are more educated are more objective and therefore more apt to provide more useful information to evaluators can lead to unconscious, unethical choices about whose voices are heard and whose voices are ignored.

Bias and unchallenged assumptions can lead to accepting definitions of success that reflect the values of the dominant group, which usually includes funders. These definitions may not reflect participant goals. For example, coauthor Patricia B. Campbell once conducted an evaluation of a multisite adult literacy program where the definition of success was increased literacy as measured by scores on a test of adult literacy. It was a good measure but not for the participants, whose definitions of success were much more practical, such as to be able to read bus schedules, letters from their children's school, job applications, and grocery store labels. The evaluation questions asked and the measures used would be quite different based on whose definition of success was used.

As was covered in Chapter 5, in the 1990s David M. Fetterman developed a new social justice evaluation paradigm, empowerment evaluation. In his Voices From the Field interview, David M. Fetterman discusses whose goals need to be considered in evaluation planning.

Voices From the Field

David M. Fetterman: Whose Goals?

All of what we are doing in evaluation is upside down and backwards. We come in as the experts in charge. We have to change who we are to become more critical friends, to support people. There should be no "I'm the expert"; it's "We are going to do it together." To do this we need to keep everyone involved and engaged including funders as well as the community, staff, and participants. If you don't have the funders involved and keep them engaged, they will be blindsided and shocked and can pull the rug out from under you.

Having goals in conflict happens all the time. The key is in finding common ground. The common denominator for most people is self-interest. For example, in one project, we brought together groups of Asian Pacific Islanders, Hispanics, and African Americans to find an area to work together on community improvement. We started with a barbeque, which is a good way to get people to come out. We asked how many people want to improve education, and hands went up. We then asked who wants to improve safety, and hands went up. When we asked who wants to improve housing, no hands went up. So we worked on the first two issues.

David M. Fetterman is president and CEO of Fetterman & Associates, an international evaluation consulting firm. He is concurrently a collaborating professor at El Colegio de Postgraduados in Mexico, Distinguished Visiting Professor at San Jose State University, and a professor of education at the University of Arkansas at Pine Bluff, as well as the director of the Arkansas Evaluation Center. He was interviewed by coauthor Patricia B. Campbell in the fall of 2018.

As discussed in Chapter 8, bias can impact definitions of who is and isn't a stakeholder and the degree to which they are involved. It can also impact who gets the results of the evaluation, who is allowed to provide feedback, and how that feedback is or isn't used. Bias can also impact the evaluator's analysis of the program's model or theory of change. It can lead to an uncritical acceptance of program models that are based on the deficit model, with its assumptions that deficiencies in the group culture are the cause of minority group member differences from dominant group members. A related corollary is that it is the individual and/or the group that needs to be "fixed"—that is, if those who are considered "other" would fit better into the values, systems of thought, and behaviors of the dominant group, things would be better, and programs and individuals would be more successful.

As shown in Chapters 11–14, bias can also impact the more technical aspects of the evaluation. For example, the quality of the data collected can be affected if the process, the language used, or even the environment facilitates **stereotype threat**. Steele and Aronson (1995) describe stereotype threat as something that occurs when individuals worry that their behavior might confirm a stereotype about a group they are part of.

For example, research has shown that Black college freshmen and sophomores performed more poorly on standardized tests than white students when their race was emphasized; however, when race was not emphasized, Black students performed better and equivalently with white students (Steele & Aronson, 1995). Two decades of research have demonstrated the harmful effects that stereotype threat can exert on a wide range of populations in a broad array of performance areas (e.g., Pennington, Heim, Levy, & Larkin, 2016; Steele, Spencer, & Arronson, 2002).

The accuracy of the ratings that people, including evaluators, give to participant behavior, attitudes, and work can also be affected by bias. Research for the past 50 years has shown that, in general, people make different judgments based on what they perceive as an individual's gender, race, and ethnicity. This happens even when raters have exactly the same information about the individuals being rated, other than a name that indicates their gender, race, or ethnicity (e.g., Eaton, Saunders, Jacobson, & West, 2019; Moss-Racusin, Dovidio, Brescoll, Graham, & Handelsman, 2012; Pheterson, Kiesler, & Goldberg, 1971). Paradoxically, people who feel that they are objective and fair are more likely to demonstrate bias, in part, because they are not on guard against subtle bias (Monin & Miller, 2001; Uhlmann & Cohen, 2007).

As was covered in Chapter 11, a belief in the importance of objectivity can impact the decisions evaluators make about the design they will use in evaluation. Rather than finding the best design for the question, there can be a bias toward designs that are considered more rigorous, such as randomized controlled trials (RCTs). While RCTs are designed to control for bias, they can instead hide it. Only in the least complex situations can all or even most variables be controlled for in RCTs. Evaluations, since they are dealing with people in context, are usually very complex. Similarly, an evaluator can be biased against RCTs, which could lead to the design not being selected when it is the best design for the question.

Acknowledging Subjectivity and Reducing Bias

There are a variety of things one can do to reduce individual bias. An important first step is to acknowledge that everyone has biases and reflect on the explicit biases we, as individuals, have. This is not an easy task. The activity that follows indicates one way to increase awareness of one's own biases, based on the highly researched and validated Implicit Association Test (IAT).

> ## Activity
> ### Take the Implicit Association Test (Optional)
>
> As was described in Chapter 1, the IAT measures attitudes and beliefs that people may be unwilling or unable to report and measures the strength of associations between concepts (e.g., Black people, gay people) and evaluations (e.g., good, bad) or stereotypes (e.g., athletic, clumsy). If you didn't take one or more of the tests before, you may want to take one or more of them now. You can take the tests at https://implicit.harvard.edu/implicit/selectatest.html. As indicated in Chapter 1, if you are unprepared to encounter interpretations that you might find objectionable, please do not take any of the tests. If you took the test as part of the Chapter 1 activities, you may want to take it again and see if your score or the experience is different this time.

It is important to remember that biases that impact evaluation decision making include areas beyond cultural and/or demographic variables. For example, a bias toward quantitative data or a bias toward qualitative data can have a strong impact on evaluation decisions made in technical areas.

Being aware of one's biases is an important first step. However, simply being aware of one's biases is not enough. To reduce one's biases, specific and tailored forms of intervention are generally needed (Tropp & Godsil, 2015). One well-validated technique is to expose one's self and others to counter-stereotypic examples and to consciously contrast negative stereotypes with specific counterexamples (Finnegan, Oakhill & Garnham, 2015; Olsson & Martiny, 2018). We become less prejudiced when we are exposed to and think about group members who have particularly positive or nonstereotypical characteristics, which can, and often does, lead to a reduction of stereotypes and biases related to those groups (Stangor, Tarry, & Jhangiani, 2014). Practice helps as well. Kawakami, Dovidio, Moll, Hermsen, and Russin (2000) found that students who practiced responding in nonstereotypical ways to members of other groups became better able to avoid activating their negative stereotypes on future occasions.

As the following case study indicates, awareness of implicit bias can help reduce bias in the short term, but over time, it is the awareness that discrimination exists that can make a difference.

> ## Case Study
> ### Scientists Avoid Bias When They Know They're Being Tested
>
> In a 2019 study, researchers examined the interactive effect of explicit and implicit gender biases on promotion decisions. The first year, promotion committees took the IAT on gender and science and were told they were part of a study to examine the impact of implicit gender bias in promotion decisions. For the second year, they were not reminded of the study.
>
> Committees with strong implicit gender biases who did not explicitly believe that external barriers hold women back promoted fewer women in year 2 (when they were not reminded of the implicit bias study) than in year 1 (when they were). For committee members who believed that women face external barriers, their implicit bias scores did not predict whether they selected more men over women either year (Regner, Thinus-Blanc, Netter, Schmakder, & Huguet, 2019). Being aware that bias and discrimination exist can make a difference.

More intergroup contact can reduce bias as well. Pettigrew and Tropp (2006) conducted a meta-analysis in which they reviewed over 500 studies that had investigated the effects of intergroup contact on group attitudes. They found that attitudes toward groups with whom they were in contact became more positive over time. Furthermore, positive effects of contact were found on both stereotypes and prejudice for many different types of contacted groups (Stangor et al., 2014). Taking the perspective of another group member has been found to increase empathy and closeness to the person and to reduce prejudice (Tropp & Godsil, 2015; Stangor et al., 2014). People, the theory proposes, will have more positive attitudes toward each other when they feel more like they are all part of one large group rather than members of separate subgroups. It is important to note that while contact can reduce prejudice, it may make it worse if it is not implemented correctly. (Stangor et al., 2014).

Confronting bias and prejudice can make a difference; however, that confrontation can be more effective when it is done by someone with more privilege. For example, Gulker, Mark, and Monteith (2013) found that confrontations of racism were met with greater acceptance when performed by a white than a Black confronter. As may be shown by participating in the activity that follows, taking action when confronted by bias or prejudice can be challenging.

Reflect and Discuss
Confronting Prejudice

Have you ever confronted or failed to confront a person who you thought was expressing prejudice or discrimination? Why did you confront (or not confront) that person, and how did doing so make you feel? (Stangor et al., 2014). Write down your responses and, if you are comfortable doing so, share them in a small group.

Building Cultural Competence

One of the major themes of the book is that evaluators need to be culturally competent. As the Centre for Research and Education on Violence Against Women and Children (CREVAWC, 2017) point out being culturally component "is more than being respectful of the cultures represented in the service or even the community. It is much more than awareness of cultural differences, more than knowledge of the customs and values of those different to our own" (para. 6). It includes fostering secure, respectful, and reciprocal relationships; partnerships; high expectations; and equity and respect for diversity. They go on to say that

> cultural competence is not static, and our level of cultural competence changes in response to new situations, experiences and relationships. The three elements of cultural competence are:
>
> - attitudes
> - skills
> - knowledge (CREVAWC, 2017, para. 13)

The following are some criteria to consider when determining cultural competence. Individuals must

- have an understanding of, and honor, the histories, cultures, languages, traditions, [and] child rearing practices;
- value [each] individual's different capacities and abilities;
- respect differences in families' home lives;
- recognize that diversity contributes to the richness of our society and provides a valid evidence base about ways of knowing;
- demonstrate an ongoing commitment to developing their own cultural competence in a two-way process with families and communities; [and]
- promote greater understanding of Indigenous ways of knowing and being engage[d] in ongoing reflection relating to their cultural competence. (CREVAWC, 2017, para. 15)

As was covered in Chapter 2, in 2011, the American Evaluation Association (AEA) issued a *Public Statement on Cultural Competence in Evaluation*, which describes cultural competence as "a stance taken toward culture, not a discrete status or simple mastery of particular knowledge and skills" (Intro., para. 3). The statement describes a culturally competent evaluator as one who is

> prepared to engage with diverse segments of communities to include cultural and contextual dimensions important to the evaluation. . . . Cultural competence in evaluation requires that evaluators maintain a high degree of self-awareness and self-examination to better understand how their own backgrounds and other life experiences serve as assets or limitations in the conduct of an evaluation. (Intro., paras. 3, 6)

One way to start to build cultural competence is by exploring one's own historical roots, beliefs, and values to help understand the pervasive role culture plays in people's lives. This can help people become aware of their own biases and want to know about other cultures (Clay, 2010). There are a number of ways to learn about other cultures, including going to conferences that include a diversity focus, attending professional development sessions that focus on developing cultural competence in evaluation, interacting with members of different cultural groups, visiting with members of different cultural groups, going to lectures, and even taking courses (Iris Center, Vanderbilt University, 2019).

Based on interviews with experts on cultural competence, Clay (2010) offers some creative suggestions on ways to increase cultural competence such as reading memoirs and novels written by members of the culture as well as reading journal articles and academic books. A second suggestion is to learn another language. Quoting Pamela Hays, one of the interviewed experts, Clay explains that

> one of the best ways to immerse yourself in another culture's worldview is to learn a second language . . . One of the most mind-expanding experiences is to learn a word or concept that doesn't exist in your own language. Plus, learning a language means you're more able to reach out and connect with people who speak that language. (p. 24)

The following four steps can help provide a road map for those who want to become more culturally competent.

- Be aware of one's own world view
- Develop positive attitudes towards cultural differences
- Gain knowledge of different cultural practices and world views
- Develop skills for communication and interaction across cultures (CREVAWC, 2017, para. 7)

The activity that follows provides an opportunity for readers to develop their own plan to increase their own cultural competence.

Activity
Building One's Cultural Competence

Cultural competence is not static, and our level of cultural competence changes in response to new situations, experiences, and relationships. Remembering that culture doesn't mean just race, ethnicity, and nationality, reflect on each of the four steps outlined earlier and write down some ways you could increase your cultural competency.

To guide the direction of areas in which evaluators need to be more culturally competent, evaluators need to be aware of the major cultural groups that may have relevance for the evaluations they are doing. For example, for an evaluation of a program to provide services to returning veterans, it may not be enough to know about the culture of the armed services, but it may be necessary to know about the different cultures of the Army, Navy, Air Force, and Marines. Similarly, if an evaluator is assessing the effectiveness of programs for prison inmates, it might be necessary to understand the different cultures of minimum-, medium-, and maximum-security facilities. In other words, it is important to recognize that there are diversities within diversity.

Understanding and becoming aware of one's own cultural values, beliefs, attitudes and judgments becomes central when we have to interact with people from different cultural backgrounds. . . . [Our] values and beliefs shape our perceptions; they define the ways we see the world. We can learn the Do's and Don'ts of other cultures trying to alter our behavior to different cultural situations[;] however, unless we are aware of the ways we perceive these situations, we will always be one step behind. (Reiche, 2012, para. 5).

As an example, the following discussion covers some of what we (coauthors Veronica G. Thomas and Patricia B. Campbell) have learned about cultural differences in levels of formality.

While in the dominant U.S. culture informality is often prized, in many other cultures more formality is an indication of respect. This includes how people are addressed by name. Levels of formality in how one addresses adults are tied to power and status. For example, doctors, lawyers, dentists, and "bosses" are traditionally addressed by their title and last name while, nurses, secretaries, and hygienists are called by their first names with no title. Culturally competent evaluators understand that

- you don't call people by their first names. Instead, you wait to be asked and, as the evaluator, use equal levels of formality with adults as they use with you;
- if a person has an honorific, such as Doctor, Officer, or Headmaster, you use that title when you address or speak about that person;
- you call people by the names they prefer. If you find the name hard to pronounce, practice. There are many online free pronunciation programs online that can help you. Search on "how to pronounce"; and
- with children, you follow the rules of the community. If children call other adults by their last name and title, be sure it is acceptable before you ask them to call you by your first name.

Martin, Martin, and Martin (2019) address cultural differences in formality of dress. They suggest people be aware of the level of formality in the dress of the adults with whom they are or will be working and reflect that level of formality in their own dress. If one's dress is seen as too casual or inappropriate, it can be interpreted as being disrespectful of the place and people being visited. In general, evaluators should be aware of and respectful of a group's folkways, informal norms, and roles.

Personalizing a Social Justice Perspective

In Chapter 5, we covered a variety of social justice definitions, issues, and related theories as well as social justice evaluation frameworks. While much work has been done in these areas, in the same way that evaluators need to reflect on and work to reduce their own biases and increase their cultural competence, they need to develop an understanding of what social justice means to them as well as to define the constructs and beliefs that are key to their own social justice frameworks.

When we examined definitions of social justice, different themes were found. Some definitions place emphasis on the individual, while others emphasize the common good and the whole community. Some definitions focus on equal treatment, while others focus on fairness, opportunity inclusion, and diversity. Definitions are useful, especially if they can help illuminate the elements of the social justice evaluation frameworks that are important to the evaluator and can cause evaluators to reflect on their attitudes and beliefs that will be translated into evaluation planning, implementation, and use.

Also in Chapter 5, we covered seven different social justice evaluation frameworks: transformative evaluation, empowerment evaluation, feminist evaluation, participatory evaluation, deliberative democratic evaluation, collaborative evaluation, and equity-focused evaluation. These frameworks do not advocate particular evaluation models, methods, designs, or approaches; rather, they can be seen as ways of thinking about evaluation. While the frameworks differ, they all acknowledge the roles power and privilege play in society as a whole and in evaluation specifically and the need to minimize the impact of those roles on the evaluation process and results. Some frameworks include a focus on achieving equitable results, others focus on increasing social justice in general, and still others focus on a specific marginalized group. In some frameworks, there is an emphasis on the importance of stakeholder involvement and empowerment, with the evaluator serving as a knowledgeable insider or coach rather than a neutral outsider. In the activity that follows, readers are provided an opportunity to think about their own social justice framework.

Reflect and Discuss
What Social Justice Means to You

Thinking about what social justice means to you, what are two or three major components, attitudes, or assumptions that you would include in your personal social justice framework?

Reflective Practice and Evaluative Thinking

As introduced in Chapter 1, the integration of reflective practice and evaluative thinking provides evaluators with a basis on which to collect information and assess beliefs and assumptions. This can help the evaluator make more informed decisions, which can lead to higher-quality evaluations. Using reflective practice, evaluators and others study their own experiences to improve the way they work. Evaluative thinking can be thought of as a reflective practice that "fully integrates systematic questioning, data, and action into an organization's work practices" (Baker & Bruner, 2012, p. 1). This, of course, can and should apply to issues of culture, bias, and social justice as well as to all evaluation decisions. With evaluative thinking, evaluators ask and reflect on why specific evaluation decisions were or are being made (IllumiLab, 2018b). As the following activity suggests, often evaluative thinking starts with asking some questions and investing in the process of answering them.

Activity
Defining Evaluation

In Chapter 1, we provided an overview of a variety of definitions of evaluation concluding with our own definition:

Evaluation is a disciplined inquiry involving the systematic, contextually responsive, and ethical application of research tools and methods to collect data that assess the effectiveness and operations of programs within the various social, political, and cultural contexts in which they operate. Evaluation's ultimate goal is to provide credible evidence that fosters greater understanding and improves decision making, all aimed at improving social conditions and promoting healthy, just, and equitable communities.

What are the concepts that you feel need to be included in your own definition of evaluation? Why did you choose these concepts and not others? What was your reasoning behind your decisions?

Applying to Practice

The first part of the chapter has focused on evaluator knowledge and attitudes and ways evaluators can help themselves to be better evaluators, including

- increasing awareness of one's own biases and steps one can take to reduce those biases;
- increasing cultural competence, not just by learning more about different cultures but also by learning what it means to be culturally component and ways one can accomplish competence for different cultures;
- reflecting on and clarifying what social justice means to the evaluator and what are the key components of social justice frameworks that need to be included in the evaluations one does; and
- including reflective thinking and evaluative practice as part of the evaluation process.

All of this is necessary but not sufficient for high-quality evaluations. As Alexandria Ocasio-Cortez points out, "it's not enough to say, 'I'm a good person.' The question is, 'Am I doing good work?'" (quoted in Washington, 2019, para. 8). To do good work, it is important to apply the knowledge and skills gained to evaluation practice.

The rest of the chapter focuses on applying that which has been learned to practice, building on a base of evaluative thinking and reflective practice and doing culturally responsive evaluations (CREs, defined in Chapter 4). CREs must take into account the culture of the program being evaluated (Frierson, Hood, & Hughes, 2002) and pay "particular attention to groups who have been marginalized seeking to bring balance and equity into the evaluation process" (Frierson et al., 2002, p. 63). It requires that evaluators critically examine culturally relevant but often neglected variables in project design and evaluation.

Making Biases Explicit

As discussed earlier, we all have biases, and those biases can impact our decision making including decision making in evaluation. While we often think about biases in terms of attitudes toward and stereotypes about people from different demographic groups and/or cultures, biases impacting evaluation decision making are much broader than encompassing favored and less favored evaluation models, methods, analyses, designs, and even reasoning. When thinking about data analysis, one may favor deductive over inductive reasoning (both described in Chapter 13) or relationship-based analysis over difference-based analysis or may be biased for or against surveys. It is key for evaluators to identify the biases most likely to affect critical decisions. Open discussion of the biases that may be undermining decision making, especially with those who may have different biases, is invaluable. It can be stimulated both by conducting postmortems of past decisions in current or previous evaluations and by asking oneself if that was the right decision or not and providing a rationale for the response.

Along with being aware of one's own biases and their potential impact, as the following activity indicates, it is important for stakeholders to be aware of an evaluator's background and potential biases.

Activity
Highlighting Potential Biases

Here are two sample personal statements from evaluators providing information that could be used by readers to assess possible biases.

> "I am an older white woman educational researcher with extensive experience in evaluation and diversity research. I am a feminist and social justice advocate who uses both qualitative and quantitative research methods."

> "I am a younger Black woman with expertise in social psychological research and culturally responsive mentoring. Critical race theory is at the core of much of my work, and my primary research methodology is quantitative."

What, if any, inferences would you make about potential biases from these statements? You are looking for possible biases but need to remember that these women may not have the biases you have inferred, and they may have other biases.

What would you include in your own personal statement?

Infusing Cultural Responsiveness in the Involvement/Engagement of Stakeholders and the Development of Evaluation Questions

As described in Chapter 8, stakeholders can be described in terms of three (non–mutually exclusive) major groups of individuals: (a) those involved in the management of program operations, (b) those served or affected by the program and (c) those who are intended users of the evaluation findings (U.S. Department of Health and Human Services Centers for Disease Control and Prevention, 2011). Another way that stakeholders can be classified is in terms of their power and interest in the project. Evaluators should not make the mistake of assuming that those individuals in leadership or decision-making positions are automatically the most important stakeholders. Evaluators also need to remember that stakeholders can play a variety of different roles at different levels in evaluations. Those roles can range from being informed to consulting, collaborating, sharing leadership, and becoming empowered through the evaluation.

Stakeholders can provide the evaluator with knowledge and context that can be key to a successful evaluation. One way to do that is to have stakeholders share their thoughts and ideas about the ways the project's philosophy compares to and interacts with the cultural values, lifestyles, and worldviews of its clients and the surrounding community. They can also provide feedback on the extent to which the project relates to the diverse groups being served by the project and the degree to which the project operates in a manner that respects local culture and traditions.

As discussed in Chapters 8, 9, and 10, in culturally responsive evaluations the involvement and engagement of stakeholders are tied to both planning the evaluation and developing evaluation questions. Evaluators should involve diverse stakeholders as part of the process of defining what success looks like. Along with the related theoretical and empirical literature, stakeholders can give evaluators input on developing meaningful indicators to assess success. Good evaluation questions reflect the multiple perspectives and take into account a number of factors. At a minimum, these factors include (a) the project's goals and objectives, (b) the project's logic model, (c) motivations for the evaluation, (d) the funder's requirements, (e) feedback from relevant stakeholders, and (f) the agreed-on focus and goals of the evaluation. To prioritize outcomes questions, the evaluator needs to think about which questions could yield outcomes (a) most useful to understanding project success and guiding program improvements, (b) most important for funders to know, and (c) most important to program participants and diverse stakeholder groups. It is equally important for the evaluator to put into place an equitable process to make sure that diverse voices are respected, heard, and acted on when prioritizing questions. This should involve critical dialogue between the evaluator and diverse stakeholders with the goal of obtaining input from as many perspectives as possible to get a more complete picture before deciding on final evaluation questions.

This can be a challenge. Developing definitions of success, evaluation questions, and indicators, ideally, is a cyclical process initially involving generating definitions of success and evaluation questions based on a knowledge of context and program and community background. This is followed by stakeholder review; refinement by the evaluator, as needed; additional stakeholder review, as needed; and joint prioritization of the questions, re-review, and reprioritization. Some stakeholders are leery to get involved in the process. Their concerns include if they have the time or the expertise to participate and if their input would be taken seriously. In addition, it can be hard for some stakeholders to see what is realistic for an evaluator to do with existing budget and time constraints. These factors should be considered and addressed as needed when developing plans to involve stakeholders from diverse groups in the evaluation.

Engaging diverse stakeholder groups, across the entire evaluation process, can be especially challenging in instances where differential power relations and cultural conflicts between/among stakeholders and evaluators might discourage engagement. In engaging stakeholders, evaluators must also deal with the reality, discussed earlier, that not all project stakeholder groups will share the same concerns or have unified opinions or priorities. Stakeholder concerns should be considered even if the evaluator is unable to be fully responsive to addressing those concerns.

Infusing Cultural Responsiveness in Decisions About Evaluation Designs

As was covered in Chapter 11, decisions about evaluation designs and analysis are often based on traditional definitions of rigor as "the strict application of the scientific method in an effort to ensure robust and unbiased experimental design, methodology, analysis, interpretation, and reporting of results" (Lauer, 2016, para. 1). In this definition, more rigorous designs are those that control for as many threats to validity as possible. Within that definition, where there is less control, there is less rigor. However, while one needs to try to control for threats to validity, high levels of control can only happen in very simple studies. In evaluation studies, we are looking at complexity and messiness.

While Riley (2017, p 11) was speaking about engineering education, her words hold for other areas, including evaluation, as well. She explains there can be an inverse relationship between traditional definitions of rigor and usefulness:

My colleagues felt the rigor of our program needed to be unassailable, and the use of this particular word—as distinct from quality, from excellence, from intellectual standards, from merit, from legitimacy, validity, or trustworthiness—reeked of a particular kind of technocratic sexism endemic to engineering. . . . Rigor refers not only to particular standards of quality for academic work, but also the problematic processes by which we discern these aspects in one another's work, or even in one another. I argue that rigor is used to maintain disciplinary boundaries, with exclusionary implications for marginalized groups and marginalized ways of knowing. (p. 11)

In evaluation, decisions about what design to use should be based on the best design to answer the questions being asked. As pointed out in Chapter 11, the best design is the one that not only can answer the questions but can do so within the budget, without compromising that which is being evaluated, while being culturally responsive and inconveniencing participants as little as possible. Some things evaluators need to keep in mind when selecting an evaluation design include

- appropriateness of the fit between the design of the program or "intervention" and the requirements of more rigorous evaluation methodologies;
- the timing of the evaluation;
- the balance between the level of investment in the evaluation and the level of investment in and the intensity of the program;
- the level of evidence expected given the nature of the intervention; and
- the strength of rival hypotheses.

Infusing Cultural Responsiveness in Decisions About Data Collection and Analysis

Data Collection

The goal of a data collection effort is to collect accurate and appropriate data and to make sure that all relevant voices are heard. To ensure that happens, as was covered in Chapter 12, it is necessary to know a great deal about participants including their preferred modes of communication, communication style, preferred language, their literacy levels, and possible issues tied to accessibility. If, for example, an evaluator is working with participants who come from an oral tradition, have learning disabilities, or are low literacy, surveys aren't going to be an effective way to collect data. If participants have visual, hearing, or mobility impairments, then data collection methods may need to be modified to accommodate them. Interviewers need to be fluent in the language(s) participants speak, and all need to be aware of and respect participants' communication styles.

In some cultures, it is disrespectful to begin an interview or focus group immediately, and it is important to begin with a conversation and getting to know each other. Some people prefer to directly answer questions; other prefer to tell stories. In some cultures, it is considered very rude to interrupt, and there can be a "wait time" of several seconds of silence before the participant is through.

As discussed earlier, the concept of stereotype threat can cause the collected data to be inaccurate and lead to false conclusions. When negative stereotypes are made salient, those who are impacted by the stereotypes perform less well. Something as seemingly small as having to indicate one's race or gender before filling out a survey or a test can increase stereotype threat and impact the responses given. As simple a change as asking demographic questions at the end of any measure can increase the quality of the data collected (Danaher & Crandall, 2008; Sinclair, Hardin, & Lowery, 2006). There are more active ways to reduce the impact of stereotype threat including, for example, telling women and girls that a math test does not show gender differences (Spencer, Steele, & Quinn, 1999) or removing physical cues that make it seem that a setting is defined by the majority group (Cheryan, Plaut, Davies, & Steele, 2009). However, evaluators need to decide, even if these actions are acceptable for programs, if they are too interventionist for evaluations.

When standardized measures are used, it is important to determine if the measures have been tested for reliability and validity on groups similar to the participants. However, that may not be enough. Culturally responsive evaluation requires that people be heard and their lived experience be included as data. That may not be possible if standardized measures are used exclusively or if they predominate. The designers of most standardized measures are generally of the dominant culture, and their assumptions may not reflect those of other cultures. The psychometric quality of measures is very important, but evaluators need to remember Tom Kibler's (personal communication, September 15, 1997) point that it is better to have a bad measure of the right thing, than a good measure of the wrong thing. Bad measures can be improved, but if the measure is of the wrong thing, it will not provide useful information.

The following activity provides an opportunity for readers to reflect on and discuss ways they can tell "the story" rather than "their story" of the program and the evaluation.

Reflect and Discuss
Spinning a Story

I realized I had been spinning a story from my science, interpreting my results, based on my conception of what should be happening instead of critically examining the facts in front of me. (Manzar, 2019, p. 514)

As an evaluator, what steps can you take to reduce the probability that you "spin a story" based on your expectations or assumptions of what should be happening?

Data Analysis

As was covered in Chapter 13, there are two basic types of reasoning that are used in analysis, deductive and inductive reasoning. Deductive reasoning starts with a possible theory or premise tied to the design of that which is to be evaluated. In deductive reasoning, one generally moves from theory to hypothesis to observation or other data collection method to confirmation. In inductive reasoning, which draws general principles from specific instances, the process is reversed. Here, one generally moves from observation to patterns to tentative hypotheses to theory (Herr, 2007). Traditionally, deductive reasoning is used when there are enough existing theories, conclusions, or results to generate hypotheses to be tested. However, in culturally responsive evaluation, before making the decision to use deductive reasoning, it is important to examine the perspectives from which the existing theories have been built and conclusions have been drawn to determine if the perspectives of marginalized people have been included. If they have not, then inductive reasoning may be a better choice.

In culturally responsive evaluation, disaggregation of data, as we discussed in earlier chapters, is a particular challenge. Breaking out the data by one characteristic—for instance, only gender—doesn't look at interactions between gender and disability or between race and age, and so on. As a result, the findings can be incomplete or inaccurate. Too, attention needs to be paid to such conceptually relevant and possibly confounding factors as socioeconomic status and individual and family educational backgrounds.

It is also important to be aware that there can be diversity within subgroups. For example, while people who are visually impaired, hearing impaired, or learning disabled are all classified as having disabilities, the differences among them are very large. Unless such differences are addressed, in any analysis, there is a great danger of generating inaccurate conclusions. There are important reasons to disaggregate the data as much as possible, but there are also statistical and privacy limitations. We have found several things that evaluators can do to determine possible levels of disaggregation, including

- using crosstabs to break down the demographic characteristics of participants to help determine where levels of disaggregation can be done;
- doing preliminary analysis of subgroup differences in areas of importance to the study; and
- reviewing the literature tied to program goals to determine if there is potential for differential project/program impact for different subgroups and therefore disaggregation would be needed.

As described here and in Chapter 13, knowing the gender, race/ethnicity, and even the first name of the person whose work is being rated has been shown to impact ratings in a variety of areas including open-ended responses, job applications, and even coursework (Anderson-Clark, Green, & Henley, 2008; Correll & Benard, 2006; Pellegrini, 2011). To reduce potential bias, evaluators need to make the coding/rating procedures as anonymous as possible, including having participants put any identifying information where coders/raters can't see that information. For interview data, bias can be reduced by transcribing the interview, having explicit codes and criteria for the analysis, and having the initial analysis done by someone other than the interviewer. Bias in observations can be reduced by having a highly scripted assessment with clear and easy-to-follow guidance for scoring and ensuring that data collectors have sufficient training—both of these make a difference (Namit & Seden, 2018).

Infusing Cultural Responsiveness in Decisions About Reports and Presentations

"To have an impact on decision-making, evaluation findings must be perceived as relevant and useful and . . . should fully reflect the different interests and needs of the many parties involved" (Organisation for Economic Co-operation and

Development, 1991, p. 7). Earlier in the book chapter, it was stressed how important it is to know about participants before designing the data collection plan. The situation is similar when evaluators are designing plans for the reporting and the dissemination of evaluation findings. Knowing different stakeholders' preferred modes of communication, preferred communication style, and preferred language and literacy levels is crucial. In addition, culturally responsive reporting attends to possibly different interpretations of the same words and images by different groups. The following are some ways that we have found evaluators can craft their findings in ways they will be used.

- Understand your stakeholders: Develop a sense of your stakeholders and use that information to craft your message.

- Do your homework: Find out as much as you can about the kinds of words commonly used and avoided by the different stakeholders and the emotions, divisions, and concepts these words and related images evoke.

- Consider your goals: Think about the findings that are particularly important and prioritize them.

- Check the language you used to make sure it reflects the tone you want (i.e., authoritative or approachable) and does not include "hot button" words that are likely to trigger negative reactions (Campbell-Kibler & Campbell, 2007).

- Add a section in the report called "Use of the Evaluation" or "Actionable Evaluation" (Davidson, 2013; Vaca, 2018).

Accessibility is the key to effective dissemination. An important first step is to find where individual stakeholder groups tend to get their information and the formats they are most comfortable with. Results should most likely be provided in different lengths and levels of readability in formats that are accessible to people with disabilities. Pilot-testing different reports and formats with a sample of stakeholders can provide important information.

Social Justice Evaluation

Throughout the book, including this chapter, the emphasis has been on what is necessary and sufficient to conduct high-quality evaluations that are accurate, useful, and used. This involves the application of a culturally responsive framework with evaluative thinking and reflective practice. These components are needed for any high-quality program evaluation, not just evaluations tied to social justice. To apply a social justice–oriented model of evaluation, as we commented in Chapter 5, these components are necessary but not sufficient. As should all program evaluations, a social justice–oriented model of evaluation should be culturally responsive, but it also needs to have a social justice aim. Additionally, this means using a strength-based perspective that focuses on uncovering assets and strengths of communities, particularly marginalized communities, rather than simply uncovering problems. A social justice–oriented evaluation includes basic assumptions and methods that help to ensure that the evaluation will have social justice implications regardless of the topic. It plans for a process of learning and not simply judging.

> Evaluators are often asked to assess the effectiveness of social programs that are designed to yield a quick "magic bullet" fix to problems derived from years of racial oppression. Here, race is and is not the problem inasmuch as racism fuels the disparities we witness. However, this reality is virtually absent in the discourse of numerous commentaries and policy makers who are quick to cite Black failure or pathology without examining the historical root causes. As a result, social programs seek to address outcomes, such as the achievement gap and health disparities, rather than the race-based structural inequalities in the social, economic, and political systems that contribute to these outcomes. (Thomas et al., 2018, p. 517)

A social justice–oriented evaluation model looks at individuals and groups but also focuses on the system. As the following fable, from coauthor Patricia B. Campbell, may help to explain, if systemic issues are not addressed, the focus of programs and of their evaluations will continue to be on fixing the broken rather than not breaking things in the first place.

> Once upon a time there were three people walking next to the Hudson River. Looking over, they saw the river was full of babies. One of the three jumped into the river and started throwing babies out to the shore; the second jumped into the river and started teaching babies to swim while the third started running upstream.
>
> "What are you doing?" cried the two in the water. "There are babies drowning in the river."
>
> "I know," said the third. "I'm going to find out who's throwing babies into the river and make them stop."

In most program evaluations, the definitions of success, the development of questions, and the resulting data collection, analysis, and interpretation of results focus on the actions of the first two people in the fable. To make change, the actions and perspectives of the person running upstream need to be addressed as well.

Politics and Evaluation

While in recent years the wall between science and politics has seemed to be breaking faster, there has always been tension between science, including evaluation, and politics, although that tends not to be acknowledged in evaluator training. In 2008, Chelimsky explained that

> because our government's need for evaluation arises from its checks and balances structure, evaluators working within that structure must deal not exceptionally, but routinely and regularly with political infringement on their independence that results directly from that structure. (p. 400)

She pointed out the irony that

> what should surprise us would be the absence of pressure on evaluators to make an agency "look good" or the lack of effort by agency managers

to try to manipulate the work of evaluators implementing legislative oversight. (p. 400)

Evaluation, as Haugem and Chouinard (2019) point out "is innately political" (p. 385). House (1995) explains that politics can have an upper hand if evaluators misunderstand their responsibilities. As discussed in Chapter 2, House describes five evaluation fallacies that evaluators need to guard against:

- *Clientism*—the fallacy that doing whatever the client requests or whatever will benefit the client is ethically correct
- *Contractualism*—the fallacy that the evaluator must follow the written contract without question, even if doing so is detrimental to the public good
- *Methodologicalism*—the belief that following acceptable inquiry methods ensures that the behavior of the evaluator will be ethical, even when some methodologies may actually compound the evaluator's ethical dilemmas
- *Relativism*—the fallacy that opinion data the evaluator collects from various participants must be given equal weight, as if there is no basis of appropriately giving the opinions of peripheral groups less priority than that given to more pivotal groups
- *Pluralism/elitism*—the fallacy of allowing powerful voices to be given higher priority because the evaluator feels they hold more prestige and potency than the powerless or voiceless. (p. 29)

Coming from a somewhat different perspective, Perrin (2019, p 356), in an article titled "How to Manage Pressure to Change Reports: Should Evaluators Be Above Criticism?" points out that "truth also is not fully owned by evaluators, nor does it arrive just through statistical analysis," and that evaluators need to be open to criticism. He further suggests that in response to pressure to make changes in reports, evaluators must "be sure you are right—and be open to making corrections when new information is presented," "specify a format for comments from stakeholders on draft reports," "be prepared to compromise," and "openly acknowledge that certain findings, conclusions or recommendations are contested" (Perrin, 2019, pp. 366–368).

Voices From the Field: Advice for New Evaluators

In their Voices From the Field interviews, six of those interviewed provided advice to new evaluators centering on values, humility, and staying current.

Katrina L. Bledsoe

As evaluators, we need to ask ourselves, "What kinds of evaluations am I interested in doing?" and "Does a proposed evaluation project fit into my core values as an evaluator?" This can help evaluators decide when we do an evaluation and when we walk away. We need to do evaluations that reflect our core values.

Donna M. Mertens

You need to clarify your own assumptions about what guides you, what are your values. You need to ask yourself serious questions: "Does my behavior as an evaluator reflect those values?" You can't do it by yourself. You need critical self-reflection, but you need to be engaged with a broad constituency and cognizant of those barriers that keep people and their experiences from being considered by others and communities with more power.

Melvin Hall

I used to tell my students, "Do not overexpect or oversell what you can do at your stage of development. If you are just starting out, recognize you will not be doing evaluation work that is as deep, as powerful, and as complex as you will be doing later in your career. Don't allow yourself to think more of what you know and what you are doing than you should." Everyone has to work at the level they are at, keeping their eyes and ears open so that they can get better at what they do. The people who read one of these books with a new evaluation model, and then go out convinced that they are doing a different type of evaluation, do themselves and their clients a disservice. That is true for people who are trying to be culturally responsive as well.

David M. Fetterman

You need to know when to use a hammer and chisel versus going in with a bulldozer or a plow. You need to listen to people and learn their issues and what they want to do and know your measures and select the right tool—one that is appropriate for the task at hand. To make people jump for metrics or approaches, for that matter, is wrong because the popular metrics or approaches might not be right for them at this time.

Karen E. Kirkhart

Familiarize yourself with the classic literature and then move it forward and integrate it in the current moment and keep in mind Jawaharlal Nehru's wisdom, "Let us be a little humble, let us think that the truth may not perhaps be entirely with us."

Ayesha S. Boyce

It's not enough to just read evaluation literature. I inform myself by staying current in work on critical race theory, feminist theory, intersectionality, and microaggressions. You need to inform yourself about what's out there and then choose what works for you.

As the book comes to an end, we would like you to reflect on what your response would be to the following situation.

Activity
Applying Cultural Competence

For a project on cultural relevance and cultural competence, the prime organization hired, without community input, an evaluator who is competent and experienced and has worked with the white principal investigator (PI) from the prime institution before, but has no experience working with people of color as supervisors or equal partners although she has collected feedback and other data from people of color. In this project co-PIs, who are people of color, questioned her about her philosophy of evaluation and asked her about her experience with and comfort with work with people of color. The white PI and other white senior staff from the prime institution said the co-PIs in their questions were being rude to the white evaluator. The evaluator suggested she, on project funds, go to each of the four sites and learn from them about their culture and community and begin to build trust.

One co-PI pointed out that what that meant was, yet again, that people of color would be asked to train white professionals about their culture and community to help the white evaluator begin to gain experience with communities of color, so that, because she is white, she will be more likely to be hired for similar evaluations than more experienced evaluators of color.

What are the ethical issues here?

What do you think the evaluator should do? Why?

How would you resolve the conflict?

A Final Thought

In a published article of his 1988 AEA keynote address, Hilliard (1989) eloquently stated that "the power to define reality is a supreme power. It must not be used casually. It must be a democratic process. It must be anchored in the truth" (p. 20). As such, as evaluators we must forge an evaluation practice that serves broad ideals of diverse participation, social justice, and equity by meaningfully engaging, understanding, and uncovering (a) the quality of the program experience for diverse participants, (b) the cultural and contextual fit of the program design and theory of change, and finally (c) the outcomes of people in programs within the context of their (oftentimes-racialized) environments.

SUPPLEMENTAL RESOURCES

Evaluative Thinking: Strategies for Reflective Thinking in Your Organization

www.cdc.gov/dhdsp/docs/CB-June2018-508.pdf

This PowerPoint presentation provides a conceptual overview of evaluative thinking as a tool for building evaluation capacity in an organization.

Practical Strategies for Culturally Competent Evaluation

www.cdc.gov/dhdsp/docs/cultural_competence_guide.pdf

This guide provides important strategies for approaching an evaluation with a critical cultural lens to ensure that evaluation efforts have cultural relevance and generate meaningful findings that stakeholders ultimately will value and use.

Beyond Rigor: Improving Evaluations With Diverse Populations

www.beyondrigor.org/index.html

This site provides easy-to-use tips to design, implement, and assess the quality of evaluations of programs and projects to improve the quality, quantity, and diversity of the STEM workforce. However, most of the tips and other information can be of use to a broad range of researchers and evaluators and those who fund them.

Appendix A

American Evaluation Association *Evaluators' Ethical Guiding Principles*

A: Systematic Inquiry: Evaluators conduct data-based inquiries that are thorough, methodical, and contextually relevant.

A1. Adhere to the highest technical standards appropriate to the methods being used while attending to the evaluation's scale and available resources.

A2. Explore with primary stakeholders the limitations and strengths of the core evaluation questions and the approaches that might be used for answering those questions.

A3. Communicate methods and approaches accurately, and in sufficient detail, to allow others to understand, interpret, and critique the work.

A4. Make clear the limitations of the evaluation and its results.

A5. Discuss in contextually appropriate ways the values, assumptions, theories, methods, results, and analyses that significantly affect the evaluator's interpretation of the findings.

A6. Carefully consider the ethical implications of the use of emerging technologies in evaluation practice.

B: Competence: Evaluators provide skilled professional services to stakeholders.

B1. Ensure that the evaluation team possesses the education, abilities, skills, and experiences required to complete the evaluation competently.

B2. When the most ethical option is to proceed with a commission or request outside the boundaries of the evaluation team's professional preparation and competence, clearly communicate any significant limitations to the evaluation that might result. Make every effort to supplement missing or weak competencies directly or through the assistance of others.

B3. Ensure that the evaluation team collectively possesses or seeks out the competencies necessary to work in the cultural context of the evaluation.

B4. Continually undertake relevant education, training or supervised practice to learn new concepts, techniques, skills, and services necessary for competent evaluation practice. Ongoing professional development might include: formal coursework and workshops, self-study, self- or externally commissioned evaluations of one's own practice, and working with other evaluators to learn and refine evaluative skills and expertise.

C: Integrity: Evaluators behave with honesty and transparency in order to ensure the integrity of the evaluation.

C1. Communicate truthfully and openly with clients and relevant stakeholders concerning all aspects of the evaluation, including its limitations.

C2. Disclose any conflicts of interest (or appearance of a conflict) prior to accepting an evaluation assignment and manage or mitigate any conflicts during the evaluation.

C3. Record and promptly communicate any changes to the originally negotiated evaluation plans, the rationale for those changes, and the potential impacts on the evaluation's scope and results.

C4. Assess and make explicit the stakeholders', clients', and evaluators' values, perspectives, and interests concerning the conduct and outcome of the evaluation.

C5. Accurately and transparently represent evaluation procedures, data, and findings.

C6. Clearly communicate, justify, and address concerns related to procedures or activities that are likely to produce misleading evaluative information or conclusions. Consult colleagues for suggestions on proper ways to proceed if concerns cannot be resolved, and decline the evaluation when necessary.

C7. Disclose all sources of financial support for an evaluation, and the source of the request for the evaluation.

D: Respect for People: Evaluators honor the dignity, well-being, and self-worth of individuals and acknowledge the influence of culture within and across groups.

D1. Strive to gain an understanding of, and treat fairly, the range of perspectives and interests that individuals and groups bring to the evaluation, including those that are not usually included or are oppositional.

D2. Abide by current professional ethics, standards, and regulations (including informed consent, confidentiality, and prevention of harm) pertaining to evaluation participants.

D3. Strive to maximize the benefits and reduce unnecessary risks or harms for groups and individuals associated with the evaluation.

D4. Ensure that those who contribute data and incur risks do so willingly, and that they have knowledge of and opportunity to obtain benefits of the evaluation.

E: Common Good and Equity: Evaluators strive to contribute to the common good and advancement of an equitable and just society.

E1. Recognize and balance the interests of the client, other stakeholders, and the common good while also protecting the integrity of the evaluation.

E2. Identify and make efforts to address the evaluation's potential threats to the common good especially when specific stakeholder interests conflict with the goals of a democratic, equitable, and just society.

E3. Identify and make efforts to address the evaluation's potential risks of exacerbating historic disadvantage or inequity.

E4. Promote transparency and active sharing of data and findings with the goal of equitable access to information in forms that respect people and honor promises of confidentiality.

E5. Mitigate the bias and potential power imbalances that can occur as a result of the evaluation's context. Self-assess one's own privilege and positioning within that context.

Source: Reprinted with permission from the American Evaluation Association, www.eval.org/p/cm/ld/fid=51.

Appendix B

Joint Committee on Standards for Educational Evaluation
Program Evaluation Standards

Utility Standards

The utility standards are intended to increase the extent to which program stakeholders find evaluation processes and products valuable in meeting their needs.

- **U1 Evaluator Credibility** Evaluations should be conducted by qualified people who establish and maintain credibility in the evaluation context.
- **U2 Attention to Stakeholders** Evaluations should devote attention to the full range of individuals and groups invested in the program and affected by its evaluation.
- **U3 Negotiated Purposes** Evaluation purposes should be identified and continually negotiated based on the needs of stakeholders.
- **U4 Explicit Values** Evaluations should clarify and specify the individual and cultural values underpinning purposes, processes, and judgments.
- **U5 Relevant Information** Evaluation information should serve the identified and emergent needs of stakeholders.
- **U6 Meaningful Processes and Products** Evaluations should construct activities, descriptions, and judgments in ways that encourage participants to rediscover, reinterpret, or revise their understandings and behaviors.
- **U7 Timely and Appropriate Communicating and Reporting** Evaluations should attend to the continuing information needs of their multiple audiences.
- **U8 Concern for Consequences and Influence** Evaluations should promote responsible and adaptive use while guarding against unintended negative consequences and misuse.

Feasibility Standards

The feasibility standards are intended to increase evaluation effectiveness and efficiency.

- **F1 Project Management** Evaluations should use effective project management strategies.
- **F2 Practical Procedures** Evaluation procedures should be practical and responsive to the way the program operates.
- **F3 Contextual Viability** Evaluations should recognize, monitor, and balance the cultural and

- political interests and needs of individuals and groups.
- **F4 Resource Use** Evaluations should use resources effectively and efficiently.

Propriety Standards

The propriety standards support what is proper, fair, legal, right and just in evaluations.

- **P1 Responsive and Inclusive Orientation** Evaluations should be responsive to stakeholders and their communities.
- **P2 Formal Agreements** Evaluation agreements should be negotiated to make obligations explicit and take into account the needs, expectations, and cultural contexts of clients and other stakeholders.
- **P3 Human Rights and Respect** Evaluations should be designed and conducted to protect human and legal rights and maintain the dignity of participants and other stakeholders.
- **P4 Clarity and Fairness** Evaluations should be understandable and fair in addressing stakeholder needs and purposes.
- **P5 Transparency and Disclosure** Evaluations should provide complete descriptions of findings, limitations, and conclusions to all stakeholders, unless doing so would violate legal and propriety obligations.
- **P6 Conflicts of Interests** Evaluations should openly and honestly identify and address real or perceived conflicts of interests that may compromise the evaluation.
- **P7 Fiscal Responsibility** Evaluations should account for all expended resources and comply with sound fiscal procedures and processes.

Accuracy Standards

The accuracy standards are intended to increase the dependability and truthfulness of evaluation representations, propositions, and findings, especially those that support interpretations and judgments about quality.

- **A1 Justified Conclusions and Decisions** Evaluation conclusions and decisions should be explicitly justified in the cultures and contexts where they have consequences.
- **A2 Valid Information** Evaluation information should serve the intended purposes and support valid interpretations.
- **A3 Reliable Information** Evaluation procedures should yield sufficiently dependable and consistent information for the intended uses.
- **A4 Explicit Program and Context Descriptions** Evaluations should document programs and their contexts with appropriate detail and scope for the evaluation purposes.

- **A5 Information Management** Evaluations should employ systematic information collection, review, verification, and storage methods.

- **A6 Sound Designs and Analyses** Evaluations should employ technically adequate designs and analyses that are appropriate for the evaluation purposes.

- **A7 Explicit Evaluation Reasoning** Evaluation reasoning leading from information and analyses to findings, interpretations, conclusions, and judgments should be clearly and completely documented.

- **A8 Communication and Reporting** Evaluation communications should have adequate scope and guard against misconceptions, biases, distortions, and errors.

Evaluation Accountability Standards

The evaluation accountability standards encourage adequate documentation of evaluations and a metaevaluative perspective focused on improvement and accountability for evaluation processes and products.

- **E1 Evaluation Documentation** Evaluations should fully document their negotiated purposes and implemented designs, procedures, data, and outcomes.

- **E2 Internal Metaevaluation** Evaluators should use these and other applicable standards to examine the accountability of the evaluation design, procedures employed, information collected, and outcomes.

- **E3 External Metaevaluation** Program evaluation sponsors, clients, evaluators, and other stakeholders should encourage the conduct of external metaevaluations using these and other applicable standards

Source: Yarbrough, D. B., Shula, L. M., Hopson, R. K., & Caruthers, F. A. (2010). *The program evaluation standards: A guide for evaluators and evaluation users* (3rd ed.). Thousand Oaks, CA: Sage. Retrieved from https://evaluationstandards.org/program/

Glossary of Terms

The terms defined in this glossary are those used in this book within the context of program evaluation from a racialized and social justice perspective. It should be noted that some of the terms may have a broader meaning or expanded definitions within other contexts. In instances where the definition of a term is taken from that of a particular individual(s), the citations for such are included within the narrative of this book where the term appears.

Ableism individual, cultural, and institutional beliefs and discrimination that systematically oppress people who have mental, emotional, and physical disabilities

Accountability demonstrated responsibility for the use of resources, activities, or decisions made in the course of a program and/or its evaluation; one of the five major quality attributes of the *Program Evaluation Standards*

Accuracy (in evaluations) extent to which an evaluation is truthful or valid in the scope and detail of what it communicates about a context, program, project, or any of their components; one of the five major quality attributes of the *Program Evaluation Standards*

Action research term, coined by Kurt Lewin, to describe comparative research on the conditions and effects of various forms of social action and research leading to social action

Actionable results can be used to make important decisions

Active consent informed agreement by adults, or in the case of children or members of vulnerable populations by their parent/guardian, to participate in a study or an evaluation

Active listening hearing a speaker and avoiding premature judgment; often involves asking questions, reflecting understanding, clarifying information by restating a paraphrased version of the speaker's message, and/or summarizing the conversation

Active voice writing where the subject acts upon its verb, as in "Over half of the participants thought the program was successful"

Activities services and tasks undertaken by the program/project

Afrocentric broadly defined as emphasizing or demonstrating the influence of African or African American history and culture

Ageism individual, cultural, and institutional beliefs and discrimination that systematically oppress young and elderly people

Alternative facts "opposite of reality" (which is delusion), or "opposite of truth" (which is untruth)

Alternative hypothesis in statistical analysis, the hypothesis based on earlier work or beliefs about the impact of a variable or treatment; it is the alternative to the null hypothesis (the hypothesis of no difference)

Alternative-form reliability degree of similarity and difference between an individual's score on different forms of a measure

American Evaluation Association (AEA) professional association of evaluators devoted to the application and exploration of program evaluation

Analysis of variance (ANOVA) statistical test that tests for differences among two or more independent samples (e.g., comparisons among people from five demographic regions)

Analysis of variance with repeated measures statistical test that tests for differences among two or more related samples (e.g., comparisons among people's responses to multiple measures over time)

Articulated program theory theory that explicitly states how a program is supposed to work

ATLAS.ti qualitative analysis software package

Axiology role and place of values in the research process

Belmont Report report provided by the National Commission for the Protection of Human Subjects of Biomedical and Behavioral Research that identifies ethical principles that must be followed in all research involving human subjects

Bias particular tendency or inclination, especially one that prevents reasonable, knowledgeable, thoughtful consideration of a question

Business entity category of type of businesses such as corporations, nonprofit organizations, and partnerships

Business plan plan developed prior to starting a business that includes a variety of components such as key resources, partners, and activities

Case study up-close, in-depth, and detailed examination of a subject of study, over time, and its related contextual conditions

CAT (Coding Analysis Toolkit) qualitative analysis software package

Causal relationship relationship where the occurrence of something such as an intervention program causes something else, such as cessation of smoking, to occur

Chi-square test nonparametric statistical test for differences among two or more independent samples (e.g., comparisons among people with bachelor's degrees and those with doctorates); the nonparametric equivalent of the independent *t*-test, because it makes no assumptions about the level of the data

Cisgender term to describe people whose gender identity reflects their birth sex

Classism institutional, cultural, and individual set of beliefs and discrimination that assigns differential value to people according to their socioeconomic class and an economic system that creates excessive inequality and causes basic human needs to go unmet

Closed-ended questions questions that are answered by ratings or other forced-choice responses

Co-construction involves evaluators collaborating and forming genuine partnerships with key stakeholder groups to conceptualize, implement, and evaluate interventions in a manner that is responsive to the project's context

Code of conduct directional document, or set of rules, that describes how its members should behave in specific situations (e.g., forbidding sexual harassment or racial intimidation)

Codebook set of codes, definitions, and examples used as a guide to help analyze qualitative data

Coding analytical process of categorizing (qualitative) or counting (quantitative) data to facilitate analysis and synthesis; in qualitative inquiry, using a word or short phrase that symbolically assigns a summative, salient, essence-capturing, and/or evocative attribute to a portion of language or visual data

Cohen's d one of the most common effect size computations that is computed by subtracting the mean score of one group from the mean score of another divided by the standard deviation

Collaborative Institutional Training Initiative (CITI) commonly used training program for the protection of human subjects required by many colleges and universities for institutional review board approval of a study

Common good shared benefit for all or most members of society including equitable opportunities and outcomes that are achieved through citizenship and collective action

Common Rule fundamental principle of human subjects protection that states that people should not (in most cases) be involved in research (or evaluation) without their informed consent, and that participants should not incur increased risk of harm from their involvement, beyond the normal risks inherent in everyday life

Comparison group group(s) similar to control groups, although some feel comparison groups are those that are not randomly assigned to participate in a program or intervention or not

Competence one of the *Evaluators' Ethical Guiding Principles* indicating that evaluators have the skills and experiences necessary to provide skilled professional services to stakeholders

Concurrent validity degree to which the results of one measure reflect the results of other measures with similar content

Conflict of interest (COI) situation in which an individual has competing interests or loyalties to more than one person or organization, which can compromise an evaluator's judgment, decisions, or actions throughout the evaluation process

Conflict theory theoretical framework that views society less as a cohesive system and more as an arena of conflict and power struggles; it argues that instead of people working together to further the societal goals, they work at achieving their will at the expense of others

Construct validity degree to which the results of a measure reflect existing theory

Constructivist approach or worldview espousing that there is not a single truth; rather, all truth is relative and constructed by the individual or society

Content equivalence degree to which an instrument's content is relevant to the cultures under consideration

Content validity degree to which a measure covers the appropriate subject matter

Context combination of factors (e.g., culture, geographic location, timing, political and social climate) that may influence project implementation or outcomes

Contract legally binding document that makes clear the evaluator's and the client's expectations as to what will be done, in what time frame, for what costs

Control group group(s) similar to comparison groups, although some feel control groups are randomly assigned to participate in a program or intervention (or not)

Copyright legal concept that gives the holder the exclusive right to print, publish, and use the developed material

Corporation independent legal entity owned by shareholders

Correlation a relationship between two sets of data (e.g., the relationship between individuals' level of participation in a program and their change)

Correlation coefficient statistical test to measure the strength of a relationship between two sets of data

Cost reimbursement payment process where invoices for costs incurred are submitted and paid or a payment structure where proportions of the total budget are paid to the evaluator upon receipt of different deliverables

Cost-benefit evaluation examines the relationship between intervention costs and outcomes in monetary terms (e.g., for every $100 spent on prenatal care for low-income mothers, savings on neonatal intensive care)

Cost-effectiveness evaluation examines the relationship between the intervention costs and gains in units of a desired outcome (e.g., one year of life gained or death prevented) for one or more interventions

Counterfactual (in evaluation) estimate of what would have happened in the absence of the intervention

Creative Commons copyright licenses and tools allow options other than the traditional "all rights reserved" under copyright law

Credibility degree to which results of evaluation are believable from the perspective of the evaluation stakeholders; shaped by the context in which it resides

Credible evidence that which is believable, reliable, and relevant to program/project stakeholders and answers evaluation questions

Critical constructivism extends and modifies constructivism; maintains that social, cultural, economic, historical, and political contexts construct individuals' perspectives on the world, self, and others; encourages the questioning of dominant systems of knowledge production and more critical awareness

Critical race theory (CRT) recognizes racism as engrained in the fabric and system of the American society and that institutional racism is pervasive in the dominant culture; CRT identifies that these power structures are based on white privilege and white supremacy, which perpetuates the marginalization of people of color

Critical theory research philosophy that assumes multiple realities and is produced through historically based social and political processes and the values associated with them; at its core, it focuses on issues of power, inequality, and social change

Cultural competence ability, skills, and knowledge to understand, communicate with, and effectively interact with people across cultures in evaluation

Cultural conflict of interest when an individual's cultural mores (social or cultural rules) are seen as the norm, the right way, or even the only way, and this perspective becomes a secondary, competing interest with the primary interest of individuals and communities different from that of the individual

Cultural humility having a humble and respectful attitude toward people of other cultures; also includes ongoing self-exploration combined with a willingness to learn from others

Cultural incongruence (in evaluation) lack of cultural similarities, expectations, values, and/or understanding between people in a relationship within the evaluation context, including between and/or among the evaluator and program staff/administrators, participants, community, and other relevant stakeholders (e.g., funders); also involves judging others by one's own cultural values, standards, and beliefs

Cultural responsiveness (in evaluation) taking into account the culture of the program that is being evaluated with the evaluation based on examination of outcomes and impacts through lenses in which the culture of the participants is considered an important factor

Culturally competent evaluator evaluator who draws on a wide range of evaluation theories and methods to design and carry out an evaluation that is optimally matched to the cultural context; the evaluator reflects the diverse values and perspectives of key stakeholder groups

Culturally responsive evaluation honors the cultural context in which an evaluation takes place and requires evaluators to critically examine culturally relevant but often neglected variables across the entire evaluation process

Culture shared values, traditions, norms, customs, arts, history, folklore, and institutions of a group of people

Data factual information (such as measurements or statistics) that is used as a basis for reasoning, discussion, or calculation

Data cleaning process of going through the submitted data, looking for inaccuracies, inconsistencies, misunderstandings, duplications, and general data anomalies

Data management process that includes acquiring, validating, storing, protecting, and processing required data to ensure the accessibility, reliability, and timeliness of the data for its users; also can include a plan regarding what will be done with the data after the evaluation study is completed

Data visualization efforts to help people understand the significance of data by placing them in a visual context, usually graphs, tables, or figures

DBA ("doing business as") name, other than their legal name, that one or more individuals give their business

De facto discrimination discrimination that is not legally mandated, but happens in fact

De jura discrimination discrimination that is legally mandated

Deductive reasoning reasoning that begins with a possible theory or premise that is tied the theory of change underlying the program to be evaluated

Deficit model assumes that there are deficiencies in the culture of a group or groups that are the cause of minority group member differences from dominant group members

Delayed treatment design participants are randomly assigned to intervention and control groups, and the same pretest and posttest data are collected from them; after the posttest, members of the control group then become intervention participants, and after their participation, additional data are collected

Deliberative democratic evaluation approach to evaluation addressing power relations through inclusion, dialogue, and deliberation and uses democratic processes to construct valid conclusions where there are conflicting views

Dependent variable that which is being measured; in evaluation, usually the outcome of interest

Descriptive design observes and describes individual and/or group behaviors without intervening or influencing those behaviors

Descriptive statistics describe and summarize numerical data using such statistics as means, frequencies, and percentages

Descriptive theories theories that describe or classify specific dimensions or characteristics of individuals, groups, situations, or events

Developmental evaluation alternative to the formative-summative paradigm as a way to address innovation and complexity in a project

Direct costs costs directly related to the project budget such as personnel, travel, payments to participants, and supplies

Direct stakeholders people or groups that have a visible role in the day-to-day activities of a project including people who utilize the services of the project or are impacted by those services

Disaggregation (of data) breaking of data into different subgroups to explore "what works for whom in what context"

Discrimination unequal allocation of goods, resources, and services, and the limitation of access to full participation in society, based on individual membership in a particular social group; reinforced by law, policy, and/or cultural norms that allow for differential treatment on the basis of identity

Dominant culture culture of the group whose members are in the majority or who wield more power than other groups

Dominant group group with power, authority, privileges, and status and that controls the value system and rewards in a particular society

Dominant paradigm values and beliefs held by those who are most powerful or dominant in a society, based on the values, or systems of thought, in a society that are most standard and widely held at a given time

Dominant positionality how individuals' identification with the dominant group influences their stance or outlook, positioning, and potential biases in relation to how they understand and view the world

Dosage how much of an intervention is delivered

Downloadable data collection templates usually spreadsheets that are downloaded, completed by whomever is reporting data, and returned to the evaluator or whomever else will be analyzing the data

Dual minority status individuals identifying or identified as belonging to multiple minority statuses such as disability, race, age, ethnicity, gender identity, and sexual orientation; sometimes referred to as multiple minority status

Effect size way of quantifying the magnitude of the difference between two groups where the differences have been found to be statistically significant

Efficiency evaluation evaluation to determine intervention costs (e.g., money, people, time, facilities, materials, and so forth) in relation to its benefits (monetary and nonmonetary)

Elevator speech short description of an idea, product, or company that explains the concept in a way such that any listener can understand it in a short period of time

Empowering Model variation of the Medical Model of Disability that focuses on having individuals with disabilities and their families, rather than the medical community, decide the course of their treatment and what services they wish to benefit from, thus turning the professional into a service provider whose role is to offer guidance and carry out clients' decisions

Empowerment evaluation type of participatory evaluation in which the evaluator's role is that of a consultant, adviser, facilitator, and coach aimed toward the development of the participating stakeholders' ability to conduct their own evaluation, to use it effectively for advocacy and change, and to foster improvement and self-determination

Epistemology study of knowledge

Equitable evaluation evaluation framework with equity at its center; it is intended to advance equity and self-determination

Equity condition of fair and just opportunities for all people to participate and thrive in society regardless of individual or group identity or difference; striving to achieve equity includes mitigating historic disadvantage and existing structural inequalities

Equity-focused evaluation evaluation focusing on judgments being made of the relevance, effectiveness, efficiency, impact, and sustainability—and, in humanitarian settings, coverage, connectedness, and coherence—of policies, programs, and projects concerned with achieving equitable development results

Equity-focused intervention intervention that seeks to redress and reduce disparities between the most and least disadvantaged groups within a population

Ethical dilemma need to choose from among two or more morally acceptable options or between equally unacceptable courses of action, when one choice prevents selection of the other; in evaluation, this might entail a conflict between two or more ethical principles (such as confidentiality vs. common good)

Ethical sensitivity ability to recognize and respond to the ethical dimensions of a situation

Ethical triggers elements that indicate potential challenges during the evaluation

Ethically grounded evaluation evaluation characterized by ongoing critical thinking, reflection, judgment, and decision making, all aimed toward protecting the rights of stakeholders and building daily ethical routines in evaluation planning, implementation, and reporting

Ethnography method that explores how people live and make sense of their lives with one another in particular places

Evaluability assessment degree to which it is possible to meaningfully evaluate a specific program at a specific time and place

Evaluand thing or entity being evaluated, typically a program, project, policy, or product

Evaluation disciplined inquiry involving the systematic, contextually responsive, and ethical application of research tools and methods to collect data that assess the effectiveness and operations of programs within the various social, political, and cultural contexts in which they operate; evaluation's ultimate goal is to provide credible evidence that fosters greater understanding and improves decision making all aimed at improving social conditions and promoting healthy, just, and equitable communities

Evaluation design determination of how, when, and from whom data will be collected and the structure of the critical comparisons that will address the questions of interest

Evaluation plan proposed details of an evaluation, generally including the evaluation's purpose, what is to be evaluated, evaluation objectives and or/questions, methodology, and how results will be reported

Evaluation theory set of coherent conceptual, hypothetical, pragmatic, and ethical principles that form a general framework to guide the study and practice of evaluation

Evaluative thinking critical thinking applied to evaluation contexts involving an ongoing process of critical reflection and appraisal of assumptions and claims made coupled with a commitment to continuous learning and willingness and ability to modify views in light of reasoned arguments and evidence

Evaluators' Ethical Guiding Principles core values of the American Evaluation Association and intended as a guide to the professional ethical conduct of evaluators

Exempt study one that has very little risk to participants; it is still subjected to human participants review, but does not need to meet all the institutional review board guidelines that are applied to expedited and full board review studies

Expedited study study that involves collection of samples and data in a manner that is not anonymous and that involves no more than minimal risk to subjects; under such circumstances, the institutional review board chairperson or one or more experienced reviewers designed by the chairperson from among members of the board can evaluate and approve the study

Experimental design where the impact of a treatment or program is assessed and compared to the impact of no treatment or another treatment, usually involving random assignment of participants to groups

Explanatory framework statements or theories used to explain a phenomenon

Explicit bias where individuals know they have a bias and accept it or try to counteract it

External evaluator evaluator from outside the program or organization being evaluated

External stakeholders people and groups from outside the project, such as funders or investors, that are affected by the consequences and outcomes of the project

External validity extent to which findings from an evaluation can be generalized to other populations, settings, treatment variables, and measurement variables

Fake news stories based on falsehoods, often spread as propaganda on social media

Family-wise error rate probability of coming to at least one false conclusion when performing multiple statistical tests; if enough tests are run, it is very likely that at least one of the statistically significant results will be false

Feminist standpoint theory frames social science research and evaluation from the standpoint of women or particular groups of women

Feminist theory shifts assumptions, analytic lens, and topical focus away from the male viewpoint and experience and toward those of women

Feasibility extent to which resources and other factors allow an evaluation to be conducted in a satisfactory manner; one of the five major quality attributes of the *Program Evaluation Standards*

Fidelity (in evaluation) extent to which the intervention's services and activities are delivered as intended

Focus groups typically composed of 5–7 people brought together by a facilitator, for periods of 30 to 60 minutes, to, collectively and individually, provide a variety of ideas about and responses to a given topic

Folkways traditional behaviors of a group or community

Formative evaluation evaluation to provide information that can guide improvement or refinement of the effort

Framework basic conceptual structures and the ideas, information, and principles that form those structures

Friedman test nonparametric statistical test that looks for differences among two or more related samples (e.g., pretest/posttest with comparison groups)

Full review study that does not fit into either the expedited or exempt category, because it is deemed to pose more than a minimal risk to participants; all aspects of the research (or evaluation) must be inspected by all members of the institutional review board

Fuzzy logic model nonlinear visual portraying the dynamic nature of systems surrounding a program/project and the fluidity and complexity of programs and projects

Gantt chart project planning and management tool consisting of a table or horizontal bar chart listing project tasks and when they are to be completed

Generalizability drawing of broad inferences from research or evaluation results

Goals broad statements of what a program/project needs to accomplish to achieve its mission or the desired results

Heterosexism belief that heterosexuality is the only normal and acceptable sexual orientation; it encompasses the individual, cultural, and/or institutional beliefs and discrimination that systematically oppress lesbian, gay, bisexual, transgender, and queer (LGBTQ) people

Hidden stakeholders individuals or groups that are unknown or ignored by funders, project administrators, and evaluators

Hybrid (or mixed) model evaluator evaluator who combines the roles of both an internal evaluator and an external evaluator

Hypothesis proposed explanation for some phenomena based on previous research and/or theory

Implementation evaluation evaluation designed to assess the extent to which the program activities are being implemented as intended; sometimes referred to as process evaluation

Implementation failure when the implementation of the program or intervention is not carried out properly

Implicit bias attitudes or stereotypes that affect individuals' understanding, actions, and decisions in an unconscious manner

Implicit program theory theory that does not explicitly articulate how the program is supposed to work, but that does include assumptions and expectations about how change should occur

Implicit stereotype stereotype that is relatively inaccessible to conscious awareness and/or control

Income inequality extreme disparity of income distributions with a high concentration of income usually in the hands of a small percentage of a population; a relatively large gap between a country's richest individuals and its poorest individuals

Independent variable variable that is changed or controlled to test the effects on the dependent or outcome variable

Indicators variables that provide evidence that a certain condition exists or certain results have, or have not, been achieved

Indigenous ethnic groups who are the original or earliest-known inhabitants of an area, in contrast to groups that have settled, occupied, or colonized the area more recently; also referred to in some regions as First Nations, First peoples, Aboriginal peoples, or Native peoples

Indigenous evaluation approaches evaluation from an Indigenous perspective and uses methods influenced by Indigenous ways of knowing, frameworks, and cultural paradigms

Indirect costs costs that are not directly tied to an individual project but are part of the costs of doing business, such as rent, utilities (including heat, electricity, telephone, and internet services such as Wi-Fi), and professional fees (including bookkeeping and tax preparation)

Indirect stakeholders people or groups that are indirectly affected by the project

Inductive reasoning reasoning that draws general principles from specific instances; moves from the collected data to patterns based on the data to tentative hypotheses to hypothesis testing to theory

Inferential statistics tests to determine the odds (probability) that the descriptive statistical results from the groups being analyzed (the sample) are real or are random, which can allow evaluators to make inferences or predictions from sample data to the population

Informed consent individual's voluntary agreement to participate in a study after learning the risks and benefits

Inputs resources, contributions, and investments that go into the program/project; including staff, volunteers, funding, materials, and facilities

Institutional review board (IRB) administrative body that reviews proposed research and evaluation plans to ensure the protection of human participants

Intellectual property original work that an individual or a group has created

Interinterviewer reliability degree to which interviewees would give the same response to the same questions posed by two different interviewers

Intermediate outcomes outcomes that are expected to result from or follow the short-term outcomes; that is, what results should occur next

Internal evaluator evaluator who is a member of the staff of the program or organization being evaluated

Internal stakeholders people or groups from within the project, such as project managers, staff, and clients, with an interest in its success and failure

Internal validity extent to which it can be confidently asserted that changes observed in the dependent variables (i.e., outcomes of interest) are due to the effects of the independent variables (e.g., intervention) and not to some other unintended variables

Interobserver reliability degree to which observer A and observer B "see" the same thing when they are observing

Interpretivism research philosophy arguing that reality is constantly renegotiated, debated, and interpreted; that is, the world exists according to how it is experienced, perceived, and interpreted by individuals

Interrater reliability degree to which different raters score or code the same response or behavior the same way

Intersectionality interconnected nature of social categorizations such as race, class, and gender, creating overlapping and interdependent systems of discrimination or disadvantage

Interval data quantitative data that are ordered with equal intervals but no true zero point (e.g., degrees on a thermometer)

Interview structured or semistructured conversations between two people, one of whom is the interviewer and the other the interviewee

Interview protocol group of interview questions to be asked and accompanying instructions

Intrarater reliability degree to which individual observers and/or raters are consistent in their own ratings or codings over time

Jim Crow laws set of repressive regulations and customs affecting virtually every section of daily life, making it legal for legislators to racially segregate groups; enacted in the late 19th and early 20th centuries after the Reconstruction period and legally enforced until 1965

Kruskal-Wallis test nonparametric statistical test for examining differences among two or more independent samples (e.g., comparisons among people from different demographic groups)

Latinx a gender-neutral or nonbinary alternative for people of Hispanic heritage

Learning objectives brief statements that describe what students will be expected to know and/or do

Legend in a figure, that which describes the different data sets

Limited liability company (LLC) hybrid type of legal structure that provides the limited liability features of a corporation and the tax efficiencies and operational flexibility of a sole proprietorship or a partnership

Logic model graphic representation of how the various components (inputs, activities, outputs, outcomes) of a program logically relate to each other and how an initiative is supposed to work

Long-term outcomes desired to occur over time resulting from the achievement of the short-term and intermediate outcomes; sometimes referred to as impacts; more distant benefits or changes that occurred as a result of the program that may take years or decades to occur

Longitudinal data data that are collected over time, usually a period of years

Macro-analysis focusing on larger structures of society such as political, legal, and economic systems

Mann-Whitney test nonparametric statistical test for differences between two independent samples (e.g., comparison between employed and unemployed people)

Marginalization when different groups of people within a given culture, context, and history are at risk of being subjected to multiple discrimination due to the interplay of different characteristics such as age, ethnicity, religion or belief, health status, disability, sexual orientation, gender identity, education or income, or living in various geographic localities

MAXQDA software package for qualitative and mixed-methods data

McNemar test nonparametric statistical test for paired nominal-level data (e.g., the number of students who passed or failed a test taken under two under different conditions)

Mean often referred to as the average, the sum of a set of numbers divided by the number of numbers in the set

Measurement validity extent to which a measure has no systematic bias and represents what it is intended and presumed to represent

Median midpoint in a set of numbers where half of the numbers are below it and half are above it

Medical Model of Disability assumes disability is an individual problem caused by disease, trauma, or another health condition and requires sustained medical care

Medicine wheel ancient symbol, whose main characteristic is a circle, that is used by almost all Indigenous peoples of North and South America

Metaevaluation evaluation of an evaluation

Methodological rigor traditionally described as a characteristic of evaluation studies that refers to the strength of the design's underlying logic and the confidence with which conclusions can be drawn

Methodology processes, procedures, and strategies of research and evaluation

Micro-analysis focus on individual or small group interaction

Microsoft Access widely available database program

Microsoft Excel widely available spreadsheet program that includes basic descriptive and inferential statistics

Mission statement describing a program/project's overall purpose for being or reason for existence

Mixed methods combination of quantitative and qualitative approaches in a single study in which each approach adds something to the understanding of the phenomenon

Mode most frequent score in a set of numbers

Moral Model of Disability holds people morally responsible for their own disability, with some associating disability with sin and shame for both the person with a disability and the person's family

Multicultural validity recognition that cultural factors shape the sensitivity of evaluation instruments and the validity of the conclusions on program effectiveness

Multiple minority status individual identification or identification by others as belonging to multiple minority statuses such as disability, race, age, ethnicity, gender identity, and sexual orientation; sometimes referred to as dual minority status

Naturalistic observations when an unobtrusive data collector observes participants interacting in a real-life setting

Needs assessment determine the most pressing needs for unserved groups and how to address such needs

Nested logic model one or more detailed logic models (or portions of models) that fit within a larger model

Net effects (program effects) changes in outcomes that can be reasonably attributed uniquely to the intervention and not to the influence of some other factors

Net impact evaluation outcome evaluation that assesses the net effect of a program or intervention e

Nominal data data without any quantitative value; labels can be numeric or alphabetic; when numbers are used as labels, they have no numeric value, but are just a unique name for the attribute (e.g., eye color, political affiliation, number on a football jersey)

Non-binary common term people whose gender is not male or female use to describe themselves

Nonparametric statistics inferential statistical tests in which data are not required to fit a normal distribution; generally used when the investigator knows that the population data do not have a normal distribution and can be used with smaller samples

Normally distributed data data set that when graphed falls into a "bell curve" with the mean, mode and median being the same and two-thirds of the data set falling between one standard deviation above and below the mean

Null hypothesis for statistical analysis, the hypothesis of no difference; if it is rejected, then the alternative hypothesis, that which is based on earlier work or beliefs about the impacts of an evaluation, is accepted

Nuremberg Code code, established in 1947, including a set of 10 research ethics principles; were established after the Nuremberg trials where Nazi doctors were convicted of the crimes committed during human experiments on concentration camp prisoners; code sought to provide clear rules about what was legal and what was not when conducting human experiments

NVivo qualitative analysis software package

Objectives precise and measurable statements of what a program/project intends to accomplish during a specific period of time to reach each goal

On spec document, in this case an evaluation design, submitted without a contract, in the hope that it will be accepted

One-tailed test statistical test for determining the possibility of a relationship or difference in one direction disregarding the possibility of a relationship or difference in the other direction; the evaluator is determining, for example, whether program A is more effective than program B

Ontology beliefs about the nature of reality, being, or existence

Open coding applying inductive reasoning to the process of breaking down and categorizing qualitative data into manageable segments

Open-ended questions questions that are answered in participants' own words or sentences

Ordinal data quantitative data that are ranked or ordered; the distance between categories is not defined, and it cannot be determined if they are equal (e.g., ranking of students as 1st, 2nd, 3rd, etc.)

Outcome evaluation assesses program results and determines the extent to which outcomes were achieved

Outcomes actual changes, benefits, and/or changes in individuals, communities, organizations, or others that occur as a result of exposure to the program/project's activities (interventions) and outputs

Outcomes-oriented objectives indicate the expected results or changes in the target population as a result of the program/project

Outputs products, goods, and services generated by the program/project

***p*-value** tool to help determine the statistical significance of observed results; it includes the probability under a specified statistical model that a statistical summary of the data (e.g., the sample mean difference between two compared groups) would be equal to or more extreme than its observed value

Paradigm distinct set of concepts or big assumptions one makes about the world; can also include a set of theories within a particular framework

Paradigm wars struggle for primacy for one research paradigm over others; particularly active in the 1980s involving qualitative and quantitative researchers

Parametric statistics powerful inferential statistics that can only be used with interval- or ratio-level data that are normally distributed

Participant observer observer who, instead of being unobtrusive, participates in whatever activities the participants are doing

Participant responsiveness participants' level of engagement in and receptivity to the program activities

Participatory evaluation partnership approach to evaluation that actively engages the stakeholders in all phases of the evaluation process; evaluator's role is that of knowledgeable insider rather than neutral outsider who facilitates the development of trust between the assessor and those being assessed

Partnership sole proprietorship with more than one owner where each partner contributes to the business and shares in the profits and losses

Passive voice writing where the subject is a recipient of a verb's action, as in "The program was thought to be successful by over half the participants"

Percentile value below which a number of the data points fall—for example, half of the scores fall below the 50th percentile

Photovoice process by which people can identify, represent, and enhance their community through a specific photographic technique

Pilot test small-scale investigation done prior to the actual study with a sample of people like those in the target population

Population entire group or data set

Positivism philosophical perspective contending that the world is external and objective and we can discover a singular truth; guided by the principles of objectivity, knowability, and deductive logic and favors the use of quantitative methods

Postmodern (postmodernism) philosophical perspective that seeks to deconstruct authority sources of power and dismantle normal ways of thinking about how meaning interpretation and reality works; argues there is no objective, knowable truth or universally true explanations but, instead, truth is always bound within historical and cultural context

Postpositivism philosophical perspective that moves away from the purely objective stance adopted by the positivist and recognizes the subjectivity of reality; argues that one can never achieve perfect knowledge because of the researcher's human limitations; favors the use of quantitative methods

Posttest-only intact group design design where no pretest data are collected from participants or comparison group members and the posttest results of the groups are compared

Pragmatism philosophy emphasizing the practical uses and effects of any conception of knowledge, ideas, beliefs, and values rather than just focusing on how this conception increases understanding of reality and truth

Predictive validity indicator of the degree to which the measure predicts what it purports to

Prescriptive theories theories that characterize what should be as opposed to simply what is

Pretest effect when taking the initial measures has an impact on how participants respond to the intervention and/or how participants and control group members respond to the posttest measures.

Primary stakeholders people or groups who stand to be directly affected, either positively or negatively, as a result of their involvement in a project

Privilege unearned access to resources that are only readily available to some people because of their group membership

Pro bono services provided at no cost

Probability likelihood or odds that an event will occur

Procedural ethics ethics mandated by an institutional review board to ensure that a study's procedures adequately address the ethical concerns of informed consent, confidentiality, right to privacy, freedom from deception, and protection of participants from harm

Process evaluation examination of the quality or efficacy of program operations; also known as implementation evaluation

Process-oriented objectives activities to be completed within a specific period of time

Program collection of projects

Program evaluation examination of a program's goals, objectives, outcomes, and impact and/or to investigate a program's structure, characteristics, activities, organization, and political and social environment; the term is often used to describe evaluation of programs and projects

Program Evaluation Review Technique (PERT) chart project management tool used to graphically schedule, organize, and coordinate tasks within a project demonstrating order in which task are to be done

Program Evaluation Standards written guidance or standards for a quality evaluation developed by the Joint Committee on Standards for Educational Evaluation

Program reach proportion of the intended priority audience that participates in the intervention

Program theory theory of change applied to a specific program

Program theory evaluation assesses whether a program is designed in such a way that it can achieve its intended outcomes

Program theory failure failure of the activities of the program to bring about the desired effects due to faulty or inadequate program conceptualization and design

Progress evaluation process to determine whether benchmarks or interim outcomes were attained at particular points in time

Project particular investigative or developmental activity funded under a program

Project evaluation evaluation focused on the value of a collection of a particular investigative or developmental activity funded under a program

Propriety (in evaluation) extent to which evaluation has been conducted in a manner that demonstrates uncompromising adherence to the highest principles and ideals (including professional ethics, civil law, moral code, and contractual agreements); one of the five major quality attributes of the *Program Evaluation Standards*

Public domain available to be duplicated and shared without permission

Qualitative data words, narrative, and/or observational data

Qualitative methods array of approaches (e.g., interviews, participant observation, case studies) that seek to understand and interpret behavior as is lived by participants in a particular social setting

Quantitative data numerical data

Quantitative methods array of approaches that use "objective" measurement in a controlled setting to gather numeric data

Quartile data divided into four equal groups by value

Quasi-experimental design where the impact of a treatment or program is assessed and compared to the impact of no treatment or another treatment, and the members of groups are not randomly assigned

Queer theory theory stressing that sexuality is a complex array of social codes and forces, forms of individual activity, and institutional power, which interact to shape the ideas of what is normative and what is deviant at any particular moment

QuickBooks one of a number of online and desktop bookkeeping programs for small businesses

R free open-source quantitative software program

Race socially constructed differences among people based on characteristics such as accent or manner of speech, name, clothing, diet, beliefs and practices, leisure preferences, places of origin, and so forth

Racial discrimination any distinction, conduct, or action, whether intentional or not, based on a person's race, that has the effect of imposing burdens on an individual or group but is not imposed upon others or that withholds or limits access to benefits available to other members of society

Racial framing persistent set of racial stereotypes, prejudices, ideologies, images, interpretations, and narratives as well as racialized inclinations to discriminate

Racialization process by which societies construct races as real, different, and unequal in ways that matter to economic, political, and social life

Racialize to impose a racial interpretation and place a person, place, or thing within a racial context

Racialized perspective perspective that pays attention, to the ways in which race shapes problem definition and solution as well as particular groups' access to opportunity

Racism individual, cultural, and institutional beliefs and discrimination that systematically oppress people of color (Blacks, Hispanics, Indigenous Peoples, and Asians).

Randomized controlled trial (RCT) design where individuals are randomly assigned to different groups to be studied; traditionally, viewed as the most rigorous and thus the best design to use

Range difference between the lowest and highest values in a data set

Rapid feedback evaluation quick assessment of program performance in terms of agreed-on objectives and indicators

Ratio data quantitative data that can be ranked, have equal intervals between data points, and have a true or absolute zero point (e.g., weight)

Raw data data that have not been processed in any way

Reach (program/project) extent to which the program attracts its target audience calculated by the numerator (top number) representing the actual number served and the denominator (bottom number) representing the number of potential participants (e.g., 50% reach if the program served 500 participants [numerator] and the target community has 1,000 potential participants who meet the inclusion criteria)

Readability indicator of the level of education needed to easily read and understand a specific piece of writing

Reflective practice way of studying one's own experiences to improve the way one works

Regression-discontinuity design pretest–posttest program-comparison group design where participants are assigned to program or comparison groups solely on the basis of a cutoff score on a preprogram measure

Relational ethics ethics whereby the evaluator situates ethical action explicitly in relationships recognizing and valuing mutual respect, dignity, and the connectedness between the evaluator and the group studied

Reliability replicability of results in quantitative assessment and the consistency of results in qualitative assessment

Research ethics core professional behaviors and institutional and federal standards by which every researcher is guided to protect the dignity, rights, and welfare of research participants

Resources things and people needed to support the program's activities; typically include money (grant funding, donations), staff, volunteers, partnerships, and collaborations

Response bias occurs when those who responded to a measure are different from those who did not

Response rate number or percentage of those who were asked to provide data and did so, regardless of whether it was completing a survey, participating in an interview or a focus group, or submitting documents

Response set bias where, possibly due to the order of items, people's response to one item biases their response to the following items

Responsive evaluation evaluation that focuses on the concerns of the stakeholders, gathered through ongoing engagement with these individuals/groups throughout the evaluation, and providing an avenue for continued communication and feedback; role of the evaluator is that of a full, subjective partner

Responsive stakeholder engagement intentional and ongoing process of relationship building and connections with multiple and diverse stakeholders whereby the evaluator pays close attention to what stakeholders are signaling as their needs (and wants) and the evaluator, to the extent feasible and ethical, conducts the evaluation in a manner that directly responds to these needs and wants

Retrospective pretest or "then-post" design (RPT) data are collected once at the end of the project where participants are asked to assess their current level of knowledge/attitudes/skills/intentions *after* an intervention (such as a professional development workshop) and then to think back to their prior knowledge/attitudes/skills/intensions *before* the intervention

Rhetorical structure as a dimension of research paradigms, consists of the language and presentation of research to the intended audience; for example, in the constructivist paradigm, language in the final report is generally more personalized and often written in the first person, while in the positivist and postpositivist paradigms, language is presented in more detached, "precise," and "scientific" manner

Rival hypothesis competing hypothesis that might plausibly explain an outcome

S corporation unlike a traditional corporation, in an S corp profits and losses are passed through to the shareholders' personal tax returns; consequently, the business is not taxed itself, only the shareholders are taxed

Sample one or more individual or data points drawn from the population

Sankofa African word roughly translated to mean "return to the source and fetch"; stresses that as we move forward into the future, we need to reach back into our past and take with us all that works and is positive

SAS (Statistical Analysis System) common quantitative statistical package

Scatter plot graphic presentation of raw data to depict relationship between two quantitative variables

Secondary stakeholders people or groups that are indirectly affected, either positively or negatively, as a result of their involvement in a project or by the project

Second-wave feminism decades-long period of feminist activities begun in the 1960s that focused on equal treatment, access, and outcomes

Self-selection bias when participants choose whether or not to participate and the group that chooses to participate is not equivalent (in terms of the criteria) to the group that opts out; self-selection can lead to biased data, as the respondents who choose or choose not to participate may not well represent the entire target population

Semantic equivalence agreement between different language versions of a measure or other pieces of writing

Sexism individual, cultural, and institutional beliefs and discrimination that systematically oppress women

Sexual minorities groups whose sexual practices, orientation, and/or identity do not reflect those of the dominant culture

Shoestring evaluation approach to evaluation under constraints of limited budget, time, and data availability

Short-term outcomes those early, most immediate changes and benefits most closely associated with the direct and immediate results of the program and are generally achievable within weeks, months, or one year

Situational ethics ethics concerning the day-to-day unpredictable, often subtle, yet ethically important periods that arise while conducting evaluation

Social constructivism (social constructivist) paradigm stressing that knowledge is socially constructed by people active in the research process and, thus, "truth varies"; further contends that researchers should attempt to understand the complex world of lived experience from the point of view of those who live it

Social Darwinism notion that certain individuals are more powerful in society because they are innately better

Social desirability bias form of response bias where individuals misrepresent their self-reported behaviors by overreporting behaviors considered socially desirable, and underreporting undesirable ones

Social intervention organized, planned efforts designed to ameliorate or improve social conditions; sometimes referred to as a social program

Social justice equitable distribution of wealth, opportunities, and privileges within a society; maintains that all individuals deserve and should have access to the same rights and resources

Social learning theory theoretical framework underlying selected program theory stressing that interventions (programs) provide knowledge, which leads to modification in individual motivation and intentions to change, which then leads to change in behavior or the desired outcome

Social Model of Disability or the Disability Model view of disability as a socially created problem; that is, what makes people disabled is not their medical condition, but the attitudes and structures of society

Social network analysis mapping and measuring of relationships and flows between people, groups, organizations, computers, URLs, and other connected information/knowledge entities

Social problem condition or behavior that has negative consequences for large numbers of people and is generally recognized as a condition or behavior that needs to be addressed

Social program coordinated activity or set of activities designed to eliminate or reduce some social problem or condition

Social programming ways that social programs and policies develop, improve, and change, especially with regard to social problems

Social-cognitive theory theoretical framework underlying selected program theory stressing that learning occurs in a social context with a dynamic and reciprocal interaction of the person, environment, and behavior; people's beliefs in their efficacy to make change is a critical component; this approach is an outgrowth of social learning theory

Sole proprietor unincorporated business owned and run by one individual with no distinction between the business and the owner; the owner is entitled to all profits and is responsible for all business debts, losses, and liabilities

Solomon four-group design involves assignment of participants to one of four groups; two groups are pretested, and two groups are not; one of the pretested groups and one of the nonpretested groups receive the intervention; all four groups receive a posttest

Spearman rank-order correlation nonparametric statistical test for correlations (e.g., the relationship between program participation and individual change)

Split-half reliability measure of consistency where the scores on half of the items in a measure are compared to the scores on the other half to determine if the test is consistently measuring the intended concept

SPSS (Statistical Package for the Social Sciences) commonly utilized quantitative statistical package

Staff competency qualifications of program staff including their level of cultural competency to work with the target population

Stakeholder person or organization invested in the program, interested in the results of the evaluation, and/or with a stake in what will be done with the results of the evaluation

Stakeholder analysis technique used to identify and assess the importance of key people, groups of people, and institutions that may influence the success of the project and the evaluation

Stakeholder engagement involvement of all stakeholders (individuals and groups) that can affect or are affected by an evaluation process and/or its findings

Standard deviation variation among individual scores in a set of numbers

Statement of Work (SOW) defines expectations and provides the evaluation team with a detailed overview of the project to be examined describing project goals, activities, expected outputs and outcomes, deliverables, and/or work plans

Statistical power probability that if there is a real effect, it will be found

Statistical regression threat to validity occurring when measures are given a second time, and there is a tendency toward pseudo-changes in outcomes, which is the lowering of extremely high scores and the raising of extremely low scores (regressing toward the average score).

Statistical significance probability that the findings are real rather than due to chance

Stereotype threat occurs when people worry that their behavior or performance on a task might confirm a stereotype about a group they are part of

Stereotypes preconceived notions, especially about a group of people, and assumptions that people have about others because of their race, sex/gender, disability, and other areas

Storyboarding (storytelling) in evaluation, a visual representation of a story about a person's or group's experience and possible transformation as a result of participation in a program/project; often used in Indigenous evaluation frameworks

Structural racism system of hierarchy and inequity, primarily characterized by white supremacy or the preferential treatment, privilege, and power for white people at the expense of Black, Hispanic, Asian, Pacific Islander, Indigenous, Arab, and other racially oppressed people; encompasses the totality of ways in which societies foster racial discrimination through mutually reinforcing systems of housing, education, employment, earnings, benefits, credit, media, health care, and criminal justice

Summative evaluation evaluation aimed at determining the worth, value, and/or success of a project, program, or product

Survey series of open- and/or closed-ended questions about a topic or topics to which the participant responds in writing

Swag free items that are given away, often at conferences, as a marketing tool to promote a business or a product

Symbolic interactionism philosophical framework that views society as the product of individuals interacting with one another and is interested in the way individuals act toward, respond to, and influence one another in society

Table of specifications matrix or two-way chart where the topics or areas to be covered are the column headers and the items or questions to be asked are the row headers

Test/retest reliability degree of similarity and difference between individuals' responses the first and the second time they respond to a measure

Theory interrelated set of concepts, definitions, and propositions that seeks to help better understand events, behaviors, or situations and provide a framework for thinking about those things

Theory of change description and graphic illustration of the processes of how and why a desired change is expected to happen in a particular context; sometimes used interchangeably with program theory

Threats to validity possible issues that can make findings of an evaluation less accurate or valid

Time and task chart chart that breaks an evaluation plan into specific tasks, determines who is going to do each task, and estimates the amount of time it will take them to do their tasks

Time-series design design where data are collected at several points prior to participation in the program and several points after

Tragedy and/or Charity Model of Disability model where people with disabilities are seen as victims of circumstance, deserving of pity

Transdiscipline disciplines that supply essential tools, scholarship, and practice for other disciplines (e.g., statistics, measurement), while retaining unique characteristics (e.g., common logic, theory), an autonomous structure, and research efforts of its own

Transferability degree to which results can be transferred to other contexts or settings

Transformative evaluation paradigmatic stance that prioritizes issues of social justice and human rights as overarching ethical principles that need to permeate all aspects of an evaluation study and directly engages the complexity encountered by researchers and evaluators in culturally diverse communities when their work is focused on increasing social justice

Transformative lens (or transformative framework) in evaluation, proposed as a means to bringing issues of social justice and human rights to the foreground in decisions about methodology, credibility of evidence, and use of evaluation findings

Triangulation process of using multiple data-gathering procedures, data sources, or multiple observers

***t*-test for dependent samples** statistical test for differences between two related samples (e.g., pretest/posttest measures of a single group)

***t*-test for independent samples** parametric statistical test for differences between two independent samples (e.g., posttest with treatment and comparison groups)

Two-tailed test test for the possibility of the relationship in either direction; for example, in a two-tailed test, the evaluator is determining if the effectiveness of program A is different from that of program B—either more or less effective

Two-way analysis of variance parametric statistical test for differences between two or more groups with two independent variables (e.g., comparisons among high- and low-income people from five demographic regions) and a single dependent variable

Type I error when an effect was concluded as real but it was not, also known as a false positive

Type II error when an effect that is real wasn't found, also known as a false negative

Uptake how much intervention is actually received by participants

Utility extent to which evaluations are aligned with stakeholders' needs such that process uses, findings' uses, and other appropriate influences are possible; one of the five major quality attributes of the *Program Evaluation Standards*

Validity accuracy in quantitative assessments and data; appropriateness in qualitative assessments and data

Variance degree to which numbers vary from the mean

vCard electronic business card attached to an email message

Weft QDA qualitative analysis software package

Wicked problem social or cultural problem (e.g., poverty) that is difficult or impossible to solve for various reasons (e.g., incomplete or contradictory knowledge, the large economic burden, changing requirements that are often difficult to recognize, the interconnected nature of these problems with other problems)

Word cloud image that shows the words used in interviews or other qualitative data in different sizes according to how often they are used

Workers' compensation system of insurance that reimburses an employer for damages that must be paid to an employee for injury occurring in the course of employment

References

Abdi, S., & Mensah, G. (n.d.). *Focus on: Logic model—A planning and evaluation tool* (p. 11). Public Health Ontario. Retrieved from https://www.publichealthontario.ca/-/media/documents/focus-on-logic-model.pdf?la=en

Abma, T. A. (2006). The social relations of evaluation. In I. F. Shaw, J. C. Greene, & M. M. Mark (Eds.), *The SAGE handbook of evaluation* (pp. 184–199). Thousand Oaks, CA: Sage.

Abma, T. A. (2000). Stakeholder conflict: A case study. *Evaluation and Program Planning, 23*(2), 199–210.

Abma, T. A., Greene, J., Karlsson, O., Ryan, K., Schwandt, T. S., & Widdershoven, G. (2001). Dialogue on dialogue. *Evaluation, 7,* 164–180.

ADA National Network. (n.d.). *What is the Americans with Disabilities Act (ADA)?* Retrieved from https://adata.org/learn-about-ada

Agency for Healthcare Research and Quality. (2014). *Advances in patient safety: Dissemination planning tool: Exhibit A from Volume 4.* Retrieved from https://www.ahrq.gov/professionals/quality-patient-safety/patient-safety-resources/resources/advances-in-patient-safety/vol4/planningtool.html

Akintunde, O. (1999). white racism, [W]hite supremacy, [W]hite privilege, & the social construction of race: Moving from modernist to postmodernist multiculturalism. *Multicultural Education, 7*(2). Retrieved from https://www.questia.com/magazine/1P3-47855587/white-racism-white-supremacy-white-privilege

Alda, A. (2019). *The Alda method.* Stony Brook, NY: Alan Alda Center for Communicating Science, Stony Brook University. Retrieved from https://www.aldacenter.org/alda-method%C2%AE

Alkin, M. C. (Ed.). (2013). *Evaluation roots: A wider perspective of theorists' views and influences* (2nd ed.). Los Angeles, CA: Sage.

Alkin, M. C. (Ed.). (2004a). *Evaluation roots: Tracing theorists' views and influences.* Thousand Oaks, CA: Sage.

Alkin, M. C. (2004b). Comparing evaluation points of view. In M. C. Alkin (2004), *Evaluation roots: Tracing theorists' views and influences* (pp. 3–11). Thousand Oaks, CA: Sage.

Alkin, M. C., & Christie, C. A. (2004). The evaluation theory tree. In M. C. Alkin (Ed.), *Evaluation roots: Tracing theorists' views and influences* (pp. 12–65). Thousand Oaks, CA: Sage.

Allen, H. G., Stanton, T. R., Di Pietro, F., & Moseley, G. L. (2013). Social media release increases dissemination of original articles in the clinical pain sciences. *PLoS One, 8*(7), e68914. Retrieved from https://journals.plos.org/plosone/article?id=10.1371/journal.pone.0068914

Altschuld, J., & Kumar, D. D. (2010). *Needs assessment: An overview* (Vol. 1). Thousand Oaks, CA: Sage.

American Association of University Women. (1995). *How schools shortchange girls: The AAUW report.* New York, NY: Marlowe & Co.

American Evaluation Association. (2018a, April 5). *AEA competencies.* Retrieved from https://www.eval.org/page/competencies

American Evaluation Association. (2018b, August). *Evaluators' ethical guiding principles.* Retrieved from https://www.eval.org/p/cm/ld/fid=51

American Evaluation Association. (2011, April 22). *Public statement on cultural competence in evaluation.* Retrieved from http://www.eval.org/ccstatement

American Evaluation Association. (n.d.). *Local affiliates.* Retrieved from https://www.eval.org/affiliate

American Psychological Association. (2013). *Disability & socioeconomic status.* Retrieved from http://www.apa.org/pi/ses/resources/publications/factsheet-disability.aspx

Anderson, M. L., & Taylor, H. F. (2013). *Sociology: The essentials.* Belmont, CA: Wadsworth.

Anderson-Clark, T., Green, R., & Henley, T. (2008). The relationship between first names and teacher expectations for achievement motivation. *Journal of Language & Social Psychology, 27*(1), 94–99.

Andrews, T. M. (2017, August 21). Jerry Lewis telethons raised billions for muscular dystrophy. Many cheered when he went off the air. *Washington Post Moring Mix.* Retrieved from https://www.washingtonpost.com/news/morning-mix/wp/2017/08/21/jerry-lewis-telethons-raised-billions-for-muscular-dystrophy-many-cheered-when-he-went-off-the-air/

Anker, M., Guidotti, R., Orzeszyna, S., Sapirie, S., & Thuriax, M. (1993). Rapid evaluation methods (REM) of health services performance: Methodological observations. *Bulletin of the World Health Organization, 71*(1), 15–21.

Anti-Defamation League. (2018). *A brief history of the disability rights movement.* Retrieved from https://www.adl.org/education/resources/backgrounders/disability-rights-movement

Aral, S., St. Lawrence, J., Dyatlov, R., & Kozlov, A. (2005). Commercial sex work, drug use, and sexually transmitted infections in St. Petersburg, Russia. *Social Science & Medicine, 60,* 2181–2190.

Archibald, T. (2018, August 3). EEE TIG Week: Tom Archibald on whose extension counts? *AEA365.* Retrieved from https://aea365.org/blog/tag/credible-evidence/

Aruffo, C. (n.d.). *Turning scientific presentations into stories.* Retrieved from http://digital.nsta.org/publication/?i=269379&article_id=2244782&view=articleBrowser&ver=html5#{%22issue_id%22:269379,%22view%22:%22articleBrowser%22,%22article_id%22:%222244782%22}

Aspen Institute Roundtable on Community Change. (n.d.). *Dismantling structural racism: A racial equity theory of change.* Retrieved from https://www.racialequitytools.org/resourcefiles/aspeninst1.pdf

Association for Women in Science. (2019). *Intersectionality: A critical framework for STEM equity.* Retrieved from https://www.awis.org/wp-content/uploads/AWIS_FactSheet_Intersectionalityv4.pdf

Astatke, Y. (2003). *Web-based foundations of mathematics course: A new approach to help identify the true math skills of freshmen engineering students while preparing them for the math placement exams.* Baltimore, MD: Morgan State University, Electrical & Computer Engineering Department.

AZ Quotes. (n.d.). *Isaac Watts: "The eyes of a man."* Retrieved from https://www.azquotes.com/quote/1157023

Azzam, T., Evergreen, S., Germuth, A. A., & Kistler, S. J. (2013). Data visualization and evaluation. In T. Azzam & S. Evergreen (Eds.), Data visualization, Part I. *New Directions for Evaluation, 139*, 7–32.

Baker, A., & Bruner, B. (2012). *Integrating evaluative capacity into organizational practice*. Cambridge, MA: Bruner Foundation. Retrieved from http://www.evaluativethinking.org/docs/Integ_Eval_Capacity_Final.pdf

Bal, A., & Trainor, A. A. (2016). Culturally responsive experimental intervention studies: The development of a rubric for paradigm expansion. *Review of Educational Research, 86*(2), 319–359.

Baldwin, J. (1961). *Nobody knows my name: More notes of a native son*. New York, NY: Dial Press.

Bamberger, M., Rugh, J., Church, M., & Fort, A. (2004). Shoestring evaluation: Designing impact evaluations under budget, time and data constraints. *American Journal of Evaluation, 25*(1), 5–37.

Bamberger, M., & Segone, M. (2011). *How to design and manage equity-focused evaluations*. New York, NY: UNICEF Evaluation Office.

Banaji, M. R., Bazerman, H., & Chugh, D. (2003). How (un) ethical are you? *Harvard Business Review, 81*(12), 3–10.

Bandura, A. (1986). *Social foundations of thought and action: A social cognitive theory*. Englewood Cliffs, NJ: Prentice Hall.

Bandura, A. (1977). *Social learning theory*. Englewood Cliffs, NJ: Prentice Hall.

Barkan, S. E. (2012). *A primer on social problems* (Version 1.0). Retrieved from https://2012books.lardbucket.org/books/a-primer-on-social-problems/s01-about-the-author.html

Barnett, C., & Camfield, L. (2016). Ethics in evaluation. *Journal of Development Effectiveness, 8*(4), 528–534.

Bartsch, D., & Belgacem, N. (2004). *Real-time evaluation of UNHCR's response to the emergency in Chad*. Geneva, Switzerland: Evaluation and Policy Analysis Unit, United Nations High Commissioner for Refugees.

Baumrind, D. (1964). Some thoughts on ethics of research: After reading Milgram's "Behavioral study of obedience." *American Psychologist, 19*(6), 421–423.

Baur, V., Abma, T. A., & Widdershoven, G. A. (2010). Participation of marginalized groups in evaluation: Mission impossible? *Evaluation and Program Planning, 33*(3), 238–245.

Bazerman, M. H., & Tenbrunsel, A. E. (2011). *Blind spots: Why we fail to do what's right and what to do about it*. Princeton, NJ: Princeton University Press.

Becker, L. A. (2000). *Effect size (ES)*. Retrieved from https://www.uv.es/~friasnav/EffectSizeBecker.pdf

Bell, B. S., & Klein, K. J. (2001). Effects of disability, gender, and job level on ratings of job applicants. *Rehabilitation Psychology, 46*(3), 229–246. Retrieved from http://digitalcommons.ilr.cornell.edu/cgi/viewcontent.cgi?article=1009&context=hrpubs

Bell, D. A. (1995). Who's afraid of critical race theory? *University of Illinois Law Review, 4*, 893–910.

Bell, D. (1992). *Faces at the bottom of the well: The permanence of racism*. New York, NY: Basic Books.

Bell, N. (2010, March). Research report on data sources: Time-to-degree for doctorate recipients. *Communicator, 1*(3) Washington, DC: Council of Graduate Schools.

Bellavita, C., Wholey, J., & Abramson, M. (1986). Performance-oriented evaluation: Prospects for the future. In J. Wholey, M. Abramson, & C. Bellavita (Eds.), *Performance and credibility: Developing excellence in public and nonprofit organizations*. Lexington, MA: Lexington Books.

Berke, J. (2019). Pathological vs. cultural point of view on deafness. *Verywell Health*. Retrieved from https://www.verywellhealth.com/pathological-view-versus-cultural-view-of-deafness-1048594

Berkin, C., Miller, C. L., Cherny, R. W., Gormly, J. L., Egerton, D., & Woestman, K. (2011). *Making America: A history of the United States* (Vol. 2). Boston, MA: Wadsworth.

Beskow, L. A. (2016). Lessons from HeLa cells: The ethics and policy of biospecimens. *Annual Review of Genomics and Human Genetics, 17*, 395–417.

BetterEvaluation. (n.d.a). *Control group*. Retrieved from http://www.beterevaluation.org/en/evaluation-options/control_group

BetterEvaluation. (n.d.b). *Cost effectiveness analysis*. Retrieved from https://www.betterevaluation.org/en/evaluation-options/CostEffectivenessAnalysis

Biesta, G. (2010). Pragmatism and the philosophical foundations of mixed methods research. In A. Tashakkori & C. Teddlie (Eds.), *Handbook of mixed methods in social and behavioral research* (2nd ed., pp. 95–117). Thousand Oaks, CA: Sage.

Blau, J. (2014). *The dynamics of social welfare policy* (4th ed.). New York, NY: Oxford University Press.

Bledsoe, K. L. (n.d.). FAQs: How is ee different from say Culturally Responsive Evaluation or any seemingly related theory or approach? *Equitable Evaluation Initiative*. Retrieved from https://www.equitableeval.org/faqs

Bloom, B. (1986). Ralph Tyler's impact on evaluation theory and practice. *Journal of Thought, 21*(1), 36–46.

Blueprints for Healthy Youth Development. (2019). *HighScope Preschool: Fact sheet*. Retrieved from https://www.blueprintsprograms.org/programs/38999999/highscope-preschool/

Bohannon, J. (2011, November). Dance vs. PowerPoint: A modest proposal. *TEDxBrussels*. Retrieved from https://www.ted.com/talks/john_bohannon_dance_vs_powerpoint_a_modest_proposal#t-193661

Bonilla-Silva, E. (2015). More than prejudice: Restatement, reflections, and new directions in critical race theory. *Sociology of Race and Ethnicity, 1*(1), 73–87.

Bonilla-Silva, E. (2018). *Racism without racists* (5th ed.). Lanham, MD: Rowman & Littlefield.

Bonilla-Silva, E., & Zuberi, T. (2008). Toward a definition of white logic and white methods. In T. Zuberi & E. Bonilla-Silva (Eds.), *white logic, white methods: Racism and methodology* (pp. 3–27). New York, NY: Rowman & Littlefield.

Bowell, T. (n.d.). Feminist standpoint theory. In S. Ayala-Lopez & S. Wurster (Eds.), *Internet encyclopedia of philosophy*. Retrieved from https://www.iep.utm.edu/fem-stan/#H5

Bowman, N. R. (2006). *Tribal sovereignty and self-determination through evaluation.* Paper presented at the National Congress of American Indians Mid-Year Session, Sault Ste. Marie, MI.

Bowman, N. R., Dodge Francis, C., & Tyndall, M. (2015). Culturally responsive indigenous evaluation: A practical approach for evaluating indigenous projects in tribal reservation contexts. In S. Hood, R. Hopson, & H. Frierson (Eds.), *Continuing the journey to reposition culture and cultural content in evaluation theory* (pp. 335–360). Charlotte, NC: Information Age.

Boykin, W. A. (2000). The Talent Development Model of Schooling: Placing students at promise for academic success. *Journal of Education for Students Placed at Risk, 5*(1&2), 3–25.

Boykin, L. L. (1958). What is evaluation? *Journal of Educational Research, 51*(7), 529–534.

Boykin, L. L. (1957). Let's eliminate the confusion: What is evaluation? *Educational Administration and Supervision, 43,* 115–121.

Boykin, L. L. (1954). Some fallacies in the evaluation and interpretation of data involving the education of Negroes in the Southern states. *Negro Educational Review, 5*(2), 52–58.

Boykin, L. L. (1950). Differentials in Negro education. *Journal of Educational Research, 43*(7), 533–540.

Boykin, L. L. (1949). The status and trends in differentials between white and Negro teachers' salaries in the Southern states: 1900–1946. *Journal of Negro Education, 18*(4), 40–47.

Brandon, P. R., & Sam, A. L. (2014). Program evaluation. In P. Leavy (Ed.), *The Oxford handbook of qualitative research* (pp. 471–497). New York, NY: Oxford University Press.

Braverman, M. T., & Arnold, M. E. (2008). An evaluator's balancing act: Making decisions about methodological rigor. In M. T. Braverman, M. Engle, M. E. Arnold, & R. A. Rennekamp (Eds.), *Program evaluation in a complex organizational system: Lessons from Cooperative Extension. New Directions for Evaluation, 120,* 71–86.

Brent, R. J. (2003). Introduction to health care evaluation. In R. J. Brent (Ed.), *Cost-benefit analysis and health care evaluation.* Northampton, MA: Edward Elgar.

Brewington, Q. L., & Hall, J. N. (2018). Givin' stakeholders the mic: Using hip-hop's evaluative voice as a contemporary evaluation approach. *American Journal of Evaluation, 39*(3), 336–349.

Brightside. (2020). What is reflective practice? *Bright Knowledge.* Retrieved from https://www.brightknowledge.org/medicine-healthcare/what-is-reflective-practice

Brown, A. (1944a). *An evaluation of the accredited secondary schools for Negroes in the South.* Unpublished PhD dissertation, University of Chicago.

Brown, A. (1944b). An evaluation of the accredited secondary schools for Negroes in the South. *Journal of Negro Education, 13*(4), 488–498.

Brown, A. (1944c). *An evaluation of the accredited secondary schools for Negroes in the South.* Chicago, IL: University of Chicago Press.

Brown, W. H. (1945). An experimental study of workshop-type professional education for Negro teachers. *Journal of Negro Education, 14*(1), 48–58.

Browne, R. B., & English, J. W. (1969). *Love my children: The education of a teacher.* New York, NY: Meredith.

Brownson, R. C., Eyler, A. A., Harris, J. K., Moore, J. B., & Tabak, R. G. (2018). Getting the word out: New approaches for disseminating public health science. *Journal of Public Health Management Practice, 24*(2), 102–111.

Bryk, A. S. (Ed.). (1983). *Stakeholder-based evaluation. New Directions for Program Evaluation, 17.* San Francisco, CA: Jossey-Bass.

Bryson, J. M., & Patton, M. Q. (2015). Analyzing and engaging stakeholders. In K. E. Newcomer, H. P. Hatry, & J. S. Wholey (Eds.), *Handbook of practical program evaluation.* (4th ed., pp. 36–61). Hoboken, NJ: Wiley Blackwell.

Bryson, J. M., Patton, M. Q., & Bowman, R. A. (2011). Working with evaluation stakeholders: A rationale, step-wise approach and toolkit. *Evaluation Program Planning, 34*(1), 1–12.

Buckley, J., Archibald, T., Hargraves, M., & Trochim, W. M. (2015). Defining and teaching evaluative thinking: Insights from research on critical thinking. *American Journal of Evaluation, 36*(3), 375–388.

Burns, D., Soward, A. C. M., Skelly, A. H, Leeman, J., & Carlson, J. (2008). Effective recruitment and retention strategies for older members of rural minorities. *Diabetes Education, 34,* 1045–1051.

BusinessDictionary. (n.d.). *Social justice.* Retrieved from http://www.businessdictionary.com/definition/social-justice.html

Cabot, P. S., deQ. (1940, June). A long-term study of children: The Cambridge-Somerville Youth Study. *Child Development, 11*(2), 143–151.

Campbell, D. T. (1994). Retrospective and prospective on program impact assessment. *Evaluation Practice, 15*(3), 291–298.

Campbell, D. T. (1969). Reforms as experiments. *American Psychologist, 24*(4), 409–429.

Campbell, D. T., & Stanley, J. C. (1963). Experimental and quasi-experimental designs for research on teaching. In N. L. Gage (Ed.), *Handbook of research on teaching* (pp. 171–246). Chicago, IL: Rand McNally.

Campbell, P. B. (2008). Evaluating youth and community programs. In A. J. Friedman (Ed.), *A framework for evaluating impacts of informal science education Projects* (pp. 69–76). Arlington, VA: National Science Foundation.

Campbell, P. B. (2006). *KISI (Keep It Simple and Interesting): Journalists' advice to researchers.* Retrieved from. http://www.fairerscience.org/kisi.html

Campbell, P. B. (2003). *Your rights and responsibilities as an evaluation client.* Groton, MA: Campbell-Kibler Associates, Inc.

Campbell, P. B. (1995). Redefining the "girl problem" in mathematics. In E. Fennema & W. Secada (Eds.), *New directions for equity for mathematics education* (pp. 225–241). New York, NY: Cambridge University Press.

Campbell, P. B. (1989). *The hidden discriminator: Sex and race bias in educational research.* Newton, MA: WEEA Publishing Center.

Campbell, P. B., & Clewell, B. C. (2008). *Building evaluation capacity: Collecting and using data in cross-project evaluations—Guide II.* Washington, DC: Urban Institute.

Campbell, P. B., Edgar, S., & Halsted, A. L. (1994). Students as evaluators: A model for program evaluation. *Phi Delta Kappan*, 76, 160–164.

Campbell, P. B., & Hill, E. (2013). *A framework for the evaluation of research projects*. A poster presented at the Annual Meeting of the American Evaluation Association, Washington, DC.

Campbell, P. B., & Hoey, L. (2000). *Equity means all: Rethinking the role of special programs in science and mathematics*. A commissioned paper for the National Institute for Science Education. Groton, MA: Campbell-Kibler Associates, Inc.

Campbell, P. B., Hoey, L., & Perlman, L. K. (2001). *Sticking with my dreams: Defining and refining youth media in the 21st century*. Groton, MA: Campbell-Kibler Associates, Inc. Retrieved from http://campbell-kibler.com/youth_media.html

Campbell, P. B., & Jolly, E. J. (n.d.a). About. *Beyond Rigor*. Retrieved from http://www.beyondrigor.org/About.html

Campbell, P. B., & Jolly, E. J. (n.d.b). Accurate data. *Beyond Rigor*. Retrieved from http://www.beyondrigor.org/PDF/BeyondRigor_Accurate Data.pdf

Campbell, P. B., & Jolly, J. (n.d.c). Coding/rating open-ended responses. *Beyond Rigor*. Retrieved from http://www.beyondrigor.org/OpenEnded.html

Campbell, P. B., & Jolly, E. J. (n.d.d). Culture. *Beyond Rigor*. Retrieved from http://www.beyondrigor.org/Culture.html

Campbell, P. B., & Jolly, E. J. (n.d.e). Each individual is diverse. *Beyond Rigor*. Retrieved from http://www.beyondrigor.org/EachDiverse.html

Campbell, P. B., & Jolly, E. J. (n.d.f). All populations are diverse. *Beyond Rigor*. Retrieved from http://www.beyondrigor.org/AllDiverse.html

Campbell, P. B., & Jolly, E. (n.d.g). Levels of aggregation and disaggregation. *Beyond Rigor*. Retrieved from http://www.beyondrigor.org/Aggregate.html

Campbell, P. B., & Jolly, E. J. (n.d.h). Money. *Beyond Rigor*. Retrieved from http://www.beyondrigor.org/Money.html

Campbell, P. B., & Kibler, T. R. (2017). *NMSU RISE to the postdoctorate (RTP) program: Fourth year evaluation report*. Groton, MA: Campbell-Kibler Associates, Inc.

Campbell, P. B., Price, T., Chubin, D. E., Carson, R., & Kibler, T. R. (2006). *Assessing what works for whom: An evaluation of the GE Foundation Math Excellence Initiative: Final Evaluation Report*. New York, NY: NACME.

Campbell, P. B., Stoll, A., & Thomas, V. (2009). Evaluating efforts to broaden participation. In B. C. Clewell & N. Fortenberry (Eds.), *Framework for evaluating impacts of broadening participation projects: Report from a National Science Foundation workshop* (pp. 64–79). Arlington, VA: Directorate for Education and Human Resources, National Science Foundation.

Campbell, P. B., Thomas, V. G., & Stoll, A. (2009). Outcomes and indicators relating to broadening participation. In B. C. Clewell & N. Fortenberry (Eds.), *Framework for evaluating impacts of broadening participation projects: Report from a National Science Foundation workshop* (pp. 54–63). Arlington, VA: Directorate for Education and Human Resources, National Science Foundation.

Campbell-Kibler, K., & Campbell, P. B. (2007). Words matter: Speaking and writing about gender and science. *FairerScience*. Retrieved from http://www.fairerscience.org/WordsMatter.html

Cato Institute. (2019). *What American think about poverty, wealth, and work: Findings from the Cato Institute 2019 Welfare, Work, and Wealth National Survey*. Washington, DC: Author.

Center for Advanced Research on Language Acquisition. (2019, April 9). *What is culture?* Minneapolis: University of Minnesota. Retrieved from https://carla.umn.edu/culture/definitions.html

Center for Assessment and Policy Development. (2013). *What special factors should a theory of change that addresses racism include?* Retrieved from https://www.racialequitytools.org/resourcefiles/What_Special_Factors_Should_A_Theory_Of_Change_That_Addresses_Racism_Include.pdf

Center for Economic and Social Justice. (2020). *Defining economic justice and social justice*. Retrieved from https://www.cesj.org/learn/definitions/defining-economic-justice-and-social-justice/

Center for Evaluation Innovation, Institute for Foundation and Donor Learning, Dorothy A. Johnson Center for Philanthropy, & Luminare Group. (2017). *Equitable evaluation framing paper*. Equitable Evaluation Institute.

Centers for Disease Control and Prevention. (2018, August). *Evaluation brief: Writing SMART objectives*. Retrieved from https://www.cdc.gov/healthyyouth/evaluation/pdf/brief3b.pdf

Centers for Disease Control and Prevention. (2014, December). *Practical strategies for culturally competent evaluation*. Atlanta, GA: U.S. Department of Health and Human Services. Retrieved from https://www.cdc.gov/dhdsp/docs/cultural_competence_guide.pdf

Centers for Disease Control and Prevention. (2013). *Good evaluation questions: A checklist to help focus your evaluation*. Retrieved from https://www.cdc.gov/asthma/program_eval/AssessingEvaluationQuestionChecklist.pdf

Centers for Disease Control and Prevention. (2008). *Introduction to process evaluation in tobacco use and prevention and control*. Atlanta, GA: U.S. Department of Health and Human Services, Centers for Disease Control and Prevention, National Center for Chronic Disease Prevention and Health Promotion, Office on Smoking and Health.

Centers for Disease Control and Prevention. (2007). Cigarette smoking among adults—United States, 2006. *Morbidity and Mortality Weekly Report*, 56(44), 1157–1161.

Centers for Disease Control and Prevention. (1999). Framework for program evaluation in public health. *Morbidity and Mortality Weekly Report*, 48(RR-11). Retrieved from https://www.cdc.gov/mmwr/PDF/rr/rr4811.pdf

Centre for Research and Education on Violence Against Women and Children. (2017). *What does it mean to be culturally competent?* Retrieved from http://makeitourbusiness.ca/blog/what-does-it-mean-be-culturally-competent

Chavez, V., Duran, B., Baker, Q., Avila, M., & Wallerstein, N. (2003). The dance of race and privilege in community-based participatory research. In M. Minkler & N. Wallerstein (Eds.), *Community-based participatory research for health: From process to outcomes* (2nd ed., pp. 81–97). San Francisco, CA: Jossey-Bass.

Chelimsky, E. (2008). A clash of cultures: Improving the "fit" between evaluative independence and the political requirements of a democratic society. *American Journal of Evaluation*, 29(4), 400–415.

Chelimsky, E. (1997). The coming transformation in evaluation. In E. Chelimsky & W. H. Shadish (Eds.), *Evaluation for the 21st century: A handbook* (pp. ix–xii). Thousand Oaks, CA: Sage.

Chelimsky, E. (1994, October 14). *Use of meta-analysis in the General Accounting Office*. Paper presented at the Science and Public Policy Seminars, Federation of Behavioral, Psychological and Cognitive Sciences, Washington, DC.

Chen, H. (1996). A comprehensive typology for program evaluation. *Evaluation Practice, 17*(2), 121–130.

Chen, H. T. (1990). *Theory-driven evaluations*. Newbury Park, CA: Sage.

Chen, J. (2018). *How to #SciComm and #StayCalm*. Retrieved from https://www.aaas.org/how-scicomm-and-staycalm

Cheryan, S., Meltzoff, A. N., & Kim, S. (2011). Classrooms matter: The design of virtual classrooms influences gender disparities in computer science classes. *Computers & Education, 57*(2), 1825–1835. Retrieved from http://dx.doi.org/10.1016/j.compedu.2011.02.004

Cheryan, S., Plaut, V. C., Davies, P. G., & Steele, C. M. (2009). Ambient belonging: How stereotypical cues impact gender participation in computer science. *Journal of Personality and Social Psychology, 97*(6), 1045–1060.

Chetty, R., Stepner, M., Abraham, S., Lin, S., Scuderi, B., Turner, N., Bergeron, A., & Cutler, D. (2016). The association between income and life expectancy in the United States, 2001–2014. *JAMA, 315*(16), 1750–1766. Retrieved from https://jamanetwork.com/journals/jama/article-abstract/2513561

Chipman, S. (1991). Content effects on word problem performance: A possible source of test bias? *American Educational Research Journal, 28*(4), 897–915.

Christie, C. A., & Alkin, M. C. (2013). An evaluation theory tree. In M. C. Alkin (Ed.), *Evaluation roots: A wider perspective of theorists' views and influences* (2nd ed., pp. 11–58). Thousand Oaks, CA: Sage.

Christie, C. A., & Alkin, M. C. (2008). Evaluation tree re-examined. *Studies in Educational Evaluation, 34*, 131–135.

Chugh, D., Bazerman, M., & Banaji, M. (2005). Bounded ethicality as a psychological barrier to recognizing conflicts of interest. In D. Moore, D. Cain, G. Loewenstein, & M. Bazerman (Eds.), *Conflicts of interest: Challenges and solutions in business, law, medicine, and public policy* (pp. 74–95). New York, NY: Cambridge University Press.

Clarke, E. H. (1972). *Sex in education or a fair chance for girls*. New York, NY: Arno Press. (Original work published 1873)

Clavijo, K. (2018, July 3). ICTIG week: Saying yes. *AEA365*. Retrieved from https://aea365.org/blog/ic-tig-week-saying-yes-by-kate-clavijo/?utm_source=feedburner&utm_medium=email&utm_campaign=Feed%3A+aea365+%28AEA365%29

Clay, R. A. (2010). How do I become culturally competent? *gradPSYCH, 8*(3), 24. Retrieved from https://www.apa.org/gradpsych/2010/09/culturally-competentHome//gradPSYCH Magazine//2010//09//

Clewell, B. C., & Campbell, P. B. (2008). *Building evaluation capacity: Guide II, Collecting and using data in cross-project evaluations*. Washington, DC: Urban Institute.

Clewell, B. C., Consentino de Cohen, C., Tsui, L., Forcier, L., Gao, E., Young, N., Deterding, N. & West, C. (2005). *Evaluation of the National Science Foundation Louis Stokes Alliances for Minority Participation Program*. Washington, DC: Urban Institute. Retrieved from https://www.urban.org/sites/default/files/publication/43766/411301_LSAMP_report_appen.pdf

Clinical and Translational Science Awards Consortium Community Engagement Key Function Committee Task Force. (2011). *Principles of community engagement* (2nd ed., NIH Publication No. 11-7782). Washington, DC: National Institutes of Health, U.S. Department of Health and Human Services.

Coe, R. (2002, September 12–14). *It's the effect size, Stupid. What effect size is and why it is important*. Paper presented at the Annual Conference of the British Educational Research Association, University of Exeter, England. Retrieved from https://www.leeds.ac.uk/educol/documents/00002182.htm

Coffman, J. (2002, Spring). A conversation with Michael Quinn Patton. *The Evaluation Exchange, 8*, 10–11.

Coffman, J. (1999). *Learning from logic models: An example of a family/school partnership program*. Cambridge, MA: Harvard Family Research Project.

Cohen, J. (1988). *Statistical power analysis for the behavioral sciences* (2nd ed.). Hillsdale, NJ: Erlbaum.

Cohen, J. (1969). *Statistical power analysis for the behavioral sciences*. New York, NY: Academic Press.

Colorado Trust. (2009). *The journey continues: Ensuring a cross-culturally competent evaluation*. Denver: Author.

Columbia University Department of Sociology. (2020). *Areas of specialization: Qualitative methodology*. Retrieved from https://sociology.columbia.edu/content/areas-specialization

Community Tool Box. (n.d.a). *Section 1. Developing a logic model or theory of change*. Retrieved from https://ctb.ku.edu/en/table-of-contents/overview/models-for-community-health-and-development/logic-model-development/main

Community Tool Box. (n.d.b). *Section 8. Identifying and analyzing stakeholders and their interests*. Retrieved from https://ctb.ku.edu/en/table-of-contents/participation/encouraging-involvement/identify-stakeholders/main

Conger, K. (2017). Of mice, men and women: Making research more inclusive. *Stanford Medicine: Sex, Gender & Medicine*. Retrieved from https://stanmed.stanford.edu/2017spring/how-sex-and-gender-which-are-not-the-same-thing-influence-our-health.html

Congressional Budget Office. (2018, March 19). The distribution of household income, 2014. Retrieved from https://www.cbo.gov/publication/53597

Conner, R. F., Fitzpatrick, J. L., & Rog, D. J. (2012). A first step forward: Context assessment. In D. J. Rog, J. L. Fitzpatrick, & R. F. Conner (Eds.), *Context: A framework for its influence on evaluation practice. New Directions for Evaluation, 135*, 89–105.

Cook, L. (2015. January 28). U.S. education: Still separate and unequal. *U.S. News & World Report*. Retrieved from https://www.usnews.com/news/blogs/data-mine/2015/01/28/us-education-still-separate-and-unequal

Cooksy, L. J., & Caracelli, V. J. (2009). Metaevaluation in practice: Selection and application criteria. *Journal of MultiDisciplinary Evaluation*, 6(11), 1–15.

Copyright.gov. (n.d.). *Copyright in general*. Retrieved from https://www.copyright.gov/help/faq/faq-general.html

Correll, S. J., & Benard, S. (2006). Biased estimators? Comparing status and statistical theories of gender discrimination. In S. R. Thye & E. J. Lawler (Eds.), *Advances in group processes* (pp. 89–116). New York, NY: Elsevier Science.

Cousins, J. B., & Whitmore, E. (1998). Framing participatory evaluation. In E. Whitmore (Ed.), *Understanding and practicing participatory evaluation. New Directions for Evaluation*, 80, 3–23.

Creative Commons. (n.d.). *About the licenses: What our licenses do*. Retrieved from https://creativecommons.org/licenses/

Crenshaw, K. W. (2017, June 8). Kimberlé Crenshaw on intersectionality, more than two decades later. New York, NY: Columbia Law School. Retrieved from https://www.law.columbia.edu/pt-br/news/2017/06/kimberle-crenshaw-intersectionality

Crenshaw, K. W. (2011, July). Twenty years of critical race theory: Looking back to move forward. *Connecticut Law Review*, 43(5), 1310–1345.

Crenshaw, K. W. (1991, July). Mapping the margins: Intersectionality, identity politics, and violence against women of color. *Stanford Law Review*, 43(6), 1241–1299.

Crenshaw, K. W. (1989). Demarginalizing the intersection of race and sex: A Black feminist critique of antidiscrimination doctrine, feminist theory and antiracist politics. *University of Chicago Legal Forum*, 140, 138–167.

Creswell, J. W. (2014). *Research design: Qualitative, quantitative, and mixed methods approaches* (4th ed.). Thousand Oaks, CA: Sage.

Creswell, J. W. (2013). *Qualitative inquiry and research design: Choosing among the five approaches*. Thousand Oaks, CA: Sage.

Cronbach, L. (1982). *Designing evaluations of educational and social programs*. San Francisco, CA: Jossey-Bass.

Cronbach, L. J., Ambron, S. R., Dornbusch, A. M., Hess, R. D., Hornik, R. C., Phillips, D. C., Walker, D. F., & Weiner, S. S. (1980). *Toward reform of program evaluation*. San Francisco, CA: Jossey-Bass.

Cronen, V. E. (2001). Practical theory, practical art, and the pragmatic-systemic account of inquiry. *Communication Theory*, 11, 14–35.

Crossman, A. (2020, February 25). Feminist theory in sociology: An overview of key ideas and issues. *ThoughtCo*. Retrieved from https://www.thoughtco.com/feminist-theory-3026624

Crowley, M. R. (1932). Cincinnati's experiment in Negro education: A comparative study of the segregated and mixed school. *Journal of Negro Education*, 1(1), 25–33.

Cummings, N. A., & Follette, W. T. (1979). Brief psychotherapy and medical utilization. In C. A. Kiesler, N. A. Cummings, & G. R. VandenBos (Eds.), *Psychology and national health insurance: A sourcebook* (p. 228–233). Washington, DC: American Psychological Association.

Cunningham, C., & Elmi, J. (2015). *Developmental evaluation and health care system interventions: A state example*. CDC Coffee Break presentation. Retrieved from https://www.cdc.gov/dhdsp/pubs/docs/cb_aug2015.pdf

Dahlbäck, N., Wang, Q. Y., Nass, C., & Alwin, J. (2007, April). Similarity is more important than expertise: Accent effects in speech interfaces. *CHI '07: Proceedings of the SIGCHI Conference on Human Factors in Computing Systems*, 1553–1556. Retrieved from http://dl.acm.org/citation.cfm?id=1240624.1240859

Dallal, G. E. (2003, October 19). Why p = .05. Retrieved from http://www.webpages.uidaho.edu/~brian/why_significance_is_five_percent.pdf

Danaher, K., & Crandall, C. S. (2008). Stereotype threat in applied settings re-examined. *Journal of Applied Social Psychology*, 38(6), 1639–1655. Retrieved from http://dx.doi.org/10.1111/j.1559-

Datta, L. (2018a, May 28). The first national Head Start evaluations. *AEA365*. Retrieved from https://aea365.org/blog/memorial-week-in-evaluation-the-first-national-head-start-evaluations-by-lois-ellin-datta/

Datta, L. (2018b). It's been a great ride. In D. D. Williams (Ed.), *Twenty-nine evaluation lives. New Directions for Evaluation*, 157, 15–20.

Datta, L. (2003). Evaluation and the government. In T. Kellaghan & D. L. Stufflebeam (Eds.), *International handbook of educational evaluation* (pp. 345–360). Dordrecht, Netherlands: Kluwer Academic.

Davenport, R. R. (1941). A Negro college examines its curricula by measuring improvement in reading. *The Journal of Negro Education*, 10(2), 178–184.

Davidson, E. J. (2013). *Actionable evaluation basics: Getting succinct answers to the most important questions* [Minibook]. New Zealand: Real Evaluation.

Davies, P. G., Spencer, S. J., & Steele, C. M. (2005). Clearing the air: Identity safety moderates the effects of stereotype threat on women's leadership aspirations. *Journal of Personality and Social Psychology*, 88(2), 276–287. Retrieved from http://www.psychology.uwaterloo.ca/~sspencer/spencerlab/articles/2005-Davies-Spencer-Steele.pdf

Davis, D., & Silver, B. D. (2003). Stereotype threat and race of interviewer effects in a survey on political knowledge. *American Journal of Political Science*, 47(1), 33–45.

Davis, R. E., Couper, M. P., Janz, N. K., Caldwell, C. H., & Resnicow, K. (2010). Interviewer effects in public health surveys. *Health Education Research*, 25(1), 14–26.

DeAngelo, R. (2011). White fragility. *International Journal of Critical Pedagogy*, 3, 54–70.

DeCuir-Gunby, J, T., Marshall, P. L., & Mcculloch, A. W. (2011, April). Developing and using a codebook for the analysis of interview data: An example from a professional development research project. *Field Methods*, 23(2), 136–155. Retrieved from https://www.researchgate.net/publication/254091978_Developing_and_Using_a_Codebook_for_the_Analysis_of_Interview_Data_An_Example_from_a_Professional_Development_Research_Project

Delgado, R., & Stefancic, J. (2001). *Critical race theory: An introduction*. New York, NY: University Press.

The Denver Foundation. (n.d.). *Example of non-discrimination statement and policy*. Retrieved from http://www.nonprofitinclusiveness.org/example-non-discrimination-statement-and-policy

Desmond, N., Allen, C., Clift, S., Justine, B., Mzugu, J., Plummer, M., Watson-Jones, D. & Ross, D. A. (2005). A typology of groups at risk of HIV/STI in a gold mining town in north-western Tanzania. *Social Science & Medicine, 60,* 1739–1749.

De Vaus, D. A. (2001). *Research design in social research.* London, England: Sage.

Diamini, T., Ebrahim, R., Evans, L., Gold, N., Ntshingila-Khosa, R., & Soobrayan, B. (1997). *Collaborative programme evaluation.* Pretoria, South Africa: U.S. Agency for International Development.

DiAngelo, R. (2018). *white fragility: Why it's so hard for white people to talk about racism.* Boston, MA: Beacon Press.

Dictionary.com. (2020a). *Alternative facts.* Retrieved from https://www.dictionary.com/e/slang/alternative-facts/?itm_source=parsely-api

Dictionary.com. (2020b). *Fake news.* Retrieved from https://www.dictionary.com/e/politics/fake-news/

Dictionary.com. (2020c). *Latinx.* Retrieved from https://www.dictionary.com/browse/latinx?s=t

DiLuzio, E. (2018). Conveying constituent voice: Two new data viz techniques to try by Elizabeth DiLuzio. *AEA365.* Retrieved from https://aea365.org/blog/dvr-tig-week-conveying-constituent-voice-two-new-data-viz-techniques-to-try-by-elizabeth-diluzio/?utm_source=feedburner&utm_medium=email&utm_campaign=Feed%3A+aea365+%28AEA365%29

Disabled World. (2019, December 6). *Models of disability: Types and definitions.* Retrieved from https://www.disabled-world.com/definitions/disability-models.php

Domenico, D., Hospes, O., & Ross, R. B. (2012). Managing wicked problems in agribusiness: The role of multi-stakeholder engagements in value creation. *International Food and Agribusiness Management Review, 15* (Special Issue B), 1–12.

Donaldson, S. I. (2007). *Program theory-driven evaluation science: Strategies and applications.* NY: Psychology Press, Taylor and Francis Group.

Donaldson, S. I. (2003). Theory-driven program evaluation in the new millennium. In S.I. Donaldson & M. Scriven (Eds.) *Evaluating social programs and problems: Visions for the new millennium* (pp. 111–142). Mahwah, NJ: Erlbaum.

Donaldson, S. I. (2001). Mediator and moderator analysis in program development. In S. Sussman (Ed.), *Handbook of program development for health behavior research and practice* (pp. 470–496). Newbury Park, CA: Sage.

Donaldson, S. I., & Lipsey, M. W. (2006). Roles for theory in evaluation practice. In I. Shaw, J. Greene, & M. Mark (Eds.), *The Sage handbook of evaluation* (pp. 56–75). Thousand Oaks, CA: Sage.

Downs, A. (1972). Up and down with ecology—the "issue-attention cycle." *The Public Interest,* 38–50.

Dozois, E., Longois, M., & Blanchet-Cohen, N. (2010, July). *DE 201: A practitioner's guide to developmental evaluation.* Montreal, Canada: J. W. McConnell Family Foundation and the International Institute for Child Rights and Development. Retrieved from https://mcconnellfoundation.ca/wp-content/uploads/2017/07/DE-201-EN.pdf

Drummond, M. F., O'Brien, B., Stoddart, G. L., & Torrance, G. (1987). *Methods for the economic evaluation of health care programmes.* Oxford, England: Oxford University Press

Duarte, N. (2012, October, 31). How to give more persuasive presentations: A Q&A with Nancy Duarte. *TEDBlog.* Retrieved from https://blog.ted.com/how-to-give-more-persuasive-presentations-a-qa-with-nancy-duarte/

DuBay, W. H. (2008). *Working with plain language: A training manual.* Costa Mesa, CA: Impact Information. Retrieved from http://www.impact-information.com/Resources/working.pdf

Duggan, C., & Bush, K. (2014). The ethical tipping points of evaluators in conflict zones. *American Journal of Evaluation, 35*(4), 485–506.

Eaton, A. A., Saunders, J. F., Jacobson, R. K., & West, K. (2019). How gender and race stereotypes impact the advancement of scholars in STEM: Professors' biased evaluations of physics and biology post-doctoral candidates. *Sex Roles, 82,* 127–141. Retrieved from http://faculty.fiu.edu/~aeaton/wp-content/uploads/2019/06/Eaton-Saunders-Jacobson-West-2019.pdf

Edelman, M. (1987). The construction of social problems as buttresses of inequalities. *University of Miami Law Review, 42*(7), 7–28.

Edwards, W. M., Guttentag, M., & Snapper, K. (1975). A decision-theoretic approach to evaluation research. In E. L. Struening & M. Guttentag (Eds.), *Handbook of evaluation research* (pp. 139–181). Beverly Hills, CA: Sage.

Eisenberg, N., & Lennon, R. (1983). Sex differences in empathy and related capacities. *Psychological Bulletin, 94*(1), 100–131.

Eitzen, D. S., Baca-Zinn, M., & Smith, E. K. (2013). *Social problems* (13th ed.). Boston, MA: Allyn & Bacon.

Ellis, C. (2007). Telling secrets, revealing lives: Relational ethics in research with intimate others. *Qualitative Inquiry, 13*(1), 3–29.

Ellis, P. D. (2010). *Effect sizes that make sense.* Retrieved from https://effectsizefaq.com/essential-guide-to-effect-sizes/

Ellison, R. (1952). *Invisible man.* New York, NY: Random House.

Energy.gov. (n.d.). *Program evaluation: Independence, conflict of interest, openness.* Retrieved from https://www.energy.gov/eere/analysis/program-evaluation-independence-conflict-interest-openness

Epley, N., Caruso, E. M., & Bazerman, M. H. (2006). When perspective taking increases taking: Reactive egoism in social interaction. *Journal of Personality and Social Psychology, 91*(5), 872–889.

Epstein, D., Goodman, L. A, & Sullivan, C. M. (2017). Beyond the RCT: Integrating rigor and relevance to evaluate the outcomes of domestic violence programs. *American Journal of Evaluation, 39,* 58–70. Retrieved from https://scholarship.law.georgetown.edu/facpub/2047/

Equitable Evaluation Initiative. (2020). *The EE framework: Principles and co-learning.* Retrieved from https://www.equitableeval.org/ee-framework

European Institute for Gender Equality. (2020). *Marginalized groups.* Retrieved from https://eige.europa.eu/thesaurus/terms/1280

FAO, IFAD, UNICEF, WFP, & WHO. (2019). *The State of Food Security and Nutrition in the World 2019. Safeguarding against economic slowdowns and downturns.* Rome, FAO. Licence: CC BY-NC-SA 3.0 IGO. Retrieved from http://www.fao.org/3/ca5162en/ca5162en.pdf

Farmer-Smith, K. (2018). Using art in evaluation. *AEA365.* Retrieved from https://aea365.org/blog/18251-2/

Feagin, J. R. (2013). *The [W]hite racial frame: Centuries of racial framing and counter framing* (2nd ed.). New York, NY: Routledge.

Fetterman, D. M. (2015). Empowerment evaluation and action research: A convergence of values, principles, and purpose. In H. Bradbury (Ed.), *The handbook of action research*. Thousand Oaks, CA: Sage.

Fetterman, D. M. (2004). Branching out or standing on a limb: Looking to our roots for insight. In M. C. Alkin (Eds.), Evaluation roots (pp. 304–318). Thousand Oaks, CA: Sage.

Fetterman, D. M. (2001). *Foundations of empowerment evaluation*. Thousand Oaks, CA: Sage.

Fetterman, D. (1998). *Empowerment evaluation: Collaboration, action research, and a case example*. Retrieved from https://pdfs.semanticscholar.org/0a34/acbaf9e87d68dcfec5f735d8cd1e8c607280.pdf

Fetterman, D. M. (1994). Empowerment evaluation. *Evaluation Practice*, 15(1), 1–15.

Fetterman, D.M. & Kaftariain, S.J. (1996). Empowerment evaluation: Knowledge and tools for self-assessment & accountability. Thousdan Oaks:, CA: Sage

Fetterman, D. M., & Wandersman, A. (2017). Celebrating the 21st anniversary of empowerment evaluation with our critical friends. *Evaluation and Program Planning*, 63, 132–135.

Fetterman, D. M., & Wandersman, A. (2007). Empowerment evaluation: Yesterday, today, and tomorrow. *American Journal of Evaluation*, 28(2), 179–198.

Few, S. (2012). *Show me the numbers: Designing tables and graphs to enlighten* (2nd ed.). El Dorado Hills, CA: Analytic Press.

Few, S. (2009). *Now you see it*. Oakland, CA: Analytic Press.

Filstead, W. J. (1979). Qualitative methods: A needed perspective in evaluation research. In T. D. Cook & C. S. Reichardt (Eds.), *Qualitative and quantitative methods in evaluation research* (pp. 33–48). Beverly Hills, CA: Sage.

Finnegan, E., Oakhill, J., & Garnham, A. (2015). Counter-stereotypical pictures as a strategy for overcoming spontaneous gender stereotypes. *Frontiers in Psychology*, 6, 1291. Retrieved from https://www.ncbi.nlm.nih.gov/pmc/articles/PMC6292925/

Fisher, R. A. (1926), The arrangement of field experiments. *Journal of the Ministry of Agriculture of Great Britain*, 33, 503–513.

FitzGerald, C., Martin, A., Berner, D., & Hurst, S. (2019). Interventions designed to reduce implicit prejudices and implicit stereotypes in real world contexts: A systematic review. *BMC Psychology*, 7(29). Retrieved from https://bmcpsychology.biomedcentral.com/articles/10.1186/s40359-019-0299-7#citeas

Fitzpatrick, J. L., Sanders, J. R., & Worthen, B. R. (2004). *Program evaluation: Alternative approaches and practical guidelines*. Upper Saddle River, NJ: Pearson Education.

Fleischer, D., & Christie, C. A. (2009). Evaluation use: Results from a survey of U.S. American Evaluation Association members. *American Journal of Evaluation*, 30(2), 158–175. Retrieved from https://www.researchgate.net/publication/243056622_Evaluation_Use_Results_From_a_Survey_of_US_American_Evaluation_Association_Members

Flick, U., Von Kardorff, E., & Steinke, I. (2004). *A companion to qualitative research*. Thousand Oaks, CA: Sage.

Forsetlund, L., Chalmers, I., & Bjørndal, A. (2007). When was random allocation first used to generate comparison groups in experiments to assess the effect of social interventions? *Economics of Innovation and New Technology*, 16, 371–384.

Fournier, D. M. (2005). Evaluation. In S. Mathison (Ed.), *Encyclopedia of evaluation* (pp. 139–140). Thousand Oaks, CA: Sage.

Francisco, V. T., Butterfoss, F. D., & Capwell, E. M. (2001). An interview with Dr. Laura Leviton, leader in the field of evaluating community health promotion initiatives. *Health Promotion Practice*, 2(3), 203–206.

Frazier-Anderson, P. N., & Bertrand Jones, T. (2015). Analysis of love my children: Rose Bultler Browne's contributions to culturally responsive evaluation. In S. Hood, R. K. Hopson, & H. Frierson (Eds.), *Continuing the journey to reposition culture and cultural context in evaluation theory and practice* (pp. 73–87). Greenwich, CT: Information Age.

Frazier-Anderson, P., Hood, S., & Hopson, R. K. (2012). Preliminary considerations of an African American culturally responsive evaluation system. In S. D. Lapan, M. T. Quartaroli, & F. J. Riemer (Eds.), *Qualitative research: An introduction to methods and designs* (pp. 347–372). San Francisco, CA: Jossey-Bass.

Frechtling, J. (Ed.). (2010). *The 2010 user-friendly handbook for project evaluation*. Arlington, VA: National Science Foundation. Retrieved from http://www.evalu-ate.org/wp-content/uploads/formidable/Doc_2010_NSFHandbook.pdf

Frechtling, J. A. (2007). *Logic modeling methods in program evaluation*. San Francisco, CA: Jossey-Bass.

Freeman, A., Stanko, P., Berkowitz, L. N., Parnell, N., Zuppe, A., Bale, T. L., & Epperson, C. N. (2017). Inclusion of sex and gender in biomedical research: Survey of clinical research proposed at the University of Pennsylvania. *Biology of Sex Differences*, 8, 22.

Frierson, H. T., Hood, S., & Hughes, G. (2002). Section IV: A guide to conducting culturally responsive evaluations. In J. Frechtling (Ed.), *The 2002 user-friendly handbook for project evaluation* (pp. 63–73). Arlington, VA: National Science Foundation. Retrieved from https://www.nsf.gov/pubs/2002/nsf02057/nsf02057_5.pdf

Frierson, H. T., Hood, S., Hughes, G., & Thomas, V. G. (2010). A guide to conducting culturally responsive evaluations. In J. Frechtling (Ed.), *The 2010 user-friendly handbook for project evaluation* (pp. 75–96). Arlington, VA: National Science Foundation. Retrieved from http://www.evalu-ate.org/wp-content/uploads/formidable/Doc_2010_NSFHandbook.pdf

Fryrear, A. (2015, July 27). What's a good survey response rate? *SurveyGizmo*. Retrieved from https://www.surveygizmo.com/resources/blog/survey-response-rates/

Full Media. (n.d.) *How do you measure readability?* Retrieved from https://www.fullmedia.com/how-do-you-measure-readability

Funnell, S. C., & Rogers, P. J. (2011). *Purposeful program theory*. San Francisco, CA: Jossey-Bass.

Gamble, J. A. A. (2006). *A developmental evaluation primer*. Montreal, Canada: J. W. McConnell Family Foundation.

Gauchat, G. (2012). Politicization of science in the public sphere: A study of public trust in the United States, 1974 to 2010. *American Sociological Review*, 77(2), 167–187.

Gazley, J. L., Remich, R., Naffziger-Hirsch, M., Keller, J., Campbell, P. B. & McGee, R. (2014). Beyond preparation: Identity, cultural capital, and readiness for graduate school in the biomedical sciences. *Journal of Research in Science Teaching*, 51(8), 1021–1048.

Geis, G., & Dodge. M. (2003). Cambridge-Somerville Youth Study. In M. D. McShane & F. P. Williams III (Eds.), *Encyclopedia of juvenile justice*. Thousand Oaks, CA: Sage.

Germuth A. (2019). Succeeding as an independent consultant: Requisite skills and attributes. In N. Martinez-Rubin, A. A. Germuth, & M. L. Feldman (Eds.), *Special Issue: Independent evaluation consulting: Approaches and practices from a growing field* (pp. 43–54). *New Directions for Evaluation*, 164.

Gerstein, J. (2016). Approaching marginalized populations from an asset rather than a deficit model of education. *User Generated Education*. Retrieved from https://usergeneratededucation.wordpress.com/2016/05/08/approaching-marginalized-populations-from-an-asset-rather-than-a-deficit-model/

Gervin, D., Kuwahara, R., Lane, R., Gill, S., Moeti, R., & Wilce, R. (2014). *Practical strategies for culturally competent evaluation: Evaluation guide*. Washington, DC: U.S. Department of Health and Human Services: Centers for Disease Control and Prevention. Retrieved from https://www.cdc.gov/dhdsp/docs/cultural_competence_guide.pdf

Gerwitz, S., & Dodge, K. (1975). Adults' evaluation of a child as a function of the sex of the adult and the sex of the child. *Journal of Personality and Social Psychology*, 32(5), 822–828.

Gilliam, W. S., Maupin, A. N., Reyes, C. R., Accavitt, M., & Shie, F. (2016). *Do early educators' implicit biases regarding sex and race relate to behavior expectations and recommendations of preschool expulsions and suspensions?* New Haven, CT: Yale University Child Study Center.

Gilligan, C. (2011). Looking back to look forward: Revisiting *In a different voice*. *Classics@* 9. Washington, DC: Center for Hellenic Studies. Retrieved from https://chs.harvard.edu/CHS/article/display/4025

Gilligan, C. (1982). *In a different voice*. Cambridge, MA: Harvard University Press.

Glass, G. V., & Ellett, F. S. (1980). Evaluation research. *Annual Review of Psychology*, 31, 211–228.

Glass, G. V., McGaw, B., & Smith, M. L. (1981). *Meta-analysis in social research*. London, UK: Sage.

Glenn, D. (2008). Huge databases offer a research gold mine and privacy worries. *Chronicle of Higher Education Section: The Faculty*, 54(35), A10.

Glover, T. (2002). *Compared to what? Purpose and method of control group selection*. Cheyenne: Wyoming Department of Employment Research & Planning. Retrieved from https://doe.state.wy.us/lmi/0602/a2.htm

Goldenberg, A., & American Anthropological Association. (2011). *Race: Human variation*. Retrieved from https://www.understandingrace.org/HumanVariation

Goldin, C., & Rouse, C. (2000). Orchestrating impartiality: The impact of "blind" auditions on female musicians. *The American Economic Review*, 90(4), 715–741. Retrieved from http://dx.doi.org/10.1257/aer.90.4.715

Goldratt, E., & Cox, J. (1986). *The goal: A process of ongoing improvement*. Great Barrington, MA: North River Press.

Great Schools Partnership. (2014, May 15). Learning objectives. *The Glossary of Education Reform*. Retrieved from https://www.edglossary.org/learning-objectives/

Greenwald, A. G., & Banaji, M. R. (1995). Implicit social cognition: Attitudes, self-esteem and stereotypes. *Psychological Review*, 102(1), 4–27. Retrieved from http://www.people.fas.harvard.edu/~banaji/research/publications/articles/1995_Greenwald_PR.pdf

Goodman, L. A., Epstein, D., & Sullivan, C. (2018). Beyond the RCT: Integrating rigor and relevance to evaluate the outcomes of domestic violence programs. *American Journal of Evaluation*, 39(1), 58–70. Retrieved from http://journals.sagepub.com/doi/full/10.1177/1098214017721008

Goodwin, L. D., Sands, D. J., & Kozleski, E. B. (1991). Estimating inter-interviewer reliability for interview schedules used in special education research. *The Journal of Special Education*, 25(1), 73–89. Retrieved from https://doi.org/10.1177/002246699102500105

Gramlich, J. (2019, April 30). The gap between the number of blacks and whites in prison is shrinking. *Pew Research Center: Fact Tank*. Retrieved from https://www.pewresearch.org/fact-tank/2019/04/30/shrinking-gap-between-number-of-blacks-and-whites-in-prison/

Green, J. W. (1995). *Cultural awareness in the human services: A multiethnic approach* (2nd ed.). Boston, MA: Allyn & Bacon.

Greene, J. C. (2015). How evidence earns credibility in evaluation. In S. I. Donaldson, C. A. Christie, & M. M. Mark (Eds.), *Credible and actionable evidence: The foundation for rigorous and influential evaluations* (2nd ed., pp. 205–220). Thousand Oaks, CA: Sage.

Greene, J. C. (2005). Context. In S. Mathison (Ed.), *Encyclopedia of evaluation* (pp. 82–84). Thousand Oaks, CA: Sage.

Greene, J. C. (2004). The educative evaluator: An interpretation of Lee J. Cronbach's vision of evaluation. In M.C. Alkin (Ed.), *Evaluation roots: Tracing theorists' values and influences* (pp. 169–180). Thousand Oaks, CA: Sage.

Greene, J. C. (2001). Dialogue in evaluation; a relational perspective. *Evaluation*, 7(2), 181–203.

Greene, J. C., Benjamin, L., & Goodyear, L. (2001). The merits of mixing methods in evaluation. *Evaluation*, 7(1), 25–44.

Greene, J. C., Boyce, A. S., & Ahn, J. (2011). *Value-engaged, educative evaluation guidebook*. University of Illinois at Urbana-Champaign. Retrieved from https://rmcresearchcorporation.com/denverco/wp-content/uploads/sites/4/2016/05/31-Values-Engaged-Educative-Guidebook-.pdf

Greene, J. C., DeStefano, L., Burgon, H., & Hall, J. (2006). An educative, values-engaged approach to evaluating STEM educational programs. *New Directions for Evaluation*, 109, 53–71.

Greene, J. C., & Hall, J. N. (2010). Dialectics and pragmatism: Being of consequence. In A. Tashakkori & C. Teddlie (Eds.), *Handbook of mixed methods in social and behavioral research* (2nd ed., pp. 113–143). Thousand Oaks, CA: Sage.

Greene, J. C., & McClintock, C. (1991). The evolution of evaluation methodology. *Theory Into Practice*, 30(1), 13–21.

Grob, G. (2015). Writing for impact. In K. E. Newcomer, H. P. Hatry, & J. S. Wholey (Eds.), *Handbook of practical program evaluation* (4th ed., pp. 739–764). San Francisco, CA: Jossey-Bass.

Guba, E. G. (Ed.). (1990). *The paradigm dialog*. Newburg Park, CA: Sage.

Guba, E. G., & Lincoln, Y. S. (2005). Paradigmatic controversies, contradictions, and emerging confluences. In N. K. Denzin & Y. S. Lincoln

(Eds.), *The Sage handbook of qualitative research* (3rd ed, pp. 191–215). Thousand Oaks, CA: Sage.

Guba, E. G., & Lincoln, Y. S. (1994). Competing paradigms in qualitative research. In N. K. Denzin & Y. S. Lincoln (Eds.), *Handbook of qualitative research* (pp. 105–117). Thousand Oaks, CA: Sage

Guba, E. G., & Lincoln, Y. S. (1989). *Fourth generation evaluation*. Thousand Oaks, CA: Sage.

Guba, E. G., & Lincoln, Y. S. (1985). *Naturalistic inquiry*. Thousand Oaks, CA: Sage.

Guba, E. G., & Lincoln, Y. S. (1982). Epistemological and methodological bases of naturalistic inquiry. *Educational Communication & Technology, 30*(4), 233–252.

Guba, E. G., & Lincoln, Y. S. (1981). *Effective evaluation*. San Francisco, CA: Jossey-Bass.

Goering, S. (2015). Rethinking disability: the social model of disability and chronic disease. *Current Reviews in Musculoskeletal Medicine, 8*(2), 134–138.

Guillemin, M., & Gillam, L. (2004). Ethics, reflexivity, and "ethically important moments" in research. *Qualitative Inquiry, 10*(2), 261–280.

Gulker, J. E., Mark, A. Y., & Monteith, M. H. (2013). Confronting prejudice: The *who*, *what*, and *why* of confrontation effectiveness. *Social Influence, 8*(4), 280–293.

Guthrie, R. V. (1976). *Even the rat was white: A historical view of psychology*. New York, NY: Harper & Row.

Guthrie, R. V. (2004). *Even the rat was white: A historical view of psychology* (2nd ed.). Boston, MA: Allyn & Bacon Classics Edition.

Habibzadeh, F., & Habibzadeh, P. (2015). How much precision in reporting statistics is enough? *Croatian Medical Journal, 56*(5), 490–492. Retrieved from https://www.ncbi.nlm.nih.gov/pmc/articles/PMC4679338/

Hall, J. N. (2020). The other side of inequity: Using standpoint theories to examine the privilege of the evaluation profession and individual evaluators. *American Journal of Evaluation, 41*(1), 20–33.

Hall, J. N. (2013). Pragmatism, evidence, and mixed methods evaluation. In D. M. Mertens & S. Hesse-Biber (Eds.), *Mixed methods and credibility of evidence in evaluation. New Directions for Evaluation, 138*, 15–26.

Hall, J., Freeman, M., & Roulston, K. (2014). Right timing in formative program evaluation. *Evaluation and Program Planning, 45*, 151–156.

Hall, M. (2018a, January 7). Building on the AEA Dialogues on Race and Class in America. *AEA365*. Retrieved from https://aea365.org/blog/mie-tig-week-building-on-the-aea-dialogues-on-race-and-class-in-america-by-melvin-hall/

Hall, M. (2018b, June). Walking the talk with Melvin Hall, PhD: Remaining alert and vigilant. *AEA Newsletter*. Retrieved from https://www.eval.org/blog/aea-newsletter-june-2018/#WalkingtheTalk

Hamburg, M. (2019, February). Transcending boundaries. *Science, 363*(6427), 563.

Hammersley, M. (2005). Should social science be critical? *Philosophy of the Social Sciences, 35*(2), 175–195.

Han, H., Kang, J., Kim, K., Ryu, J., & Kim, M. (2007). Barriers to and strategies for recruiting Korean Americans for community-partnered health promotion research. *Journal of Immigrant and Minority Health, 9*, 137–146.

Handford, M., Van Maele, J., Matous, P., & Maemura, Y. (2019, April). Small culture, big changes. *Prism*, 45.

Hanisch, C. (1969, February). The personal is political. Retrieved from http://www.carolhanisch.org/CHwritings/PIP.html (Originally published in *Notes from the Second Year: Women's Liberation* in 1970)

Hanman, N. (2013, August 22). Eve Kosofsky Sedgwick and Judith Butler showed me the transformative power of the word queer. *The Guardian*. Retrieved from https://www.theguardian.com/commentisfree/2013/aug/22/judith-butler-eve-sedgwick-queer

Hannum, K. (2018, September 30). NPF TIG Week: Finding meaning in the "post-truth" era. *AEA365*. Washington, DC: American Evaluation Association. Retrieved from https://aea365.org/blog/npf-tig-week-finding-meaning-in-the-post-truth-era-by-kelly-hannum/?utm_source=feedburner&utm_medium=email&utm_campaign=Feed%3A+aea365+%28AEA365%29

Harding, S. (1987). Introduction is there a feminist method? In S. Harding (Ed.), *Feminisim and methodology* (pp. 1–14). Bloomington: Indiana University Press.

Harding, S., & O'Barr, J. F. (1987). *Sex and scientific inquiry*. Chicago, IL: University of Chicago Press.

Harmon, L. W. (1973). Sexual bias in interest measurement. *Measurement and Evaluation in Guidance, 5*(4), 496–501.

Harrison, E. C. (1950). An evaluation of industrial education programs in secondary schools for Negroes in Louisiana. *The Journal of Negro Education, 19*(1), 38–46.

Hastings, T. (1976). *A portrayal of the changing evaluation scene*. Keynote address delivered at the Annual Meeting of the Evaluation Network, St. Louis, MO.

Hatchett, B. F., Holmes, K., Duran, D. A., & Davis, C. (2000). African Americans and research participation: The recruitment process. *Journal of Black Studies, 30*, 664–674.

Hatcher, D. L. (2016). *The poverty industry: The exploitation of American's most vulnerable citizens*. New York: New York University Press.

Hatry, H. P. (2015). Using agency records. In K. E. Newcomer, H. P. Hatry, & J. S. Wholey (Eds.), *Handbook of practical program evaluation* (4th ed., pp. 325–343). Hoboken, NJ: Wiley.

Hatry, H. P., & Newcomer, K. E. (2015). Pitfalls in evaluations. In K. E. Newcomer, H. P. Hatry & J. S. Wholey (Eds.), *Handbook of practical program evaluation* (4th ed., pp. 701–724). San Francisco, CA: Jossey-Bass.

Hauck, K., Smith, P. C., & Goddard, M. (2004). *The economics of priority setting for health care: A literature review*. HNP discussion paper series. Washington, DC: World Bank.

Haugen, J. S., & Chouinard, J. A. (2018). Transparent, translucent, opaque: Exploring the dimensions of power in culturally responsive evaluation contexts. *American Journal of Evaluation, 40*(3), 376–394.

Heiner, R. (2016). *Social problems: An introduction to critical constructionism* (5th ed.). New York, NY: Oxford University Press.

Heiner, R. (2013). *Social problems: An introduction to critical constructionism* (4th ed.). New York, NY: Oxford University Press.

Hengen, T. (2013). *Medicine wheel model of mental health*. Victoria, BC, Canada: Friesen Press.

Henry, G. T., Smith, A. A., Kershaw, D. C., & Zulli, R. A. (2013). Formative evaluation: estimating preliminary outcomes and testing rival explanations. *American Journal of Evaluation*, 34(4), 465–485.

Hernandez, M. (2000). Using logic models and program theory to build outcome accountability. *Education & Treatment of Children*, 23(1), 24–41.

Herr, D. (2007). Deductive reasoning. *The sourcebook for teaching science*. Retrieved from http://www.csun.edu/science/ref/reasoning/deductive_reasoning/index.html

Hilliard, A. G., III. (1989). Kemetic (Egyptian) historical revision: Implications for cross-cultural evaluation and research in education. *Evaluation Practice*, 10, 7–23.

Hoit, R. (2019). Democracy's plight. *Science*, 363(6426), 433

Hollo, T. (2017, July 11). Musk's big battery brings reality crashing into a post-truth world. *Taipei Times*. Retrieved from http://www.taipeitimes.com/News/editorials/archives/2017/07/11/2003674312

Hood, S. (2017). Continuing the exploration of African Americans in the early history of evaluation in the United States: Contributions of Ambrose Caliver in the U.S. Office of Education. *American Journal of Evaluation*, 38(2), 262–274.

Hood, S. (2005). Culturally responsive evaluation. In S. Mathison (Ed.), *Encyclopedia of evaluation* (pp. 96–100). Thousand Oaks, CA: Sage.

Hood, S. (2001). Nobody knows my name: In praise of African American evaluators who were responsive. *New Directions for Evaluation*, 92, 31–44.

Hood, S. (1998). Responsive evaluation Amistad style: Perspectives of one African American evaluator. In R. Davis (Ed.), *Proceedings of the Stake Symposium on Educational Evaluation* (pp. 101–112). Urbana-Champaign: University of Illinois.

Hood, S., & Hopson, R. K. (2008). Evaluation roots reconsidered: Asa Hilliard, a fallen hero in the "Nobody knows my name" project, and African education excellence. *Review of Educational Research*, 78(3), 410–426.

Hood, S., Hopson, R., & Frierson, H. (Eds.). (2015). *Continuing the journey to reposition culture and cultural context in evaluation theory and practice*. Greenwich, CT: Information Age.

Hood, S., Hopson, R., & Frierson, H. (Eds.). (2005). *The role of culture and cultural context: A mandate for inclusion, the discovery of truth and understanding in evaluation theory and practice*. Greenwich, CT: Information Age.

Hood, S., Hopson, R. K., & Kirkhart, K. E. (2015). Culturally responsive evaluation: Theory, practice, and future implications. In K. E. Newcomer, H. P. Hatry & J. S. Wholey (Eds.), *Handbook of practical program evaluation* (4th ed., pp. 281–317). Retrieved from http://journals.sagepub.com/doi/full/10.1177/1098214017721008

Hopkins, W. G. (2000). A new view of statistics. Reviewed from http://www.sportsci.org/resource/stats/errors.html

Hopson, R. (2009). Reclaiming knowledge at the margins: Culturally responsive evaluation in the current evaluation moment. In K. E. Ryan & J. B. Cousins (Eds.), *The Sage international handbook of educational evaluation* (pp. 429–446). Thousand Oaks, CA: Sage.

Hopson, R., & Cram, F. (2018). Tackling wicked problems in complex evaluation ecologies. In R. Hopson & F. Cram (Eds.), *Problems in complex ecologies* (pp. 3–25). Stanford, CA: Stanford University Press.

Hopson, R., & Hood, S. (2005). An untold story in evaluation roots: Reid E. Jackson and his contributions toward culturally responsive evaluation at three quarters of a century. In S. Hood, R. Hopson, & H. Frierson (Eds.), *The role of culture and cultural context in evaluation* (pp. 87–104). Greenwich, CT: Information Age.

Hopson, R. K., & Kirkhart, K. E. (2011, June). *Strengthening evaluation through cultural relevance and cultural competence*. Workshop delivered at the AEA/CDC (American Evaluation Association/Centers for Disease Control) Summer Evaluation Institute.

Horn, K., & Dino, G. (2011). A. How do you engage the community when there are cultural differences (race or ethnicity) between the community and the researchers? In Clinical and Translational Science Awards Consortium Community Engagement Key Function Committee Task Force, *Principles of community engagement* (2nd ed., NIH Publication No. 11-7782). Washington, DC: National Institutes of Health, U.S. Department of Health and Human Services.

Horsch, K. (1997). *Indicators: Definition and use in a results based accountability system*. Cambridge, MA: Harvard Family Research Project.

House, E. R. (2017). Evaluation and the framing of race. *American Journal of Evaluation*, 38(2), 167–189.

House, E. R. (2016, November 15). *Reducing biases in evaluation*. Paper presented to the New Mexico Evaluators, Albuquerque.

House, E. R. (2011). Conflict of interest and Campbellian validity. *New Directions for Evaluation*, 130, 68–80.

House, E. R. (1995). Principled evaluation: A critique of the AEA Guiding Principles. *New Directions for Program Evaluation*, 66, 27–34.

House, E. R. (1987). The evaluation audit. *Evaluation Practice*, 8(2), 52–56.

House, E. R. (1983). Assumptions underlying evaluation models. In G. F. Madaus, M. S. Scriven, & D. L. Stufflebeam (Eds.), *Evaluation models: Viewpoints on educational and human services evaluation* (pp. 45–64). Boston, MA: Kluwer-Nijhoff.

House, E. (1980). *Evaluating with validity*. Thousand Oaks, CA: Sage.

House, E. R., & Howe, K. R. (2003). Deliberative democratic evaluation. In T. Hellaghan & D. L. Stufflebeam (Eds.), *International handbook of educational evaluation: Part one* (pp. 79–100). Dordrecht, Netherlands: Kluwer Academic.

House, E. R., & Howe, K. R. (2000a). Deliberative democratic evaluation. In K. E. Ryan & L. DeStefano (Eds.), *Evaluation as a democratic process: Promoting inclusion, dialogue, and deliberation* (pp. 3–12). *New Directions for Evaluation*, 85.

House, E. R. & Howe, K. R. (2000b). Deliberative democratic evaluation checklist. *Evaluation checklist project*. Ann Arbor: University of Western

Michigan. Retrieved from https://wmich.edu/sites/default/files/attachments/u350/2018/DD-eval-House%26Howe.pdf

Howe, K. R., & Ashcraft, C. (2005, October). Deliberative democratic evaluation: Success and limitations of an evaluation of school choice. *Teachers College Record, 107*(10), 2275–2298.

Hubbard, R., & Armstrong, J. S. (1992, Summer). Are null results becoming an endangered species in marketing? *Guiding Principles for Evaluators, 66*, 27–34. Retrieved from http://repository.upenn.edu/marketing_papers/110

Huberty, C. J., & Olejnik, S. (2006). *Applied MANOVA and discriminant analysis* (2nd ed.). Hoboken, NJ: Wiley-Interscience.

Hudson, L., & Ozanne, J. (1988). Alternative ways of seeking knowledge in consumer research. *Journal of Consumer Research, 14*(4), 508–521.

Huff, D. (1954). *How to lie with statistics.* New York: Norton.

HuffPost. (2014, February 26). These 12 everyday words used to have completely different meanings. Retrieved from https://www.huffpost.com/entry/words-that-have-changed-meaning_n_4847343

Hughes, G. B. (2000). Discussion highlights. In *Workshop proceedings. The cultural context of educational evaluation: The role of minority evaluation professionals* (pp. 8–12). Arlington, VA: National Science Foundation, Directorate for Education and Human Resources, Division of Research, Evaluation, and Communications.

Human Rights Campaign. (2020). Repeal of "Don't Ask, Don't Tell." Retrieved from https://www.hrc.org/resources/the-repeal-of-dont-ask-dont-tell

Hummel, K., Candel, M. J. J. M., Nagelhout, G. E., Brown, J., van den Putte, B., Kotz D., . . . de Vries, H. (2018, September). Construct and predictive validity of three measures of intention to quit smoking: Findings from the International Tobacco Control (ITC) Netherlands Survey. *Nicotine & Tobacco Research, 20*(9), 1101–1108.

Hutchinson, K. (2015, March 25). Logic Models Week: Kylie Hutchinson on logic models in the age of systems thinking. *AEA365.* Retrieved from https://aea365.org/blog/logic-models-week-kylie-hutchinson-on-logic-models-in-the-age-of-systems-thinking/

IllumiLab. (2018a, April 9). *Evaluative thinking: The heart of (meaningful, useful) evaluation.* Retrieved from https://www.insightsintoimpact.com/evaluative-thinking-the-heart-of-meaningful-useful-evaluation/

IllumiLab. (2018b, April 23). *Encouraging & practicing evaluative thinking.* Retrieved from https://www.insightsintoimpact.com/encouraging-practice-evaluative-thinking/

Ingersoll, G. (1982). Experimental methods. In H. Mitzel (Ed.), *Encyclopedia of educational research* (5th ed., pp. 624–631). New York, NY: Free Press.

Ingraham, C. (2017, July 12). A brief history of DARE, the anti-drug program Jeff Sessions wants to revive. *Washington Post.* Retrieved from https://www.washingtonpost.com/news/wonk/wp/2017/07/12/a-brief-history-of-d-a-r-e-the-anti-drug-program-jeff-sessions-wants-to-revive/

Institute of Education Sciences. (2003, December). *Identifying and implementing educational practices supported by rigorous evidence: A user friendly guide.* Retrieved from https://ies.ed.gov/ncee/pubs/evidence_based/randomized.asp

Institute of Medicine Board on Global Health. (2014). *Evaluation design for complex global initiatives: Workshop summary. Mapping Data Sources and Gathering and Assessing Data.* Washington, DC: National Academies of Science, Engineering, and Medicine.

Internal Revenue Service. (2019). *SEP plan FAQs.* Retrieved from https://www.irs.gov/retirement-plans/retirement-plans-faqs-regarding-seps

Internal Revenue Service. (n.d.). *Employee (common-law employee).* Retrieved from https://www.irs.gov/businesses/small-businesses-self-employed/employee-common-law-employee

International Association for Public Participation. (n.d.). *What is the spectrum of public participation? Sustaining community: Families, communities, the environment.* Retrieved from https://sustainingcommunity.wordpress.com/2017/02/14/spectrum-of-public-participation/

International Development Research Center. (2012). 10 data visualization tips. *Evaluating IDRC results: Communicating research for influence.* Retrieved from https://www.idrc.ca/sites/default/files/sp/Documents%20EN/Quick-tips-English-22-May-2012.pdf

International Program for Development Evaluation Training. (2009). *Module 14: Guiding the evaluator: Evaluation ethics, politics, standards, and principles.* Retrieved from http://www.dww.cz/docs/module14.pdf

Iris Center, Vanderbilt University. (2019). *Cultural responsiveness.* Retrieved from https://iris.peabody.vanderbilt.edu/module/clde/cresource/q1/p02/

Iskarpatyoti, B. S., Sutherland, B., & Reynolds, H. W. (2017). *Getting to an evaluation plan: A six-step process from evidence to engagement. A Workbook.* Chapel Hill, NC: Measure Evaluation.

Jackson, J. F. L., & O'Callaghan, E. M. (2011). Understanding employment disparities using glass ceiling effects criteria: An examination of race/ethnicity and senior-level position attainment across the academic workforce. *Journal of the Professoriate, 5*(2), 67–99.

Jackson, K. M., Pukys, S., Catro, A., Hermosura, L., Menhez, J., Vohra-Gupta, S., Padilla, Y., & Morales, G. (2018), Using the transformative paradigm to conduct a mixed methods needs assessment of a marginalized community: Methodological lessons and implications. *Evaluation and Program Planning, 66*, 111–119.

Jackson, R. E. (1940a). An evaluation of educational opportunities for the Negro adolescent in Alabama, I. *Journal of Negro Education, 9*(1), 59–72.

Jackson, R. E. (1940b). An evaluation of educational opportunities for the Negro adolescent in Alabama, II. *Journal of Negro Education, 9*(2), 200–207.

Jackson, R. E. (1938). *A critical analysis for educating secondary school teachers in Negro colleges in Alabama.* Unpublished doctoral dissertation, The Ohio State University.

Jackson, R. (1936). Status of education of the Negro in Florida, 1929–1934. *Opportunity, 14*(11), 336–339.

Jackson, R. (1935). The development and present status of secondary education for Negroes in Kentucky. *Journal of Negro Education, 4*(2), 185–191.

Jank, S., & Owens, L. (n.d.). *Inequality in the United States.* Stanford University. Retrieved from https://inequality.stanford.edu/sites/default/files/Inequality_SlideDeck.pdf

Jenkins, S., Robinson, K., & Davis, R. (2015). *Adapting the medicine wheel model to extend the applicability of the traditional logic model in evaluation research*. Proceedings of the 2015 Federal Committee on Statistical Methodology (FCSM) Research Conference (p. 7).

Johnson, B., & Onwuegbuzie, A. (2004). Mixed methods research: A research paradigm whose time has come. *Educational Researcher, 33*(7), 14–26.

Johnson, E. C., Kirkhart, K. E., Madison, A. M., Noley, G. B., & Solano-Flores, G. (2008). The impact of narrow views of scientific rigor on evaluation practices for underrepresented groups. In N. L. Smith & P. R. Brandon (Eds.), *Fundamental issues in evaluation* (pp. 197–218). New York, NY: Guilford Press.

Johnston, L., O'Malley, P., & Bachman, J. (2002). *Monitoring the future national survey results on drug use, 1975–2002*. NIH Publication No. 03-5375. Bethesda, MD: National Institute on Drug Abuse.

Jones, J. (2018, October 30). Black unemployment is at least twice as high as white unemployment at the national level and in 12 states and D.C. *Economic Policy Institute*. Retrieved from https://www.epi.org/publication/2018q3_unemployment_state_race_ethnicity/

Jones, R. L. (1996). *Handbook of tests and measurements for black populations*. Hampton, VA: Cobb & Henry.

Jones, T. M. (1991). Ethical decision making by individuals in organizations: An issue contingent model. *Academy of Management Review, 16*(2), 366–395.

Jorgensen, D. L. (1989). *Participant observation: A methodology for human studies*. Newbury Park, CA: Sage.

Kaplan, D. (n.d.). The definition of disability. *The Center for an Accessible Society*. Retrieved from http://www.accessiblesociety.org/topics/demographics-identity/dkaplanpaper.htm

Kaplan, S. A., & Garrett, K. E. (2005). The use of logic models by community-based initiatives. *Evaluation and Program Planning, 28*, 167–172.

Kawakami, K., Dovidio, J. K., Moll, J., Hermsen, S., & Russin, A. (2000). Just say no (to stereotyping): Effects of training in the negation of stereotypic associations on stereotype activation. *Journal of Personality and Social Psychology, 78*(5), 871–888. Retrieved from https://www.ncbi.nlm.nih.gov/pmc/articles/PMC6292925/

Keene, M., & Metzner, C. (2011, September). *Fuzzy logic models*. American Evaluation Association Coffee Break Demonstration Webinar.

Kellaghan, T., Stufflebeam, D. L., & Wingate, L. A. (2003). Introduction. In T. Kellaghan & D. L. Stufflebeam (Eds.), *International handbook of educational evaluation* (pp. 1–6) Dordrecht, Netherlands: Kluwer Academic.

King, M. F., & Bruner, G. C. (2000). Social desirability bias: A neglected aspect of validity testing. *Psychology and Marketing, 17*(2), 79–103.

Kirby, D. (2004). *BDI logic models: A useful tool for designing, strengthening, and evaluating programs to reduce adolescent sexual risk-taking, pregnancy, HIV and other STDs*. ERT Associates. Retrieved from http://recapp.etr.org/recapp/documents/BDILOGICMODEL20030924.pdf

Kirkhart, K. E. (2010). Eyes on the prize: Multicultural validity and evaluation theory. *American Journal of Evaluation, 31*(3), 400–413.

Kirkhart, K. E. (2005). Through a cultural lens: Reflections on validity and theory in evaluation. In S. Hood, R. K. Hopson, & H. T. Frierson (Eds.), *The role of culture and cultural context: A mandate for inclusion, the discovery of truth, and understanding in evaluative theory and practice* (pp. 21–39). Greenwich, CT: Information Age.

Kirkhart, K. (1995). 1994 conference theme: Evaluation and social justice seeking multicultural validity: A postcard from the road. *American Journal of Evaluation, 16*(1), 1–12.

Kirkpatrick, D. L. (1994). *Evaluating training programs: The four levels*. Emeryville, CA: Berrett-Koehler.

Kirkpatrick, J. D., & Kirkpatrick, J. W. (2016). *Kirkpatrick's four levels of training evaluation*. Alexandria, VA: ATD Press.

Kistler, S. (2010, July 26). Michael Quinn Patton on developmental evaluation. *AEA365*. Retrieved from https://aea365.org/blog/michael-quinn-patton-on-developmental-evaluation-applying-complexity-concepts-to-enhance-innovation-and-use/

Kitchener, K. S., & Kitchener, R. F. (2009). Social science research ethics: Historical and philosophical issues. In D. M. Mertens & P. E. Ginsberg (Eds.), *The handbook of social research ethics* (pp. 5–22). Thousand Oaks, CA: Sage.

Klages, M. (2006). *Literary theory: A guide for the perplexed*. London, UK: Bloomsbury.

Klempin, S., & Mincy, R. B. (2009). *Process analysis: Child support intervention services with African American men. The Center for Urban Families' Baltimore Responsible Fatherhood Program*. Conducted by the Center for Research on Fathers, Children and Family Well-Being. Retrieved from http://crfcfw.columbia.edu/files/2012/09/CFUF-Final-Report_final.pdf

Klugman, B. (2018, September 5). Six conditions that increase the likelihood and effectiveness of evaluators speaking truth to power by Barbara Klugman. *AEA365*. Retrieved from https://aea365.org/blog/six-conditions-that-increase-the-likelihood-and-effectiveness-of-evaluators-speaking-truth-to-power-by-barbara-klugman/?utm_source=feedburner&utm_medium=email&utm_campaign=Feed%3A+aea365+%28AEA365%29

Knowlton, L. W., & Phillips, C. C. (2013). *The logic model guidebook: Better strategies for great results* (2nd ed.). Thousand Oaks, CA: Sage.

Kochhar, R., & Cilluffo, A. (2017). How wealth inequality has changed in the U.S. since the Great Recession, by race, ethnicity and income. *FactTank: Pew Research Center*. Retrieved from https://www.pewresearch.org/fact-tank/2017/11/01/how-wealth-inequality-has-changed-in-the-u-s-since-the-great-recession-by-race-ethnicity-and-income/

Kosofsky Sedgwick, E. (1990). *Epistemology of the closet*. Berkeley: University of California Press.

Krause, H. (2018, March 6). FIE TIG Week: So you think math is an objective science? Think again. *AEA365*. Retrieved from http://aea365.org/blog/fie-tig-week-so-you-think-math-is-an-objective-science-think-again-by-heather-krause/?utm_source=feedburner&utm_medium=email&utm_campaign=Feed%3A+aea365+%28AEA365%29

Krebs, V. (n.d.). Social network analysis: An introduction. *Orgnet*. Retrieved from http://www.orgnet.com/sna.html

Kuhn, T. S. (1984). Revisiting Planck. *Historical Studies in the Physical Sciences, 14*(2), 231–252.

Kuhn, T. S. (1962). *The structure of scientific revolutions*. Chicago, IL: University of Chicago Press.

Kukolic, S. (2017). We see them as we are. *HuffPost*. Retrieved from https://www.huffpost.com/entry/we-see-them-as-we-are_b_590cab8ae4b056aa2363d461

Kurzius, R. (2018, November 5). Is it Meridian Hill Park or Malcolm X Park? Your answer is meaningful. *Washington Post*. Retrieved from https://www.washingtonpost.com/lifestyle/magazine/is-it-meridian-hill-park-or-malcolm-x-park-your-answer-is-meaningful/2018/11/02/610af0e2-d07e-11e8-b2d2-f397227b43f0_story.html?utm_term=.e4c299d3b018

Kushner, S. (2009). Own goals: Democracy, evaluation, and rights in millennium projects. In K. E. Ryan & J. B. Cousins (Eds.), *The SAGE international handbook of educational evaluation* (pp. 413–428). Thousand Oaks, CA: Sage.

Kushner, S. (2000). *Personalizing evaluation*. London, UK: Sage.

Ladson-Billings, G. (2006). From the achievement gap to the education debt: Understanding achievement in U.S. schools. *Educational Researcher*, 35(7), 3–12.

Ladson-Billings, G. (1997). It doesn't add up: African American students' mathematics achievement, *Journal for Research in Mathematics Education*, 28(6) 697–708.

LaFrance, J. (2004). Culturally competent evaluation in Indian Country. In M. Thompson-Robinson, R. Hopson, & S. SenGupta (Eds.), *In search of cultural competence in evaluation: Toward principles and practices. New Directions for Evaluation*, 102, 39–50.

LaFrance, J., & Nichols, R. (2010). Reframing evaluation: Defining an indigenous evaluation framework. *Canadian Journal of Evaluation*, 23(2), 13–31.

LaFrance, J., &, Nichols, R. (2009). *Indigenous evaluation framework: Telling our story in our place and time*. Alexandria, VA: American Indian Higher Education Consortium (AIHEC).

LaFrance, J., Nichols, R., & Kirkhart, K. E. (2012). Culture writes the script: On the centrality of context in indigenous evaluation. *New Directions for Evaluation*, 135, 59–74.

Lambert, E. Y., & Wiebel, W. W. (Eds.). (1990). *The collection and interpretation of data from hidden populations*. Washington, DC: National Institute on Drug Abuse. Retrieved from http://www.drugabuse.gov/pdf/monographs/download98.html

Lariviere, V., Ni, C., Gingras, Y., Cronin, B., & Sugimoto, C. R. (2013). Bibliometrics: Global gender disparities in science. *Nature*, 504, 211–213.

Lauer, M. (2016). Scientific rigor in NIH grant applications. *Extramural Nexus*. Retrieved from https://nexus.od.nih.gov/all/2016/01/28/scientific-rigor-in-nih-grant-applications/

Lave, J., & Wenger, E. (1990). *Situated learning: Legitimate peripheral participation*. Cambridge, UK: Cambridge University Press.

Law.com. (n.d.). *Conflict of interest*. Retrieved from https://dictionary.law.com/Default.aspx?selected=292

Lawrence, C. R. (1995). The word and the river: Pedagogy as scholarship as struggle. In K. Crenshaw, N. Gotanda, & G. Peller (Eds.), *Critical race theory: The key writings that formed the movement* (pp. 336–351). New York, NY: New Press.

Lawrence, K., & Keleher, T. (2004). Structural racism. *Race and Public Policy Conference: Chronic Disparity: Strong and Pervasive Evidence of Racial Inequalities: Poverty Outcomes*. Retrieved from https://www.racialequitytools.org/resourcefiles/Definitions-of%20Racism.pdf

Lee, T., & Price, M. (1995). Indicators and research methods for rapid assessment of a tuberculosis control programme: Case study of a rural area in South Africa. *Tubercle and Lung Disease*, 76(5), 441–449.

Leeuw, F. L., & Donaldson, S. I. (2015). Theory in evaluation: Reducing confusion and encouraging debate. *Evaluation*, 21(4) 467–480.

Leuchtenburg, W. E. (n.d.). Franklin D. Roosevelt: The American franchise. Miller Center, University of Virginia. Retrieved from https://millercenter.org/president/fdroosevelt/the-american-franchise

Leung, L. (2015). Validity, reliability, and generalizability in qualitative research. *Journal of Family Medicine and Primary Care*, 4(3), 324–327.

Levin, H. (1975). Cost-effectiveness analysis in evaluation research. In M. Guttentag & E. L. Struening (Eds.), *Handbook of evaluation research* (Vol. 2, pp. 89–122). Beverly Hills, CA: Sage.

Leviton, L. C., & Lavizzo-Mourey, R. (2013). A research network to prevent obesity among Latino children. *American Journal of Preventive Medicine*, 44(3), S173–S174.

Leviton, L. C., & Melichar, L. (2016). Balancing stakeholder needs in the evaluation of healthcare quality improvement. *BMJ Quality & Safety*, 10, 803–807.

Leviton, L. C., & Schuh, R. G. (1999). The importance of a discovery capacity in community-based health and human service program evaluation. In J. Telfair, L. C. Leviton, & J. C. Merchant (Eds.), *Evaluating health and human service programs in community settings* (pp. 17–35). *New Directions for Evaluation*, 83. San Francisco, CA: Jossey-Bass.

Lewin, K. (1946). Action research and minority problems. *Journal of Social Issues*, 2(4), 34–46.

Lexico.com. (2020a). *Evaluation*. Retrieved from https://www.lexico.com/en/definition/evaluation

Lexico.com. (2020b). *Intersectionality*. Retrieved from https://www.lexico.com/definition/intersectionality

Lincoln, Y. S. (1991). The arts and sciences of program evaluation. *Evaluation Practice*, 12(1), 1–7

Lincoln, Y., & Guba, E. (1985). Research, evaluation and policy analysis: Heuristics and disciplined inquiry. *Policy Studies Review*, 5(3), 546–565.

Lindenberg, C. S., Solorzano, R. M., Vilaro, F. M., & Westbrook, L. O. (2001). Challenges and strategies for conducting intervention research with culturally diverse populations. *Journal of Transcultural Nursing*, 12, 132–139.

Linn, E. L. (1997). Evaluating the validity of assessments. The consequences of use. *Educational Measurement*, 16(2), 14–16.

Liptak, A. (2015, June 26). Supreme court ruling makes same-sex marriage a right nationwide. *New York Times*. Retrieved from https://www.nytimes.com/2015/06/27/us/supreme-court-same-sex-marriage.html

Liston, M., & Peoples, L. (2018, January 8). MIE TIG Week: Lessons learned as evaluators in urban education. *AEA365*. Retrieved from http://aea365.org/blog/mie-tig-week-lessons-learned-as-evaluators-in-urban-education-part-1-by-monique-liston-and-leah-peoples/

Lorde, A. (1984). The master's tools will never dismantle the master's house. In *Sister outsider: Essays and speeches* (pp. 110–114). Berkeley, CA: Crossing Press. Retrieved from https://collectiveliberation.org/wp-content/uploads/2013/01/Lorde_The_Masters_Tools.pdf

Mabry, L. (2004). Commentary: "Gray skies are gonna clear up." *American Journal of Evaluation, 25*(3), 385–390.

Mabry, L. (1999). Circumstantial ethics. *American Journal of Evaluation, 20*(2), 199–212.

MacDonald, B. (1976). Evaluation and the control of education. In D. Tawney (Ed.), *Curriculum evaluation today: Trends and implications* (pp. 125–134). London, UK: Macmillan.

Mackenzie, N., & Knipe, S. (2006). Research dilemmas: Paradigms, methods and methodology. *Issues in Educational Research, 16*(2), 1–11.

Madaus, G. F. (2004). Ralph W. Tyler's contribution to program evaluation. In M. C. Alkin (Ed.), *Evaluation roots: Tracing theorists' views and influences* (pp. 69–79). Thousand Oaks, CA: Sage.

Madaus, G. F., & Stufflebeam, D. L. (2000). Program evaluation: A historical overview. In D. L. Stufflebeam, G. F. Madaus, & T. Kellaghan (Eds.), *Evaluation models: Viewpoints on educational and human services evaluation* (2nd ed., pp. 3–18). Norwell, MA: Kluwer Academic.

Madaus, G. F., & Stufflebeam, D. L. (Eds.). (1989). *Educational evaluation: The classic works of Ralph W. Tyler.* Boston, MA: Kluwer-Nijhoff.

Madison, A. M. (2000). Language in defining social problems and in evaluating social programs. In R. Hopson (Ed.), How and why language matters in evaluation. *New Directions in Evaluation* (pp. 17–28). San Francisco, CA: Jossey-Bass.

Madison, A. M. (Ed.). (1992). Minority issues in program evaluation. *New Directions for Program Evaluation, 53*. San Francisco, CA: Jossey-Bass.

Make It Our Business. (2017, June 22). *What does it mean to be culturally competent?* London, ON, Canada: Centre for Research & Education on Violence Against Women & Children. Retrieved from http://makeitourbusiness.ca/blog/what-does-it-mean-be-culturally-competent

Maniccia, D. M., & Leone, J. M. (2019). Theoretical framework and protocol for the evaluation of Strong Through Every Mile (STEM), a structured running program for survivors of intimate partner violence. *BMC Public Health, 19*, 692.

Manzar, G. (2019, August 2). Seeing my science clearly. *Science, 365*(6452), 514.

Marin, G., & Marin, B. (1991). *Research with Hispanic populations.* Newbury Park, CA: Sage.

Mark, M. M. (2011). New (and old) directions for validity concerning generalizability. In H. T. Chen, S. I. Donaldson, & M. M. Mark (Eds.), *Advancing validity in outcome evaluation: Theory and practice. New Directions for Evaluation, 130,* 31–42.

Mark, M. M. (2003). Toward an integrative view of the theory and practice of program and policy evaluation. In S. I. Donaldson & M. Scriven (Eds.), *Evaluating social programs and problems: Visions for the new millennium* (pp. 183–204). Mahwah, NJ: Erlbaum.

Mark, M. M., Donaldson, S. I., & Campbell, B. (2011). The past, the present, and possible futures of social psychology and evaluation. In M. M. Mark, S. I. Donaldson, & B. Campbell (Eds.), *Social psychology and evaluation* (pp. 4–28). New York, NY: Guilford Press.

Mark, M. M., Greene, J. C., & Shaw, I. F. (2006). Introduction: The evaluation of policies, programs and practices. In I. F. Shaw, J. C. Greene, & M. M. Mark (Eds.), *The Sage handbook of evaluation* (pp. 1–30). Thousand Oaks, CA: Sage.

Marsh, K. (2010). Economic evaluation of criminal justice interventions: A methodological review of the recent literature. In K. Roman, .T. Dunworth, & K. Marsh (Eds.), *Cost-benefit analysis and crime control* (pp. 1–28). Washington, DC: Urban Institute Press.

Martin, D., Lee, C. D., & Bang, M. (2014, October 1). Point of view affects how science is done: Gender and culture influence research on a fundamental level. *Scientific American.* Retrieved from https://www.scientificamerican.com/article/point-of-view-affects-how-science-is-done/

Martin, J., Martin, N., & Martin, J. (2019, August 13). Miss Manners: If others wear jeans must I follow suit? *Washington Post: Advice.* Retrieved from https://www.washingtonpost.com/lifestyle/advice/miss-manners-if-others-wear-jeans-must-i-follow-suit/2019/08/11/8077f720-aff0-11e9-bc5c-e73b603e7f38_story.html

Martinez, A., Running Wolf, P., Big Foot, D., Randal, C., & Villegas, M. (2018). The process of becoming: A roadmap to evaluation in Indian country. In F. Cram, K. Tibbetts, & J. LaFrance (Eds.), *Indigenous evaluation. New Directions for Evaluation, 159,* 33–45

Mastroianni, A. C., Faden, R., & Federman, D. (Eds.). (1994). *Women and health research: ethical and legal issues of including women in clinical studies* (Vol. 1). Washington, DC: National Academies Press.

Mathison, S. (2007, October). *Ethical issues in evaluation.* Paper presented at the International Symposium on Evaluation, National Autonomous University of Mexico (UNMA), Ciudad Universitaria, Mexico.

Mathison, S. (1999, Summer). Rights, responsibilities, and duties: A comparison of ethics for internal and external evaluators. *New Directions for Evaluation, 82,* 25–34.

Mattlin, B. (1991, September 1). Personal perspective: An open letter to Jerry Lewis: The disabled need dignity, not pity. *Los Angeles Times.* Retrieved from https://www.latimes.com/archives/la-xpm-1991-09-01-op-2249-story.html

Maxwell, J. A. (2010). Using numbers in qualitative research. *Qualitative Inquiry, 16*(6), 475–482. Retrieved from https://www.researchgate.net/publication/258181991_Using_Numbers_in_Qualitative_Research

McCord, J. (1978). A thirty-year follow-up of treatment effects. *American Psychologist, 2,* 284–289.

McDavid, J. C., Huse, I., & Hawthorn, L. R. L. (2013). *Program evaluation and performance measurement: An introduction to practice* (2nd ed). Los Angeles, CA: Sage.

McDonald, G., Starr, G., Schooley, M., Yee, S. L., Klimowski, K., & Turner, K. (2001). Chapter 1: Engage stakeholders. *Introduction to program evaluation for comprehensive tobacco control programs.* Atlanta, GA: U.S. Department of Health and Human Services, Centers for Disease Control and Prevention

McDonald, J. H. (2014). Small numbers in chi-square and G-tests. *Handbook of biological statistics.* Retrieved from http://www.biostathandbook.com/small.html

McGarrell, E. F., & Sabath, M. J. (1994). Stakeholder conflict in an alternative sentencing program. *Evaluation and Program Planning, 17*(2), 179–186.

McHugh, M. C., Koeske, R. D., & Frieze, I. H. (1986, August). Issues to consider in conducting nonsexist psychological research: A guide for researchers. *American Psychologist, 41*, 879–890. Retrieved from https://www.researchgate.net/profile/Maureen_Mchugh2/publication/232521777_Issues_to_Consider_in_Conducting_Nonsexist_Psychological_Research_A_Guide_for_Researchers/links/5a089969aca272ed279ff20c/Issues-to-Consider-in-Conducting-Nonsexist-Psychological-Research-A-Guide-for-Researchers.pdf

McKillup, S. (2012). *Statistics explained: An introductory guide for life scientists* (2nd ed.). Cambridge, UK: Cambridge University Press.

McLaughlin, J. A., & Jordan, G. B. (2015). Using logic models. In K. E. Newcomer, H. P. Hatry, & J. S. Wholey (Eds.), *Handbook of practical program evaluation* (pp. 62–87). Hoboken, NJ: Wiley

McLaurin v. Oklahoma State Regents, 339 U.S. 637 (1950).

McNall, M., & Foster-Fishman, P. (2007). Methods of rapid evaluation, assessment, and appraisal. *American Journal of Evaluation, 28*(2), 151–168.

MDRC. (n.d.). *Opening doors*. Retrieved from https://www.mdrc.org/project/opening-doors#overview

Meleady, R., & Seger, C. R. (2016). Imagined contact encourages prosocial behavior towards outgroup members. *Group Processes & Intergroup Relations, 20*(4), 447–464.

Meriam Library. (2010, September 17). *Evaluating information: Applying the CRAAP Test*. California State University, Chico. Retrieved from https://library.csuchico.edu/sites/default/files/craap-test.pdf

Merriam-Webster. (2020a). Data. Retrieved from https://www.merriam-webster.com/dictionary/data

Merriam-Webster. (2020b). Framework. Retrieved from https://www.merriam-webster.com/dictionary/framework

Merriam-Webster. (2020c). Paradigm. Retrieved from https://www.merriam-webster.com/dictionary/paradigm

Merriam-Webster. (2020d). Standpoint. Retrieved from https://www.merriam-webster.com/dictionary/standpoint

Mertens, D. M. (2020). *Research and evaluation in education and psychology: Integrating diversity with quantitative, qualitative, and mixed measures* (5th ed.). Thousand Oaks, CA: Sage.

Mertens, D. M. (2013). What does a transformative lens bring to credible evidence in mixed methods evaluations? In D. M. Mertens & S. Hesse-Biber (Eds.), *Mixed methods and credibility of evidence in evaluation* (pp. 27–35). *New Directions for Evaluation, 138*.

Mertens, D. M. (2012). Transformative mixed methods: Addressing inequitites. *American Behavioral Scientist, 56*(6), 802–813.

Mertens, D. M. (2010). Transformative mixed methods research. *Qualitative Inquiry, 16*(6), 469–474.

Mertens, D. M. (2009). *Transformative research and evaluation*. New York, NY: Guilford Press.

Mertens, D. M. (2007). Transformative paradigm: Mixed methods and social justice. *Journal of Mixed Methods Research, 1*(3), 212–225.

Mertens, D. M. (2005). *Research and evaluation in education and psychology: Integrating diversity with quantitative, qualitative, and mixed methods* (2nd ed.). Thousand Oaks, CA: Sage.

Mertens, D. M. (2001). Inclusivity and transformation: Evaluation in 2010. *American Journal of Evaluation, 22*(3). 367–374.

Mertens, D. M. (2000). Deaf and hard of hearing people in court: Using emancipatory perspective to determine their needs. In C. Truman, D. M. Mertens, & B. Humphries (Eds.), *Research and inequity* (pp. 111–125). London, UK: Taylor & Francis.

Mertens, D. (1999). Inclusive evaluation: Implications of transformative theory for evaluation. *American Journal of Evaluation, 20*(1), 1–14.

Mertens, D. T., & Hesse-Biber, S. (Eds.). (2013). Mixed methods and credibility of evidence in evaluation. *New Directions for Evaluation, 138*, 5–13.

Mertens, D. M., Sullivan, M., Bledsoe, K., & Wilson, A. (2010). Utilization of mixed methods for transformative purposes. In C. Teddlie & A. Tashakkori (Eds.), *Handbook of mixed methods research* (2nd ed., pp. 193–214). Thousand Oaks, CA: Sage.

Mertens, D. M., & Wilson, T. (2019). *Program evaluation theory and practice: A comprehensive guide* (2nd ed.). New York, NY: Guilford Press.

Mertens, D. M., & Zimmerman, H. (2015). A transformative framework for culturally responsive evaluation. In S. Hood, R. Hopson, & H. Frierson (Eds.), *Continuing the journey to reposition culture and cultural context in evaluation theory and practice* (pp. 275–288). Charlotte, NC: Information Age.

Metz, S. S., Donohue, S., & Moore, C. (2012). Spatial skills: A focus on gender and engineering. In B. Bogue & E. Cady (Eds.), *Apply Research to Practice (ARP) resources*. http://www.engageengineering.org/associations/11559/files/ARP_SpatialSkills.pdf

Miles, B., & Huberman, A. M. (2009). *Qualitative data analysis*. Thousand Oaks, CA: Sage.

Minkler, M. (2004). Ethical challenges for the "outside" researcher in community-based participatory research. *Health Education & Behavior, 31*(6), 684–697.

Miron, G. (2004). *Evaluation report checklist*. Retrieved from https://wmich.edu/sites/default/files/attachments/u350/2014/evaluation-reports.pdf

Monin, B., & Miller, D. T. (2001). Moral credentials and the expression of prejudice. *Journal of Personality and Social Psychology, 81*, 33–43.

Moore, D., & Tananis, C. A. (2009). Measuring change in a short-term educational program using a retrospective pretest design. *American Journal of Evaluation, 30*(2), 189–202.

Morewedge, C. K., Yoon, H., Scopelliti, I., Symborski, C. W., Korris, J. H., & Kassam, K. S. (2015). Debiasing decisions improved decision making with a single training intervention. *Policy Insights From the Behavioral and Brain Sciences, 2*(11), 129–140.

Morgan, D. L. (2014). Pragmatism as a paradigm for social research. *Qualitative Inquiry, 20*, 1045–1053.

Morgan, K. P. (1996). Describing the emperor's new clothes: Three myths of educational in)equity. In Ann Dillan (Ed.), *The gender question in education: Theory, pedagogy, & politics* (pp. 105–122). Boulder, CO: Westview Press.

Morra-Imas, M., & Rist, R. (2009). *The road to results: Designing and conducting effective development evaluations*. Washington, DC: World Bank.

Morris, M. (2015). Research on evaluation ethics: Reflections and an agenda. In P. R. Brandon (Ed.), *Research on evaluation. New Directions for Evaluation, 148*, 31–42.

Morris, M. (Ed.). (2008). *Evaluation ethics for best practice: Cases and commentaries*. New York, NY: Guilford Press.

Morris, M., & Cohen, R. (1993). Program evaluators and ethical challenges: A national survey. *Evaluation Review, 17*, 621–642.

Morris, M., & Jacobs, L. R. (2000). You got a problem with that? Exploring evaluators' disagreements about ethics. *Evaluation Review, 24*(4), 384–406.

Mosavel, M., & Sanders, K. (2011). Needs of low-income African American cancer survivors: Multifaceted and practical. *Journal of Cancer Education, 26*(4), 717–723.

Moss-Racusin, C. A., Dovidio, J. F., Brescoll, V. L., Graham, M. J., & Handelsman. J. (2012). Science faculty's subtle gender biases favor male students. *PNAS Early Edition*, 1–6.

Mosteller, F. (1981, February 27). Innovation and evaluation. *Science, 7*(*4485*), 881–886.

Munteanu, C., Molyneaux, H., Wendy, M., Romero, M., O'Donnell, S., & Vines, J. (2015). Situational ethics: Re-thinking approaches to formal ethics requirements for human-computer interaction. *Proceedings of the 33rd Annual ACM Conference on Human Factors in Computing Systems* (pp. 105–114).

Murphy, M. C., Steele, C. M., & Gross, J. J. (2007). Signaling threat: How situational cues affect women in math, science, and engineering settings. *Psychological Science, 18*(10), 879–885.

Myrdal, G. (1944). *An American dilemma: The Negro problem and modern democracy*. New York, NY: Harper & Bros.

Nage, E. (1961). *The structure of science*. New York, NY: Harcourt, Brace and World.

Namit, K., & Seden, J. (2018, July 30). Reducing data collection bias in education research. *World Bank Blogs*. Retrieved from https://blogs.worldbank.org/education/reducing-data-collection-bias-education-research

National Academies of Science, Engineering, and Medicine. (2017). *Principles and practices for federal program evaluation: Proceedings of a workshop*. Washington, DC: National Academies Press.

National Center for Education Statistics. (2017). *The condition of education: Disability rates and employment status by educational attainment*. Retrieved from https://nces.ed.gov/programs/coe/indicator_tad.asp

National Center for Transgender Equality. (2018, October 5). *Understanding non-binary people: How to be respectful and supportive*. Retrieved from https://transequality.org/issues/resources/understanding-non-binary-people-how-to-be-respectful-and-supportive

National Commission for the Protection of Human Subjects of Biomedical and Behavioral Research. (1978). *The Belmont Report: Ethical principles and guidelines for the protection of human subjects of research*. Bethesda, MD: Author.

National Conference for Community and Justice. (2020). Social justice definitions. Retrieved from https://www.nccj.org/resources/social-justice-definitions

National Constitutional Center. (2019, June 12). On this day: Supreme Court rejects anti-interracial marriage laws. *Constitutional Daily*. Retrieved from https://constitutioncenter.org/blog/today-in-supreme-court-history-loving-v-virginia

National Council of Nonprofits. (n.d.). *Conflicts of interest*. Retrieved from https://www.councilofnonprofits.org/tools-resources/conflicts-of-interest

National Institutes of Health. (2019). *Exempt human subjects research: 8 exemptions*. Retrieved from https://grants.nih.gov/sites/default/files/exemption_infographic_v7_508c-3-21-19.pdf

National Institutes of Health. (2003, February 26). *Data sharing brochure*. Retrieved from https://grants.nih.gov/grants/policy/data_sharing/data_sharing_brochure.pdf

National Institutes of Health. (2003, March 5). *Data sharing policy and implementation guidance*. Retrieved from https://grants.nih.gov/grants/policy/data_sharing/data_sharing_guidance.htm

National Institutes of Health. (n.d.a). *Enhancing reproducibility through rigor and transparency*. Bethesda, MD: NIH Policy & Compliance. Retrieved from https://grants.nih.gov/reproducibility/index.htm

National Institutes of Health. (n.d.b). *Human subjects research—home page*. Retrieved from https://grants.nih.gov/policy/humansubjects.htm

National Science Foundation. (2014, December 26). *Chapter II. Proposal preparation instructions*. Retrieved from https://www.nsf.gov/pubs/policydocs/pappguide/nsf15001/gpg_2.jsp#IIC2j

National Science Foundation. (n.d.). *Dissemination and sharing of research results*. NSF data sharing policy. Retrieved from https://www.nsf.gov/bfa/dias/policy/dmp.jsp

Needle, R., Trotter, R., Singer, M., Bates, C., Page, G., Metzger, D. & Marcelin, L. H. (2003). Rapid assessment of the HIV/AIDS crisis in racial and ethnic minority communities: An approach for timely community interventions. *American Journal of Public Health, 93*(6), 970–979.

Nelson, A. (2002). Unequal treatment: Confronting racial and ethnic disparities in health care. *Journal of the National Medical Association, 94*(8), 666–668.

Nelson-Barber, S., LaFrance, J., Trumbull, E., & Aburto, S. (2005). Promoting culturally reliable and valid evaluation practice. In S. Hood, R. Hopson, & H. Frierson (Eds.), *The role of culture and cultural context: A mandate for inclusion, the discovery of truth, and understanding in evaluative theory and practice* (pp. 61–85.). Greenwich, CT: Information Age.

Neuman, L. W. (2000). *Social research methods: Qualitative and quantitative approaches* (4th ed.). Needham Heights, MA: Allyn & Bacon.

Newcomer, K. E., Hatry, H. P., & Wholey, J. S. (Eds.). (2015). *Handbook of practical program evaluation* (4th ed.). Hoboken, NJ: Jossey-Bass.

Newman, D., & Brown, R. (1996). *Applied ethics for program evaluation*. Thousand Oaks, CA: Sage.

Niemann, Y. F. (2015). The problem with the phrases "women and minorities" and "women and people of color." University of Colorado Press. Retrieved from https://upcolorado.com/about-us/news-features/item/2843-the-problem-with-the-phrases-women-and-minorities-and-women-and-people-of-color

Norris, A. L., Marcus, D. K. & Green, B. A. (2015). Homosexuality as a discrete class. *Psychological Science, 26*(12), 1843–1853.

Novak, M. (2009, December 29). *Social justice: Not what you think it is*. Heritage Foundation. Retrieved from https://www.heritage.org/poverty-and-inequality/report/social-justice-not-what-you-think-it

NPC & Clinks. (n.d.). *Improving the evidence: Using comparison group approaches to understand impact*. Retrieved February 13, 2018, from https://www.clinks.org/sites/default/files/UsingControlGroupApproachesToIdentifyImpact.pdf

Nyren, E. (2017, December 5). Beyoncé presents Colin Kaepernick with SI Muhammad Ali Legacy Award. *Variety*. Retrieved from https://variety.com/2017/music/news/beyonce-colin-kaepernick-si-muhammad-ali-legacy-award-1202631812/

Oak, V. V. (1938). Evaluation of business curricula in Negro colleges. *The Journal of Negro Education, 7*(1), 19–31.

Office for the Protection of Human Subjects. (2014). *Informed consent in human subjects research*. Los Angeles: University of Southern California.

Oliver, M. (1996). A sociology of disability or a disablist sociology? In L. Barton (Ed.), *Disability and society: Emerging issues and insights* (pp. 18–42). Harrow, UK: Longman.

Olsson, M., & Martiny, S. E. (2018). Does exposure to counterstereotypical role models influence girls' and women's gender stereotypes and career choices? A review of social psychological research. *Frontiers in Psychology, 9*, 2264. Retrieved from https://www.ncbi.nlm.nih.gov/pmc/articles/PMC6292925/

Oluo, I. (2019, March 28). Confronting racism is not about the needs and feelings of white people. *The Guardian*. Retrieved from https://www.theguardian.com/commentisfree/2019/mar/28/confronting-racism-is-not-about-the-needs-and-feelings-of-white-people?fbclid=IwAR2HZL8tU0QeKfiGlwAPFpq3a71vhLFLvtlIQv_PRNWBVPZe-xkZOHcmiLE

Ontario Human Rights Commission. (n.d.). *Racial discrimination, race and racism (fact sheet)*. Retrieved from http://www.ohrc.on.ca/en/racial-discrimination-race-and-racism-fact-sheet

Oral History Project Team. (2009). The professional development of Eleanor Chelimsky. *American Journal of Evaluation, 30*(2), 232–244.

Oral History Project Team. (2004). The professional development of Lois-Ellin Datta. *American Journal of Evaluation, 25*(2), 243–253.

Oregon State University. (n.d.). *Comparison: Characteristics of human subject research vs. other project types*. Retrieved from https://research.oregonstate.edu/sites/research.oregonstate.edu/files/irb/comparison_research_v_non_research_v01292018.pdf

Orfield, G., & Frankenberg, E. (2014, May 15). *Brown at 60: Great progress, a long retreat and an uncertain future*. The Civil Rights Project. University of California, Los Angeles. Retrieved from https://civilrightsproject.ucla.edu/research/k-12-education/integration-and-diversity/brown-at-60-great-progress-a-long-retreat-and-an-uncertain-future

Organisation for Economic Co-operation and Development. (1991). *Principles for evaluation of development assistance*. Paris, France: Author. Retrieved from https://www.oecd.org/dac/evaluation/50584880.pdf

Osterwalder, A., & Pigneur, Y. (2010). *Business model generation: A handbook for visionaries, game changers, and challengers*. New York, NY: Wiley.

O'Sullivan, R. G. (2012). Collaborative evaluation within a framework of stakeholder-oriented evaluation approaches. *Evaluation and Program Planning, 35*(4), 518–522. Retrieved from https://www.ncbi.nlm.nih.gov/pubmed/22364849

O'Sullivan, R. (2004). *Practicing evaluation: A collaborative approach*. Thousand Oaks, CA: Sage.

O'Sullivan, R. G., & D'Agostino, A. (2002). Promoting evaluation through collaboration with community-based programs for young children and their families. *Evaluation, 3*, 372–387.

Oxendine, J. K. (2014, April 8). *Native American medicine wheel: Comparison in life*. Retrieved from http://www.powwows.com/2014/04/08/native-american-medicine-wheel-comparison-in-life/#ixzz3yqMJkAOe

Oxford University Press. (2016). *Word of the Year 2016*. Retrieved from https://en.oxforddictionaries.com/word-of-the-year/word-of-the-year-2016

Palumbo, D. J., & Hallett, M. A. (1993). Conflict versus consensus models in policy evaluation and implementation. *Evaluation and Program Planning, 16*, 11–23.

Pannucci, C. J., & Wilkins, E. G. (2010). Identifying and avoiding bias in research. *Plastic and Constructuive Surgery, 126*(2), 619–625. Retrieved from https://www.ncbi.nlm.nih.gov/pmc/articles/PMC2917255/

Parker, L. (2004). Commentary: Can critical theories of or on race be used in evaluation. In V. G. Thomas & F. I. Stevens (Eds.), *Co-constructing a contextually responsive evaluation framework: The Talent Development Model of School Reform* (pp. 85–93). New Directions for Evaluation, 101.

Parlee, M. (1975). Psychology. *Signs: A Journal of Women in Culture and Society, 1*, 119–138. Retrieved from http://www.scielo.org.za/pdf/hts/v74n1/06.pdf

Parsons, B. (2013). *ZIPPER: A mnemonic for systems-based evaluation*. Ft. Collins, CO: InSites. Retrieved from http://insites.org/resource/zipper-a-mnemonic-for-systems-based-evaluation/

Parsons, B. (2010). *Using complexity science concepts when designing system interventions and evaluations*. Ft. Collins, CO: InSites. Retrieved from http://www.insites.org

Parsons, B., Jessup, P., & Moore, M. (2016). *A complex-systems evaluation orientation to support a culture of health*. Ft. Collins, CO: InSites.

Patterson, E. (2018a, March 3). Tyranny of quantification. *Realize Engineering*. Retrieved from https://realizeengineering.blog/2018/03/07/tyranny-of-quantification/

Patterson, E. (2018b, November 28). Epistemic triage. *Realize Engineering*. Retrieved from https://realizeengineering.blog/tag/julian-baggini/

Patterson, E. A., Busch-Vishniac, I., Campbell, P. B., & Guillaume, D. W. (2011, June). The effect of context on student engagement in engineering. *European Journal of Engineering Education, 36*(3), 211–224.

Patton, M. Q. (2012). *Essentials of utilization-focused evaluation*. Thousand Oaks, CA: Sage.

Patton, M. Q. (2011). *Developmental evaluation: Applying complexity concepts to enhance innovation and use*. New York, NY: Guilford.

Patton, M. Q. (2010). On developmental evaluation. *AEA365*. Retrieved from https://aea365.org/blog/michael-quinn-patton-on-developmental-evaluation-applying-complexity-concepts-to-enhance-innovation-and-use/

Patton, M. Q. (2008). *Utilization-focused evaluation* (4th ed.). Thousand Oaks, CA: Sage.

Patton, M. Q. (2006). Evaluation for the way we work. *The Nonprofit Quarterly, 13*(1), 28–33.

Patton, M. Q. (2003). *Qualitative evaluation checklist*. Retrieved from http://wmich.edu/evaluation/checklists

Patton, M. Q. (2002). Qualitative evaluation and research methods. Newbury Park, CA: Sage.

Patton, M. Q. (2000). Overview: Language matters. In R. Hopson (Ed.), *How and why language matters in evaluation* (pp. 5–16). San Francisco, CA: Jossey-Bass.

Patton, M. Q. (1999). Some framing questions about racism and evaluation: Thoughts stimulated by Professor John Stanfield's "Slipping through the front door." *American Journal of Evaluation, 20*(3), 437–443.

Patton, M. Q. (1997). *Utilization-focused evaluation: The new century text* (3rd ed.). Thousand Oaks, CA: Sage.

Patton, M. Q. (1996). A world larger than formative and summative. *Evaluation Practice, 17*(2), 131–144.

Patton, M. Q. (1980). *Qualitative evaluation methods*. Beverly Hills, CA: Sage.

Patton, M. Q. (1978). *Utilization-focused evaluation*. Beverly Hills, CA: Sage.

Pawson, R., & Tilley, N. (1997). *Realistic evaluation*. London, England: Sage.

Pellegrini, A. D. (2011). "In the eye of the beholder": Sex bias in observations and ratings of students' aggression. *Educational Researcher, 40*(6), 281–286.

Pennington, C. R., Heim, D. L., Levy, A. R., & Larkin, D. T. (2016). Twenty years of stereotype threat research: A review of psychological mediators. *PLoS ONE*. Retrieved from https://journals.plos.org/plosone/article?id=10.1371/journal.pone.0146487

Peoples, B. K., Midway, S. R., Sackett, D., Lynch, A., & Cooney, P. B. (2016). Twitter predicts citation rates of ecological research. *PLoS ONE*. Retrieved from https://journals.plos.org/plosone/article?id=10.1371/journal.pone.0166570

Perrin, B. (2019). How to manage pressure to change reports: Should evaluators be above criticism? *American Journal of Evaluation, 40*(3), 354–375.

Perrin, B. (2000). Donald T. Campbell and the art of practical "in-the-trenches" program evaluation. In L. Bickman (Ed.), *Validity & social experimentation: Donald Campbell's legacy* (pp. 267–282). Thousand Oaks, CA: Sage.

Pétervári, J. (2017). *Dance your PhD 2017: Building up creativity*. Retrieved from https://www.youtube.com/playlist?list=PLybCEj22itwAaf-OQNmxmmMeF1fXnAGv1

Pettigrew, T. F., & Tropp, L. R. (2006). A meta-analytic test of intergroup contact theory. *Journal of Personality and Social Psychology, 90*(5), 751–783.

Pheterson, G. I., Kiesler, S. B., & Goldberg, P. A. (1971). Evaluation of the performance of women as a function of their sex, achievement, and personal history. *Journal of Personality and Social Psychology, 19*(1), 114–118.

Phillips, G., Lindeman, P., Adames, C. N., Bettin, E., Bayston, C., Stonehouse, P., . . . Greene, G. J. (2019). Empowerment evaluation: A case study of citywide implementation within an HIV prevention context. *American Journal of Evaluation, 40*(3), 318–334.

Phillips, D. (2019, March 13). New rule for transgender troops: Stick to your birth sex, or leave. *New York Times*. Retrieved from https://www.nytimes.com/2019/03/13/us/transgender-troops-ban.html

Phillips, D. I., & Clancy, K. J. (1972). Some effects of "social desirability" in survey studies. *American Journal of Sociology, 77*(5), 921–940.

PlainLanguage.gov. (n.d.). *What is plain language?* Retrieved from https://www.plainlanguage.gov/about/definitions/

Polit, D. F., & Beck, C. T. (2011). Generalization in quantitative and qualitative research: Myths and strategies. *International Journal of Nursing Studies, 47*, 1451–1458

Ponterotto, J. G. (2005). Qualitative research in counseling psychology: A primer on research paradigms and philosophy of science. *Journal of Counseling Psychology, 52*(2), 126–136.

Porter, S. (2018, September 6). Leaving no one behind in our evaluation practice. *Oxfam Views and Voices*. Retrieved from https://views-voices.oxfam.org.uk/2018/09/leaving-no-one-behind-in-our-evaluation-practice/

Posavac, E. J., & Carey, R. G. (1980). *Program evaluation*. Englewood Cliffs, NJ: Prentice-Hall.

Powell, J., Heller, C. C. & Bundalli, F. (2011, June). *Systems think and race* (Workshop summary). Los Angeles: The California Endowment.

Powers, E. (1951). *An experiment in the prevention of delinquency*. New York, NY: Columbia University Press.

Preskill, H., & Beer, T. (2012). *Evaluating social innovation*. Washington, DC: FSG and the Centre for Evaluation Innovation. Retrieved from http://www.evaluationinnovation.org/sites/default/files/EvaluatingSocialInnovation.pdf

Preskill, H., & Jones, N. (2009). *A practical guide for engaging stakeholders in developing evaluation questions*. Princeton, NJ: Robert Wood Johnson Foundation.

Preskill, H., & Lynn, J. (2016, February 1). Redefining rigor: Describing quality evaluation in complex, adaptive settings. *FSG: Reimagining Social Change*. Retrieved from https://www.fsg.org/blog/redefining-rigor-describing-quality-evaluation-complex-adaptive-settings

Project Implicit. (2011a). About the IAT. Cambridge, MA: Harvard University. Retrieved from https://implicit.harvard.edu/implicit/iatdetails.html

Project Implicit. (2011b). Frequently asked questions. Cambridge, MA: Harvard University. Retrieved from https://implicit.harvard.edu/implicit/faqs.html

Pruitt, S. (2018, August 22). US military lifts ban on women in combat. *History.com*. Retrieved from https://www.history.com/news/u-s-military-lifts-ban-on-women-in-combat

Purdie-Vaughns, V., Steele, C. M., Davis, P. G., Ditlmann, R., & Crosby, J. R. (2008). Social identity contingencies: How diversity cues signal threat or safety for African Americans in mainstream institutions. *Journal of Personality and Social Psychology, 94*(4), 615–630. Retrieved from http://www.yale.edu/intergroup/PurdieVaughns.Steele.Davies.Ditlmann.Crosby.pdf

Purdue Online Writing Lab. (n.d.). *Active versus passive voice*. Retrieved from https://owl.purdue.edu/owl/general_writing/academic_writing/active_and_passive_voice/active_versus_passive_voice.html

Regner, I., Thinus-Blanc, C., Netter, A., Schmakder, T., & Huguet, P. (2019). Committees with implicit biases promote fewer women when they do not believe gender bias exists. *Nature, 3*, 1171–1179. Retried from https://www.nature.com/articles/s41562-019-0686

Reichardt, C. S., & Rallis, S. F. (1994). Qualitative and quantitative inquiries are not incompatible: A call for a new partnership. *New Directions for Program Evaluation, 61*, 85–91.

Reiche, S. (2012, December 5). *Want to become more culturally competent? Start with your cultural self-awareness*. IESE Business School, University of Navarra. Retrieved from https://blog.iese.edu/expatriatus/2012/12/05/want-to-become-more-culturally-competent-start-with-your-cultural-self-awareness/

Resnik, D. B. (2015, December 1). What is ethics in research & why is it important? *Research*. Bethesda, MD: National Institute of Environmental Health Sciences. Retrieved from https://www.niehs.nih.gov/research/resources/bioethics/whatis/index.cfm

Retief, M., & Letšosa, R. (2018). Models of disability: A brief overview. *HTS Teologiese Studies/Theological Studies, 74*(1), 1–8.

Reynolds, M. (2007). Evaluation based on critical systems heuristics. In B. Williams & I. Imam (Eds.), *Systems concepts in evaluation: An expert anthology* (pp. 101–122). Point Reyes, CA: Edge Press.

Rice, L. (2019, February 15). Long before redlining: Racial disparities in homeownership need intentional policies. *Shelterforce*. Retrieved from https://shelterforce.org/2019/02/15/long-before-redlining-racial-disparities-in-homeownership-need-intentional-policies/

Riley, D. (2017): Rigor/us: Building boundaries and disciplining diversity. *Journal of Engineering Studies, 9*(3) 249–265.

Rittel, H. W. J., & Webber, M. M. (1973). Dilemmas in the general theory of planning. *Policy Sciences, 4*, 155–169.

Robinson, S. (2014, January 18). Ask a brilliant question, get an eloquent answer. *Blog*. Retrieved from https://www.sheilabrobinson.com/2014/01/18/ask-a-brilliant-question-get-an-elegant-answer/

Robles, J., Venkateswaran, N., & Feldman, J. (2018, October 3). NPF TIG Week: Stakeholders come first: Reflecting on lessons learned from prioritizing truth in evaluations. *AEA365*. Retrieved from https://aea365.org/blog/npf-tig-week-stakeholders-come-first-reflecting-on-lessons-learned-from-prioritizing-truth-in-evaluations-by-jessica-robles-nitya-venkateswaran-and-jay-feldman/

Robson, C. (2000). *Small-scale evaluation*. Thousand Oaks, CA: Sage.

Rog, D. J., Fitzpatrick, J. L., & Conner, R. F. (2012). Editor's notes. In D. J. Rog, J. L. Fitzpatrick, & R. F. Conner (Eds.), *Context: A framework for its influence on evaluation practice. New Directions for Evaluation, 135*.

Rosenstein, B., & Syna, H. D. (2015). Editors' notes. In B. Rosenstein & H. D. Syna (Eds.), *Evaluation and social justice in complex sociopolitical contexts* (pp. 3–8). *New Directions for Evaluation, 146*.

Rosenstock, I. (1974). Historical origins of the health belief model. *Health Education & Behavior, 2*(4), 328–335.

Ross, L., & Cronbach, L. (1976). Handbook of evaluation research: Essay review. *Educational Researcher, 5*(10), 9–19.

Rossi, P. H., & Berk, R. A. (1990). *Thinking about program evaluation*. Newbury Park, CA: Sage.

Rossi, P. H., & Freeman, H. E. (1979). *Evaluation: A systematic approach*. Beverly Hills, CA: Sage.

Rossi, P. H., Lipsey, M. W., & Freeman, H. E. (2004). *Evaluation: A systematic approach* (7th ed.). Newbury Park, CA: Sage.

Rossi, P. H., Lipsey, M. W., & Henry, G. T. (2019). *Evaluation: A systematic approach* (8th ed.). Thousand Oaks, CA: Sage.

Rossi, P. H., & Wright, J. D. (1984). Evaluation research: An assessment. *Annual Review of Sociology, 10*, 331–352.

Rothman, J. (1977). Action evaluation and conflict resolution training: Theory, method and case study. *International Negotiation, 2*, 451–470.

Rougier, N. P., Droettboom, M., & Bourne, P. E. (2014). Ten simple rules for better figures. *PLOS Computational Biology*. Retrieved from https://journals.plos.org/ploscompbiol/article?id=10.1371/journal.pcbi.1003833 sharable

Rouse, M. (2012). Data visualization. *Essential Guide*. Retrieved from https://searchbusinessanalytics.techtarget.com/definition/data-visualization

Royse, D., Thyer, B., & Padgett, D. (2010). *Program evaluation: An introduction* (5th ed.). Belmont, CA: Wadsworth Cengage Learning.

Rubington, E., & Weinberg, M. S. (2010). *The study of social problems: Seven perspectives* (7th ed.). New York, NY: Oxford University Press.

Ryan, A. G. (1988). Program evaluation within the paradigms: Mapping the territory. *Knowledge: Creation, Diffusion, Utilization, 10*(1), 25–47.

Ryan, K. (2005). Democratic evaluation approaches for equity and inclusion. *Evaluation Exchange, XI*, 3, 1.

Ryan, P., & Dundon, T. (2008). Case research interviews: Eliciting superior quality data. *International Journal of Case Method Research & Application, 4*, 443–450.

Ryan, W. (1976). *Blaming the victim* (Rev. ed.). New York, NY: Vintage Books.

Salabarría-Peña, Y., Apt, B. S., & Walsh, C. M. (2007). *Practical use of program evaluation among sexually transmitted disease (STD) programs*. Atlanta, GA: Centers for Disease Control and Prevention.

Saldana, J. (2008). *The coding manual for qualitative researchers*. Thousand Oaks, CA: Sage. Retrieved from https://www.sagepub.com/sites/default/files/upm-binaries/24614_01_Saldana_Ch_01.pdf

Salkind, N. J. (2008). Cultural deficit model In N. J. Salkind (Ed.), *Encyclopedia of educational psychology*. Thousand Oaks, CA: Sage. Retrieved from http://sk.sagepub.com/reference/educationalpsychology/n60.xml

Salsberg, R., & Kastanis, A. (2018). Analysis: Blacks largely left out of high-paying jobs, government data shows. *USA Today: Money*. Retrieved from https://www.usatoday.com/story/money/2018/04/02/analysis-blacks-largely-left-out-high-paying-jobs-government-data-shows/477845002/

Samuels, M., & Ryan, K. (2011). Grounding evaluations in culture. *American Journal of Evaluation, 32,* 183–198.

Sandison, P. (2003). *Desk review of real-time evaluation experience.* New York, NY: UNICEF.

Sanzone, L. A., Lee, J. Y., Divaris, K., DeWalt, D. A., Baker, A. D., & Vann, W. F., Jr. (2013). A cross sectional study examining social desirability bias in caregiver reporting of children's oral health behaviors. *BMC Oral Health,* 13–24.

Schuetz, J. (2017, December 8). Metro areas are still racially segregated. Washington, DC: Brookings Institution. Retrieved from https://www.brookings.edu/blog/the-avenue/2017/12/08/metro-areas-are-still-racially-segregated/

Schuller, S. K., Yaffee, S. L., Higgs, S. K., Mogelgaard, K., & DeMattia, E. A. (2006). *Evaluation sourcebook: Measures of progress for ecosystem- and community based projects.* Ecosystem Management Initiative. Ann Arbor: University of Michigan. Retrieved from http://seas.umich.edu/ecomgt/evaluation/pdf/EMI_SOURCEBOOK_August_2006.pdf

Schweitzer, I. (2017). What is women's and gender studies? In D. Rockmore (Ed.), *What are the arts and sciences: A guide for the curious* (pp. 328–338). Hanover, NH: Dartmouth College Press.

Scriven, M. (1996). The theory behind practical evaluation. *Evaluation, 2*(4), 393–404.

Scriven, M. (1994). Evaluation as a discipline. *Studies in Educational Evaluation, 20,* 147–166.

Scriven, M. S. (Ed.). (1993). Hard-won lessons in program evaluation. *New Directions for Evaluation, 58.*

Scriven, M. (1991). *Evaluation thesaurus* (4th ed.). Thousand Oaks, CA: Sage.

Scriven, M. (1969). An introduction to metaevaluation. *Educational Products Report, 2,* 36–38.

Scriven, M. (1967). The methodology of evaluation. In R.W. Tyler, R. M. Gagne, & M. Scriven (Eds.), *Perspectives of curriculum evaluation* (pp. 39–83). Chicago, IL: Rand McNally.

Segone, M. (2012). Evaluation to accelerate progress toward equality, social justice and human rights. In *Evaluation for equitable development results* (pp. 2–12). New York, NY: UNICEF Evaluation Office.

Seidel, J. V. (1998). *Qualitative data analysis.* Retrieved from www.qualisresearch.com (Originally published as Qualitative data analysis. In *The ethnograph v5.0: A users guide, Appendix E.* Colorado Springs, CO: Qualis Research.

Seigart, D. M., & Brisolara, S. (Eds.). (2002). Feminist evaluation: Explorations and experiences. *New Directions in Evaluation, 96.*

Sen, A. (2011). *The idea of justice.* Cambridge, MA: Harvard University Press.

SenGupta, S., Hopson, R., & Thompson-Robinson, M. (2004). Cultural competence in evaluation: An overview. *New Directions for Evaluation, 2004*(102), 5–19. Retrieved from https://onlinelibrary.wiley.com/doi/abs/10.1002/ev.112

Sezer, O., Gino, F., & Bazerman, M. H. (2015). Ethical blind spots: Explaining unintentional unethical behavior. *Current Opinion in Psychology, 6,* 77–81.

Shadish, W. R. (1998). Evaluation theory is who we are. *American Journal of Evaluation, 19*(1), 1–19.

Shadish, W. R., Cook, T. D., & Leviton, L. C. (1991). *Foundations of program evaluations: Theories of practice.* Newbury Park, CA: Sage.

Shadish, W. R., & Epstein, R. E. (1987). Patterns of program evaluation practice among members of the Evaluation Research Society and Evaluation Network. *Evaluation Review, 11,* 555–590.

Shadish, W. R., & Luellen, J. (2005). History of evaluation. In S. Mathison (Ed.), *Encyclopedia of evaluation* (pp. 184–186). Thousand Oaks, CA: Sage.

Shadish, W. R., & Luellen, J. K. (2004). Donald Campbell: The accidental evaluator. In M. Alkin (Ed.), *Evaluation roots: Tracing theorists' views and influences* (pp. 80–87). Thousand Oaks, CA: Sage.

Shakeshaft, C., Baker, G., Campbell, P., Dwyer, C., Guerrer, T., & Murphy, R. (1985). AERA guidelines for eliminating race and sex bias in educational research and evaluation. *Educational Researcher, 14*(6), 16–17.

Shapiro, J. S. (1988). Participatory evaluation: Towards a transformative assessment for women's studies programs and projects. *Educational Evaluation and Policy Analysis, 10,* 191–199.

Shedlin, M. G., Decena, C. U., Mangadu, T., & Martinez, A. (2011). Research participant recruitment in Hispanic communities: Lessons learned. *Journal of Immigrant and Minority Health, 13,* 352–360.

Sheltzer, J. M., & Smith, J. C. (2014). Elite male faculty in the life sciences employ fewer women. *Proceedings of the National Academy of Sciences, 111,* 10107–10112.

Shetterly, M. L. (2016). *Hidden figures: The American Dream and the untold story of the Black women mathematicians who helped win the space race.* New York, NY: HarperCollins.

Siegel, S. (1956). *Nonparametric statistics for the behavioral sciences.* New York, NY: McGraw-Hill.

Sielbeck-Bowen, K. A., Brisolara, S., Deigart, D., Tischler, X., & Whitmore, E. (2002). Exploring feminist evaluation: The ground from which we rise. In D. M. Seigart & S. Brisolara (Eds.), *Feminist evaluation: Explorations and experiences. New Directions in Evaluation, 96,* 3–8.

Sielbeck-Mathes, K., & Selove, R. (2014). FIE TIG Week: Kathryn Sielbeck-Mathes and Rebecca Selove on feminist evaluation and framing. *AEA365.* Retrieved from https://aea365.org/blog/fie-tig-week-kathryn-sielbeck-mathes-and-rebecca-selove-on-feminist-evaluation-and-framing/

Silverman, M., Ricci, E. M., & Gunter, M. J. (1990). Strategies for increasing the rigor of qualitative methods in evaluation of health care programs. *Evaluation Review, 14*(1), 57–74.

Siminoff, L. A., & Step, M. M. (2011). A comprehensive observational coding scheme for analyzing instrumental, affective, and relational communication in health care contexts. *Journal of Health Communication, 16*(2), 178–197. Retrieved from https://www.ncbi.nlm.nih.gov/pmc/articles/PMC3147015/

Sinar, E. (2016, February 14). Data visualization types you should be using more (and how to start). *Medium.* Retrieved from https://medium.com/@EvanSinar/7-data-visualization-types-you-should-be-using-more-and-how-to-start-4015b5d4adf2

Sinclair, S., Hardin, C. D., & Lowery, B. S. (2006). Self-stereotyping in the context of multiple social identities. *Journal of Personality and Social Psychology*, 90(4), 529–542. Retrieved from https://psych.princeton.edu/psychology/research/sinclair/pubs/self%20stereo%20and%20multiple%20identities.PDF 8/30, 2019

Sipuel v. Board of Regents, 332 U.S. 631 (1948).

Skloot, R. (2010). *The immortal life of Henrietta Lacks*. New York, NY: Crown.

Small Business Administration. (n.d.a). *Choose a business structure*. Retrieved from https://www.sba.gov/starting-business/choose-your-business-structure/sole-proprietorship

Small Business Administration. (n.d.b). *Write your business plan*. Retrieved from https://www.sba.gov/business-guide/plan-your-business/write-your-business-plan

Smith, L., & Kliene, P. F. (1986). Qualitative research and evaluation: Triangulation and multimethods reconsidered. *New Directions for Program Evaluation*, 30, 55–71.

Smith, M. F. (2005). Evaluability assessment. In S. Mathison (Ed.), *Encyclopedia of evaluation* (pp. 136–139). Thousand Oaks, CA: Sage.

Smith, N. L. (2010). Characterizing the evaluand in evaluating theory. *American Journal of Evaluation*, 31(3), 383–389.

Smith, N. L. (1994). Clarifying and expanding the application of program theory-driven evaluations. *Evaluation Practice*, 15(1), 83-87.

Smith, N. L., & Brandon, P. R. (Eds.). (2008). *Fundamental issues in evaluation*. New York, NY: Guilford Press.

Smith, V. S. (2013). Data dashboard as evaluation and research communication tool. *New Directions for Evaluation*, 140, 21–45

Social Security Administration. (2019). *OASDI and SSI program rates & limits, 2019*. Retrieved from https://www.ssa.gov/policy/docs/quickfacts/prog_highlights/RatesLimits2019.html

Solano-Flores, G. (2011). Assessing the cultural validity of assessment practices: An introduction. In M. R. Basterra, E. Trumbull, & G. Solano-Flores (Eds.), *Cultural validity in assessment*. Bethesda, MD: MidAtlantic Equity Coalition.

Solórzano, D. G. (1997). Images and words that wound: Critical race theory, racial stereotyping, and teacher education. *Teacher Education Quarterly*, 24, 5–19.

Solórzano, D. G., & Yosso, T. J. (2002). Critical race methodology: Counter-storytelling as an analytical framework for education research. *Qualitative Inquiry*, 8(1), 23–44.

SparkNotes. (2020). *Society and culture: Hierarchy of cultures*. Retrieved from https://www.sparknotes.com/sociology/society-and-culture/section6/

Spaulding, D. T. (2014). *Program evaluation in practice: Core concepts and examples for discussion*. San Francisco, CA: Jossey-Bass.

Spencer, S. J., Steele, C. M., & Quinn, D. M. (1999). Stereotype threat and women's math performance. *Journal of Experimental Social Psychology*, 35, 4–28.

Staats, C., Capatosto, K., Tenney, L., & Mamo, S. (2017). Preface. *State of the Science: Implicit Bias Review*. Columbus: Kirwan Institute for the Study of Race and Ethnicity, The Ohio State University. Retrieved from http://kirwaninstitute.osu.edu/wp-content/uploads/2017/11/2017-SOTS-final-draft-02.pdf

Stake, R. E. (2005). Qualitative case studies. In N. K. Denzin & Y. S. Lincoln (Eds.), *The Sage handbook of qualitative research* (p. 443–466). Thousand Oaks, CA: Sage.

Stake, R. E. (1976). A theoretical statement of responsive evaluation. *Studies in Educational Evaluation*, 2(l), 19–22

Stake, R. (1975). To evaluate an arts program. In R. Stake (Ed.), *Evaluating the arts in education: A responsive approach* (pp. 13–31). Columbus, OH: Merrill.

Stake, R. E. (1974). *Nine approaches to educational evaluation*. Urbana: University of Illinois.

Stame, N. (2010). What doesn't work? Three failures, many answers. *Evaluation*, 16(4), 371–387.

Stanfield, J. H. (1993). African American traditions of civic responsibility. *Nonprofit and Voluntary Sector Quarterly*, 22(2), 137–153.

Stanfield, J. H. (1999). Slipping through the front door: Relevant social scientific evaluation in the people of color century. *American Journal of Evaluation*, 20(3), 415–431.

Stangor, C., Tarry, H., & Jhangiani, R. (2014). *Principles of social psychology* (1st international ed.). Retrieved from https://ecampusontario.pressbooks.pub/socialpsychology1interntl/

Stanovich, K. E. (2010). *Decision making and rationality in the modern world*. New York, NY: Oxford University Press.

Statistics How To. (2016, September 17). *Familywise error rate (alpha inflation): Definition*. Retrieved from https://www.statisticshowto.datasciencecentral.com/familywise-error-rate/

Steele, C. M., & Aronson, J. (1995). Stereotype threat and the intellectual test performance of African Americans. *Journal of Personality and Social Psychology*, 69(5), 797–811.

Steele, C. M., Spencer, S. J., & Arronson, J. (2002). Contending with group image. The psychology of stereotype and social identity threat. *Advances in Experimental Social Psychology*, 62(34), 379–440.

Stevens, F. L. (2000). Reflections and interviews: Information collected about training minority evaluators of math and science projects. In *The cultural context of educational evaluation: The role of minority professionals. Workshop proceedings* (pp. 41–46). Alexandria, VA: National Science Foundation, Directorate for Education and Human Resources, Division of Research, Evaluation and Communication.

Stevens, S. S. (1946). On theory of scales of measurement. *Science*, 103(2684), 677–680.

Stewart, D. W., Shamdasani, P. N, & Rook, D. W. (2002). *Focus groups: Theory and practice*. Thousand Oaks, CA: Sage.

Stone, C., Trisi, D., Sherman, A., & Taylor, R. (2018, March 15). *A guide to statistics on historical trends in income inequality*. Washington, DC: Center on Budget and Policy Priorities.

Streuning, E., & Guttentag, M. (1975). *Handbook of evaluation research*. Beverly Hills, CA: Sage.

Stufflebeam, D. (2004). The 21st-century CIPP model: origins, development, and use. In M. C. Alkin (Ed.), *Evaluation roots* (pp. 245–266). Thousand Oaks, CA: Sage.

Stufflebeam, D. L. (2001a). Evaluation models. *New Directions for Evaluation, 89*.

Stufflebeam, D. L. (2001b). The metaevaluation imperative. *American Journal of Evaluation, 22*(2), 183–209.

Stufflebeam, D. L. (1971). The relevance of the CIPP evaluation model for educational accountability. *Journal of Research and Development in Education, 5*, 14–28.

Stufflebeam, D. L., & Coryn, C. L. S. (2014). *Evaluation theory, models, and applications* (2nd ed.). San Francisco, CA: Jossey-Bass.

Stufflebeam, D. L., & Shinkfield, A. J. (2007). *Evaluation theory, models, and applications*. San Francisco, CA: Jossey-Bass.

Stufflebeam, D. L., & Shinkfield, A. J. (1988). *Systematic evaluation: A self-instructional guide to theory and practice* (3rd ed.). Norwell, MA: Kluwer Academic.

Stufflebeam, D. L., & Zhang, G. (2017). *The CIPP evaluation model: How to evaluate for improvement and accountability*. New York, NY: Guilford Press.

Substance Abuse and Mental Health Services Administration. (2019, June). *A guide to SAMHSA's strategic prevention framework*. Retrieved from https://www.samhsa.gov/sites/default/files/20190620-samhsa-strategic-prevention-framework-guide.pdf

Substance Abuse and Mental Health Services Administration. (2015). Retrieved from https://www.samhsa.gov/capt/tools-learning-resources/reporting-evaluation-results

Suchman, E. A. (1967). *Evaluative research: Principles and practice in public service and social action programs*. New York, NY: Russell Sage Foundation.

Sulewski, J. S., & Gothberg, J. (2013). *Universal design for evaluation checklist* (4th ed.). Retrieved from http://comm.eval.org/HigherLogic/System/DownloadDocumentFile.ashx?DocumentFileKey=8afd48c6-39c3-4dad-9629-1ed7c2654f3f&forceDialog=0

Sullivan, G. M. (2011). Getting off the "Gold Standard": Randomized controlled trials and education research. *Journal of Graduate Medical Education, 3*(3), 285–289.

Sullivan, G. M., & Feinn, R. (2012). Using effect size-or why the *p* value is not enough. *Journal of Graduate Medical Education, 4*(3), 279–282. Retrieved from https://www.ncbi.nlm.nih.gov/pmc/articles/PMC3444174/

Swanson, T. (2016). Time-series methods in experimental research. *Association for Psychological Sciences*. Retrieved from https://www.psychologicalscience.org/observer/time-series-methods-in-experimental-research

Sweatt v. Painter, 339 U.S. 629 (1950).

Sydor, A. (2013). Conducting research into hidden or hard-to-reach populations. *Nursing Research, 20*(3), 33–37.

Symonette, H. (2004). Walking pathways toward becoming a culturally competent evaluator: Boundaries, borderlands, and border crossings. In M. Thompson-Robinson, R. Hopson, & S. SenGupta (Eds.), *In search of cultural competence in evaluation* (pp. 95–109). *New Directions for Evaluation, 102*.

Tatsuoka, M. M. (1982). Statistical methods. In H. Mitzel (Ed.), *The encyclopedia of educational research* (pp. 1780–1808). New York, NY: Macmillan.

Taylor, P. J., Russ-Eft, D. F., & Taylor, H. (2009). Gilding the outcomes by tarnishing the past: Inflationary biases in retrospective pretests. *American Journal of Evaluation, 30*(1), 31–43.

Tashakkori, A., & Teddlie, C. (1998). *Mixed methodology: Combining qualitative and quantitative approaches*. Thousand Oaks, CA: Sage.

Teddlie, C., & Tashakkori, A. (2003). Major issues and controversies in the use of mixed methods in the social and behavioral sciences. In A. Tashakkori & C. Teddlie. (Eds.), *Handbook of mixed methods in the social and behavioral science* (pp. 3–30). Thousand Oaks, CA: Sage.

Tenbrunsel, A. E., & Messick, D. M. (2004). Ethical fading: The role of self-deception in unethical behavior. *Social Justice Research, 17*(2), 223–236.

Tenney, L. (2017). Author reflection. *State of the Science: Implicit Bias Review*. Columbus: Kirwan Institute for the Study of Race and Ethnicity, The Ohio State University. Retrieved from http://kirwaninstitute.osu.edu/wp-content/uploads/2017/11/2017-SOTS-final-draft-02.pdf

Thomas, V. G. (2011). Cultural issues in evaluation: From margin toward center. *American Journal of Evaluation, 34*(4), 578–582.

Thomas, V. G. (2009). Critical race theory: Ethics and dimensions of diversity in research. In D. M. Mertens & P. E. Ginsberg (Eds.), *The handbook of social research ethics* (pp. 54–68). Thousand Oaks, CA: Sage.

Thomas, V. G. (2004). Building a contextually responsive evaluation framework. In V. G. Thomas & F. I. Stevens (Eds.), *Co-constructing a contextually responsive evaluation framework: The Talent Development Model of school reform* (pp. 3–24). *New Directions for Evaluation, 101*.

Thomas, V. G., & Campbell, P. B. (2017). *Cultural conflicts of interest: Definition, description, and avoidance*. A think tank presented to the annual meeting of the American Educational Research Association, Washington, DC.

Thomas, V. G., & Madison, A. (2010). Integration of social justice into the teaching of evaluation. *American Journal of Evaluation, 31*(4) 570–583.

Thomas, V. G., Madison, A., Rockcliffe, F., DeLaine, K., & Lowe, S. M. (2018). Racism, social programming, and evaluation: Where do we go from here? *American Journal of Evaluation, 39*(4), 514–526.

Thomas, V. G., & Parsons, B. (2017). Culturally responsive evaluation meets systems-oriented evaluation. *American Journal of Evaluation, 38*(1), 7–28.

Thomas, V. G., & Smith, V. (2013, October). *Using dashboards to Improve Understanding and Use of Results: Tracking and Evaluation Strategies from the Georgetown-Howard Universities Center for Clinical Translational Science (GHUCCTS)*. Paper presented at the Annual Meeting of the American Evaluation Association Meeting, Washington, DC.

Thomas, V. G., & Stevens, F. I. (Eds.). (2004). Co-constructing a contextually responsive evaluation framework: The talent development model of school reform. *New Directions for Evaluation, 101*.

Thompson-Robinson, M., Hopson, R., & SenGupta, S. (Eds.). (2004). *In search of cultural competence in evaluation: Toward principles and practices. New Directions for Evaluation, 102*.

Tobin, M. J. (2003). Conflict of interest and AJRCCM: Restating policy and a new form to upload. *American Journal of Respiratory and Critical Care Medicine, 167*, 1161–1164.

Torgovnick May, K. (2012, October 31). How to give more persuasive presentations: A Q&A with Nancy Duarte. *TED Blog*. Retrieved from https://blog.ted.com/how-to-give-more-persuasive-presentations-a-qa-with-nancy-duarte/

Traffis, C. (n.d.). Active vs. passive voice. *Grammarly*. Retrieved from https://www.grammarly.com/blog/active-vs-passive-voice/

Trainor, A. A., & Bal, A. (2014). Development and preliminary analysis of a rubric for culturally responsive research. *Journal of Special Education, 47*, 203–216.

Travis, J. (2020, February 14). Watch the winner of this year's "Dance Your Ph.D." contest. *Science*. Retrieved from https://www.sciencemag.org/news/2020/02/watch-winner-year-s-dance-your-phd-contest

Trevisan, M. S. (2007). Evaluability assessment from 1986 to 2006. *American Journal of Evaluation, 28*(3), 290–303.

Trochim, W. M. K. (2008). The regression-discontinuity design. In *The research methods knowledge base*. Cincinnati, OH: Atomic Dog. Retrieved from https://socialresearchmethods.net/kb/regression-discontinuity-design/

Trochim, W. M. K. (1998). An "evaluation" of Michael Scriven's "Minimalist theory: The least theory that practice requires." *American Journal of Evaluation, 19*(2), 243–249.

Tropp, L. R., & Godsil, R. D. (2015). Overcoming implicit bias and racial anxiety Fighting subconscious bias takes effort—but it can be done. *Psychology Today*. Retrieved from https://www.psychologytoday.com/us/blog/sound-science-sound-policy/201501/overcoming-implicit-bias-and-racial-anxiety

Tucker, M. (2014, August 13). Education research: Reflections on the "Gold Standard." *Education Week*. Retrieved from http://blogs.edweek.org/edweek/top_performers/2014/08/education_research_reflections_on_the_gold_standard.html

Tufte, E. R. (2001). *The visual display of quantitative information* (2nd ed.). Cheshire, CT: Graphics Press. Retrieved from http://sphweb.bumc.bu.edu/otlt/MPH-Modules/BS/DataPresentation/DataPresentation3.html

UCLA Institute for Digital Research and Education Statistical Consulting Group. (n.d.). *FAQ: What are the differences between one-tailed and two-tailed tests?* Retrieved from https://stats.idre.ucla.edu/other/mult-pkg/faq/general/faq-what-are-the-differences-between-one-tailed-and-two-tailed-tests/

UCLA School of Public Affairs. (2009, June). *What is critical race theory?* Retrieved from https://spacrs.wordpress.com/what-is-critical-race-theory/

Uhlmann, E. L., & Cohen, G. L. (2007, December). "I think it, therefore it's true": Effects of self-perceived objectivity on hiring discrimination. *Organizational Behavior and Human Decision Processes, 104*(2), 207 223.

USAID Office of Learning, Evaluation, and Research. (2013). *Checklist for defining evaluation questions Version 1.0*. Retrieved from https://usaidlearninglab.org/sites/default/files/resource/files/2-checklist_for_defining_evaluation_questions.pdf

U.S. Department of Agriculture. (2019). *Definitions of food security*. Retrieved from https://www.ers.usda.gov/topics/food-nutrition-assistance/food-security-in-the-us/definitions-of-food-security.aspx

U.S. Department of Health and Human Services. (n.d.a). *Research Initiative for Scientific Enhancement (RISE) (R25)*. Retrieved from https://grants.nih.gov/grants/guide/pa-files/PAR-16-361.html

U.S. Department of Health and Human Services. (n.d.b). *Text version of OHRP decision charts*. Retrieved from https://www.hhs.gov/ohrp/regulations-and-policy/decision-trees-text-version/index.html#ch01

U.S. Department of Health and Human Services, Centers for Disease Control and Prevention. Office of the Director, Office of Strategy and Innovation. (2011, October). *Introduction to program evaluation for public health programs: A self-study guide*. Atlanta, GA: Centers for Disease Control and Prevention. Retrieved from https://www.cdc.gov/eval/guide/CDCEvalManual.pdf

U.S. Department of Health and Human Services, Office for Human Research Protections. (2016, March 18). Federal policy for the protection of human subjects ("Common Rule"). Retrieved from https://www.hhs.gov/ohrp/regulations-and-policy/regulations/common-rule/index.html

U.S. Department of Health and Human Services, Office of Research Integrity. (n.d.). *Definitions: ORI Introduction to RCR: Chapter 3. The protection of human subjects*. Retrieved from https://ori.hhs.gov/content/chapter-3-The-Protection-of-Human-Subjects-Definitions

U.S. Department of Justice. (2015). *Disabilities among prison and jail inmates, 2011–2012*. Washington, DC: Office of Justice Programs, Bureau of Justice.

U.S. Government Accountability Office. (2012). *Designing evaluations* (rev.). Washington, DC: Retrieved from https://www.gao.gov/assets/590/588146.pdf

USLegal. (2019). Social justice law and legal definition. Retrieved from https://definitions.uslegal.com/s/social-justice/

University of California Davis. (n.d.). *The 30 second elevator speech*. Retrieved from http://sfp.ucdavis.edu/files/163926.pdf

University of Cincinnati Office of Research. (n.d.). *Levels of reviews*. Retrieved from https://www.research.uci.edu/compliance/human-research-protections/researchers/levels-of-review.html

University of Illinois Library. (2020, March 10). *Queer theory: Background*. Retrieved from https://guides.library.illinois.edu/queertheory/background

University of New Hampshire Office of Community, Equity and Diversity. (2020). *SJE concepts defined*. Retrieved from https://www.unh.edu/inclusive/trainings-news-events/social-justice-educator-training/sje-concepts-defined

University of South Australia. (n.d.). *Overview of statistical software packages*. Retrieved from https://lo.unisa.edu.au/mod/book/view.php?id=631718

Usabilla. (n.d.). How to design for color blindness. *Usability by Survey Monkey*. Retrieved from https://usabilla.com/blog/how-to-design-for-color-blindness/

Vaca, S. (2018). Facilitating the use of evaluations by Sara Vaca. *AEA365*. Retrieved from https://aea365.org/blog/facilitating-the-use-of-evaluations-by-sara-vaca/

Vallas, R. (2016). *Disabled behind bars: The mass incarceration of people with disabilities in America's jails and prisons*. Washington, DC: Center for American Progress.

VeneKlasen, L., & Miller, V. (2006, May). Dynamics of power, inclusion and exclusion. *Nonprofit Online News Journal*, 38–56.

Vincent, N., Allsop, S., & Shoobridge, J. (2000). The use of rapid assessment methodology (RAM) for investigating illicit drug use: A South Australian experience. *Drug and Alcohol Review*, 19, 419–426.

VisionAware. (n.d.). *Tips for making print more readable*. Retrieved from https://careerconnectprod.azurewebsites.net/wp-content/uploads/sites/3/2019/12/afb_visionaware_printreadable_flyer_accessible_final.pdf

Vocabulary.com. (n.d.). *Stereotype*. Retrieved from https://www.vocabulary.com/dictionary/stereotype

Waapalaneexkweew [Bowman-Farrell, N. R.]. (2018). Looking backward but moving forward: Honoring the sacred and asserting the sovereign in Indigenous evaluation. *American Journal of Evaluation*, 39(4), 543–568.

Waapalaneexkweew [Bowman, N.], & Dodge-Francis, C. (2018). Culturally responsive indigenous evaluation and tribal governments: Understanding the relationship. In F. Cram, K. A. Tibbetts, & J. LaFrance (Eds.), *Indigenous evaluation. New Directions for Evaluation*, 159, 17–31.

Waldick, L. (2011, February 9). *In conversation: Michael Quinn Patton*. International Development Research Centre. Retrieved from https://www.idrc.ca/en/article/conversation-michael-quinn-patton

Wang, C., & Burris, M. A. (1997). Photovoice: Concept, methodology and use for participatory needs assessment. *Health Education & Behavior*, 24. 369–387. Retrieved from http://strive.lshtm.ac.uk/sites/strive.lshtm.ac.uk/files/wang%20concept%20and%09%20methodology.pdf

Washington, K. (2019, September 5). A no-nonsense conversation between Alexandria Ocasio-Cortez and Kerry Washington. *Interview*. Retrieved from https://www.interviewmagazine.com/culture/a-no-nonsense-conversation-between-alexandria-ocasio-cortez-and-kerry-washington

Wasserstein, R. L., & Lazar, N. A. (2016, March 7). The ASA's statement on p values: Context, process and purpose. *The American Statistician*, 70(2), 129–133.

Waters, G. A. (1998). Critical evaluation for education reform. *Education Policy Analysis Archives*, 6(20), 1–38.

Watts, I. (1821). *The improvement of the mind*. London, England: Chiswick.

Wauchope, B. (2001). *Using logic models in a multi-site, multi-level evaluation*. Paper presented at the Annual Meeting of the American Evaluation Association, St. Louis, MO.

Web Accessibility Initiative. (2019). *Introduction to web accessibility*. Retrieved from https://www.w3.org/WAI/fundamentals/accessibility-intro/

Weiss, C. H. (2004a). On theory-based evaluation: Winning friends and influencing people. *The Evaluation Exchange*, IX (4), 1–5.

Weiss, C. (2004b). Rooting for evaluation: A cliff notes version of my work. In M. C. Alkin (Ed.), *Evaluation roots* (pp. 153–168). Thousand Oaks, CA: Sage.

Weiss, C. H. (1997). Theory-based evaluations: Past, present, and future. *New Directions for Evaluation*, 76, 41–55.

Weiss, C. H. (1995). *Nothing as practical as good theory*. Washington, DC: Aspen Institute.

Weiss, C. (1993). Where politics and evaluation research meets. *Evaluation Practice*, 14(1), 93–106.

Weiss, C. H. (1986). The stakeholder approach to evaluation: Origins and promise. In E. House (Ed.), *New directions in educational evaluations* (pp. 145–157). London, England: Falmer.

Weiss, C. (1983). Toward the future of stakeholder approaches in evaluation. In A. S. Bryk (Ed.) *Stakeholder-based evaluation*. (pp. 83-96). San Francisco: Jossey-Bass

Weiss, C. (1972). *Evaluation research: Methods of assessing program effectiveness*. Upper Saddle River, NJ: Prentice-Hall.

West, S. L., & O'Neal, K. K. (2004). Project D.A.R.E. Outcome effectiveness revisited. *American Journal of Public Health*, 94(6), 1027–1029. Retrieved from https://www.ncbi.nlm.nih.gov/pmc/articles/PMC1448384/

Westley, F., Zimmerman, B., & Patton, M. Q. (2006). *Getting to maybe. How the world is changed*. Canada: Random House.

White, D. E. (2017). What is African American studies? In D. Rockmore (Ed.), *What are the arts and sciences: A guide for the curious* (pp. 1–22). Hanover, NH: Dartmouth College Press.

White, J. M. (2017). The evolution of federal evaluation. In *Principles and practices for federal program evaluation: Proceedings of a workshop* (Chapter 2). Washington, DC: National Academies Press. Retrieved from https://www.nap.edu/read/24831/chapter/3

White, J., Drew, S., & Hay, T. (2009). Ethnography vs case study: Positioning research and researchers. *Qualitative Research Journal*, 9(1) 18–27.

Whitesell, N. R. (2018). *Setting the stage: Building strong evidence in challenging contexts*. Centers for American Indian & Alaska Native Health, University of Colorado Anschutz Medical Campus. Retrieved from https://opremethodsmeeting.org/docs/2016/Whitesell_BuildingStrongEvidenceInChallengingContexts.pdf

Whitesell, N. R., Sarche, M., Keane, E., Mousseau, A. C., & Kaufman, C. E. (2018). Advancing scientific methods in community and cultural context to promote health equity: Lessons from intervention outcomes research with American Indian and Alaska Native communities. *American Journal of Evaluation*, 39(1), 42–57.

Wholey, J. S. (2015). Exploratory evaluation. In K. E. Newcomer, H. P. Hatry, & J. S. Wholey (Eds.), *Handbook of practical program evaluation* (4th ed., pp. 88–107). Hoboken, NJ: Jossey-Bass.

Wholey, J. S. (1996). Formative and summative evaluation: Related issues in performance measurement. *Evaluation Practice*, 17(2), 145–149.

Wholey, J. (1983). *Evaluation and effective public management*. Boston, MA: Little, Brown.

Wholey, J. S. (1979). *Evaluation: promise and performance*. Washington, DC: Urban Institute.

Wholey, J. S. (1977). Evaluability assessment. In L. Rutman (Ed.), *Evaluation research methods: A basic guide* (pp. 41–56). Beverly Hills, CA: Sage.

Whyte, W. F. (1955). *Street corner society* (2nd ed.). Chicago, IL: University of Chicago Press.

Whyte, W. F. (1943). *Street corner society*. Chicago, IL: University of Chicago Press.

Wikibooks. (2020, January 3). *Statistics/testing data/t-tests*. Retrieved from https://en.wikibooks.org/wiki/Statistics/Testing_Data/t-tests

Wikipedia. (2020a, March 19). *Social justice*. Retrieved from https://en.wikipedia.org/wiki/Social_justice

Wikipedia. (2020b, April 16). *Case study*. Retrieved from https://en.wikipedia.org/wiki/Case_study

Wilkens, T. B. (1962). Ambrose Caliver: Distinguished civil servant. *Journal of Negro Education, 31*(2), 212–214.

Williams, B. (n.d.). *Qualitative data analysis*. Retrieved from http://www.bobwilliams.co.nz/ewExternalFiles/analysis2.pdf

Williams, C. C. (2006). The epistemology of cultural competence. *Families in Society: The Journal of Contemporary Social Service, 87*(2), 209–220.

Wilson, B. D. M., Jordan, S.P., Meyer, I. H., Flores, A. R., Stemple, L., & Herman, J. L. (2017). Disproportionality and disparities among sexual minority youth in custody. *Journal of Youth and Adolescence, 46*(7), 1547–1561. Retrieved from https://www.ncbi.nlm.nih.gov/pubmed/28093665

Wingate, L., & Schroeter, D. (2016). *Evaluation questions checklist for program evaluation*. Retrieved from https://wmich.edu/sites/default/files/attachments/u350/2018/eval-questions-wingate%26schroeter.pdf

Winter, N. (2008). *How ideas about race and gender shape public opinion*. Chicago, IL: University of Chicago Press.

Wolf, A., Turner, D., & Toms, K. (2009). Ethical perspectives in program evaluation. In D. M. Mertens & P. E. Ginsberg (Eds.), *The handbook of social research ethics* (pp. 170–184). Thousand Oaks, CA: Sage.

Workforce Council. (2015). *Fact sheet: Social justice and health*. Retrieved from https://www.checkup.org.au/icms_docs/182820_15_FACTSHEET_Social_Justice_and_Health.pdf

W. K. Kellogg Foundation. (2017a). *The step-by-step guide to evaluation: How to become savvy evaluation consumers*. Battle, MI: Author. Retrieved from https://www.wkkf.org/resource-directory/resource/2010/w-k-kellogg-foundation-evaluation-handbook

W. K. Kellogg Foundation. (2017b). *WKKF online application: Important information, questions & related helper text*. Retrieved from https://wrm.wkkf.org/uWebRequestManager/UI/Application_Questions_HelperText.pdf

W. K. Kellogg Foundation. (2004). *W. K. Kellogg Foundation logic model development guide*. Battle, MI: Author.

Wright, M. T. (1945). Book review of *An Evaluation of the Accredited Secondary Schools for Negroes in the South*. *Journal of Negro Education, 14*(2), 209–211.

The Writing Center, University of North Carolina at Chapel Hill. (n.d.). *Figures and charts*. Retrieved from https://writingcenter.unc.edu/figures-and-charts/

Yarbrough, D. B., Shulha, L. M., Hopson, R. K., & Caruthers, F. A. (2011). *The program evaluation standards: A guide for evaluators and evaluation users* (3rd ed.). Thousand Oaks, CA: Sage.

Yates, B. T. (2009). Cost-inclusive evaluation: A banquet of approaches for including costs, benefits, and cost-effectiveness and cost-benefit analyses in your next evaluation. *Evaluation and Program Planning, 32*, 54–56.

Ye Hee Lee, M. (2015, July 8) Donald Trump's false comments connecting Mexican immigrants and crime. *Washington Post*. Retrieved from https://www.washingtonpost.com/news/fact-checker/wp/2015/07/08/donald-trumps-false-comments-connecting-mexican-immigrants-and-crime/

Yin, R. K. (1984). *Case study research: Design and methods*. Thousand Oaks, CA: Sage.

Young, E. (2019). How do blind people who've never seen colour, think about colour? *British Psychological Association: Research Digest*. Retrieved from https://digest.bps.org.uk/2019/03/28/how-do-blind-people-whove-never-seen-colour-think-about-colour/

Zahra, F. (2018). MIE TIG Week: Much ado about privilege by Fatima Zahra. *AEA365*. Retrieved from https://aea365.org/blog/mie-tig-week-much-ado-about-privilege-by-fatima-zahra/

Zimmer, B. (2017, January 26). A clash of "alternative" and "facts." *Wall Street Journal*. Retrieved from https://www.wsj.com/articles/a-clash-of-alternative-and-facts-1485454691

Zlotnick, D. M. (2001). The Buddha's parable and legal rhetoric. *Washington and Lee Law Review*. Retrieved from http://www.contemplativemind.org/admin/wp-content/uploads/2012/09/Zlotnick.pdf

Zukoski, A., & Luluquisen, M. (2002, April). Participatory evaluation: What is it? Why do it? What are the challenges? *Community-Based Public Health Policy & Practice, 5*, 1–6.

Index

Note: Figures and Tables are indicated by 'f' and 't' following the page number.

Ableism, 11t
Abma, T., 260
Accountability, 57, 504
Accreditation, 68
Accuracy, 57, 503–504
Actionable, 415
Action research movement, 75
Active consent, 30
Active listening, 45
Active voice, 422
Activities
   analyzing group and individual differences, 396–397
   applying codes and coding, 406
   applying cultural competence, 497
   applying paradigms to evaluation study, 115
   attitude scales, ordinal or interval data, 390
   building one's cultural competence, 484
   categorizing evaluation studies, 125
   choosing designs, 350
   data mapping, 379
   defining evaluation, 6, 486
   defining success, 289
   design your own project, 224
   determining levels of data, 388–389
   developing and using codes, 408–409
   developing business plan, 473
   developing marketing plan, 460
   developing stakeholder engagement communications plan, 268–269
   developing time and task chart, 463, 463t
   draft logic model, 232–233
   ethical "blind spots" in evaluation, 44–45
   evaluation requirements, 461
   evaluation tools, 456
   evaluative thinking, 8–9
   exempt, expedited, full review, or not research, 375
   generating and prioritizing evaluation questions, 316
   generating types of evaluation questions, 321–322
   highlighting potential biases, 488
   identify potential stakeholder conflict, 262
   Implicit Association Test, 15
   improving data collection techniques, 378
   influential 20th-century evaluator, 98–99
   interface among social science theory, social programming, and evaluation, 117
   justifying using control or comparison groups, 336
   planning a formative evaluation, 186
   privilege and oppression, 139
   school violence reduction program theory of change, 118–119
   SMART, 222
   take the implicit association test (optional), 481
   testing readability, 422
   thinking about conflicts of interest, 455
   trying translation software, 423
   using inductive or deductive reasoning, 388
   using word and excel to make tables, 429
   validating "truth," 23
   wicked problems, 208
   Williams's four steps, 409–410
   working with white people and antiracism, 17
African American Culturally Responsive Evaluation System for Academic Settings, 235
Afrocentric-centered logic models, 234–236
Ageism, 11t
Alkin, M. C., 76, 122, 125, 128
Alternative facts, 1, 21
Alternative-form reliability, 368
Alternative hypothesis, 398
American Educational Research Association (AERA), 35, 143
American Evaluation Association (AEA), 28, 34, 40–41, 75, 150, 236
   Evaluators' Ethical Guiding Principles, 150, 499–501
   Public Statement on Cultural Competence, 40–41, 129–130
American Indian Higher Education Consortium, principles, 237–238
American Journal of Evaluation, 36
American Nurses Association (ANA), 34
American Psychological Association (APA), 34, 143
American Sociological Association (ASA), 34
Americans with Disabilities Act (ADA), 145
Analysis of variance (ANOVA), 394t, 395
   with repeated measures, 394t
Archibald, T., 326
Arnold, M. E., 325, 330
Articulated program theory, 118
Ashcraft, C., 161
ATLAS.ti, 411
Axiology, 110

Baggini, J., 22
Bailey, Thomas R., 336
Baker, A., 7
Bal, A., 111
Baldwin, J., 77
Baltimore Responsible Fatherhood Project (BRFP), 234, 235f
Bamberger, M., 162, 164, 217, 293
Baumrind, D., 33
Bazerman, M. H., 44
Behavioral modification program, 185
Belief systems, 11t
"Bell curve," 393
Bell, Derrick, 141
Belmont Report, 29, 33
   beneficence, 33, 34
   justice, 33
   respect for persons, 33, 34
Bias, 13
   explicit, 13
   impact on evaluation, 478–480
   implicit, 14–15
   reducing, 16–17, 480–482
Black Lives Matter, 144
Bledsoe, Katrina L., 332
Bohannon, J., 442
Bookkeeping, 472
Boyce, Ayesha S., 147
Boykin, Leander L., 81–82
Boykin, W. A., 81
Braverman, M. T., 325, 330
Brown, A., 39
Brown, Aaron A., 80–81
Browne, Rose Butler, 79–80
Brown v. Board of Education, 78, 81, 82, 83–84
Bruner, B., 7
Buckley, J., 7
Budget making
   additional costs, 464–465
   direct and indirect costs, 465
   personnel costs, 463–464, 463t, 465t
   sample time and task chart, 463, 463t
   for small program evaluation, 466t
Bunche, Ralph, 75, 83
Bureau of the Budget (BOB), 71–72
Burris, M. A., 357
Business entity
   bookkeeping and record keeping, 472
   corporation/S corporation, 471

employee, 470
limited liability company (LLC), 471
nonprofit organization, 471–472
partnership, 471
sole proprietor, 470
Business evaluation
contracts, 466–467
developing business plan, 472–473
ethics, 451–455
financially viable, 468–469
knowledge and skills, 455–460
making a budget, 462–466
marketing, 455–460
preparing a proposal, 460–462
sample knowledge and experience table, 456t
perspectives on, 449–450
selecting business entity, 469–472
Business plan, 472–473

Caliver, Ambrose, 78–79
The Cambridge-Somerville Youth Study
example of experimental evaluation in 1930s, 73–74
Campbell, Donald T., 88, 338, 348
"accidental evaluator," 87
Campbell, P. B., 149, 288, 291, 338
Caracelli, V. J., 197
Case studies
accidental design, 345, 394
broadening participation indicators, 292
The Cambridge-Somerville Youth Study, 1930s, 73–74
CDC cost-effectiveness evaluations, 193
classifying stakeholders, 248–249
components of sample project, 223–224
comprehensive qualitative coding process, 411
compromised evaluator, 45
credible evidence, 306
developmental evaluation of leadership program, 199
equity-focused evaluation case studies, 164
ethical challenges by evaluators, 51–52
evaluation activities, CDC, 101
evaluation making difference, 446
evaluation report, 48
evaluation results vs. politicians, 20–21
evaluators' ethical guiding principles, 54–55
FACES sample process, outcomes, and impact questions, 320
gaining consensus on evaluation purpose, 286
generating hypotheses, 386
global food insecurity, 208
handling stakeholder conflict, 261
identifying hidden agendas and ethical land mines, 36–37
impact of comparison groups on data interpretation, 333–334
of inclusion, democratic participation, and social justice in evaluation, 253
issue of racism, 43
Jerry Lewis Muscular Dystrophy Telethon, 146
marketing tips from the AEA365 Blog, 457–458, 459
messiness and value of stakeholder engagement, 264
moving beyond past experience, 40
opening doors, 340
political power plays, 60
process evaluation of teen pregnancy and parenting program, 184
Project DARE (Drug Abuse Resistance Education), 21
rapid evaluations, 195
scientists avoid bias, 481
simple Gantt chart for planning evaluation of PD project, 297
social network analysis, 400
social science paradigms, 114–115
21st Century Community Learning Centers, 20
strong through every mile program, 188
students as evaluators, 160
summarizing data, 391
summary of conclusions and recommendations, 418
talent development evaluation framework, 282
using control and comparison groups, 335
CAT (Coding Analysis Toolkit), 411
Causal relationship, 338
Center for Advanced Research on Language Acquisition (CARLA), 18
Center for Culturally Responsive Evaluation and Assessment (CREA), 102, 236
Center for Research on the Education of Students Placed at Risk (CRESPAR), 276
Centers for Disease Control and Prevention (CDC) approach, 101, 175, 313, 313t–314t
Chelimsky, E., 175
Chelimsky, Eleanor, 94–95
Chen, H. T., 120
Chen, J., 425
Chi-square test, 394t
Chouinard, J. A., 495
Christie, C. A., 76, 125, 128, 445
Circular logic models, 233, 234f
Cisgender, 138
Clark, Kenneth, 83
Clark, Mamie, 83
Classifying evaluations
for accountability, 175
approaches and theories, 123–129
for development, 175
formative and summative evaluations
classification overview of, 171–173
distinguishing and coupling, 174–175
impact evaluations, 175
for knowledge, 175
net impact evaluation, 175
outcome evaluations, 175
performance evaluations, 175
process or implementation evaluations, 175
transdiscipline, 170
Classism, 11t
Clewell, Beatriz Chu, 98
Clientism, 58, 495
Clinton, Bill, 101
Closed-ended questions, 358
Co-construction, 225, 255
Codebooks, 405–408, 407, 407t
Code of conduct, 35
Coding, 405–408
Coffman, J., 225
Cohen's d, 395, 396t
Collaborative evaluation, 162, 163t
Collaborative Institutional Training Initiative (CITI), 374
Common good, 53, 501
Common Rule, 372
Community-Based Mentoring (CBM) program, 306
Community, evaluation
appreciation, 94
cultural analysis, 94
dealing with people very different from ourselves, 94
"hearing secret harmonies," 94
judgment, 93–94
Comparison groups, 333–336
Competence, 53, 499–500
Conclusions and recommendations, summary of, 418
Concurrent validity, 364
Conflict of interest (COI), 49–51, 451–452
Conflict theory, 210
Constructivist, 93
Construct validity, 364
Content equivalence, 367
Context, 184
Context questions, 317
Contracts, 437
components, 466–467
intellectual property, 467
Contractualism, 58, 495
Control groups, 333–336

on data interpretation, 333–334
ethical issues, 334
ethical use, 334–336
Cooksy, L. J., 197
Copyright, 440
Corporation, 471
Correlation, 399
Correlation coefficient, 394t
Corruptibility, evaluation
conflict of interest, 58
inducements, 58
not honoring commitments, 58
prejudices and biases, 58
unsubstantiated opinions, 58
Coryn, C. L. S., 120, 123
Cost-benefit evaluations, 191–192
Cost-benefit questions, 320–321
Cost-effectiveness evaluation
CDC, 193
efficiency evaluations, 194
outcomes, 192–193
policymakers and stakeholder groups, 193
Cost-effectiveness questions, 320–321
Cost reimbursement, 467
Counterfactual, 190
Cousins
practical participatory evaluation, 75
Cousins, J. B., 75
Cox, J., 478
CRAAP test, 22–23
accuracy, 22
authority, 22
currency, 22
purpose, 22
relevance, 22
Craig Method, 80
Creative Commons, 467
Credibility, 301, 306–307
Credible evidence, 6
Crenshaw, K., 400
Crenshaw, K. W., 140, 141, 142
Critical constructivism, 210
Critical race feminism, 114
Critical race theory (CRT), 141–142
Critical theory paradigm, 113–114
Cronbach, L. J., 91
Crowley, M., 83
Cultural attitudes, 18t
Cultural competence, 1, 18–19, 40–43, 129, 151–152
culturally incongruent settings, 41
ethical dimension of racial bias, 42–43
Evaluators' Ethical Guiding Principles, 40–41
procedural ethics, 41–42
relational ethics, 42
situational ethics, 42
Cultural conflict of interest (COI), 150

Cultural humility, 45
Culturally competent evaluator, 40
Culturally incongruent settings, 41
Culturally relevant logic models, 233
Culturally responsive evaluation (CRE), 119, 153, 176
Cultural relevance, 152
Cultural responsiveness, 1, 18–19, 151–152
data collection, 490–491
evaluation designs, 489–490
in involvement/engagement of stakeholders, 487–488
reports and presentations, 492–493
Culture, 18, 184

D'Agostino, A., 162
Danish International Development Agency (DANIDA), 196
Darden, Christine, 76
Dashboards, 436–437, 438f
Data
definition, 353
qualitative, 353
quantitative, 353
Data analysis
deductive and inductive reasoning, 385–388
qualitative analysis, 404–411
quantitative analysis, 388–404
Data cleaning, 381
Data collection
accessibility, 377–378
mapping to project goals and objectives, 379
Data management, 380
electronic controls and data cleaning, 381
plans, 382
privacy, 381–382
timing, 380
Data Management Plan (DMP), 382
Data maps, 298, 298t
Data quality
pilot-testing, 370
reliability, 368–369
response rates, 370–372
validity, 362–368
Data visualization
chart preferences, 433f
dashboards, 436–437, 438f
diversity resources, 428t
figures, 430–436
graph, 431f, 432f
participant presentations vs. publications, 434f
presentations of data, 435f, 436f
student-centered learning, 429t–430t
tables, 428–430
Datta, L., 96, 97

Davidson, E. J., 308, 421
DBA ("doing business as"), 470
Decision error, 397–398, 398t
Deductive reasoning, 385–388
De facto discrimination, 12
Deficit models, 149–150
De jura discrimination, 12
Delayed treatment design, 340
Deliberative democratic evaluation, 160–162, 251
Democratic evaluation, 251–253
Democratization
of evaluation process with stakeholders, 251–253
Dependent variable, 386
Descriptive statistics, 391–392
Descriptive theories, 120
Designs, evaluation
best design for question, 349–350, 349t–350t
case studies/ethnography, 346–348
control and comparison groups, 333–336
definition, 325
experimental designs, 338–341
longitudinal data, 336–338
pretest/posttest designs, 343–344
quasi-experimental designs, 341–343
retrospective pretest designs, 344–345
rigor, 326–333
rival hypotheses and threats to validity, 348–349
Developmental evaluations
complex and dynamic, 199
evaluator's role, 200
feedback, 200
innovations and standard projects and programs, 198
of leadership program, 199
monitoring, 198
questioning and learning, 200
scope of work, 200–201
and traditional evaluation, difference between, 198–199
Direct costs, 465
Direct stakeholders, 248, 248t
Disability model, 146
Disability rights movement, 146–147
Disability theory, 145–147
Disaggregation, 141
Discrimination, 11
Dissemination, 437
dissemination plans, 437, 439
effective dissemination strategies, 443
interesting, 442
modes, creative, 442
sharing information, 439
simple, 441–442
using mainstream media, 441

using websites and social media, 439–441
working with others, 442–443
Diverse stakeholder groups, 245
Domenico, D., 207
Dominant culture, 10
Dominant paradigm, 10
Dominant positionality, 170
Donaldson, S. I., 116, 120
Dosage, 184
Downloadable data collection templates, 377
Downs, A., 211
Du Bois, W. E. B., 83
Dundon, T., 369
Edelman, M., 210
Educational accreditation, 68
Educational Testing Service (ETS) Test Link, 375
Edwards, W. M., 90
Effectiveness evaluations. *See* outcome evaluations
Effect size, 395, 396, 396t
Efficiency evaluations
board members of private foundation, 191
cost-benefit evaluations, 191–192
cost-effectiveness evaluation, 192–194
in criminal justice, 190–191
government agency, 190
policymakers, 190
Eisenhower, Dwight D., 74
Eitzen, D. S., 216
Electronic controls, 381
Elementary and Secondary Education Act (ESEA), 85, 95, 96
Elevator speech, 417
Ellett, F. S., 65
Employee, 470
Employer Identification Number (EIN), 472
Empowering model, 145–146
Empowerment evaluation, 147, 157–158
Epistemology, 110
Equitable evaluation (EE), 153
Equity, 501
Equity-based social programming, 217
Equity-focused evaluation, 162–164
Equity-focused interventions, 217
Ethical considerations in evaluation, 57
Ethical decision making, factors, 46
Ethical dilemmas
handling ethical dilemmas, 47–49
sources, 46–47
arise from doing evaluation, 46
conducting the evaluation, 47
context of evaluand, 47
created by evaluator, 46–47
Ethically grounded evaluations, 28
Ethical sensitivity, 44–51
Ethical thinking, 39

Ethical triggers, 34
Ethics, 27–28
challenges and dilemmas, 51–52
conflict of interest (COI), 49–51, 451–452
cultural competence, 40–43
cultural respect, 454–455
decision making and behavior, 37–38
"ethically important moments," 38
in evaluation, 34–40
evaluation corruptibility and fallacies, 58–59
evaluator role, power, politics, and ethics, 59
guidelines, 34–35
individual and professional levels, 38
interplay of politics and ethics, 59–60
nondiscrimination, 453–454
organization's code of conduct, 35
principles and standards, 52–57
protection of human participants, 452–453
research ethics, 29–34, 35–36
responsibility of evaluators, 37
sensitivity and dilemmas, 44–51
sources of ethical thinking, 39–40
Ethnography, 347
European Institute for Gender Equality, 137
Evaluability assessments, 182–183
Evaluand, 44
Evaluation
approaches, 120–122, 123, 130, 130t–131t
five-category classification, 123–124
Mertens and Wilson's four-branch tree, 126–129, 127t, 128f
Stufflebeam and Colleagues' classification, 124t
definition, 4–6, 65–66
models, 120–122, 123
phases of, 5t
program, 5
types
culturally responsive evaluation, 176
efficiency evaluations, 190–194
formative and implementation evaluations, 179–183
impact evaluations, 186, 190
metaevaluations, 196–198
outcome evaluations, 186–189
process evaluations, 183–185
progress evaluations, 185–186
rapid evaluations, 194–196
summary, 176, 177t–178t, 179
summative evaluation, 186
value, 5
Evaluation fallacies
clientism, 58, 495
contractualism, 58, 495
methodologicalism, 58, 495
pluralism/elitism, 59, 495

relativism, 59, 495
Evaluation plan, 219
Evaluation Questions Checklist for Program Evaluation, 308
Evaluation report, 48
Evaluation results, 443–445
Evaluative Research: Principles and Practices in Public Service and Social Action Programs (Weiss), 85–86
Evaluator
ethical sensitivity, 45–46
program activities, 223
program goals, 221
program mission, 220
program objectives, 221–223
program resources, 223
Evaluator Competencies, 28
Evaluators' Ethical Guiding Principles, 40, 52–53, 75, 276
application of
data analysis and interpretation, 55
data collection, 54–55
dissemination and utilization of results, 55
entry, contracting, and design, 54
evaluation context, 54
common good and equity, 53, 501
competence, 53, 499–500
integrity, 53, 500
respect for people, 53, 500–501
systematic inquiry, 53, 499
Every Student Succeeds Act (ESSA), 95
Exempt study, 373
Existing measures
assessing existing measures, 376
measuring complex concepts, 376–377
sources of measures, 375–376
Expedited studies, 373
Experimental designs
causal relationship, 338–341
delayed treatment design, 340
feasibility of implementation, 340–341
methodological strengths, 339
pretest effect, 341
qualitative data, 339
Solomon four-group design, 341
Explanatory framework, 120
Explicit bias, 13
External evaluator, 294
External stakeholders, 248, 248t
External validity, 348

Fake news, 1
Family-wise error rate, 393
Farmer-Smith, K., 357
Feasibility, 56, 502–503
Feedback reports, 419–420
sample qualitative summary, 419
sample quantitative summary, 419–420

Feminist evaluation, 158–159
Feminist research and theory, 142–144
Feminist standpoint theory, 143
Feminist theory, 143
Fetterman, David, 75, 157
   empowerment evaluation, 75
Fidelity, 184
Figures, 430–436
FitzGerald, C., 16
Fitzpatrick, J. L., 58
Five-category classification, 123–124
Fleischer, D., 445
Flick, U., 404
Focus groups, 355–356
Folkways, 485
Formal educational program evaluation, 68
Formative evaluations, 171–172, 179–183
   evaluability assessments, 182–183
   needs assessments, 179–181
Forward/backward translation (FBT), 367
Foucault, Michael, 144
Foundations for Evidence-Based
      Policymaking Act, 101
Frameworks, 478
Frazier-Anderson, P. N., 235
Frazier, E. Franklin, 83
Frechtling, J., 225
Freeman, Howard E.
   Evaluation: A Systematic Approach Handbook of Evaluation Research, 86
Friedman test, 394t
Frierson, Henry T., 176
Fryrear, A., 370
Full evaluation report, 416–417
Full review, 373
Funnell, S. C., 225
Future, evaluations of
   characteristics, 6–7
   definitions, 4–6
   evaluative thinking, 7–9
Fuzzy logic models, 233

Gantt charts, 296, 297
Garrett, K. E., 225
General Accounting Office (GAO), 71
Generalizability, 361
Germuth, A., 450
Gilliam, W. S., 38
Glass, G. V., 65
Goals, 221
Goldratt, E., 478
Goodman, L. A., 327, 377
Gothberg, J., 366
Government Accountability Office, 2004, 71
Government Performance and Results Act
      (GPRA), 101, 179
Graph, 431f, 432f
Great Depression, 72
Great Society programs, 91

Greene, J. C., 282, 306
Greene, Jennifer C., 262
Grob, G., 421
Guba, E., 5
Guba, E. G., 247, 265
Guiding Principles for Evaluators, 87
Guillemin, M., 38
Gulker, J. E., 482
Gunnar Myrdal, 75
Guttentag, Marcia
   Handbook of Evaluation Research, 86

Hall, J., 144
Hall, M., 6, 477
Hannum, K., 13
Harding, S., 143
Hatcher, D. L., 216
Hatry, H. P., 300, 360
Hauck, K., 192
Haugen, J. S., 495
Health Services Center (HSC), 36
Heiner, R., 210
HeLa Story: 1950s and beyond, 32
Henrietta, 32
Heteronormativity, 144
Heterosexism, 11t
Hidden stakeholders, 249–250
Hood, S., 66, 76–77, 79, 81, 369
Hoover, Herbert, 78
Hopson, R., 66, 79, 208, 365
House, E. R., 136, 147, 148, 160, 251, 495
Howe, K. R., 160, 161
Huberman, A. M., 404
"Human computers," 76
Human participants, protection of,
      372–374
Hybrid (or mixed) model, 294
Hypothesis, 385–386

Images matter, 426–427
Impact evaluations, 175, 190
Impact questions, 319–320
Implementation evaluations, 175, 179–183
Implementation failure, 120
Implicit bias
   characteristics, 14
   Implicit Association Test, 15
   implicit stereotypes, 15
Implicit program theory, 118
Implicit stereotypes, 15
Income inequality, 206
Independent variable, 386
Indicators
   guidelines for selecting, 290
   identifying, 289–290
   levels of, 291–292
      broadening participation
         indicators, 292
      funder-level, 291–292

      individual-level, 291, 292
      institutional-level, 291, 292
   multiple, 289
   types of, 290–291
      input indicators, 290–291
      outcome indicators, 291
      output indicators, 291
      process indicators, 291
Indigenous communities, 236–237
Indigenous evaluation, 237
Indigenous evaluators, 238
Indirect costs, 465
Indirect stakeholders, 248, 248t
Inductive reasoning, 386–387
   using, 387–388
Inferential statistics, 392
Informed consent, 372–373
Input indicators, 290–291
Institutional review board (IRB), 373
Integrity, 53, 500
Intellectual property, 467
Interconnections and practical implications
   advice for new evaluators, 495–496
   analysis data collection, 490–491
   building cultural competence, 482–485
   cultural responsiveness
      data collection, 490–491
      evaluation designs, 489–490
      in involvement/engagement of
         stakeholders, 487–488
      reports and presentations, 492–493
   data analysis, 491–492
   development of evaluation questions,
      488–489
   making biases explicit, 487
   objectivity and bias, 478–482
   personalizing social justice perspective,
      485–486
   politics and evaluation, 494–495
   reflective practice and evaluative
      thinking, 486
   social justice evaluation, 493–494
Interinterviewer reliability, 369
Intermediate outcomes, 188
Internal evaluator, 294
Internal stakeholders, 248, 248t
Internal validity, 348
Interobserver reliability, 369
Interpretivism, 112–113
Interrater reliability, 369
Intersectionality, 12, 140
Interval level, 388
Interview, 354–355
Interview protocol, 354

Jackson, Mary, 76
Jackson, Reid E., 78, 79
Jenkins, S., 240
Jim Crow laws, 72

Johnson, James Weldon, 83
Johnson, Katherine, 76
Johnson, Lyndon B., 84
Joint Committee on Standards for Educational Evaluation
  Program Evaluation Standards, 502–504
Jolly, Eric, 137
Jones, Camara Phyllis, 141
Jones, N., 267
Jones, T. M., 46
Jordan, G. B., 225, 228
Journal of Negro Education and Founding (Charles H. Thompson), 82–84
Juvenile justice program, 187

Kaplan, S., 225
Kawakami, K., 481
Keene, M., 233
Kennedy, John F., 84
Key stakeholders, 249, 266t
Kirkhart, K., 362
Kirkhart, K. E., 365
Knowlton, L. W., 225, 226
Kosofsky Sedgwick, E., 141
Krause, H., 327
Kruskal-Wallis test, 394t
Kuhn, T., 108, 327
Kushner, S., 213

LaFrance, 238
LaFrance, J., 238, 424
Latinx, 425
Learning objectives, 2
Leeuw, F. L., 116
Legend, 430
Lesbian, gay, bisexual, transgender, or queer (LGBTQ), 145
Leung, L., 361
Levin, H., 193
Leviton, Laura, 97–98
Leviton, L. C., 264
Lewin, Kurt, 74–75, 108
  action research perspective, 75
  father of social psychology, 75
  Social Psychology and Evaluation, 74
Limited liability company (LLC), 471
Lincoln, Y., 5
Lincoln, Y. S., 93–94, 247, 265
Lipsey, M. W., 116, 120
Locke, Alain, 83
Logic models
  African American Culturally Responsive Evaluation System for Academic Settings, 236, 237f
  afrocentric-centered, 234–236
  American Indian Higher Education Consortium, principles, 237–238
  benefits for program planning, 225–226
  circular, 233, 234f
  components of, 227–229
    inputs, 228
    outcomes, 228–229
    outputs, 228
  culturally relevant, 233
  and evaluation planning, 227–233, 228t
  evaluation processes, 238
  fuzzy, 233
  indigenous communities, 240
  indigenous evaluation, 237
  from indigenous framework, 236–240
  limitations, 226–227
  nested, 231–233
  outcomes column, 229
  progression of program logic, 230, 230f
  simple, 229–230, 229f
  story creation, goal of, 238–239
  and theory of change, 239
  types and look of, 229–230
Long-term outcomes, 188
Luellen, J., 66, 88

MacDonald, B., 135
Macro-analysis, 209
Madaus, G. F., 66
Mann-Whitney test, 394t
Marginalization, 137
Marginalized groups
  fixing the group *vs.* fixing the system, 139–141
  impacts of marginalization, 138–139
Mark, M. M., 4, 75, 392
Martin, D., 13
Martin, J., 485
Martin, N., 485
Mathison, S., 47
MAXQDA, 411
Maxwell, J. A., 387, 411
McLaughlin, J. A., 225, 228
McNemar test, 394t
Mean, 391
Measurement validity, 301
Median, 391
Medical model of disability, 145
Medicine wheel, 240
Mertens and Wilson's four-branch tree
  branches (or essential elements), 127
  evaluation approaches and theories, 128f
  mapping of major paradigms to Christie and Alkin's (2013) Evaluation Tree, 127t
  social justice, 127–128
Mertens, D. M., 126, 127, 128, 145, 154, 155, 281, 307
Metaevaluations
  definition, 196–197
  professional obligation of evaluators, 197
  qualitative procedures, 197
  quality of evaluation, 197–198
  reports and sources, 197
Methodologicalism, 58, 495
Methodological rigor, 330
Methodology, 110
Metzner, C., 233
Micro-analysis, 209
Microsoft Access, 377–378
Microsoft Excel, 403
Miles, B., 404
Milgram, Stanley, 32
Milgram Study of 1963, 32–33
Miller, Kelly, 83
Mission, 220
Mixed methods, 101
Mode, 391
Moral model of disability, 146
Morewedge, C. K., 16
Morgan, D. L., 129
Mosteller, F., 68
Multicultural validity, 364–365
  consequential, 366
  experiential, 365
  interpersonal, 365
  methodological, 365
  theoretical, 365
Multiple forward translations (MFTs), 367
Multiple-minority status, 250
Myrdal, Alva, 75
Myrdal, Gunnar, 75
  An American Dilemma, 75

Nage, E., 13
National Aeronautics and Space Administration's (NASA) Langley Research Center, 76
National Assessment of Educational Progress (NAEP), 76
National Association of Social Workers (NASW), 34
National Center for Education Statistics (NCES), 337
National Center for Science and Engineering Statistics (NCSES), 337
National Defense Education Act of 1958, 74
National Research Act of 1974, 33–34
National Science Foundation (NSF), 95, 337
  Louis Stokes Alliances for Minority Participation (LSAMP) program, 98
  projects, 376
National Society of Professional Engineers (NSPE), 34
Naturalistic observations, 356
Needs assessments
  case study, 180
  conceptualization and design of programs, 180–181
  definition, 179

organizations, 179
  program planners and decision makers, 181
Nested logic models
  advantage, 232
  examples of, 231, 231f–232f
  organization, program, and project level, 231–232
Net effects, 88, 175
Net impact evaluation, 175
Newcomer, K. E., 300
New Deal programs, 72
New Jersey Agricultural Experiment Station, 359
Newman, D., 39
Nichols, 238
Nichols, R., 238, 424
1970s–1990s, influential women in evaluation
  Beatriz Chu Clewell, 98
  Carol H. Weiss, 92–93
  Eleanor Chelimsky, 94–95
  Floraline I. Stevens, 95–96
  Laura Leviton, 97–98
  Lois-Ellin Datta, 96–97
  Yvonna S. Lincoln, 93–94
1960–2000 evaluation
  establishment of professional societies, 86
  establishment of standards and codes of conduct, 86–87
  federal legislation and great society programs, 84–85
  graduate training and professional development, 86
  growth of evaluation scholarship, 85–86
  methodological approaches and paradigm wars, 87
  1960s–1970s, influential scholars' contributions
    Donald T. Campbell, 88
    Lee J. Cronbach, 88–89
  professionalization of field, 85
Nobody Knows My Name project, 77
Nominal level, 388
Non-binary, 11
Nondiscrimination, 453–454
Nongovernmental organizations (NGOs), 162
Nonparametric statistics, 393, 394t
Nonprofit organization, 471–472
Normally distributed, 393
Null hypothesis, 398
Nuremberg Code of 1947, 29–30
Nutrition evaluation study, 68
NVivo, 411

Obama, Barack, 101
Objective element of social problems, 209
"Objective process," 163

Objectives, 221–223
Objectivity, 13, 478–482
Observations, 356
  naturalistic observations, 356
  participant observer, 356
Office of Management and Budget (OMB), 72
One-page bullet point summary, 417–418
One-tailed test, 392
Online Evaluation Resource Library, 376
On spec, 468
Ontology, 110
Open coding, 406
Open-ended questions, 358
Oral presentations, 420
Ordinal level, 388
O'Sullivan, R. G., 162
Outcome evaluations
  expensive and time-consuming, 188
  intermediate outcomes, 188
  juvenile justice program, 187
  long-term outcomes, 188
  professional development (PD) workshop, 188
  short-term outcomes, 188
  smoking cessation program, 187
  STEM Program Model, 188, 189f
  summative evaluations, 186–187
  of teen pregnancy and parenting program, 187
Outcome indicators, 291
Outcomes-oriented objectives, 222
Outcomes questions, 318–319
Output indicators, 291

Paradigms, 107
  constructivism, 112, 114–115, 125
  dimensions, 110, **110**
  evaluation study, 115
  interpretivism, 112, 114–115
  "paradigm wars," 110
  positivism, 112, 114
  postpositivism, 112, 114, 125
  pragmatism, 112, 115, 125
  way of framing, 109, 110
Paradigm wars, 87
Parametric statistics, 393, 394t
Parker, L., 150
Participant-generated visual data, 356–357
Participant observer, 356
Participant presentations *vs.* publications, 434f
Participant responsiveness, 184
Participatory evaluation, 159–160, 240
Partnership, 471
Passive voice, 422
Patterson, E., 22
Patton, Michael Q.
  developmental evaluation, 75

Utilization-Focused Evaluation, 86
Patton, M. Q., 75, 87, 197, 199
Percentile, 391
Performance evaluations, 175
Perry Preschool Project, 89–90
Personnel Evaluation Standards, 87
Pettigrew, T. F., 482
Pew Research Center, 359
Phillips, C. C., 225, 226
Phillips, G., 253
Photovoice, 357
Pilot-testing, 370
Planning evaluation
  activities, listing of, 279, 280, 280t
  analysis of context, 282–283, 283t–284t
  context analysis guide, 283t–284t
  culturally responsive evaluations, 277–278
  dealing with power imbalances, 274–277
  evaluation team, assembling, 293–296
  hidden and invisible sources of power, 275
  hypothetical STEM project, 279
  inclusiveness and racial equity, 277–278
  and management visualization tools, 296–298
  overcoming pitfalls, 300–301
  project goals, identifying and clarifying, 284–285
  purpose(s) of evaluation, identifying, 285–287
  resource needs, identifying, 293
  social justice-oriented evaluations, 277–278
  stakeholders, identifying and involving, 280–281
  success definitions, 287–292
  timelines, developing, 293
  written evaluation plan, developing, 299–300
Plessy v. Ferguson, 78
Pluralism/elitism, 59, 495
Politics
  and evaluation, 494–495
  impact of, 20–21
Ponterotto, J. G., 110
Population, 392
Positivism, 112
Post-facts, 21
Postmodern views, 346
Postpositivism, 112, 125
Posttest-only intact group design, 342
Post-truth culture, 21–22
Pragmatism, 113, 125
Predictive validity, 364
Prescriptive theories, 120
Preskill, H., 267
Pretest effect, 341
Pretest/posttest designs, 343–344

Primary stakeholders, 248, 248t
Privilege, 11
Probability, 392
Pro bono evaluation, 468
Procedural ethics, 41
Process evaluations, 175
   aspects of project implementation, 183, 184
   implementation failure, 185
   of teen pregnancy and parenting program, 184
   theory failure, 185
Process indicators, 291
Process-oriented objectives, 223
Process questions, 317–318
Professional development (PD) project, 188, 297
Professional evaluators, 27
Program evaluation, 5, 219
   complaints about evaluation research, 1970s, 90, 91t
   history of evaluation, 77
   influential 20th-century evaluator, 98–99
   1960–2000 evaluation, 84–89
   1970s–1990s evaluation, 92–98
   rethinking role of evaluation, 89–91
   20th-century evaluation, 67–84
   21st-century evaluation, 99–103
   through social justice lens, 66
Program Evaluation Review Technique (PERT) charts, 297–298, 297f
Program Evaluation Standards, 56–57, 86–87, 121, 305
   accountability standards, 57, 504
   accuracy standards, 57, 503–504
   feasibility standards, 56, 502–503
   propriety standards, 56, 503
   utility standards, 56, 502
Program reach, 184
Program theory failure, 120
Program theory of change, 111, 117–120
   evaluating, 119–120
Program theory questions, 316–317
Progress evaluations, 185–186
Project, 219
Project DARE (Drug Abuse Resistance Education), 21
Project evaluation, 219
Propriety, 56, 503
"Pseudo-evaluations," 123
Public domain, 467
Purpose, evaluation
   evaluator's priorities, 287
   funder's priorities, 286–287
   project administrators' priorities, 287
   stakeholders perspectives, 286
P-value, 392

Qualitative data, 353–360
   coding and codebooks, 405–408
   sample qualitative analysis models, 409–411
   sources of, 354
   sources of qualitative data, 405
   strengths and weaknesses of, 360–362
Qualitative methods, 87
Quality standards, 52–57
Quantitative data, 353–360
   decision error and statistical power, 397–398
   descriptive statistics, 391–392
   difference-based and relationship-based analysis, 399–400
   disaggregating data, 400–404
   effect size, 394–397
   hypothesis testing, 398
   inferential statistics, 392
   levels of quantitative data, 388–390, 389t
   parametric and nonparametric statistics, 393–394, 394t
   sources of
      records and archival data, 359–360
      surveys and other structured questionnaires, 358–359
   statistical significance, 392–393
Quantitative methods, 87
Quartile, 391
Quasi-experimental designs
   feasibility of implementation, 342–343
   posttest-only intact group design, 342
   pretest/posttest version, 341
   regression-discontinuity, 343
   self-selection bias, 342
Queer theory, 144–145
Questions, evaluation
   asking questions, 314–315
   characteristics of, 307–310
   critical functions, 304
   for diverse audiences, 311–312
   factors, 305
   good evaluation questions
      align with funder's requirements, 308
      are clear, specific, and well Wdefined, 309
      are realistic considering contexts and project realities, 310
      are reasonable in number and scope, 310
      are researchable (or answerable), 309–310
      characteristics of, 307–310
      issues, 308–309
      local needs, 309
   inclusion/exclusion criteria, 312–314
   meet information needs of diverse users, 305
   power and privilege issues, 307
   set stage for collection of credible evidence, 306
   sources of, 310–311
   steps to identifying, formulating, and prioritizing questions, 314–315
   types of, 322t
      context questions, 317
      cost-benefit and cost-effectiveness questions, 320–321
      impact questions, 319–320
      outcomes questions, 318–319
      process questions, 317–318
      program theory questions, 316–317
      relevance questions, 318
      sustainability questions, 321
QuickBooks, 472

R, 404
Race, 9, 42
Racial discrimination, 9
Racial framing, 214
Racialization, 9
Racialized perspective, 1–2, 10
Racism, 9–10, 11t, 42
   critical race theory, 114
   impact of, 148
   principles, 10
Radiation Studies of 1940–1960, 32
Randomized controlled trial (RCT), 327
Range, 391
Rapid Early Action for Coronary Treatment (REACT), 262
Rapid evaluations
   advantages, 195
   cases of, 195
   feedback evaluations, 194
   formative or summative, 194
   methods of, 194
   program life cycle, 196
   public health initiatives, 195–196
Rapid feedback evaluation, 194
Ratio level, 388
Raw data, 421
Reach, 230
Readability, 421–424
Record keeping, 472
Reducing bias, 16–17
Reflective practice, 7
Regression-discontinuity, 343
Relational ethics, 42
Relativism, 59, 495
Relevance questions, 318
Reliability, 301, 368–369
   alternative-form, 368
   interinterviewer, 369
   interobserver, 369
   interrater, 369
   intrarater, 369
   of qualitative data, 369
   of quantitative data, 368–369
   split-half, 368–369
   test/retest, 368

Reporting results, 416t
  feedback reports, 419–420
  full evaluation report, 416–417
  one-page bullet point summary, 417–418
  oral presentations, 420
  sharing of raw data, 421
  stand-alone summaries, 417
  summary of conclusions and recommendations, 418
Reports and presentations
  images matter, 426–427
  readability, 421–424
  words matter, 424–426
Research ethics
  HeLa Story: 1950s and beyond, 32
  importance of, 34
  Milgram Study of 1963, 32–33
  National Research Act of 1974, 33–34
  Nuremberg Code of 1947, 29–30
  Radiation Studies of 1940–1960, 32
  Tuskegee Syphilis Study of 1932–1972, 30
Resnik, D. B., 34
Resources, 223
Respect for people, 53, 500–501
Response rates, 370–372
Response set bias, 370
Responsive evaluation, 255
Responsive stakeholder engagement
  barriers to, 259–262
  benefits of, 262–264
  communicating with stakeholders, 268–269
  democratizing evaluation process, 251–253
  diverse stakeholder engagement, 245–246
  misuse of, 257
  from nonresponsive to responsive, 257–259
  relationships and values, 254
  responsive stakeholder engagement, 255–257
  right stakeholders, 246–251, 263t
  six-step process, 265–268
    step I: diverse stakeholder engagement, 265
    step II: diverse stakeholders, 265, 266t
    step III: key stakeholders, 266–267
    step IV: stakeholders' values, needs, motivations, interests, and concerns, 267
    step V: key stakeholders fall on stakeholder continuum, 267
    step VI: ongoing stakeholder engagement, 267–268
  stakeholders, 243–244
  valuing stakeholders, 245–246
Retrospective pretest design (RPT), 344–345

Rhetorical structure, 110
Rice, Joseph Mayer, 68
Rigor
  bias, 327
  definition of, 326
  epistemological politics, 327
  methodological rigor, 330
  myth of, 332–333
  practical considerations, 328–330
  program quality and/or effectiveness, 326–327
  randomized controlled trial (RCT), 327
  redefinition of, 331–332
  theoretical and cultural considerations, 330–333
  traditional definitions of, 149
Riley, D., 330, 331, 489
Rittel, H. W. J., 206
Rival hypothesis, 329
Robles, J., 424
Rogers, P. J., 225
Roosevelt, Franklin D., 72, 78
Rossi, Peter H., 68, 87
  Evaluation: A Systematic Approach Handbook of Evaluation Research, 86
Rossi, P. H., 5, 179, 190, 247, 316
Ross, L., 91
Rothman, J., 75
  action evaluation research, 75
Rougier, N. P., 428
Ryan, P., 369

Saldana, J., 407
Sample, 392
Sankofa, 236
SAS (Statistical Analysis System), 404
Scatter plot, 434
School violence intervention program theory, 118–119
Schroeter, D., 308
Science, technology, engineering, and mathematics (STEM) fields, 378
Scientific paradigms and theories
  guiding and improving evaluation practice, 111
  nature of scientific paradigms, 108–111
S corporation, 471
Scriven, M., 123, 171, 196–197
Secondary stakeholders, 248, 248t
Second-wave feminism, 139
Segone, M., 162, 164, 217
Seidel, J. V., 410
Self-selection bias, 342
Semantic equivalence, 367
SenGupta, S., 19, 151
Sexism, 11t
  critical feminist theory, 114
Sexual minorities, 139

Shadish, W. R., 66, 88, 120
Shapiro, J. S., 159
Shetterly, M. L., 77
Shinkfield, A. J., 122, 123, 171
Shoestring evaluation, 293
Short-term outcomes, 188
Sielbeck-Bowen, 158
Situational ethics, 42
SMART, 221, 222t
Smith, N. L., 122
Smoking cessation program, 187
Social-cognitive theories, 116
Social constructivism, 113
Social Darwinism, 211
Social desirability bias, 368
Social experiments
  with scurvy, 68–69
  in U.S., wartime activities of 1800s, 69
Social interventions, 255
Social justice, 10–12, 135–136
  challenges, 149–150
    cultural conflict of interest, 150
    deficit models, 149–150
    traditional definitions of rigor, 149
  definitions of, 136–137, 136t
  efforts to reduce the impact of racism on evaluation, 150–152
    cultural competence and cultural responsiveness, 151–152
  evaluation models and social justice, 153–154
  frameworks and paradigms, 154–164, 155t
    collaborative evaluation, 162
    deliberative democratic evaluation, 160–162
    empowerment evaluation, 157–158
    equity-focused evaluation, 162–164
    feminist evaluation, 158–159
    participatory evaluation, 159–160
    transformational evaluation, 155–157
  marginalized groups, 137–141
  privilege and oppression, 140t
  race, racism, and evaluation, 147–149
  theories
    critical race theory, 141–142
    disability theory, 145–147
    feminist research and theory, 142–144
    queer theory, 144–145
  Word Cloud, 137f
Social justice evaluation, 493–494
Social justice lens, 66
  social programs, 213–214
  See also historical evolution of program evaluation
Social learning theories, 116
Social model of disability, 146
Social network analysis, 399
Social problems
  definition, description, and theoretical underpinnings, 209

economic nature, 216
equity-based social programming, 217
fluid nature, 212
objective element, 209
political perspectives, 215–216
power, 215
social programs, 213–214
sources of, 211–212
sources of problem, 216–217
subjective element, 209–211
wicked problems, 206–209
Social programming, 27
 components of, 205–206
 evaluations vs. project evaluations, 219, 220f
 key program/project components, 219–225
 logic models, 225–240
 program and evaluation planning, integrating, 218–219
 social problems, 206–217
 structural racism, 217–218
Social science paradigms, 111–115
Social science theories, 111, 116, 117
Social transformative lens, 213–214
Sole proprietor, 470
Solomon four-group design, 341
Spearman rank correlation, 394t
Split-half reliability, 368–369
SPSS (Statistical Package for the Social Sciences), 403–404
Sputnik, 74
Staff competency, 184
Stakeholder analysis, 265
Stakeholder engagement, 245
 from nonresponsive to responsive, 257, 258t–259t, 259
Stakeholders
 to clarify project goals, 284–285
 classifications, 247–249
 communicating with, 268–269
 definition, 243
 democratizing evaluation process, 251–253
 direct stakeholders, 248, 248t
 diverse, 245–246
 engaging with respect, honesty, and trust, 254
 external stakeholders, 248, 248t
 forms of, 243–244
 identifying and classifying right, 246–251
 indirect stakeholders, 248, 248t
 internal stakeholders, 248, 248t
 involving, 281
 key and hidden, 249–251
 perspectives on evaluation goals and priorities, 286
 and potential role(s), 280–281
 primary stakeholders, 248, 248t
 secondary stakeholders, 248, 248t

for selected program type, 244, 244t
 valuing, 245–246
Stake, R., 255
Stake, R. E., 123, 346
Stame, N., 185
Stand-alone summaries, 417
Standard deviation, 391
Stanfield, J. H., 111
Stanley, J. C., 338, 348
Statement of Work (SOW), 308
Statistical power, 397–398
Statistical regression, 400
Statistical significance, 361
STEM Program Model, 188, 189f
Stereotypes, 12
Stereotype threat, 480
Stevens, F. L., 95
Stevens, Floraline I., 95–96
Storyboarding (storytelling), 238–239
Strong through every mile program (STEM), 188, 189f
Structural racism (or race-based inequalities), 217–218
 social programming and evaluation, 217–218
Struening, Elmer L.
 Handbook of Evaluation Research, 86
Student-centered learning, 429t–430t
Student Evaluation Standards, 87
Stufflebeam and Colleagues' classification, 124t
Stufflebeam, D. L., 66, 120, 122, 123, 171
Subjective element of social problems, 209–211
 critical constructivism, 210
 "issue-attention cycles," 211
 social constructivist viewpoint, 209–210
Subjectivity, acknowledging, 480–482
Success definitions
 beyond quantitative definitions, 288–289
 identifying indicators, 289–290
 levels of indicators, 291–292
 problem with "parity," 288
 understanding different types of indicators, 290–291
Suchman, E. A., 87
Suchman, Edward, 85
Summative evaluations, 172–173, 186–187
Survey, 358
SurveyMonkey, 359
Sustainability questions, 321
Swag, 459
Symbolic interactionism, 210
Systematic inquiry, 53, 499

Table of specifications, 363
Tables, 428–430
Talent development evaluation framework, 282

Team, evaluation
 and good evaluator, 295–296
 internal vs. external evaluators, 294–296
 advantages and disadvantages, 295t
 roles and responsibilities, identifying, 294
Tenbrunsel, A. E., 44
Tenney, L., 17
Test/retest reliability, 368
Theories, evaluation, 107, 111, 130, 130t–131t
 care about, 120–122
 within cultural context, 129–130
 elements
  evaluation practice, 121
  knowledge construction, 120
  knowledge use, 121
  social programming, 120
  valuing, 121
 evaluation tree, 125–126
 five-category classification, 123–124
 models and approaches, distinction among, 122–123
 Stufflebeam and Colleagues' classification, 124t
Theory of change, 117
Thomas, V. G., 9, 20, 142, 369
Thompson, Charles H., 78, 82–84
Threats to validity, 348–349
Time and task charts, 298, 298t
Time-series design, 344
Tragedy and/or charity model, 146
Trainor, A. A., 111
Transdiscipline, 170
Transferability, 301
Transformational evaluation, 155–157
Transformative evaluation, 147
Transformative framework, 307
Transformative lens, 213
Translation by committee (TBC), 367
Tree, evaluation, 125–126
 branches
  methods theories, 125
  use theories, 125
  values-based theories, 125
 roots
  epistemology, 125
  social accountability, 125
  social inquiry, 125
Trevisan, M. S., 182
Triangulation, 87
Trochim, W. M. K., 386
Tropp, L. R., 482
"Truth," validating, 22, 23
T-test for dependent samples, 394t
T-test for independent samples, 394t
Tufte, E., 436
Tuskegee Syphilis Study of 1932–1972, 30
Tuskegee Timeline, 30–31

20th-century evaluation
  Alva and Gunnar Myrdal, 75
  Cambridge-Somerville Youth Program
    Evaluation, 73
  evaluation-related events during, 69,
    69t–71t, 71
  hidden figures and histories, 76–84
    Aaron A. Brown, 80–81
    Ambrose Caliver, 78–79
    Charles H. Thompson, 78, 82–84
    Leander L. Boykin, 81–82
    Reid E. Jackson, 78, 79
    Rose Butler Browne, 79–80
  Kurt Lewin, 74–75
  in 1900–1950s, 71–72
  in 1930s–1950s, 72–73, 74
  prior to modern times, 67–69
    early social experiments, 68–69
    evaluation-related events, 67t
    intersection between education and
      evaluation pre-20th
      century, 68
    Old Testament, 68
  Ralph W. Tyler, 75–76
  Sputnik's impact on the growth of
    evaluation, 74
21st-century evaluation
  evaluation-related events, 100t
  federal level, strengthening evaluation
    at, 101
  increased emphasis on social justice and
    diversity, 102
  shift in quantitative-qualitative debate, 101
  support for capacity building, 102–103
Two-tailed test, 392–393
2005–2014, "age of global and
  multidisciplinary
  expansion," 99
Two-way analysis of variance, 394t
Tyler, Ralph W.
  educational evaluation, 75–76
  variety in evaluation procedures, 76
Type I error, 397
Type II error, 397

United Nations High Commissioner for
  Refugees (UNHCR), 196
Universal Declaration of Human Rights, 30
Universal Design for Evaluation
  Checklist, 367
Uptake, 184
U.S. Agency for International Development
  (USAID) approach, 312–313
U.S. Department of Health and Human
  Services Centers for Diseases Control
  and Prevention, 243
U.S. Department of Labor's Comprehensive
  Employment and Training Act
  programs, 85
Utility, 56, 502

Vaca, S., 445
Validity, 361, 362–368
Variance, 391

Vaughan, Dorothy, 76
VCard, 457

Wandersman, A., 157
Wang, C., 357
War on Poverty/Great Society programs, 84
Webber, M. M., 206
Weft QDA, 411
Weiss, Carol H., 85, 87, 92–93
Weiss, C. H., 92, 93, 108, 245
White, J., 346
Whitesell, N. R., 349
Whitmore
  practical participatory evaluation, 75
Whitmore, E., 75
Wholey, J. S., 182, 183, 194
Wicked problems
  cause-effect relationships, 207
  characteristics of, 206, 207f
  "complex ecologies of evaluation," 208
  global food insecurity, 208
  income inequality, 206
  marginalization of individuals, 207
  micro-analysis and macro-analysis, 209
Williams, Patricia, 141
Wilson, B. D. M., 126, 127, 128, 145, 154
Wingate, L., 308
Word cloud, 436
Words matter, 424–426
Workers' compensation, 464

Yates, B., 190